Equine Stud Farm
Medicine and Surgery

Commissioning Editor: *Joyce Rodenhuis*
Development Editor: *Zoë Youd*
Project Manager: *Derek Robertson*
Design Direction: *Andy Chapman*

Equine Stud Farm Medicine and Surgery

Derek C Knottenbelt BVM&S, DVM&S,

DipECEIM, MRCVS

Philip Leverhulme Hospital,
University of Liverpool,
Liverpool, UK

Reginald R Pascoe AM, BVSc, DVSc, FACVSc, FRCVS

Director, Oakey Veterinary Hospital,
Oakey, Queensland,
Australia

Cheryl Lopate MS, DVM

Diplomate, American College of Theriogenologists,
Maple Valley, WA
USA

Michelle M LeBlanc DVM

Diplomate, American College of Theriogenologists,
Road and Riddle Equine Hospital,
Lexington, KY,
USA

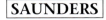
SAUNDERS

An imprint of Elsevier Science

Edinburgh • London • New York • Oxford • Philadelphia • St Louis • Sydney • Toronto • 2003

SAUNDERS

An imprint of Elsevier Science Limited

First published 2003

ISBN 07020 2130 X 1005096898

British Library Cataloguing in Publication Data
A catalogue record for this book is available from the British Library

Library of Congress Cataloging in Publication Data
A catalog record for this book is available from the Library of Congress

Note
Medical knowledge is constantly changing. As new information becomes available, changes in treatment, procedures, equipment and the use of drugs become necessary. The authors and the publishers have taken care to ensure that the information given in this text is accurate and up to date. However, readers are strongly advised to confirm that the information, especially with regard to drug usage, complies with the latest legislation and standards of practice.

Printed in China

your source for books, journals and multimedia in the health sciences

www.elsevierhealth.com

The publisher's policy is to use **paper manufactured from sustainable forests**

CONTENTS

PREFACE

Equine stud medicine has become an increasingly important veterinary specialty over the last 40 years. There has been a new understanding that careful stud management can have a significant benefit in improving fertility and thereby the commercial viability of equine breeding establishments. Stud veterinarians across the world form a vital part of the team that sustains the viability of stud farms and they have the responsibility to provide the best possible service to their clients. However, there is little that generates greater emotion in horse owners than problems with the breeding of their horses. Failure of a mare to conceive should probably be accepted but, because many mares are expensive, and certainly most high-quality stallions carry expensive stud fees, there is a general perception that if enough science can be brought to bear every mare will prove fertile and every foal will become a star performer. Often, in reality, neither of these is possible. Nevertheless, careful stud management can maximize the chances of a mating resulting in a healthy normal foal, which in turn may develop into a useful performance horse. Where problems develop, the stud veterinarian needs to be able to investigate the origin of the difficulty and then provide useful advice and/or treatment. We hope that this book will at least provide a basis to allow such investigations to be scientifically and logically developed. The book follows the outstanding Equine Stud Farm Medicine by Peter Rossdale and Sidney Ricketts. Since that book was published in 1980, it has served veterinarians and owners alike as a standard reference and we hope that our attempt to follow it will also serve the same function.

In the production of this book we set out to provide sufficient basic information for effective stud practice. We have avoided description of advanced diagnostic, medical and surgical procedures that require specialized facilities or experience. Surgical procedures are usually adequately described in specialized surgical texts, therefore the procedures included in this book are for the most part the basic ones that form routine stud medicine practices. We have included some flow charts which we hope will provide a useful diagnostic protocol for some of the more significant problems facing stud veterinarians. The text is referenced with limited numbers of relevant literature reports, which may provide readers with further useful information.

We hope that this book will be a useful asset to senior veterinary students and those veterinarians who are developing an interest in equine stud medicine. Furthermore, we hope that it will also be of interest to stud owners and owners of brood mares.

The first three chapters of the book are dedicated to the stud farm and routine stud procedures. We set out to provide some useful help to stud owners based upon areas where, in our experience, problems are relatively frequent. These chapters have been difficult to construct because facilities and management vary widely in different geographical and economic circumstances, but at least the general principles are often similar. Owners of stud farms may ask for veterinary input when they are designing or changing facilities and it is always important to consult widely before construction starts.

Chapter 4 deals with the stallion. In spite of their importance in breeding, there remains a common impression that most stallions always perform well and always remain fertile despite less than perfect management. Without a healthy stallion, free of significant disease, fertility will inevitably suffer. Previous breeding practices with stallion books of up to 40–60 mares have in the case of some stallions been increased to 100–150 mares, which means that an individual stallion will have a considerable influence on the succeeding foal crop and indeed the genetic structure of female blood lines. Genetic defects and venereal infections can be significant risks if the stallion is not properly managed and prepared for the stud season. The increasing use of chilled semen and improved artificial insemination techniques have in some instances helped overcome increasing pressures on some performance stallions not bred for racing. However, the results of artificial insemination with frozen semen in horses still lags well behind those of the ruminant species and much further research into the cryopreservation of semen needs to be undertaken to improve them. Furthermore, there are still prejudices against the use of artificial insemination in some breeds, but the perceived disadvantages are probably balanced by significant potential advantages.

The mare's role is of course pivotal. Her health and well-being is critical and there is little that causes more acrimony between owners, stud managers and veterinarians than a mare's failure to produce a normal healthy foal. Failure to conceive, abortion, stillborn or weak/non-surviving foals represent serious financial loss to any owner, be they small or large horse enterprises. It has always been common practice in the Thoroughbred industry in particular to attempt to breed mares as early in the breeding season as possible. Unfortunately, in the past, this has always been a time when fertility has been naturally low, but stud management procedures such as increased daylight with artificial lighting, etc. have largely overcome these problems. Inevitably there are mares in the earliest parts of the breeding season that have low fertility for other reasons and these continue to present difficulties. Older mares may often be sent to stud at the end of long and distinguished performance careers only to be found to be inherently less fertile than younger (often unproven) mares. Nevertheless, a proven record is often the major force behind the selection of brood mares and special stud precautions may need to be taken to maximize their fertility. New techniques, such as embryo transfer and gamete intrafallopian transfers, are becoming more feasible, but this area in horses lags behind that in other species. It is the high-value foals that drive most of the research effort and these also carry the greatest veterinary challenges. A more natural approach to breeding could reap considerable rewards, but this is unlikely to be accepted in Thoroughbred breeding at least.

Following the delivery of a healthy foal, the mare needs to continue to nurture the foal. The health of the mammary gland, in the provision of both good-quality colostrum and adequate supplies of milk for up to 6 months or more, is vital for the foal. We have included a section on the mammary gland because we view this as a very important aspect of stud medicine that frequently fails to generate its deserved attention.

Orphaned foals are widely regarded as a serious problem in both the short and the long term, so special measures need to be taken to maximize growth and minimize the behavioral difficulties that accompany these foals.

The role of the placenta during gestation and the information it can provide after its delivery has not received enough attention in the past. We have attempted to provide some new information in this chapter which we hope will generate further interest and understanding. We are sure that more information can be gained from prepartum placental assessment and from postpartum examination. The placenta should always be examined systematically because it can provide an early warning system for postnatal problems in the foal.

We have limited the foal medicine component because neonatal medicine has become a specialty in its own right, although it is of course impossible to separate the foal from the practice of stud medicine. The concept of 'risk status' of foals is one of the cornerstones of stud management and provides the stud team with pre-emptive information on the likely health of the foal. Most stud managers and owners of breeding mares will be more than capable of making a neonatal assessment of the foal. However, it is important that foals are always examined by a veterinarian between 12 and 24 hours of birth, with earlier examinations given to premature or weak foals, which hopefully will have been classified as high risk. This will surely result in increased survival rates.

We commend this text to the reader in the hope that it will be a useful reference and will also encourage and nurture greater interest in stud farm medicine in veterinarians, stud managers and horse owners alike.

Derek C Knottenbelt, Michelle LeBlanc, Cheryl Lopate, Reg R Pascoe, 2003

ACKNOWLEDGEMENTS

We would like to thank all those who have made contributions in either illustrations, comments or other assistance. Without this help we would not have managed to produce this book. In particular, we are grateful to Woody Asbury who stepped in at the last minute to provide wonderful assistance with the project. Barrie Edwards, John Cox, Nicky Holdstock, Jonathan Pycock and Katherine Whitwell have provided images that add richly to the text and we are grateful to them in particular. Rebecca Christian gave us enormous help with the illustrations and we extend our gratitude to her.

We also pay tribute to the founders of the stud medicine specialty, including, of course, Dr Peter Rossdale, Newmarket, UK, who has by common consent been the founding father of equine stud farm medicine. The current universally accepted status of the specialty is due to the continued efforts of many hundreds of veterinarians and stud managers across the world who have pushed back the barriers and broken down many of the myths associated with horse breeding. We accept, however, that there remain considerable problems that will need to be addressed by succeeding generations of stud veterinarians.

We would also like to pay tribute to our mentors who encouraged each of us to develop a particular interest in stud medicine; without their encouragement we would probably not be so intimately involved is this exciting, ever-changing and challenging field of veterinary medicine.

Finally we would like to thank the editorial team at Elsevier Science for their support. A project like this inevitably has difficulties, but they have maintained a sense of humor with a sharp administrative edge and encouraged us to its conclusion.

DEDICATION

This book is dedicated to the next generation of stud veterinarians across the world. They hold the key to the development of the horse in modern society.

It is also dedicated to the horse itself – this wonderful, elegant and versatile creature to which we all owe our all. The horse has willingly and (usually) without enmity provided essential and nonessential services to mankind for many centuries and we can count ourselves privileged to be custodians of their health and their future. We cannot and will not shirk this responsibility.

> *The start of a new life remains a miracle of nature*
> *and we take it for granted at our peril.*

I think that a general thank you to all of our mentors, colleagues, clients and patients is in order. Horses have made our lives fuller and more exciting and we appreciate their presence and to be lucky enough to work on them on a daily basis. A thank you also to our publishers for asking us to do the work.

Cheryl Lopate, MS, DVM

I want to thank all those individuals that have entered my life and taught me about the amazing mysteries of the horse. I also want to thank my loving husband, Kevin Anderson, who has tolerated my computer illiteracy with humor and grace.

Michelle Le Blanc

Chapter 1
DESIGN AND CONSTRUCTION OF A BREEDING FARM

Reg Pascoe, Woody Asbury

Although many breeders assert that a very good horse can only be bred in a few places in the world, horses are extremely adaptable and reproduce successfully in almost all regions and climates. In general, horses do well in both cold and hot climates. They tolerate high altitudes and deserts, flatlands and mountainous terrain. Furthermore, they reproduce in feral bands with no management at all in some countries.

It is unrealistic, therefore, to provide breeders with definitive directions for farm facilities, layouts and fencing that are suitable for any location. Moreover, it is probably too simplistic to prescribe definitive plans for the development of stud farms because there are so many possible variations. The basic concepts will apply in the majority of areas, and local information on building materials and methods will be utilized in the adaptation of these to local conditions. Also, it is recognized that ingenuity applied to management may be more important than defined structures that conform to accepted standards.[1] Use of good proven designs from existing facilities can often eliminate mistakes.

Climatic conditions and economic constraints have profound influences on the construction and management of the stud farm. The detailed requirements will vary markedly throughout the world. Although in some areas horses require to be stabled throughout the breeding season, in other areas this is not only undesirable but may be impractical. In areas without the rigors of periods of cold weather, drought and heat play a major role in the breeding industry and are significant factors in the running costs. As a general philosophy for horse management, horses are healthier when they spend longer outside. Clearly, however, the management and the quality of the pastures, paddocks and fencing will have a profound influence on the best circumstances under any particular conditions. Larger holdings with more equitable weather lead to fewer farm personnel being required than for the labor-intensive housing in barns in the winters of the northern hemisphere.

In planning and developing a facility to manage horses, safety for both the animals and their handlers must be a primary focus. In spite of the perception that there are more ways for a horse to injure itself than could ever be described, careful planning and management will prevent most avoidable injuries to both man and horse. A thorough understanding of equine behavior, careful thought about the procedures to be undertaken and focused concentration on the job at hand by the handlers should enable a stud to function safely and economically. Nevertheless, many facilities are adapted from previous farming facilities and here the dangers can be much higher. Before any detailed planning is started, and certainly before any building is undertaken, it is useful to visit as many other facilities as possible and discuss the advantages and disadvantages of individual systems.

The general outlines in this chapter apply to all horse-breeding areas in the world. Most countries have their own unique methods of handling, holding, feeding and rearing horses. However, there are many principles that can provide ideas for additional improvement and which may enhance the quality of the environment for horses.

Suggested references to broaden the reader's scope appear at the end of this chapter. For the purposes of covering as many aspects of the subject as possible, it will be assumed that the reader intends to develop a breeding farm from the ground up. Realistically, many stud farms have been developed from existing agricultural facilities and this will inevitably introduce limitations of adaptation and difficulties of use that will need to be overcome. Obviously the purchase of a 'turn-key' facility changes the scenario, but the principles of sound, safe and efficient construction still apply and will influence that purchase.

FEATURES OF SUCCESSFUL FARM DESIGN

All farm designs should be aimed at ease of use and safety for the horses and their handlers. Problems are introduced by financial limitations, lack of understanding of the requirements of horse and handler safety, and the failure of some horse-management systems to take account of the fact that horses are living creatures, not just figures in a financial statement.

Hobby farms are seldom built to any recognizable standard of either economy or safety; frequently, they grow and adapt without conscious long-term design planning. Most restrictions are based upon financial considerations and where these are of no material concern it may be possible to construct the ideal facility for the specific place and time.

The management structures of commercial breeding farms are largely dictated by economic considerations, ease of management and safety aspects. There should always be contingency plans for expansion or recession. The investment in the land and all the subsequent developments must be put into context with the goals of the operation. In all but the most exceptional circumstances the economic aspects of the venture are also important. Hobby farms may not be subject to economic limitations and the biggest operations may also be run without regard for financial aspects. Most investors, however, are seeking some financial return or tax relief from their operation, if not always serious profits. Therefore, what is paid for the land, the level of property tax assessment and other operational costs are important. Furthermore, perhaps the most critical pressure is the appreciation potential of the property. Increasing population pressure exerts an upward pressure on land values. Should the horse-breeding venture be terminated, it would be some consolation to realize a gain from the investment in land and improvements. Careful planning at the outset should improve the chances of this.

Traditional approaches to housing mares and stallions were for two independent sets of quarters, isolated from each other to minimize excitement. However, recent equine behavioral research suggests that integrating stallions and mares in common facilities may have important benefits for the operation.[2] The so-called 'harem effect', resulting from interactions of sight and sound, produces a calming effect on both sexes, similar to the behavior of a band of mares running with a stallion. It is believed that both behavior and fertility are positively affected. No specific guidelines for facilities are offered, but the obvious first step is to house a stallion in a barn with mares.

Considerations of climate and local conditions are important in designing the farm and can significantly affect the layout. In subtropical regions, for example, housing requirements may be completely different from those in more temperate regions. The need for barn space will be significantly less if horses can remain outside all the time. Separation for feeding can be accomplished with small portable pens, or with simple 'feeding barns', which can double as holding spaces for routine examinations or extended day-length lighting systems (Fig. 1.1).

SITE SELECTION

The selection of one type of site over another is based almost entirely on the prevailing climate. Before developing a farm in an unfamiliar area, it is important to consult with local agricultural extension services. Additional input from existing horse farm managers will also be helpful. The breeding records for particular areas may be helpful in establishing the best areas for horse breeding, but most established properties have adapted and altered their environmental features significantly over many years. Most breeders agree on the benefits of grass, whether it is naturally or artificially irrigated.

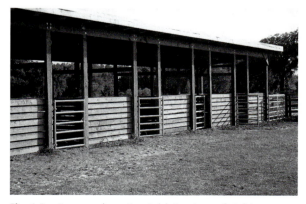

Fig. 1.1 An open barn 'portable' system of stables allowing easy access and good air hygiene.

Horse farms are based on three types of space:

- Pastures watered exclusively by rainfall.
- Partially or supplementally irrigated pastures.
- Dry-lot areas in which there is effectively no pasture.

- For example, a desert property could be either irrigated pasture or dry-lot. The cost of water, an irrigation system and the labor to operate it would be significant factors in this decision. Commercial breeding farms usually opt for the dry-lot in this situation, providing forage with high-quality hay that can be grown efficiently where water is cheaper.

Water

Planning for water usage is critical to the consideration of a farm site. Regardless of its source, the quantity and quality of water are important and should be considered together with the potential to construct a reliable distribution system. Failure of free-choice water supplies, through prolonged subfreezing weather or extended droughts, for example, is potentially disastrous. In very cold climates the provision of warmed water is good management, and will spare labor in hauling bulk water. Brackish or salty water is usually poorly tolerated by horses and can result in poor condition and poor breeding.

Water may be available by access to natural watercourses, but care should be exercised when inspecting small watercourses that they are in fact permanent rather than temporary. More frequently, water is supplied by an extensive underground piped distribution system of water troughs with automatic floats to regulate the level and prevent overflow.

- Daily or twice-daily routine water checks for every situation are a critical part of stud farm management.

Sufficient water space must be provided for larger groups of horses. Moreover, it is essential that the water is clean and, in summer, that it is in such volume as to be cool, rather than hot from too small a volume. Automatic water troughs in stables are often too small and rarely allow a thirsty horse to have an uninterrupted drink before the water level becomes too low. A more satisfactory volume of 20–30 liters should be provided, usually in buckets.

Paddock water troughs should have a secure drainage plug to allow ease of cleaning. Regular cleaning is essential to prevent build-up of algae and decayed matter. Volume-controlling float valves should be protected from interference by the horses, either by guards or by being out of reach. Horses will play with accessible floats, often causing loss of water, muddy surrounds and, if undetected, severe loss from the main water supply. Long or round troughs provide the best cool water for horses and plenty of room for them to move around.

Continuous fresh water supplies are also essential if pastures are to be irrigated effectively; shortages of supply can be particularly harmful to a stud operation.

Topography

Rolling land has an advantage over flat land in that sites for barns, gates, roads, etc. can be sited away from storm water run-off areas, thus avoiding excessive mud in areas with high levels of traffic. It is important to observe the land after major rainfall. Moderately hilly or rolling terrain, such as the Epsom Downs in England, is often favored by growers of athletic breeds of horses on the basis that exercising on that type of land favors the development of bone, muscle and condition.

Soil or land type

The productivity of the soil is important for growing quality forage. Aspects such as depth of the topsoil, organic matter in the soil and drainage are significant.

Although a sandy loam soil is widely regarded as the ideal for growing grass and horses, it is, unfortunately, also ideal for many arable crops. Market pressures force the cost of this land higher than might be justified by the commercial return on horses.

Large amounts of rock or shale in the soil, which are not conducive to healthy feet, and very heavy clay soils that impede drainage are undesirable soil types and are often poor forage producers.

Trees and natural shelter

Shade from trees is beneficial in hot climates. However, in many circumstances, particularly if there are feed shortages (i.e. roughage), horses will destroy the trees by eating the bark (Fig. 1.2). Simple trunk protectors may be effective in preventing this. Furthermore, some trees are potentially poisonous. In the UK, many older properties have ancient trees that are very dangerous (e.g. yew, red oak, and laburnum).

Trees in areas prone to severe thunderstorms are potentially lethal lightning conductors. Fencing off the areas concerned is more difficult if there is to be any benefit from the trees in terms of shade or shelter provision. Lightning conductors are effective measures to reduce the risks.

Properties that have few effective shade or shelter trees are seldom used for stud farms unless there is the potential to grow them. Fast-growing eucalyptus, poplar or conifer trees can provide shelter within a few years. There are also esthetic aspects of stud farming that depend on trees.

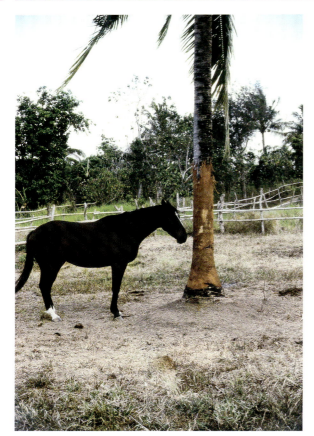

Fig. 1.2 Boredom and lack of roughage often lead to horses causing severe damage to tree trunks, such as this ring-barked tree in the paddock.

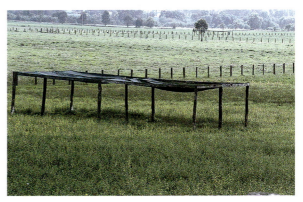

Fig. 1.4 Simple sun shelter constructed of upright posts supporting a shade cloth roof.

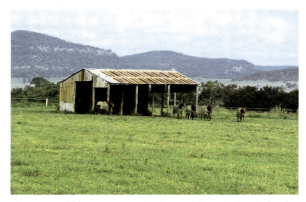

Fig. 1.5 Old hay-storage shed, providing shelter in both winter and summer.

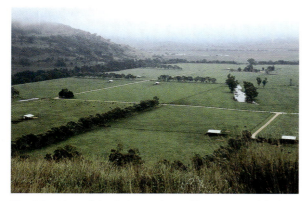

Fig. 1.3 Line of shade trees planted between paddocks.

A row of trees can be planted as a windbreak outside a fence line (Fig. 1.3) and horses will appreciate the protection they afford in the worst weather conditions.

Shade houses/field shelters

These can be simple constructions of four posts with a shade cloth roof in dry climates (Fig. 1.4), or an iron-roofed, more solid waterproof construction of wooden panels or sheet and brick, in which the feeding and water facilities are placed. The protection afforded by shelters is also helpful where *Musca* flies and culicoides midges are a problem as these invade darkened shade areas less frequently than open-air paddocks with no cover.

Where prevailing winter winds are severe, shelters also provide protection from inclement weather. Old hay-storage sheds are often converted into low-cost shelters against, heat, cold and wet conditions (Fig. 1.5).

ROADS AND ACCESS

Consideration should be given to access to the farm by the services that will be required. Delivery of construction materials, maintenance needs, service personnel and eventually transportation of animals and foodstuffs require decent hard-surfaced roads with reasonable access to the farm for suitable vehicles. In the UK, small country lanes can be a serious limitation for modern transporters, but by compensation they afford some sense of security. Careful planning of access roads, which should be kept wide enough for vehicles capable of moving horses (particularly mares, foals and young horses) is very important to allow ease of access to all points of the farm. Roads can be used to separate paddocks and so may act as effective quarantine barriers in case of disease outbreaks. They also allow planting of shade trees and installation of water conduits without having to interfere with the fields themselves. Free movement of feed vehicles and farm machinery, and the transfer of mares/foals to other locations on the farm without entry to other occupied paddocks, are also important advantages of a carefully planned road structure.

The movement of horses (possibly stallions or mares with foals at foot) by leading them should not be unduly risky; crossing main traffic routes or railway lines is fraught with danger and increases the risks to man and horse. Consideration should be given to possible escaped horses: gates and other restrictive measures such as walls and fences should ultimately allow the animals to be recaptured easily.

Connections to basic utilities such as water, electricity and gas need to be planned. Drainage and handling of waste must also be considered carefully if disease is to be limited.

Buildings

The basic requirements include adequate space for exercise, secure fencing, shelter according to the climatic conditions and special requirements of the operation, and a workable layout dedicated to safe and efficient execution of the intended functions.

Facilities are functionally the same for any size of operation, with the need for:

- Stallion boxes (and exercise yards).
- Mare boxes (for mares due for service, pregnant mares and mares with foals).
- Exercise yards and paddocks.
- 'Hospital' facilities comprising loose boxes for mares with sick foals.
- Facilities to hold and store feed (grains, chaff and hay) and bedding.

Farm layout

Before the specific layout of the operation is designed, careful regard to the functions required of the facility is essential. The plan must be carefully made before the first post hole is dug. Basic questions include:

- Will stallions be standing at the stud with their own 'book' of mares or will they simply be used for artificial insemination?
- If stallions are to be used, how many will be kept and what is their expected 'book'?
- Will outside mares be brought in for breeding and, if so, how many and over what period?

- Will mares be visiting the stud to foal in order to get better supervision and foal care and to maximize the use of the foal heat?
- Will there be permanently resident mares on the farm and will these take precedence over visiting mares?
- Will weanling foals and yearlings be held on the premises? If so, will they be in contact with other outside horses or will they be kept segregated?
- Will a high level of veterinary attention be expected (will a veterinarian live on the farm?) or will this be more casual?
- Should there be isolation facilities for new animals? This is a very important aspect, and should be discussed in careful detail with the consulting veterinarian.
- How long will mares (with or without foals at foot) remain on the stud after covering?

These questions should yield a list of the facilities that are required immediately and for future developments. Ultimately, the safety of personnel and the well-being of the animals must be paramount in the design and construction of a stud farm. The nature of horses is such that their management is inherently dangerous and a full understanding of the potential hazards will limit the problems.

> The basic requirements include:
> - A stallion barn.
> - Mare barn(s).
> - Foaling facilities.
> - Teasing facilities.
> - Hay/feed storage.
> - Office.
> - Housing for staff.
> - Veterinary examination area and laboratory facilities.
> - Pastures and exercise paddocks for stallion(s), mares and foals, barren and pregnant mares, and yearlings/weanlings.

With the essential structures in mind, a plan should be developed for the relationship of each unit to pastures, paddocks, roads, water lines, utility connections, etc. so that the whole facility will be coordinated. Each unit should be able to function independently from the others.

- The breeding unit might contain mare and stallion housing, a breeding area, mare examination stocks/chute, laboratory, loading and unloading facilities, feed and hay storage and equipment sheds.
- An isolation facility for new arrivals should be located so that farm traffic will not cross-contaminate other portions of the farm (a separate drug-treatment area should be kept and made secure).

- A separate, self-contained unit is indicated for weaning and for longer-term housing of weanlings. Weaning is a stressful event for both mares and foals and injuries are commonplace even when facilities are ideal.

The underlying threat of infectious disease should not ever be overlooked. The potential catastrophe that can follow from the speed of spread and the economic damage from an outbreak of an infectious disease such as contagious equine metritis should not be forgotten. Serious economic danger from possible outbreaks of virus abortion and strangles creates the necessity for quarantine facilities (yards, stables, and paddocks) that are separate and distinct from the main farm area. Quarantine facilities should work on the principle of an 'all-in all-out' policy. Simply, this means that a group of horses held in quarantine for the required time must be kept separate from any new arrivals because of the possibility of cross-contamination in both directions if they are mixed. On large farms, this can mean very complex horse-holding facilities with enforceable management methods that prevent the breakdown of quarantine.

Visiting walk-in mares should be carefully segregated from home farm or live-in mares. Head collars, bridles, etc. must be thoroughly cleaned and/or sterilized if any suspected problems arise, and gear that is used in pre-entry (quarantine) areas should not be used elsewhere in order to minimize disease spread.

Strict control of stray dogs, cats and vermin such as foxes, rats and mice is necessary, especially if virus abortion erupts. Serious spread to adjoining paddocks can occur when dogs and carrion-eating birds spread infected aborted material.

FENCING

Safe fencing is essential on a stud farm. The horses on the facility, whether highly valuable Thoroughbred or other purebred horses or animals of lesser value, provide the raw material on which the stud functions. Their safe restraint is vital. All fences have some measure of danger: the more secure and solid the fence, the more solid fracture-type injuries occur; with star posts and wire, there are leg injuries from the wire and body injury from the pickets. When panicked by storms, etc., horses may break, or become entangled in, any type of fencing.

A survey of fence-related injuries[3] supported the contention that no fence is horse-proof and free of potential hazard. The survey pointed out that the highest rate of serious injury occurred with barbed wire fencing, followed by high-tensile steel wire and page wire. Wooden fences (post and rail, and post and board) had high rates of injury, but those injuries were less severe than those related to wire. Although these results are not surprising, the fact that barbed wire fencing on metal posts is the most economical in terms of both materials and installation means that these fences will probably not disappear.

Selecting and building fencing for horses is an exercise in compromise. First, it must be recognized that there are no totally safe fences for horses. The animal's basic nature is to run from real or perceived danger. If that flight is blocked by anything, a collision is a strong possibility. The options are to attempt to run through or jump over the fence. The results may vary from escape to serious injury from splintered fence boards or unyielding posts or wire. Moreover, the consequences of escape, whether in one piece or not, may produce further injury. Another cause for concern is the altercation between horses that can occur at the right-angled corners of a fence, in which the aggressors pin the recipient in the corner and settle the dispute. The dilemma, then, is whether to select a solid unbreakable fence or one that will fall apart on contact. In both cases there is ample opportunity for injury.

The cost of fencing is a significant factor on all horse farms, particularly for those in excess of 300–500 hectares. Many large stud farms are over 3000 hectares and the quality and type of fencing is an important financial and management consideration.

Installation costs will depend largely on the methods used to install posts and on the rock content of the soil.

Fence height should be a minimum of 5 feet for light-horse breeds, with variations recommended for young horses or stallions. Wire or boards should be installed inside the posts, or closest to the horses. This arrangement offers an unobstructed plane, preventing injury to knees and shoulders when horses run along the fences (Fig. 1.6).

A disadvantage of this arrangement is that horses pushing on boards midway between posts will raise the nail heads enough to cause a problem. All fences need regular maintenance in order to avoid accidental injuries. With better constructed fences, rails are either bolted or fastened with heavy wire to overcome this problem. Another disadvantage of placing posts out-

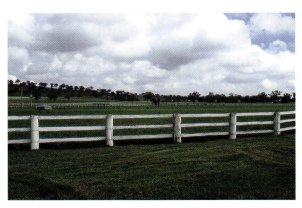

Fig. 1.6 Rails placed on the inside of the paddock prevent injury from exposed posts when horses gallop up and down fence lines.

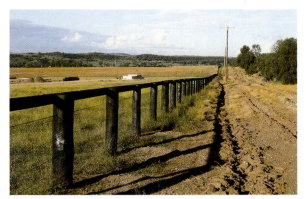

Fig. 1.7   A safe fence for mares and foals; note top rail inside the paddock and strong wire mesh netting fastened inside the posts.

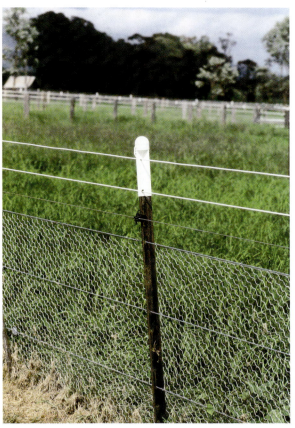

Fig. 1.8   Star picket with safety cap, two 'highlight' wires and heavy-gauge wire netting.

side the fence is noticed in wire mesh applications. It is difficult to make a curved corner without pulling the wire off the posts, or causing the posts to lean inwards. Posts and boards can be used to modify the problem by cutting across the corners.

Fencing can take many forms, and varies in different parts of the world. Larger areas (50–100 hectares) in Australia or America are usually fenced with plastic-coated wire with or without a top rail. For security purposes, these should be at least 1.75 m (5 feet) high (Fig. 1.7).

Wire-based fencing

Fences constructed with wire and/or starred metal posts can be dangerous for horses due to the rigidity of the pickets, causing damage to any horse that runs into them. This problem can be partially minimized by the use of plastic caps to cover the tops of the pickets (Fig. 1.8), or they may carry standard wire, or electric tape, which is used as a temporary measure to create laneways, etc. (Fig. 1.9). No barbed or razor wire or large open-mesh 'sheep' wire should ever be used for the construction of horse-holding fences (Fig. 1.10). All wire should be correctly tensioned so as to avoid animals becoming tangled up in loose sections. Severe, often life-threatening, damage is common with poorly constructed wire fences.

A very common safe fence has two or three top wires with posts at intervals of 3–4 m (12–15 feet), with the bottom filled with strong chain (diamond) wire mesh. On well-established farms, the posts are regularly coated with bituminous paint (creosote), which preserves the wood and prevents termite damage or rot.

Well-spaced posts 4–6 m (15–20 feet) apart strung with four or five strands of plastic-coated 6G wire is a common fencing method; posts are often painted white for safety and esthetic reasons. A strong plastic band containing two wires with a plastic strip between the wires is often used to top the fence.

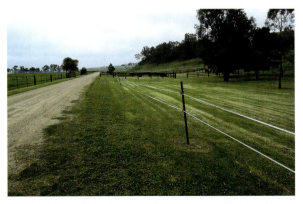

Fig. 1.9   Use of electric tape for temporary fencing to form laneways.

Diamond mesh wire stretched on pressure-treated wooden posts, set on 2.5-m centers, with a top rail (Fig. 1.11) is probably the most expensive fencing system, principally due to the cost of the wire. Advantages include the inability of horses of all ages to get a foot into the apertures in the wire. This type of fencing has the longest useful life of any of those listed and requires the least maintenance. Diamond

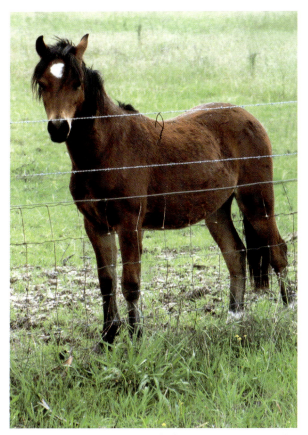

Fig. 1.10 Example of an unsafe fence; barbed wire and large sheep mesh cause many injuries.

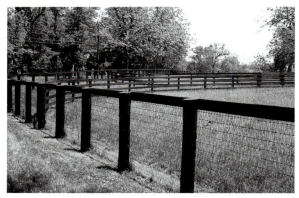

Fig. 1.11 Example of a post and rail fence with a diamond mesh 'infill'.

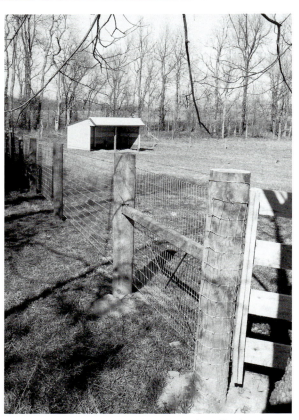

Fig. 1.12 Woven or welded mesh can be effective, but the top strands should be multiple or made visible.

mesh wire, and the 5 × 10 cm mesh listed below, are best placed so that the wire is clear of the ground by at least 6 inches to deter rusting. Any closer to the ground may cause a foot to be trapped under the wire. The top rail is generally nailed, bolted or wired to the posts after the wire has been tensioned and attached to the posts. This makes replacing the boards in the top rail easier, but also allows easier chewing of the boards.

Oak planks are harder to chew, but determined horses will eat them in time.

Woven wire mesh (5 × 10 cm) stretched on posts, with either 2.5- or 5-m centers, can have either a top rail, a multiple-strand smooth wire top or a highly visible tape at the top (Fig. 1.12). If a top rail is used, posts should be on 2.5-m centers.

Wooden fencing

Three- or four-board fencing on 2.5-m centered posts (Fig. 1.13) is a traditional standard fencing method for stud premises. A space of 15–35 cm underneath the bottom board is suggested because there is less scope for feet to get caught in this much space. A post and board fence can be curved to eliminate square corners. Maintenance costs are highest for this type of fence, due to weathering of the wood and chewing by the animals. The older established farms use hardwood rails (10–20 × 5 cm) set on the inside of the posts. These are very expensive but, by way of compensation, true hardwoods are fairly resistant to both termite and wood rot. They do not require the constant applications of preservatives or paint to limit termite and wood rot that are needed to preserve softer timber. The rails can be substituted with tannalized

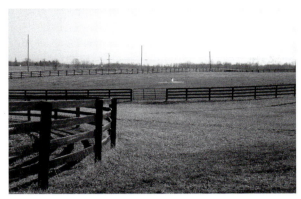

Fig. 1.13   Board and post fencing is a safe, common and attractive fencing method.

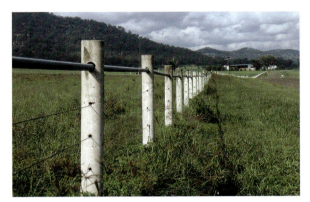

Fig. 1.14   Concrete upright posts are very strong but require regular checking and can be rough.

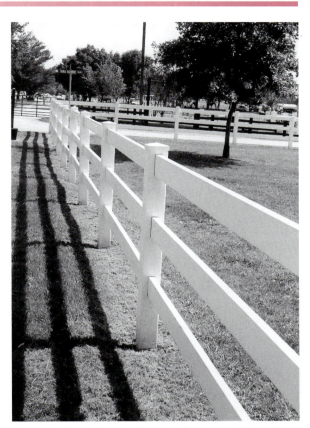

Fig. 1.15   Plastic fencing is safe, effective and attractive. It is virtually maintenance free but is very expensive.

(chromium-based wood preservative) softwood, but these are more prone to chewing damage.

Plastic or concrete fencing

Concrete posts with a 25–30-cm top rail, or complete four-rail plastic fences, are also used but must be strictly maintained to prevent injury from broken posts or rails (Fig. 1.14). In the UK, plastic (PVC) post and rail fencing that is not subject to damage by chewing or rot is becoming commonplace (Fig. 1.15). This type of fence has a much longer life than wooden fences, but a higher initial cost. Repairs are easily made by replacing segments. Some brands are reported to be brittle at very low temperatures, resulting in jagged breaks in posts or rails; others are adversely affected by strong sunlight. Clearly, extensive horse farms would need to invest heavily for this type of material.

Electric fencing

Electric fencing (Fig. 1.16) is widely used throughout the world but there are very mixed opinions on its safety and value. Usually a single strand is used and

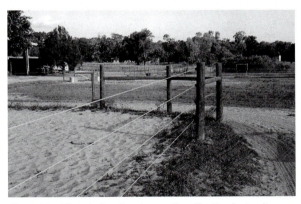

Fig. 1.16   Electric fencing is usually effective but relies upon recognition of the 'danger'. The wires are thin and could cause serious injury.

the effect is dependent on the recognition by the horse of the 'danger'. Recently developed versions feature wide tapes or braided nylon ropes containing the conductive wire. These provide better visibility than single wires. Horses learn quickly to stay away from these fences. Posts can be spaced much further apart than for board fencing, thus reducing installation time. Temporary electric fencing has the advantage of being moveable with relative ease, allowing use of pasture to be maximized with little disruption.

Natural fencing methods

Hedgerows are a safe and environmentally friendly fencing material that horses understand, but they also have hidden dangers. Hedgerows are common in the UK and Ireland in particular, but they carry the risk of eye injuries and their care is much more difficult.

Stonewalls and dykes are sometimes used in areas where wind and rain are likely to cause damage to fences. In the UK and Ireland they are common features of countryside establishments and provide secure restraint. They do, however, have dangers relating to collapse and decay/breakdown.

Fence corners and gate openings

Gates and corners where horses crowd when being handled, teased or fed can be dangerous. Horses also tend to congregate around gates and water troughs, making muddy conditions worse. The locations and types of gates installed in fence lines therefore deserve careful consideration. Fencing off the corner of a field is a useful management tool. The planner should visualize the potential traffic areas in and out of the fenced enclosures, and locate gates so as to minimize the risks. Care in selection of gate positions to allow easy access and easy movement of horses when being driven, or herded, is essential.

Gates should be located in areas of the fence line that drain well. Spreading gravel in gate openings may be beneficial.

Gate openings may have two or three panels of rails to direct the horses through the gateway. Gate placement towards or at the corner rather than in the middle of a line of fencing helps horse movement but adds risks.

Gates should be large enough for all future traffic; 3.5 m is a safe span for most equipment. If much of the traffic will be horses led on foot, smaller gates may make sense in some locations. Every gate, however, is a potential escape route if it is inadvertently left unlatched; this leads most farms to minimize the number of gates.

Ideally, gates will be constructed to avoid sharp edges or places where feet can be caught. Tubular metal gates, either commercially built or custom welded, are favored in most areas. There should be sufficient horizontal bars to keep the spacing small enough to discourage horses from sticking their heads between them.

Although there are many types of gates, some are safer than others. Horses seem to have an ability (and inclination) to get heads and legs caught in gate openings. All gates should be closed flush with gate posts if possible, and should not allow feet to become caught either between the gate post and gate or through the gate, forcing the gate away from the gate post on either the top or bottom hinge. Gates closing into recessed gate posts increase the safety but they should have sufficient adjustment to allow any sagging to be corrected to facilitate ease of opening and closing.

Gate and yard catches

Many types of latches are available but none of them are perfect. The simpler designs are usually better because it is more likely that personnel will close them properly. Particular attention should be given to main gates that connect the farm roads to the outside. Regardless of the latch, each gate should be equipped with a chain and snap as a supplementary safety feature.

Types of catches include:

- The simple lock catch. These require chain fittings that go around the post so that a horse's weight does not pull out bolts or staples that are just holding a short chain.
- Chain and eye, to drop over an angle bolt in the gate post. Care must be taken to position the bolt so that horses running through the gate are not injured.

PASTURES AND PADDOCKS

'Good horses and good pastures go together'.[4] Horse owners whose mares fail to breed have often reported an improvement when they have access to good-quality pastures. This may partly explain why conception rates are highest when the grass is at its best.

Pasture management has several important features, including proper fertilization, irrigation and/or drainage, and regular rotational grazing patterns to ensure that rank grasses do not dominate the better species. The specific methods for these procedures are described in standard texts on pasture management. Important aspects of the control of pasture quality include consideration of:

- The soil type and fertility.
- The type of pasture grasses used (single or multi-species, new or old leys, and grazing patterns).
- Watering methods (natural/irrigation).
- Season and natural levels of trace elements.

These factors will inevitably influence the types of pasture that can be grown in particular localities, but horses are very adaptable and can thrive in apparently adverse conditions. Legume-based pastures can be used for all types of breeding horses but can have laxative effects at certain times of the year.

The parasite burden on stud farm pastures is an important factor; it is generally accepted that collection of droppings and the control of the development of 'roughs and lawns' are essential. Regular monitoring of parasite infestation from pasture counts and from fecal counts is now normal practice (see p. 37).

The location of paddocks and pastures should fit with the overall needs of the farm, although the topographical features may dictate the basic structure. For example, multiple small paddocks may be indicated immediately adjacent to a foaling barn. This arrangement allows mares with young foals to get outside by themselves yet remain within sight of the farm buildings, which is a good management plan. Larger paddocks that are suitable for several mares and their foals should be nearby, and pastures housing six or more pairs could be further out. Weather conditions in early spring may dictate that all foals under 4–6 weeks of age come into the barn at night, so this will dictate the proximity and convenience of paddocks to barns.

When individual animals or groups are held in adjacent paddocks or pastures, there is always a tendency for them to communicate with or, worse, combat with the neighboring horses. It is therefore desirable to have double fencing with adequate separation between paddocks or pastures. This arrangement significantly adjusts fencing costs upwards and to keep the grass down in the lanes adds to labor costs. Nevertheless, this system reduces injuries, and that is a worthy goal in any farm operation.

Round yards and exercise yards

These may be constructed from post and rail fencing using four or six rails, or may have conveyor belting stretched tightly around the inside perimeter (Fig. 1.17). These constructions are very safe, as horses can run into the walls with a much lower risk of injury than from wooden or plastic rails, or from wire mesh bolted onto the inside of a rail fence. Careful attention needs to be paid to the cut edge of the conveyor belting as horses can chew (and swallow) long lengths of the fiber with catastrophic results. Any

mare that is inclined to chew this material should be removed from access.

The environmental safety of the pastures is important. This involves consideration of the type and quality of the fencing and gating, and care to avoid nails, iron or glass, which are potential sources of injury.

BARNS

Buildings or other structures designed for specific functions are usually required for breeding farms. These include barns for brood mares, foaling facilities, stallion quarters, a breeding shed or barn, and combinations of all of the above. Dedicated facilities for teasing, mare examination and van loading should be considered, in addition to the normal support structures such as hay barns and equipment sheds.

Barns and stables are required because of the need for:

- Shelter from inclement weather. The need to shelter horses from weather varies greatly with the geographic area. In areas of extreme cold, the need for protection against wind and rain depends on the age and health of the animals. Mature horses with good winter hair coats can tolerate subfreezing weather quite well, assuming that they have access to decent roughage at all times. Windbreaks or run-in sheds may be just as efficient as barns in such weather, although very young foals are clearly better off in a stall during severe winter weather. In very hot climates, shade from one source or another is desirable for some horses. Again, very young or very old animals need more protection from the direct heating effect of the sun.
- Separation of individual animals for individual management such as feeding.
- Treatment and control of disorders or routine inspections away from a paddock environment.
- Convenience for some management activities such as weaning of foals.

Construction

Barns are typically either of concrete block or wood frame construction. The increased cost of a brick or block construction is offset somewhat by the lower fire hazard these afford.

The main approaches to the floor plan include the following:

- The center aisle barn (Fig. 1.18). This provides more protection from severe winter weather and can easily be air-conditioned in hotter climates. Feeding and cleaning can be more efficient. Sliding aisle doors should open to the width of the aisle (4 m or greater) to allow maximum air circulation. This system has the added advantages

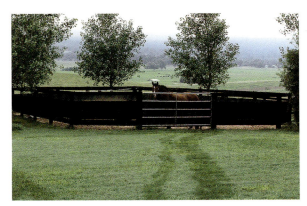

Fig. 1.17 Safe holding yards using top rail and heavy-duty conveyor belting bolted to the inside of heavy yard posts.

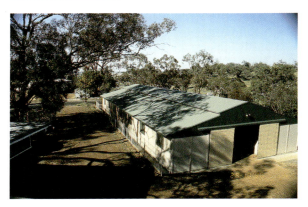

Fig. 1.18 Covered center aisle with boxes on both sides.

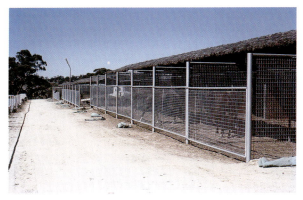

Fig. 1.20 Shedrow-type stables back to back with open exercise yards.

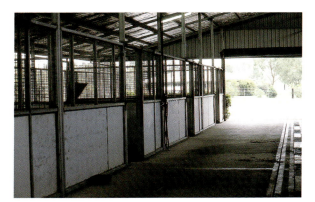

Fig. 1.19 Open style stables used in yearling barns in Australia.

80% shade cloth approximately 12 feet (4 m) high. Such a facility for temporary accommodation (e.g. for use as temporary quarantine boxes) is very useful because of ease of removal and re-assembly.

Ventilation

Notwithstanding the perceived benefits of stabling, the goal of best horse management based on health and economics should be to maintain horses outside whenever possible. There is ample evidence to support this concept. Ensuring adequate ventilation is probably the most important single factor in the design and construction of horse barns and stables. Regardless of how well the barn is designed and built, its ventilation is inevitably worse than an outdoor environment. In addition, when hay and straw are used in feeding and bedding, contaminants in the air and the build-up of ammonia in stalls from urine-soaked bedding are known to be harmful. Chronic obstructive pulmonary disease is almost unheard of where horses are never stabled, and affected horses are invariably better when they are outside. It is impossible to harm a horse with too much ventilation; reduced ventilation is always much more harmful. Warm, humid, non-circulating airflows are probably the worst of all and may also predispose to respiratory infections.

When summer heat is a serious problem, overhead sprinkler systems to physically wet both horses and surroundings can be installed to lower the temperature during the day. The same system is sometimes used to reduce the concentration of airborne particles in cooler climates where pollen, fungal spores and dust induce upper respiratory tract problems.

Air quality in barns can also be improved dramatically by not storing hay and straw in the same building as the horses. Overhead lofts are especially detrimental, as considerable dust is circulated when hay is dropped to floor level for feeding. The dust of hay and straw is associated with many types of mold

of ease of observation for foaling mares. A major disadvantage is the potential spread of infectious disease from horse to horse by common air space and by common drainage, as well as common access corridors. Clearly, if these drawbacks can be overcome by careful design, the system is potentially more efficient. This open style of center aisle is also favored in Australia as a yearling barn (Fig. 1.19).

- The shedrow style. These barns are more commonly found in milder climates and training facilities. The stalls are usually back-to-back and open to the outside, under an overhanging shed roof, and may have attached fenced exercise yards (Fig. 1.20). The open stable yard in which the stables are arranged in rows or around an open rectangular yard is widely used in the UK. Management is somewhat less efficient than with the center aisle barn system, but there is less risk of contagion. Direct sunlight and rainfall on the common passages and pathways reduce the major areas of risk in this system.
- Portable steel stables with shade cloth roof. These are constructed in panels and connected to form a row of loose boxes. They are covered by a roof of

and fungi, which are thought to contribute to chronic obstructive pulmonary disease. Even smaller farms should endeavor to provide a completely separate structure for hay storage.

Guidance must be sought from experienced architects who specialize in barn design, from barn builders and from experienced operators of breeding farms who have learned from experience.

> 'The principle of ventilation is not a complex one. Hot air rises. The problem is making sure it has a place to escape out of the barn and that cooler, fresh air is continually pulled into the structure.'[5]

A factor critical to the efficiency of the 'stack effect' is a steep pitch to the roof, with vents along the roof ridges and louvered ventilators through windows, dormers, cupolas, etc. The orientation of barns should take account of the direction of the prevailing winds.

- In hot climates the prevailing wind can be a critical cooling factor; the barn should therefore be aligned so that the maximum amount of air can circulate. High ceilings keep the hottest air above horse level. The use of fans to increase air movement is valuable in the summer; large exhaust fans or individual stall-front fans are options. Overhead water sprayers, such as permanently mounted garden sprays with the spray directed downwards, are another option for cooling.
- In cold climates, it may be wiser to avoid direct placement of the stables into the prevailing winds.

The herd instinct prevails, even inside a barn, and so design should take this into account. Visual contact is very important in most herd species. Direct contact between horses may be beneficial but increases the risk of spread of disease.

Individual stable/loose box construction

These are largely similar across the world, being based on a required size and shape. Stall sizes range from 4 × 4 m (12 × 12 feet) up to 5 × 5 m (16 × 16 feet). The larger stables are usually used for foaling mares, mares with foals at foot, and for stallions.

Stall doors that slide to open are favored for their minimal obstruction of the aisle space. They must be securely fastened when closed to prevent accidental forced opening (Fig. 1.21).

Stall dividers should be high enough to prevent a horse from putting a foot over the top. Windows or Dutch doors on the back wall of the stall are an asset

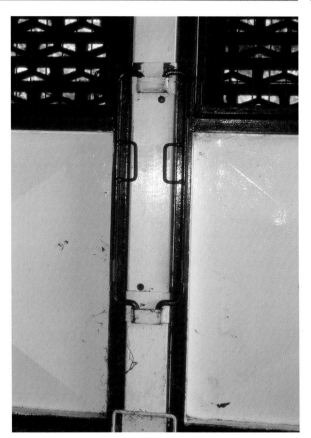

Fig. 1.21 Sliding doors with secure double latches and floor stays to prevent accidental forced opening and possible injury.

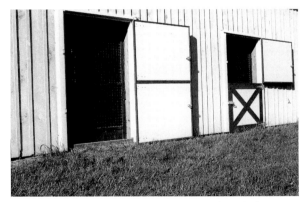

Fig. 1.22 Metal screening doors to guard mesh doors.

for enhancing cross-ventilation. Heavy metal screens should be used to guard these openings (Fig. 1.22).

Flooring materials

Stall flooring is of major concern in barns that are used for housing horses. There must be a substantial base to support the animals, to which adequate bedding can be added for comfort and moisture absorption. Regardless of frequency of cleaning, excess moisture from feces and urine must be considered in the management of the stall. A wide variety of flooring is used, with different means of handling the problem.

The most common and least expensive approach is a base of packed material, which will absorb the moisture over time. For example, a 6–10-inch layer of clay or crushed rock, particularly limestone, is packed over a layer of larger stones. The bedding is applied directly over the base and the moisture filters through to the deeper levels. This type of stall must be refurbished periodically by digging out and replacing portions of the base when moisture is no longer absorbed adequately. This will probably be necessary at least annually if the stall is used heavily.

Solid stall floors can be installed, using concrete or asphalt. In these situations, extra-heavy bedding is needed to prevent injury to the horses. Moisture is handled by removing all of the bedding and washing down the surface. The floor must have a suitable slope, preferably towards the door.

Drains in the stall are a problem if bedding clogs the drain.

Bedding and surfacing materials

There are several different systems, each with advantages and disadvantages based on convenience, cost and secondary effects.[6] For example, straw- and grass-based bedding is inclined to be dusty, whereas slatted rubber floors often appear to be inhospitable to the horse. In any case, bedding must not be harmful to either the mare or the foal. It should provide suitable insulation and cushioning both for the mare during foaling and for the foal.

Suitable materials include:

- Woven rubber matting/rubber chips set into an impervious rubber matrix. In recent years many different styles of rubber or other synthetic mats have become popular. Solid or perforated mats (typically in rectangles 4 × 6 feet) are placed over the base flooring. Moisture works down around the edges or through the perforations, and the mats can be removed for periodic cleaning. Probably the best flooring materials are the rubber pavers and bricks that can be laid down as flooring. Initial costs are quite high for these materials, but maintenance costs are minimal.
- Cinders/sand/peat. These are conventional bedding materials in many places, but are sometimes viewed as inhospitable for foals. However, they are almost free of dusty particles and can be highly absorptive of fluid. They are often difficult to clean out because of the extra weight involved.

- Straw/shavings. These are widely used in arable areas of the world. Wheat or barley straw is widely available as a by-product of cereal farming and there may be little alternative use in many places so prices are usually low and the supply abundant. Unfortunately, straw has a rather bad reputation for diseases of the airways, but this is possibly not much worse than shavings (a by-product of sawmill timber operations). In either case, deep litter systems are not as hygienic as the use of regular cleaning. Shavings are often more expensive than the equivalent amount of straw. Disposal of both straw and shavings requires the construction of a midden or muck heap to permit rotting down.
- Paper, cardboard chippings and other waste and by-products. These materials are hygienic and easily available in most places. They have a low dust rating. Paper products tend to felt together and, if they are not turned twice daily, can be extremely difficult to cut up and remove, so disposal can be a problem.

Fastenings on stable doors

Stable doors may be either sliding or swinging; the former may be safer and take less space in the aisles of barn systems. In both types, double drop latches with floor-level slots/kick bars (Fig. 1.21) reduce the risk to horses, when cast or pawing at the door, of getting feet caught between the door and the door jamb.

Breeding barn/service area

Many large commercial breeding farms standing more than four stallions follow almost universal design protocols. However, many studs use a well-grassed lawn area kept for the purpose of covering mares out in the open. The area is situated away from contact with the general population of mares but may be close to the stallion-holding stables.

An adjacent small area where an individual stallion can tease the mare for service provides an important part of the breeding process.

- It ensures that the mare is in full estrus and will readily accept the stallion. Mares that react badly at this stage may need a recheck, sedation, or possibly additional restraint during mating.
- It allows some arousal of the stallion, which is sometimes an important part of the mating ritual.
- Although it is recognized in breeding terms that collection from stallions for artificial insemination can be managed with well-trained horses on phantom or dummy mares, even these stallions can be easily upset by changes to routine. Care to maintain a quiet orderly progression of accustomed events usually keeps most stallions active and eager workers.

Feeding systems

The specific total requirements for feed storage on a stud farm will depend on the management systems employed and the number of horses on the property at any one time. Storage facilities will almost inevitably include suitable bulk forage storage (lucerne hay, hay or haylage) and smaller storage facilities for concentrate feeds and individual foodstuffs ('straights'). Access to (irrigated) growing pastures reduces the need for large storage barns. The commercial aspects of bulk purchases need to be set against the losses from spoilage and the availability of seasonal foods.

Special provisions

Increasing the length of daylight hours

The provision of adequate facility to alter the (day)light hours to which a mare is exposed is critical to modern stud farm management. If mares are stabled, this can be accomplished by means of artificial overhead lighting. In areas where stabling is not the norm (e.g. in parts of Australia), yard facilities provided with water and hay feeders have overhead light towers (see p. 164). Automatic gate openers have been installed on some farms to allow mares to return to normal paddocks at the shutdown of light, usually around 11.00 p.m.

In drier subtropical climates, most farms have the majority of their mares and mares/foals out at pasture for most of the year, so there is less requirement for expensive barn space and stables.

Stocks/mare-handling facilities

Examination crushes (stocks, chutes) can range from fairly simple, even primitive, to a sophisticated construction allowing many procedures to be performed. Overall dimensions are extremely important as a crush that is oversize can be dangerous to both horse and operator. Simple examination crushes are basically four posts, side rails, front rail, and a gate at the back. Where larger numbers of mares are examined, a partly enclosed crush with a safety opening side gate is both safe and useful (Fig. 1.23). Another useful design for rapid through-put is the use of a sliding door crush as part of an overall yard system (Fig. 1.24). Where large numbers of mares are being examined, a flow pattern centered on a central examination area is important and has been used very successfully for many years.

- A more sophisticated examination crush has the advantage of holding the foal in front of the mare. This has a calming effect, whereas separation and movement of the foal outside the mare's immediate vision may cause serious behavioral difficulties.

Foaling facilities

- Individual foaling boxes of up to 6–10 boxes with closed-circuit television systems installed, etc.
- Small foaling paddocks under floodlights.

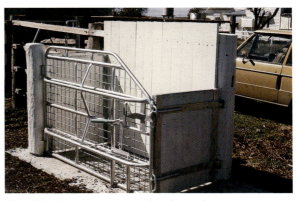

Fig. 1.23   Simple secure steel and wood mare examination stocks; side and back gates can be easily disengaged if the mare goes down.

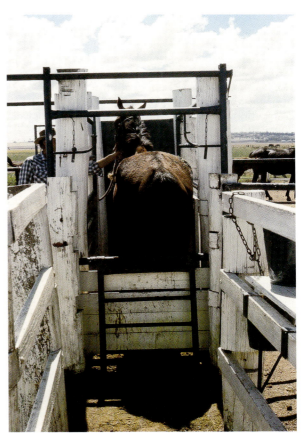

Fig. 1.24   Walk-through stocks with sliding gates, useful for examining large numbers of mares.

Although there are systems that are helpful in setting off alarms for mares that are foaling (see p. 272), these are largely unreliable and most large studs prefer to observe the foaling mares directly or via continuous closed-circuit television. All the systems require direct 24-hour supervision without any noticeable interference. The observer needs to have immediate access to suitably qualified assistance when foaling is seen to be imminent, so telephone and alarm points must be to hand.

Foaling barns

Foaling barns in which mares are housed during the last week or so of gestation and in the immediate post-foaling period are constructed with stalls that are larger than normal. Keeping all the imminent mares in one barn/block provides efficiency of observation; moreover, at the time of delivery, all the necessary equipment is close at hand. However, the mare must be moved first to the foaling barn and back again to her regular stall after foaling; this can be stressful for her and the foal. On large farms in temperate climates, where every foaling mare is housed at night, there is merit to this objection. In warmer climates, however, the foaling area might be a clean grass paddock close by a barn, equipped with good lights. Then, a mare might only be stalled if there is a problem.

A more specialized facility dedicated to foaling mares has been used to advantage on some large farms, particularly in the western USA. The concept is based on having a clean location for foaling, often utilizing an impervious padded flooring instead of conventional bedding. Mares are housed in adjacent conventional stalls in the same building. They are discreetly observed until the second stage of labor begins, and are then moved to the foaling stall to deliver. The absence of straw or shavings in this environment is felt to reduce the contamination to both mare and foal, but the unusual environment might worry the occasional mare.

Breeding barn

It is advantageous to have a covered breeding barn, whether natural service or artificial breeding programs are employed. Adequate space to handle stallions and mares safely is a basic necessity. The building requires an adequate ceiling height, ideally about 5 m (16 feet). The breeding behavior of some stallions suggests that a quiet, undisturbed environment is an advantage.

The floor should be of a material that provides a good foothold for both the stallion and the mare and should provide some cushioning in case an animal slips and falls. Rubber mats or shredded rubber are excellent flooring materials provided they do not get slippery when wet. Tanbark, shavings or their equivalents are common choices for the floor covering, but dust can be a problem in some conditions. Although the hygiene of the area may be a secondary consideration to convenience and safety, it should always be borne in mind.

A conveniently located dust-proof laboratory space is essential, and a set of stocks for mare preparation is useful. If artificial breeding programs are in use, a similar clean service area must be maintained and the use of a phantom or dummy mare is utilized for semen collection. Such an area must have laboratory facilities for semen evaluation and processing in close proximity. Multiple-purpose races (Fig. 1.25) make for easy fast insemination of larger numbers of mares.

Teasing facilities

There are many variations in teaser facilities that are understood by individual stud farm managers. If 'teaser stallions' are kept as a management tool (see p. 77), they can be used in a variety of ways. Some farms have small (6 m², 20 square feet) four-railed paddocks within the mare paddocks into which teaser stallions are introduced. They provide fairly long daily contact to allow mares to quietly approach the teaser when in season. This system often works well with occasional dominant mares; timid mares will not approach the teaser, even when in full estrus. It is also valuable in post-service and pregnant mare paddocks to detect mares returning early, or suffering early pregnancy loss. Similarly, these same small yards can be used adjacent to the breeding yards.

With single mare operations, it is rarely a problem as often there is not the means to tease the mare.

Use of a teasing board or railed fence

The teaser stallion is positioned behind a solid rail with a solid lower section; mares are then led individually up to the teaser and pushed against the rail to allow the teaser to nuzzle and 'talk' to the mare to determine whether or not the mare is showing estrus. Teasing over a rail fence is not as safe a procedure as over a teasing board. Both the teaser and the mare can injure their legs through a two-railed fence. The behavior of the mare should always be carefully observed (see p. 214).

Use of teasing races

Some farms with stock horses use long teasing races that hold between 6 and 50 mares, with several teasers being led along the race to tease the mares. Care must be exercised as anestrous mares often kick out, possibly causing injury to their legs.

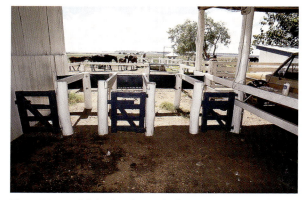

Fig. 1.25 Multiple simple stocks for insemination of multiple mares in artificial insemination programs; open plan allows ease of use.

Feeding facilities

Hay feeding

Bulk forage in the form of hay, haylage or lucerne (alfalfa) hay is frequently fed to brood mares and mares with foals at foot, from steel or wooden hay feeders. There are many different feeding systems in use, but the overriding requirement is for safe access to the feed. Foals should not be able to get into the feeders; they will of course quickly begin to eat small amounts of the feed and are soon better fed with better quality feed by means of creep feeders. Thus both accessibility and quality must be considered.

Paddock feeders

These can be simple, individual feeders, galvanized or heavy-duty plastic buckets. Half oil drums (202 liters, 44 gallons), with the bottom two-thirds filled with cement to prevent horses rolling them around, are widely used.

A 3-m (10-foot) feeder trough (Fig. 1.26) can safely accommodate four horses, if they are placid and compatible, but is the minimum for two less compatible mares. Some feeders have a roof covering, others are open to the weather, and many have sled skids on the ground under leg supports to allow easier transfer when the surrounding ground is muddy.

Stacked tractor and truck tires are also commonly used for feeding horses in yards and small paddocks. They are usually safe as far as leg injury goes, but must be carefully checked to ensure that the wall-reinforcing wires are not exposed; horses can swallow the fine strands of high-tensile wire and this can lead to bowel wall penetration and possibly even death. While on balance they are probably not advisable, they are often better than ground feeding in times of severe drought.

All of these feeders can cause potential injury to mares and foals; this can be compounded if over-crowding occurs (Fig. 1.27).

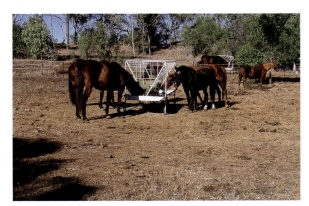

Fig. 1.26   Three-meter (10-foot) feeders can safely accommodate four quiet horses, but may only cater for two incompatible horses.

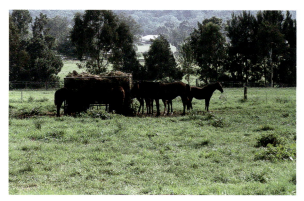

Fig. 1.27   Injuries usually occur with over-crowding at hay and other feeders.

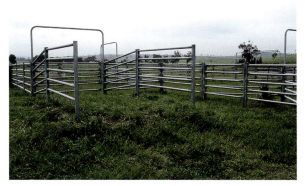

Fig. 1.28   Simple steel yards with loading bay.

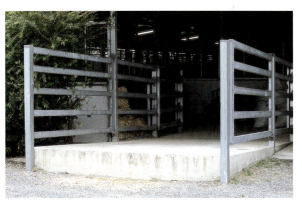

Fig. 1.29   Simple minimal loading ramp allows easy loading of young horses.

Horse-loading facilities

The provision of loading ramps and chutes is an essential part of all stud farm facilities. They are useful for safe loading of young, partially or untrained horses, and horses with poor loading tolerance, which often refuse to walk into horse transporters of any type. Loading ramps need not be complex (Figs 1.28, 1.29), but safety is paramount. Low earth banks can be used to reduce the slope of the wagon ramp. More complex systems using gates and fences designed to accommodate a variety of horse trailer arrangements prevent the horse being loaded from constantly running sideways away from the transport. It also allows foals that have not been taught to lead to be loaded more easily and safely (Fig. 1.30).

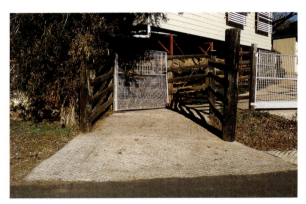

Fig. 1.30 Loading complex with varying height and race widths to allow for variation in transport sizes.

Veterinary treatment (hospital) area

The veterinary facility is a pivotal part of any equine breeding operation. It needs to provide the basic necessities, but many include more impressive facilities such as a lockable drug-storage room, laboratory, office, and examination areas. The facility usually contains at least one set of stocks within individual paddocks, adjacent to the stallion service barn. There are usually additional paddocks where covered mares are held for observation after service.

The outbreak of contagious equine metritis in 1977 made it abundantly clear that casual examination of mares over a stable door and around door posts was no longer safe or acceptable. Veterinary examination areas have improved over the last 20 years with the provision of more covered areas with stocks suitable for using ultrasound scanners. Previously, lack of suitable examination areas, often with insufficient lighting mechanisms, made accurate scan diagnosis less than satisfactory. Mistakes arising from a poor working environment were very disappointing.

Larger stud farms often have a small dust-proof, air-conditioned laboratory with various types of technical equipment, refrigerator, and washing facilities. This important area allows immediate processing of mare swabs, semen evaluation, and microscopic examination of smears from swabs and cultures. More sophisticated facilities for bacterial cultures are sometimes available, but the existence of the space and equipment does not necessarily equate with the technical skills needed to make use of it.

RECORD-KEEPING

Health and breeding records should be kept in the veterinary facility.[7] The records for the stud must be kept fully up to date. Failure to do so can lead to continued confusion and often to acrimony.

Current developments in computer technology mean that records are easily stored and analyzed from data accumulated over long or short periods. Modern computers can readily store digital ultrasound images, and image analysis systems can be used to follow the pregnancy and management procedures. Breeding records stored over a full season will allow accurate analysis of efficiency and may easily identify problems that might not be obvious with conventional study. Feeding analysis and medical records are helpful both to the stud and to the owner's veterinary surgeon who might need to consider these at other times.

Computer-generated recording of admission, services, examinations, and other treatments are essential for both stud and owner confidence in the daily running of the breeding procedure. Also, financial aspects of service, holding and handling fees can be more easily managed and readily available to owners at any time.

Retrospective records are often helpful in understanding problems and, perhaps more importantly, can be used in legal matters relating to stud procedures.

The well-managed stud farm will always have good detailed and complete records that are kept fully up to date. Data should be input directly from the procedures; it is unwise to rely on later memory. Day sheets with action lists for the following 24 hours provide stud managers with an effective tool for improving efficiency. The attending veterinarian can be made aware of the likely workload before arrival so that adequate equipment can be brought to the stud farm.

Notwithstanding the clear advantages of computer records, there are some excellent manual systems in operation, but the extraction of suitable information may be time-consuming and open to errors. With careful data input, computers will provide:

- Accurate data on the individual pregnancy rates for each stallion.
- Detailed data on the cyclicity of mares and the likely optimum service times with supportive medication advice.
- Pregnancy monitoring through image analysis of ultrasound scans.
- Critical assessment of the efficacy of therapeutic measures, such as hormone treatments, uterine therapy, and other procedures.
- Comparative data from successive breeding seasons.
- Financial status.

REFERENCES

1. Taylor JL. Joe Taylor's complete guide to breeding and raising racehorses. Nenah, WI: The Russell Meerdink Co.; 1993.
2. McDonnell S. Understanding horse behavior. Lexington, KY: The Blood Horse, Inc.; 1993.
3. Briggs K. Safe and secure fencing. In: The horse, your guide to equine health care, Vol. XVI, No. 4. Lexington, KY: The Blood Horse, Inc.; 1999:68–74.
4. Cunha TJ. Pasture for horses. In: Horse feeding and nutrition. 2nd edn. San Diego, CA: Academic Press; 1991:274–293.
5. McFarland C. Barn ventilation the natural way. Thoroughbred Times 1998; 14(10):28–29.
6. McFarland C. The floor beneath their feet. Thoroughbred Times 1999; 15(10):28–30.
7. Pascoe DR. Computer use for improved farm efficiency. Proceedings of the Nineteenth Bain-Fallon Memorial Lectures. Australian Veterinary Association 1997:127–131.

Chapter 2
FEEDING AND EXERCISE

Reg Pascoe,
Derek Knottenbelt

STALLIONS

Feeding

There is little information on the specific needs of breeding stallions, but most resting stallions and those with less reproductive demand ('small book') require little more than the normal maintenance requirements for all nutritional components. There is no evidence to suggest a link between stallion fertility and diet, but it is reasonable to suppose that a good healthy diet results in a healthy horse with breeding vigor. A suitable maintenance ration for a 500-kg stallion should provide the amounts shown in Table 2.1.

The total requirement must be supplied within the possible appetite for the individual horse. A good rule is that a stallion can consume up to 1.5–1.8% of its bodyweight per day in dry matter terms. This equates with about 1.5 kg of good-quality hay per 100 kg of bodyweight. Access to good-quality pasture is widely regarded as essential for good health and exercise, but this may not be absolutely necessary.

During the nonbreeding season a good-quality pasture should provide sufficient nutrition, but access to minerals should be allowed, possibly using a general mineral block or a self-feed variety (cafeteria system).

Before the start of the breeding season the stallion should receive a small concentrate feed so that his weight increases slightly. Stallions with a heavy reproductive demand or those in inclement (cold) conditions will inevitably need at least some concentrate feed. Regular accurate weight measurement is probably a very useful management procedure. Working stallions should not be overweight; indeed, there is probably some merit in maintaining a body condition score of 3.5–4.5 (on a scale of 10) during the breeding season. Obesity may result in lowered daily sperm output (see p. 51). Similarly, a stallion that is underweight will probably not be a long-term vigorous breeder. Dietary supplementation with vitamins and minerals does not seem to be helpful in the face of a good, balanced roughage diet based on high-quality hay or pasture. In particular, vitamins A and E do not seem to be needed in extra supply for normal fertility and libido,[1,2] but the provision of the extra diet usually results in increases in supply in any case.

Table 2.1 The normal feeding requirements for a 500-kg stallion (DCP, digestible crude protein)

Nutrient	Maintenance	Stud season
Energy (mJ)	420–450	500–550
Protein (g DCP)	650	820
Calcium (g/day)	20	25
Phosphate (g/day)	14	18
Vitamin A (IU/day)	15,000	22,000

Exercising

Moderate daily exercise is probably essential for working stallions, but during this time they are at some risk of self-trauma or escape. Suitable facilities must be provided for safe exercise, either on grass paddocks or in well-protected yards. Access to good pasture should be encouraged to allow free movement and the stimulation of sunshine and grass, but excessive exercise should be avoided.[3]

MARES

Feeding

Nutritionally, the most important part of gestation is the last 3 months, during which the foal is growing very quickly; up to 60–65% of its birth weight will be gained during this time.[4] The extra demand on the mare during early gestation is regarded as insignificant (but not unimportant as mares that lose weight in early lactation have a lower chance of conception). The total weight gain in the full-term mare is around 12% of her bodyweight. Thus, the nutritional demand on the mare is high during the later stages of gestation; the increase in energy demand in the ninth month of gestation is around 10% and this rises to 20% in the eleventh month of gestation (see Table 2.2). In some cases, reliance on forage alone is poor practice because the mare cannot possibly ingest enough food to maintain her own condition and that of the fetus. Furthermore, the appetite/feeding capacity of the mare falls from 1.8% of bodyweight (dry matter terms) to 1.4% at full term.[5]

Mares do not respond to the flushing system (beginning with a thin mare and providing high nutritional planes) prior to breeding that is used in farm animals.[6] Body condition is probably linked to cyclicity of the ovary. Mares in poor body condition appear to have less ovarian activity than control mares at grass.[7] A low plane of nutrition and weight loss during prebreeding and breeding periods reduces reproductive efficiency. Thin mares (with body condition score <2.5 on a scale of 10) have reduced ovulation, reduced conception rates and a higher rate

of early embryonic loss[8,9] (see p. 253). Increasing the energy intake by 50% has no effect on its own on ovulation or cyclicity, but mares with body condition scores of over 3 (on a scale of 10) have increased follicular activity.[10] Optimal reproductive efficiency is probably achieved when the body condition score is around 3.5–4 (on a scale of 10). High planes of nutrition (gradual increase in energy intake and weight gain) are probably therefore beneficial to fertility.

β-Carotenes may affect the fertility of mares; mares that do not have access to pasture (or other green foods) may benefit significantly from increased dietary supplementation or from injections of vitamin A.

During early gestation little or no concentrate needs to be fed (unless, of course, the mare is lactating at the same time) and from around 6–7 months a small but increasing amount of concentrate is added to her diet. Suitable concentrates are available commercially and these are usually excellent, balanced rations. In the last 90 days some 25–35% of the total intake should be concentrate. The diet should have an overall protein content of 12%. This means that the concentrate should contain 13–14% protein. Although the protein content is less significant than might be expected, most diets supplied to pregnant mares are in excess of requirements. However, if the mare is lactating at the same time, the additional protein and energy requirements are much greater, and diets with up to 35% concentrate feeds with a protein of 17% may be required to supply the needs. Low dietary protein levels (less than 8%) have a deleterious effect on conception rates; conception rates are highest with diets that contain between 11% and 12% protein.

> - A nonlactating Thoroughbred mare weighing 550–600 kg in the last month of gestation should therefore receive 3–3.5 kg of concentrate with sufficient hay or pasture *ad libitum* to provide 12% of protein and 120% of maintenance energy intake.

The mineral requirements of the pregnant (and lactating) mare are critical and must always be considered when calculating a ration for mares.

The lactational demands are far greater than for the early growing fetus (see Table 2.3). The combined demands of recovery from pregnancy, parturition and lactation and the need to conceive again soon after delivery are considerable. Protein and carbohydrate/energy are the major factors, of course, but intake of minerals and vitamins is probably as important. Mares that lose weight or that are nutritionally compromised in any aspect of their food intake are far more likely to fail to conceive than mares that are well fed. Overweight is probably just as bad as underweight. Mares that are gaining weight slightly during the breeding

Table 2.2 The normal feeding requirements for a pregnant mare (DM, dry matter)

Nutrient	Maintenance	Ninth month	Eleventh month
Digestible energy (mJ/kg bodyweight)	8.4	9.45	10.08
Protein (% of diet DM)	8.0	10.00	10.60
Calcium (% DM)	0.24	0.43	0.43
Phosphate (% DM)	0.17	0.32	0.32
Vitamin A (IU/kg)	1837		3650

Table 2.3 The normal feeding requirements for a lactating mare (DM, dry matter)

Nutrient	Maintenance	Lactation
Energy (mJ/kg bodyweight)	8.4	10–11
Protein (% DM)	8.0	11–13
Calcium (% DM)	0.24	0.36–0.52
Phosphate (% DM)	0.17	0.22–0.34
Vitamin A (IU/kg DM)	1830	1250–1370

season have a higher fertility than mares that are either too fat or are losing weight. Mares that are in dietary deficit during early lactation also tend to produce foals that grow more slowly.[11]

During the first 3 months of lactation the appetite will increase to 1.7–2.0% of bodyweight; this is a significant increase over the depressed appetite of the late gestation stage. The extra demand on the mare's protein, energy and mineral metabolism requires that the diet should contain up to 35% concentrate and that the protein content of the diet as a whole should be 12.5–14%. The quality of the forage is clearly important and regular weighing of both mare and foal is probably the best indicator of nutritional adequacy. Careful observation of the mare and the foal may make downward adjustments necessary, particularly if the mare is seen to gain weight or the foal suffers from production/growth abnormalities such as osteochondrosis or contracted tendons. The growth rate of the foal is often an excellent indicator of the mare's nutritional status because during the first 3 months of life its major source of nutrition is mare's milk.

Prolonged dietary deprivation in mares in poor body condition will decrease milk production but will have no material effect on milk composition.[12] Excessive dietary intake resulting in weight gain only appears to have an effect in obese mares when the milk production will decrease (although the composition will be unaffected).[13] The implications for the drop in milk production mainly relate to the foal. Reductions in milk production are sometimes sought as a therapeutic measure for foals with angular and flexural deformities arising from over-nutrition.

Minerals should always be available to lactating mares on a self-feed basis. The calcium/phosphate balance of the ration is probably a critical factor, but the other trace elements and vitamins must always be considered. Some commercial concentrates contain added minerals and some forages are higher in minerals than others (e.g. alfalfa is high in calcium). For the most part, a good balanced ration will supply all the mineral and vitamin needs of the mare and the foal (and the developing fetus) during the first 3 months of lactation.

In the later stages of lactation (3 months to weaning), the volume of milk gradually falls and the foal's reliance on milk falls as more forage is taken.

Nevertheless, there is little doubt that foals grow better 'on the mare', although this may be due to many other social factors. It is generally accepted that foals should not grow too fast and should not appear to be fat or out of condition. A slim, energetic and inquisitive foal is the ideal! Over this period the mare's diet can be adjusted downwards to take account of increasing forage quality and decreasing demand, so that between 5 and 8 months of gestation the diet may comprise forage (pasture ideally or good-quality hay) alone. For mares on a self-feed system, minerals should probably always be available.

Exercising

The healthy pregnant mare benefits from natural free exercise in social groups. Pregnant mares can probably be safely quietly ridden up to 6–7 months of gestation. Thereafter, the mare should be allowed to exercise freely up to and including the last days of pregnancy. There is little proven risk from any natural movement.

FOALS AND WEANLINGS

Feeding

The weaning process is a traumatic event for both mare and foal. The nutritional stress is probably minor compared with the psychological stress because the foal will have derived little nutrition from the milk over the 5–6-month period. Some breeders wean foals as late as possible (often up to 7–9 months) to take advantage of the perceived nutritional value of the milk. However, it is common practice in some areas to wean foals at an earlier stage (often as early as 3 months); it is then important to ensure the supply of a suitable palatable creep feed so that at the point of weaning the foal has less overall stress. Early weaning should not be carried out unless management is excellent. Sometimes, of course, there are reasons beyond control, but in any case early weaning requires extra management input if problems are to be avoided. The feeding of weaning foals is an important management procedure if errors are to be avoided. There are significant dangers in over-feeding (osteochondrosis, physitis/physeal dysplasia, cervical instability syndromes/wobbler foals, and contracted tendons) and also with undernourishment (deficiency problems with calcium/phosphate ratios and poor health/growth). The latter are probably less significant than the former.

Weanlings grow very fast, often going through a growth spurt at around 6–7 months. During this time they develop much extra bone and muscle and this requires a significant dietary input. Shortly before weaning the foal should be taking about 0.3–0.5 kg of concentrate feed per 100 kg bodyweight; after weaning this should be increased to 0.6–0.75 kg per 100 kg bodyweight. Forage intake should be encouraged and the body condition should be kept within the 3.5–5.5 band (on a scale of 0–10). The foals will therefore appear to be slightly thinner than expected. Overweight is potentially much more dangerous than underweight, assuming that the basic nutritional requirements are met. However, Thoroughbred weanlings being pushed on for racing careers are often given much more food and are often in much heavier condition at the yearling sales. There is much controversy over the ideal condition for maximal growth without danger.

Commercial creep and weanling rations and formulations for older growing foals are usually excellent and make calculations of requirements redundant; however, careful examination and regular weight checks are essential to identify the individuals that do not tolerate one or more of these or the management system that supplies them.

Exercising

Foals and weanlings grow best when raised on grass in social groups. Free exercise is critical to their development. Exercise is needed to stimulate muscular and skeletal fitness. Foals may exercise very hard but will naturally regulate themselves when fatigue sets in. Forced exercise is potentially harmful to developing bone and cartilage in particular.[14] There is little to be gained from confining normal foals in stables, small yards or lots. Nevertheless, there are dangers from accidental injuries and nutritional anonymity when the foals are not noticed among the group. Dominant foals may grow faster while less dominant ones may lose weight and fail to thrive. Regular individual handling and checking is essential.

REFERENCES

1. Ralston SL, et al. The effect of vitamin A supplementation on seminal characteristics and vitamin A absorption in stallions. Journal of Equine Veterinary Science 1986; 6:203–207.
2. Rich GA, et al. Effect of vitamin E supplementation on stallion seminal characteristics and sexual behavior. In: Proceedings of the International Congress on Animal Reproduction and Artificial Insemination 1984:111–163.
3. Dinger JE, Norles EE. Effect of controlled exercise on libido in 2-year-old stallions. Journal of Animal Science 1986; 62:1220–1224.
4. Platt H. Growth of the equine foetus. Equine Veterinary Journal 1984; 16:247–249.
5. Hintz HF, Baker JP, Jordan RM, et al. Nutrient requirement of horses. Washington, DC: National Academy of Science/National Research Council; 1978.
6. National Research Council. Description of individual condition scores. In: Nutrient Requirements of Horses. 5th edn. Washington, DC: National Academy Press; 1989:39–49.
7. Ginther OJ. Anovulatory season: nutrition. In: Ginther OJ, ed. Reproductive biology of the mare. 2nd edn. Cross Plains, WI: Equiservices; 1979:241–245.
8. Henneke DR, Potter GD, Kruder JL. Body condition during pregnancy and lactation and reproductive efficiency rates of mares. Theriogenology 1984; 21:897–899.
9. Potter TJ, Kreidler JL, Potter GD. Embryo survival during early gestation in energy deprived mares. In: Proceedings of the 9th Equine Nutrition and Physiology Society Symposium 1985:293–298.
10. Morris RP, Rich GA, Ralton SL. Follicular activity in transitional mares as affected by body condition and dietary energy. In: Proceedings of the 9th Equine Nutrition and Physiology Society Symposium 1987:93–99.
11. Pagan JD, Hintz JF. In: Proceedings of the 7th Equine Nutritional Physiology Symposium 1981:121–124.
12. Banach MA, Evans JW. Effects of inadequate energy during gestation and lactation on the oestrous cycle and conception rates and their foals weights. In: Proceedings of the 7th Equine Nutritional Physiology Symposium 1981:97–100.
13. Kubiak JR, Evans JW, Potter GD. Milk production and composition in the multiparous mare fed to obesity. In: Proceedings of the 11th Equine Nutritional Physiology Symposium 1989:295–299.
14. Squires EL, Todter GE, Berndtson WE, et al. Effect of anabolic steroids on reproductive function of young stallions. Journal of Animal Science 1982; 54:576–579.

Chapter 3
ROUTINE STUD MANAGEMENT PROCEDURES

Derek Knottenbelt,
Reg Pascoe

GENERAL PROCEDURES

Weight and condition

Regular recording of the weight of stallions, mares and foals should be performed on the stud. The ideal is to maintain the animals in a good (but not overweight) body condition that takes account of their production. Production for a stallion is considerably different in nutritional demand from that of a pregnant, lactating mare or young growing foal.

The body score system can be used in addition to the weight; the ideal adult body condition score should remain between 4 and 6 (on a scale of 10).[1]

Foot care

Routine foot care by a skilled farrier is essential for adult breeding animals and foals. Brood mares can easily be forgotten during the busiest times of the year. Minor corrective measures can be taken to control limb deviations (angular and flexural) in foals either by careful rasping of the foot or by the application of surgical shoes with extensions.

Dental care

Dental examinations must be performed at least at 6-monthly intervals in older breeding stock (particularly stallions). Routine dental procedures include:

- Examination of the whole mouth using a gag and a suitable light source; it is best to use a head light during this examination.
- Rasping ('floating') of sharp enamel edges.
- Corrective dentistry such as hook removal or extractions. These procedures are described in standard texts.[2]

Identification procedures

One of the most essential aspects of stud farm management is the effective identification of mares, particularly those visiting animals that are not well known to the stud staff. Unfortunately, this is an area that is sometimes neglected and can then cause considerable problems.

There are a number of effective means of identification, each with some advantages and some disadvantages. Failure to identify a mare correctly at a stud can have catastrophic financial implications. Stallions are usually relatively simple to identify because they are generally managed in an individual fashion, whereas the mare population on a stud may vary markedly.

The methods available for identification of the animals include several visible means, some hidden means and some that rely on documentation. Most of the effective methods are permanent, but temporary identification can be useful under some conditions (e.g. short-term movement to a stud farm).

Hoof branding

Hoof branding (Fig. 3.1) is a semi-permanent method of identification, but of course the marks are lost as the hoof grows out. Also, it is possible to tamper with the marks by altering the figures to some extent. Nevertheless, it is a reasonably effective way that is painless (hopefully) and will certainly be identifiable for some 4–6 months. It can be repeated as many times as necessary.

Usually a postcode/zipcode or telephone number is used, which can be spread over all four hooves.

What does it involve?

A red-hot iron is applied briefly to the hoof capsule to create an easily identifiable mark. Usually a combination of numbers or letters is used.

Advantages
- Reasonable duration of marking (it usually takes at least 4–6 months to grow out completely).
- Painless.
- Quick.

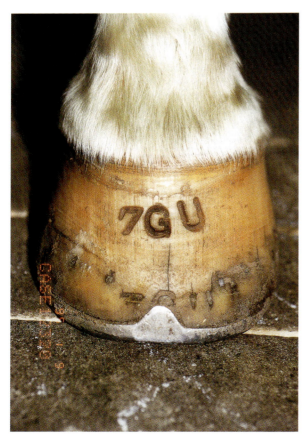

Fig. 3.1 A hoof brand.

- Cheap.
- Difficult if not impossible to delete, but can be altered.

Disadvantages
- Temporary. It relies on some identification held elsewhere (e.g. at the owner's home address: postcode/zipcode or telephone number).
- Possibly alterable within limits.
- Needs to be repeated as required.

Tattoo (lip/gum or ear)

A tattoo is a recognized way of identifying horses that relies upon the ancient art of permanent skin coloring. Usually the tattoo is applied to the soft pink lining of the inside of the lip. This enables the dark-colored pigment to be easily recognized. The shape of the lip, however, makes it difficult to apply the tattoo with a consistent degree of accuracy and so experience is required.

What does it involve?

A needle punch is loaded with stencils of an appropriate number/letter configuration and then the skin is wiped with the ink. Clamping the punch onto the lip (or ear, or gums) drives the needles into the mucous membrane (or skin). This carries a small amount of the ink into the skin and this remains as a permanent colored 'scar'. The color of the ink can be altered but invariably it is much more difficult to see when it is applied to the skin rather than on the pink mucosal surface of the inside of the upper or lower lip.

Advantages
- Clear, permanent and definite.
- Little specialist equipment needed (often Indian ink is used).
- Cheap.
- Very difficult to erase/tamper with.

Disadvantages
- Painful.
- Messy.
- Not visible from a distance.
- Not easily visible in dark skin.
- Liable to be irregular (not every needle takes in the same amount of dye and some foci will not take up the dye).
- Many are difficult to read accurately.

Freeze marking

Freeze marking (Fig. 3.2) has been used for many years as a means of identification. It relies upon the change in color of the hair from body color to white when the skin is subjected to a defined cycle of freezing. The freezing is not enough, however, to cause serious freezing leading to ulceration of the skin. In gray horses the method requires a harder freeze because the

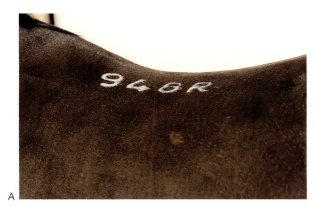

A

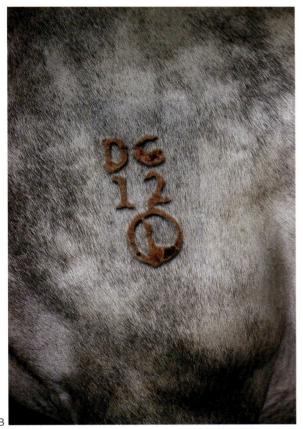

B

Fig. 3.2   (A) A freeze brand. (B) A freeze brand can suggest both identity and a possible insurance history.

intention is to create a hairless mark rather than just a change in the color of the hair coat. A white mark on a white-haired horse would probably not be obvious! In many cases the freeze mark is not very obvious until the area is clipped, but most freeze marks are obvious from a distance.

What does it involve?

This is a simple procedure that is usually performed without the need for sedation. It is seldom if ever uncomfortable for the horse; most just continue to eat while it is being done. The technicians who are skilled

at doing the procedure have a standard freeze protocol for gray and nongray horses. Usually an obvious site is chosen. The procedure involves clipping and removal of an area of hair where the brand is to be placed, spraying the area with 70% alcohol and applying the chilled brand (the brand is placed in liquid nitrogen until 'boiling' ceases) to the area of application. Foals require 10–12 seconds of contact, yearlings 15–18 seconds, adults 20–25 seconds. These times can vary if incorrect brands are used.

Advantages

- Simple method.
- Painless.
- Cheap.
- Definite; no scope for tampering.
- Visible from a distance (thieves will be less inclined to steal a horse with a visible freeze mark).

Disadvantages

- Requires a skilled technician.
- Loss of cosmetic appearance due to presence of numbers.
- Not always clearly visible (differences in gray horses).

Hot branding

Hot branding (Fig. 3.3) commonly takes two forms. The first is a standard identification mark that is used for specific breeds of horse. The second is some form of specific identification; historically, this was used to identify the owner of the horse or its origin, but it could equally be used to add numbers and letters in combination so that the animal can be identified permanently. The brand is usually applied at an early age (when restraint is more practicable). The effect is obtained by creating an obvious, defined shaped scar. No hair grows on the scar and it is therefore visible from a distance and regardless of the hair coat status (winter/summer).

What does it involve?

The brand is invariably applied by a red-hot iron, either as a single preformed 'trade mark' or as a series of numbers/letters. The resultant burn causes scarring of the skin and hair loss over the area. The scar is usually black and thinner than the normal skin. Some operators will try to use a lower temperature and create a lesser scar. Over the passage of time the scar may become distorted and so may be less recognizable. Hot branding is no longer permitted in some circumstances (e.g. in Thoroughbred and Standardbred horses in Australia and New Zealand).

Advantages

- Permanent markings are easily identified as being applied on purpose rather than as accidental scars.

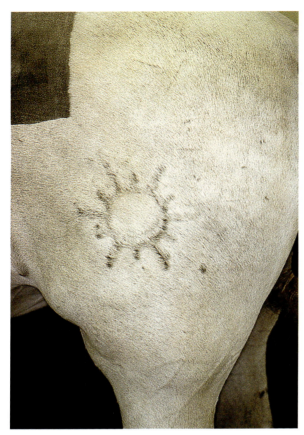

Fig. 3.3 This example of a hot brand simply identifies a breed or type.

- Categorical identification should be possible.
- Little opportunity for tampering with them.

Disadvantages
- Very painful, rather brutal, procedure.
- Causes significant skin destruction.
- Scars can distort over time and will in any case inevitably shrink, making the mark less clear.
- 'Lightly' branded horses may be impossible to identify accurately by the brand.

Microchip identification

Microchip identification of horses is gaining much credibility as more and more chips become available and more and more microchip readers are held by police, slaughter houses, customs, and welfare and charitable institutions. Although there are the usual horror stories of nasty injection reactions and migrating chips, these are extremely rare; indeed, they may be less common than physical injury to the exact site of the chip placement.

What does it involve?

The procedure is relatively simple with a single sub-cutaneous injection, usually on the side of the neck.

The procedure is usually (but not always) virtually painless.

Advantages
- Definite.
- Permanent.
- Tamper-proof.
- Minor cost.
- Little pain involved in insertion.
- Can be read from a distance with the appropriate reader gun (e.g. from outside a truck or by a reader placed by the roadside during an event).

Disadvantages
- Invasive procedure.
- Invisible.
- May move/migrate.
- The occasional horse may require sedation or twitching.
- Occasional abscess formation with loss of chip.
- Detection relies on possession of a 'reader'.
- Reader must be passed over the chip.
- Not all readers read all chips.

Identification by natural markings/scars
(permanent alterations)

This has been used for many years as a means of categorical identification. It relies upon the accurate and detailed sketching and written description of all naturally occurring white marks and hair whorls. Often it includes certain permanent acquired markings.

What does it involve?

A written description and a sketch that corresponds exactly have considerable advantages in that there should be no debate thereafter that the horse is the one described. However, it does rely on a suitable piece of paper/document and this is not always filled in completely or legibly. Furthermore, after regular handling the document may become difficult to read. A passport that contains a photocopy of the original identifies Thoroughbred horses and certain other breeds. This is over-stamped to ensure that there is no possibility of tampering with the sketch or the narrative.

Advantages
- Usually completed by a veterinary surgeon with a signature to support its veracity.
- Text and sketch should correspond exactly making tampering difficult/impossible.

Disadvantages
- A very time-consuming, and therefore expensive, procedure if performed properly by a veterinary surgeon. Most breed societies will only accept certificates of identification if they are signed by a veterinary surgeon.

- The passport or ID form is required for comparison.
- Open to abuse if blank forms fall into the wrong hands. Forged signatures and false sketches and narratives are easy to prepare.
- Some difficulties with colors, especially in bay/chestnut foals that subsequently turn gray.

Photographic identification

Photographic identification has not gained the reputation or universal application it perhaps deserves. There is scope for the inclusion of color pictures in a sealed tamper-proof plastic sheath. However, photographic quality varies and in some cases it may not be helpful at all. For example, almost all Fell ponies are a very similar uniform color and so a photograph might not be helpful. Similarly, gray horses and Appaloosa horses will often not retain either the same color or the same pattern distribution. Some foals are born bay or chestnut and change to gray.

What does it involve?

A simple series of photographs taken from the left, right, front and rear with a close-up of the head will identify a horse definitively so long as the markings are obvious on the photographic plate.

Advantages

- Easy.
- Cheap.
- Very positive (color is exact).
- Cannot be tampered with (some exceptions with modern computer technology).

Disadvantages

- Lack of credibility with respect to the individual horse unless accompanied by a certificate of authenticity signed by a veterinary surgeon.
- Some breeds such as the Fell pony have few if any identification marks apart from whorls and these may be difficult/impossible to see on a photograph.
- Will depend heavily on photographic quality. In many cases it is impossible to see whorls or small marks/scars clearly.
- New scars or skin damage from injury, etc. may change the appearance significantly from that in the photograph.

Blood typing (gene/DNA mapping)

Blood typing is helpful in establishing parentage but on its own does not help to identify an individual horse.

Tissue typing can, in theory, be performed from any body tissue, including clippings, hair, blood, semen or even cells taken from the cheek lining. In practice, it is usual to use hair or blood. The tissues can be stored indefinitely and the technology is becoming more readily available and cheaper with advancing scientific methods.

The genetic make-up of the tissue cells of an individual is totally unique. However, gene mapping is really an advanced form of tissue typing and provides no more information than the tissue type with respect to identification.

What does it involve?

A single sample of a body tissue is all that is required. Commonly, this is frozen whole blood but could equally be hair or hoof clippings. Every cell and its remnants will carry the unique genetic code for that particular individual and this could (at least theoretically) be used to identify the original animal categorically for eternity.

Advantages

- Categorical method of identification.
- Permanent.

Disadvantages

- Invisible.
- Only applies when there is other tissue to compare it with (i.e. 'is this my horse for which I have tail or mane hairs or a blood sample').
- Expensive technology at present.

Vaccination

Routine vaccination is usually performed for a variety of diseases according to local disease-control requirements. For an effective immunologic response the animal needs to be healthy and have an active immune system. Stress, debility, illness or malnutrition can influence the response to a vaccine. All vaccines have a defined protocol that enhances the protective response in the vaccinated animal, but although most are regarded as beneficial some do have potential harmful effects and some are much less efficacious than others. Thus, the vaccine for tetanus is regarded as excellent protection whereas that for influenza can be less predictable. The nature of the disease and the organism itself has an influence on the efficacy of a vaccine.

Tetanus

In general, all horses are vaccinated routinely against tetanus using a standard routine. This involves a primary course of two intramuscular injections of tetanus toxoid followed by a booster vaccination after one year and then every alternate year.

Foals are usually considered to be effectively covered for up to 6–8 weeks of age through colostral transfer of antibody (see p. 374) provided that the mare received a booster vaccination in the last trimester of pregnancy. If a mare has not been vaccinated for between 1 and 2 years before foaling the duration of transferred immunity is probably inadequate.

If there is any doubt about either the effectiveness of the vaccination of the mare or the efficiency of colostral (passive) transfer of immunity (see p. 377) it is common practice to administer a single or repeated doses of between 1500 and 6000 IU of tetanus antiserum. This will usually confer effective protection for up to 12 weeks of age.[3]

The administration of a tetanus toxoid at, or shortly after, birth is controversial, but in theory at least there should be no particular problem with vaccination at 2–4 weeks of age.[4] However, most authorities do not recommend vaccination at birth of a foal that has effective passive transfer on the basis that passive antibodies will interfere with active immunity for a primary vaccination. Repeated vaccination during this time may indeed result in poor long-term immunologic response to the vaccine, and in some cases there may be no effective response. However, some authorities consider that active vaccination in the face of passive maternal immunity is effective.[5]

Influenza

Vaccination against influenza viruses (equine influenza A, types 1 and 2) is common practice in most areas of the world. However, there are a few places where the disease does not appear to exist and vaccination is not practiced (e.g. Australia and New Zealand).

There are several different combinations of virus strains in commercial vaccines. The natural antigenic drift means that vaccination is not likely to confer certain and complete protection. Rather it serves to modify the course and severity of the infection. Vaccines are regularly up-dated to include the most recent strains so that the conferred immunity is as near to the field virus as possible.

Immunity to the adjuvanted vaccines is reported to be around 6–9 months, but the immune-stimulating complex vaccines provide protective antibody for 12–14 months.

Passive immunity is transferred to the foal via the colostrum and is probably protective for up to 6–8 weeks.

Primary vaccination for a foal is instigated at around 5–6 months of age. Vaccination is repeated at 30 and 150 days after the initial vaccination. Annual boosters are usually given, with stud mares receiving a booster some 3–5 weeks pre-term.

Equine herpesvirus 1 and 4 (rhinopneumonitis)

Infection with equine herpesvirus 1 is a serious cause of abortion, neurological disease in adult horses and neonatal death in foals. Vaccination has become more widely used since the quality of protection has improved. Infection with equine herpesvirus 4 is probably less serious but can cause abortion.

The vaccines do not appear to prevent the development of the neurological form of the disease.

There are three types of vaccine available:

- A killed oil-based vaccine that has been used for many years to prevent abortion. The vaccine is administered to pregnant mares at 3, 5 and 7 months of gestation. Stallions are vaccinated as for nonpregnant mares (i.e. by annual booster).
- Modified live virus vaccine. Although this vaccine does confer good immunity against both virus strains, it should not be used in pregnant mares.
- Killed bivalent vaccine with immune stimulating complex. These vaccines are widely available and are effective in controlling abortion as well as respiratory disease.

Usually three doses are administered at 3–4-week intervals with 6-monthly boosters thereafter, but individual vaccines may have particular requirements for the various classes of stud animals. It should be noted that for maximum protection all in-contact horses must be regularly vaccinated.

Equine viral arteritis

This disease causes abortion, infertility, upper respiratory tract disease and arteritis (see p. 259). It has a worldwide distribution, but some areas are free of the disease. Vaccines are effective in preventing the disease but do not result in the cure of an infected carrier stallion (see p. 259).

An annual booster dose is given to all breeding stock at least 3 weeks before breeding.

Responses to vaccination cannot be distinguished from natural infection, thus serological investigation should precede the vaccine. This ensures that carriers and potential carriers (usually stallions) will not be used for breeding unless proven to be clear of the disease.

Equine viral encephalitis

Various types of equine viral encephalitis are prevalent in different areas of the world but large areas are free of infection and so vaccination is not practiced.

Most types of encephalitis are spread by blood-feeding insects (usually mosquitoes and midges). The disease therefore tends to be seasonal, but can be spread by fomites (e.g. needles and blood products).

Vaccination is usually by an inactivated bivalent or trivalent vaccine and the conferred immunity from a primary course is probably less than 6–9 months.[5] The first dose of vaccine for foals is usually administered at 4–6 months of age.

Rabies

Stud mares and stallions are probably not at major risk of rabies infection but vaccination is quite properly used in endemic areas where the horses are exposed to possible wildlife vectors.

The primary vaccination course is two doses given 3–4 weeks apart; seroconversion is then measured and vaccination repeated until a protective level is achieved. Annual or bi-annual boosters are usually given.

Passive immunity is probably conferred for 12 weeks but little is known about this.

African horse sickness

This disease is restricted to Africa and has a highly seasonal prevalence based upon the presence of the vector (*Culicoides imicola*).

The vaccines comprise eight major strains of the live virus (covering over 40 subtypes). Vaccine is administered 2–3 months prior to the onset of the risk (rainy) season. An initial 'weak' vaccine is administered intramuscularly about 4 weeks before the stronger vaccine. Booster vaccines are given to protected or vaccinated horses by a single injection of the combined strains 4–6 weeks before the risk season starts.

Foals are passively immune for 10–12 weeks and are usually first vaccinated at around 8 months of age.

Potomac horse fever (equine ehrlichiosis; *Ehrlichia risticii*)

This disease is limited to some areas of North America and vaccination is used routinely in these areas.

Primary vaccination comprises two doses 3 weeks apart. Annual boosters are given 2–4 weeks before foaling.

Strangles

The current vaccines are based on whole bacterin or M-protein components of the bacterium. A new intranasal vaccine may be a significant advance.

The vaccines are not highly effective and side-effects such as purpura hemorrhagica have been reported. There is also a high rate of injection site reactions.

Botulism

Botulism is a rare disease in adult horses, but the toxic/infectious form is encountered from time to time in foals (Shaker foal syndrome). Endemic areas do occur where the organisms (particularly *Clostridium botulinum* type B) live in the soil, and losses can occur regularly in unvaccinated horses and particularly in foals.

Primary vaccination comprises three doses 4 weeks apart with the last dose 3–4 weeks before foaling. Annual boosters are given at 3–4 weeks before foaling. Passive immunity is considered to be good.

Unfortunately, the vaccine is not universally available.

Routine control measures for infectious diseases

There are protocols for the control of:

- Contagious equine metritis (see p. 193).
- *Klebsiella pneumoniae* infection (see p. 182).
- *Pseudomonas aeruginosa* infection (see p. 182).
- Equine herpesvirus infection (abortion/ respiratory/neurological) (see p. 257).
- Equine viral arteritis (see p. 259).
- Dourine (*Trypanosoma equiperdum* infection) (see p. 196).

Parasite control

See below, p. 37.

PARASITIC DISEASES

Strongyloidosis

Etiology

- Infestation with *Strongyloides westeri*.
- *Strongyloides westeri* is host-specific for the horse.[6]
- This parasite causes diarrhea, usually in the first weeks of life, but cases have been reported in foals as old as 16 weeks.
- Most parasites of this class are not pathogenic; skin penetration causes the most obvious signs.
- This parasite can undergo its full life-cycle as free-living stages in the environment, but under certain circumstances third-stage larvae can penetrate the skin and parasitize the small intestine. Most serious infestations, however, arise from the lactogenic route. Populations of parthenogenic females can survive in the gut of foals, and the larval stages can survive in contaminated soil and bedding, especially when there is increased humidity.
- Significant intestinal infestations seldom (if ever) develop in animals over 6 months of age.
- Larvae that penetrate the skin accumulate there and then migrate to the mammary gland in late pregnancy and early lactation. Larvae may also penetrate the placenta to cause prenatal infection.

Clinical signs

- Heavy infestations can cause mild enteritis and diarrhea in foals.
- Possible dermatitis, especially of lower limbs/coronary bands. This can be severe when collecting yards are heavily infested, and foals may show bizarre behavior patterns resembling colic. These signs abate when the foals are removed from the source of the worms. The signs are attributable to a massive and very irritating penetration of the skin by larvae.

Diagnosis

- Clinical signs and massive egg burdens in feces (often several thousand or more per gram of feces). Look for small thin-walled eggs, but note that the worm egg count is not an index of clinical significance.

- Larvae may be found in washings taken from the skin of heavily contaminated foals.

Differential diagnosis

Other causes of ill-thrift and diarrhea:

- Rotavirus.
- *Rhodococcus equi* infection (enteric form).
- Ascaridiasis.
- Foal heat diarrhea.
- Lactose intolerance.
- Overfeeding.
- Ingestion of sand or foreign body.

Treatment

- Anthelmintics are very effective. The adult worms are susceptible to a single dose of fenbendazole or ivermectin.

Note:
- Diarrhea can quickly lead to dehydration in young foals so appropriate measures should be taken to ensure that the foal remains properly hydrated.
- Other serious causes of diarrhea should be eliminated.

Prognosis

- Good. Spontaneous resolution is the norm.

Control

- Deworming the mare shortly after foaling can significantly reduce the extent of infection.[7]
- Ivermectin in mares during pregnancy reduces the burden of worms migrating to the udder.
- Good hygiene of stable and pastures is important.
- On studs where this has become a problem, foals can be wormed routinely at 2 weeks of age.

Ascaridiasis

Etiology

- *Parascaris equorum* has an extensive hepato-pulmonary migration route.
- Infestation occurs only by eating embryonated eggs from the environment (i.e. from pasture). High levels of immature worms in the small intestine can lead to obstructions (Fig. 3.4).
- There is no evidence of prenatal or transmammary infection.
- The eggs hatch in the gastrointestinal tract; the larvae reach the liver within 48 hours of ingestion and are found in the lung by 7 days post infection. The parasites are then found in the intestine some 4 weeks later; they are only 2 mm

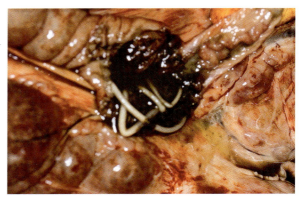

Fig. 3.4 Impaction of *Parascaris equorum* ascarid in the jejunum of a young foal. Note that coarse fibrous food and ascarids can cause impaction. The foal had pica and ate coarse food without much chewing.

long at first and then grow rapidly (males up to 25 cm long, females up to 50 cm long). The prepatent period is approximately 10 weeks. Thus, ascarid eggs are found in foals of about 80 days old if infection occurs soon after birth.
- 30–60% of foals are infested with this parasite.

Clinical signs

Clinical signs are attributable to massive infestation, which causes two major syndromes:

1. Respiratory signs.
   - These appear 3–4 weeks post infection and are associated with the pulmonary stage of migration.
   - Mucoid tracheal exudate.
   - Cough.
   - Nasal discharge (mucoid or mucopurulent).
2. Intestinal signs.
   - These are attributable to the hepatic and intestinal phases of migration and maturation.
   - Signs of chronic ill-thrift, poor condition, weight loss, diarrhea. Appetite remains good.
   - Occasionally, more serious signs of colic are seen; these are associated with the massive simultaneous death of parasites in the distal jejunum or ileum. Anthelmintics or spontaneous immune rejection at or around 6 months of age can cause this. Intestinal obstruction/ intussusception can cause signs of severe nonstrangulating colic.

Note:
- Intussusceptions can be misleading and peritoneal fluid may not reveal the severity of the strangulating condition.
- Ultrasonographic examination is very useful.

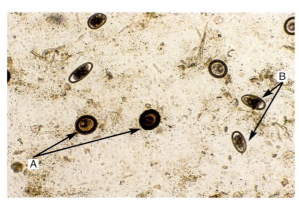

Fig. 3.5   Ascarid eggs (A) and strongyle eggs (B) in feces.

Diagnosis

- Clinical signs and epidemiological factors.
- Worm eggs are usually very prominent (Fig. 3.5). However, eggs may not be detectable in feces during the prepatent period and this is especially relevant in cases with respiratory signs.
- Tracheal washes may show eosinophilia.

Differential diagnosis

- Other causes of coughing:
  ❑ Viral respiratory infections.
  ❑ Bacterial pneumonia (including *Rhodococcus equi* and secondary bacterial pneumonia).
  ❑ Inhalation of food/milk.
- Other causes of ill-thrift:
  ❑ Rotavirus diarrhea.
  ❑ Strongylosis.
  ❑ Strongyloidosis.
  ❑ Immunocompromising conditions.
  ❑ Lactose intolerance.
  ❑ Foal heat diarrhea.
  ❑ Malnutrition/malabsorption syndromes.

Treatment

- Anthelmintic treatments: efficacy claims against *Parascaris equorum* are given for pyrantel, moxidectin (this should NOT be used in foals less than 4 months of age), and fenbendazole.
- Immunity is thought to be age-related and, by 18 months to 2 years of age, young horses acquire a solid immunity to ascarids. This immunity is truly age-related and does not depend on prior exposure; therefore, when ascarids are identified in older horses, their immune status should be examined.

Prognosis

- Good if diagnosis is made early and appropriate anthelmintics are given.
- Poor if present as acute colic due to massive parasite death.

Control

- Eggs are very resistant and difficult to eliminate from contaminated premises/stables.
- Ascarid infections are essentially passed from foal to foal so, if possible, do not allow foals to graze pasture that was grazed by foals and yearlings the previous season.
- Start routinely worming the foal at 6 weeks of age (i.e. before the worms start egg-laying), to avoid contamination of the environment.

Strongylosis (see Table 3.1)

Etiology

- *Strongylus* spp., including *S. vulgaris*, *S. edentatus* and *S. equinus*. The latter two species are rare.
- Migrating larvae cause most of the clinical problems.
- The prepatent period is about 9 months and adult worms are rare in foals.
- Hypobiosis (arrested development) is not well defined.
- Adult worms are blood feeders: *S. edentatus* and *S. equinus* are more avid blood feeders than *S. vulgaris*, but their larvae are not nearly so pathogenic.[8]
- *S. edentatus* and *S. equinus* are more difficult to remove with anthelmintic therapy.
- Can be a significant cause of debility in immunocompromised foals.
- The parasite is becoming less common as larvicidal doses of fenbendazole and the avermectin/milbemycin class of anthelmintics are being used more frequently.

Note:
- There are no known reports of large strongyle resistance to these classes of anthelmintic (cf. cyathostomes, below).

Note:
- Patent infections are rare in foals under 3–4 months of age because of the long prepatent period of these parasites, but arteritis lesions are possible.

Clinical signs

- Vascular/arterial signs are prominent in foals under 6 months of age.
- Minor arteritis lesions at the root of the cranial mesenteric artery may cause minor or major episodes of occlusive/thromboembolic colic.

Table 3.1 Strongyle prepatent periods, migration routes and clinical disease

Parasite	Prepatent (months)	Target organ	Notes
Strongylus vulgaris	6–9	Arterial walls	Cause of arteritis and infarctive colic
Strongylus edentatus	5–7	Liver via hepatic portal vein to the peritoneal and subperitoneal tissues of the flank and return to mesentery by tissue migration and thence into wall of large intestine gut wall	Rarely causes clinical disease. Can cause significant colic and rarely causes problems associated with aberrant migration to other organs
Strongylus equinus	5–12	Liver via peritoneum and subperitoneal tissues of the flank and return to mesentery by tissue migration and thence into the wall of the large intestine	Rarely causes clinical disease

- Larger emboli can cause catastrophic nonstrangulating vascular obstructive colic. In either case, peritonitis is common; the peritoneal fluid is turbid, yellow-orange, contains increased numbers of red and white cells, and has a high protein content. Clinical signs of colic can be persistent and unremitting.
- Anemia and ill-thrift due to heavy burdens of adult worms, which are plug feeders. Hemorrhage can occur from ulcerated sites of attachment on the mucosa.
- Occasional cases show rupture of major vessels (e.g. aorta, cranial mesenteric artery or renal artery).

> Note:
> - Relationship to future development of iliac thrombosis is equivocal.
> - Intestinal motility disorders are rare and diarrhea is not a feature.

Diagnosis
- History of a poor anthelmintic control program, especially if grazing is on poorly maintained pastures with older horses.
- The mature worms are visible to the naked eye.

Differential diagnosis
- Other forms of colic and other causes of ill-thrift and weight loss.

Treatment
- Standard dose of ivermectin or moxidectin (horses over 4 months) or a 5-day course of fenbendazole (see Table 3.2).

Prognosis
- Fair if treated early.
- Verminous aneurysms are rare.
- Colic is a far more important sign of serious infection in young foals.

Control
- Full anthelmintic control program with prophylactic anthelmintic drugs started by 6–8 weeks of age.
- Intensity of program varies with likely challenge.
- Foals grazing in mixed-age groups over the summer may be wormed at least every 8 weeks with fenbendazole.
- There is no known resistance to the current anthelmintics, but the possibility should be considered if the diagnosis is confirmed and the treatment fails to resolve the problem.

> Note:
> - These parasites flourish in exactly the same conditions that are conducive to the survival of cyathostomes, so over-use of fenbendazole may quickly lead to benzimidazole-resistant cyathostomes. Thus, it may be better (especially in the summer months) to routinely monitor the fecal egg output of all grazing horses and treat only those animals with a positive egg count (i.e. more than 100 eggs per gram of feces).

- Some foals are left with long-term intestinal or vascular problems from heavy burdens.

Table 3.2 Current worming remedies against equine intestinal parasites and the recommended interval between doses

Drug	Recommended frequency of dosing for adult horses (weeks)	Efficacy against cyathostomes and tapeworms
Fenbendazole	6 or 26–52 (for 5-day course)	• Will kill adult small redworms, their eggs and some immature stages • Some small redworms are resistant to this drug • 5-day course effective against inhibited mucosal stages of small redworms • No efficacy against tapeworms
Mebendazole	6	• Will kill adult small redworms • Some small redworms are resistant to this drug • No efficacy against tapeworms
Oxibendazole	6–8	• Will kill adult small redworms and their eggs • Some small redworms are resistant to this drug • No efficacy against tapeworms
Febantel	Occasional	• Will kill adult small redworms • No efficacy against tapeworms
Pyrantel embonate	4–6	• Will kill adult small redworms • Not effective against encysted mucosal stages • Double dose will kill tapeworms • Use anti-tapeworm dose every 6–12 months • No efficacy against *A. mamillana*
Ivermectin	8–10	• Highly effective against adult small redworms; limited effect against inhibited mucosal stages • No efficacy against tapeworms
Moxidectin	13	• High efficacy against adult and developing small redworms • Persistent effect • No efficacy against tapeworms
Praziquantel	Occasional	• Efficacy against tapeworms, including *Anoplocephela mamillana* • Veterinary surgeons can administer solution by stomach tube (NOT INJECTION) • No efficacy against roundworms

Note: Efficacy against strongyles (*Parascaris equorum and Oxyuris equi*) is assumed unless stated otherwise.

Aberrant larval migration

Etiology

- Most often *Strongylus vulgaris* larvae (also *Draschia megastoma, Hypoderma bovis, Setaria digitata*).
- Rare in very young foals.[9] Usually affects older horses.

Clinical signs

- Acute onset of convulsions and progressive asymmetric gait abnormality.
- Signs may remain stable for a few days before advancing again (possibly because of the irregular behavior of the migrating parasite). Generally the signs get worse with time.
- Cranial nerve or behavioral problems can develop, but signs are dependent upon number, location and activity of the parasite (very unpredictable).

Diagnosis

- Eosinophils and macrophages in the cerebrospinal fluid.
- Rarely any peripheral eosinophilia and very rarely correlated to parasite eggs in feces.

Differential diagnosis

- Cranial trauma.
- Central nervous system infections, including bacterial/viral encephalitis/meningitis, equine protozoal myeloencephalopathy.
- Cervical vertebral instability/malformation syndromes.

Treatment

- Larvicidal anthelmintics (may take up to 10 days to have any effect):
  ❑ Ivermectin.
  ❑ Moxidectin, in animals more than 4 months of age.
  ❑ Fenbendazole (5-day course).
- Systemic corticosteroids and nonsteroidal anti-inflammatory drugs:
  ❑ Dexamethasone at 0.1–0.5 mg/kg intravenously or orally every 12 hours.
  ❑ Flunixin/phenylbutazone helpful in some cases but there may be serious side-effects on the gastric mucosa so these should not be used without due care.
  ❑ Dimethylsulfoxide (1 g diluted to 10–20% solution in 5% dextrose saline) by slow intravenous injection.

Prognosis

- Slow recovery.
- Some animals have residual neurological deficits (variable).
- If mentation is affected prognosis is poor.

Control

- Adequate worming regimens.

Cyathostomosis

Etiology

- Cyathostomes (of which there are more than 40 species) invade the intestinal mucosa and then return to the gut lumen (Fig. 3.6). There is no tortuous migration through tissues.
- The prepatent period is thought to be 2–4 months, but can be extended to at least several months when the third-stage larvae undergo inhibited development in the mucosa. Inhibition of development (also known as larval arrest) is a prominent feature of the life-cycle of these parasites and there can be massive accumulation of mucosal-stage larvae over the autumn and winter, leading to dramatic reactivation and maturation in winter/spring. This leads to clinical signs of larval cyathostomosis.
- Cyathostomosis is most common in weanlings and yearlings and these are the most vulnerable groups. However, larval cyathostomosis is also seen in 'elderly' horses.
- Epidemiologically, the occurrence of larval cyathostomosis is particularly associated with previous hot dry summers, when infective third-stage larvae do not translate to the pasture until a wetter period in the autumn. Not only will low summer challenge interfere with the development of any immunity, but the high autumn challenge will predispose to high levels of mucosal (and probably inhibited) larvae which may activate synchronously in early winter through to spring to cause larval cyathostomosis. Hospital surveys show that full-blown larval cyathostomosis carries an approximately 50% case fatality rate.
- Young foals are seldom affected except when they become infected by high challenges from older horses (prepatent period of 2–8 months minimum).

Clinical signs

- Poor condition, ill-thriving, starry-coated foal.
- Pot-bellied appearance may be present.
- Diarrhea (not always present).
- Rarely colic.
- Dependent edema (associated with low plasma albumin).

Diagnosis

- Larvae in feces, often in the absence of eggs. Often, however, there are no obvious parasitic stages in the feces, especially in the early stages of larval reactivation. Recent treatment with anthelmintics, especially adulticidal drugs such as pyrantel and ivermectin, may promote clinical signs. It is thought that, by killing any adults in the intestinal lumen or later developing larval stages in the mucosa, there is a reduction in possible 'negative feedback' from these later

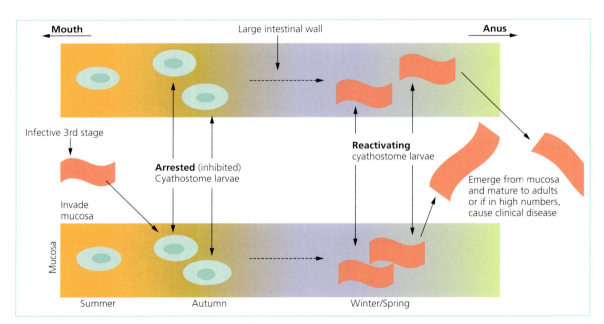

Fig. 3.6 Schematic representation of the cyathostome life-cycle.

developmental stages, which stimulates the inhibited larvae to reactivate en masse.
- Often dramatic diarrhea with acute onset after some stress factor.

Differential diagnosis
- Nutritional deficiencies (absolute starvation, poor-quality diet).
- Dental problems.
- Rotavirus.
- Strongyloidosis.
- Lactose intolerance.

Treatment
- Best not to use adulticidal drugs such as pyrantel and ivermectin for reasons outlined above. Best treatment is probably still a 5-day course of fenbendazole. The other option is moxidectin, which has a licensed claim for adults and developing larvae but, as yet, no licensed claim for inhibited larvae. Care must be taken when using the latter drug in very thin horses and in foals; the dose should be calculated as accurately as is possible.
- Severe damage can result in chronic diarrhea and permanently reduced intestinal absorption. These (and overt clinical cases of larval cyathostomosis) may be treated with prednisolone by mouth (starting at 1 mg/kg every 24 hours, continued to effect and reduced slowly to establish a minimal effective daily dose).
- Nutritional support.
- Antidiarrheal doses of codeine phosphate can help but cannot cure the condition.

Prognosis
- Fair, but some remain 'poor-doers' (possibly due to permanent intestinal wall damage/malabsorption).
- Persistent low plasma albumin and peripheral/ventral edema carry a poor prognosis.

Control
- Worm control programs should start in foals when they go onto pasture.
- Beware of multi-age grazing groups.
- Pasture management is essential.

PARASITE CONTROL STRATEGIES IN YOUNG HORSES

Worm control is one of the most important aspects of stud management. Failure to control parasitic infestation and pasture build-up renders all other stud procedures largely irrelevant.

The main factors leading to infection are:

- High stocking density.
- Over-grazed pasture; horses forced to graze close to fecal pats.

- Use of the same pasture by mixed-age groups.
- Presence of horses with high fecal egg counts.
- Presence of young horses (which tend to be more heavily infected).
- Warm, damp weather.

Simple management practices are important in minimizing the source of infection:

- Not over-stocking.
- Resting heavily grazed pasture.
- Use of cultivation tillage and cropping.
- Mixed-species grazing.
- Avoiding turn-out of horses with high fecal egg counts.

Management control measures decrease the force of infection by minimizing pasture contamination. The most effective way of achieving this is by regular removal of feces from the pasture; twice weekly is the suggested frequency. Experimental studies have demonstrated that, when performed correctly, pasture hygiene is an extremely effective method of suppressing fecal egg counts in grazing horses. A disadvantage is that it is labor-intensive.

As in all types of equine management, the main aim of control is to prevent transmission of infective stages via the pasture, especially during the summer months. Reduction in transmission can be achieved in a number of ways, either in concert (preferably) or individually:

- Anthelmintic treatment (see section on chemotherapeutic control, below).
- Reducing translation of parasites to pasture by dung removal.
- Reducing year-to-year transmission by controlled grazing and management practices, including resting pasture.

A veterinary surgeon with a detailed knowledge of management practices on a premises will be able to evaluate the degree of risk associated with grazing. This knowledge is important in assessing the likely need for additional chemotherapy. Of even greater significance are the results of coprological (or serological) diagnosis to identify heavily infected animals. Repeated evaluation of intestinal parasite status, particularly at high risk times of year, will allow rational advice to be given about anthelmintic use and will allow the efficacy of management control to be monitored.

Chemotherapeutic control

The use of anthelmintic drugs to suppress fecal egg output has been the mainstay of strongyle control for many years. The rationale behind the use of anthelmintics was to kill the egg-laying adult parasites and thereby minimize pasture contamination. For the reasons discussed above, such a strategy can no longer be totally relied upon.

Anthelmintic drugs can be used in a number of different ways:

1. Interval dosing
   This strategy involves the administration of a specific drug at regular time intervals during the high-risk summer grazing period. Some horse owners continue to dose their animals at the same frequency during the low-risk winter period or when stabled for most of the day. This is expensive and unnecessary. Furthermore, many horse owners use anthelmintics at inappropriate intervals (e.g. the monthly use of ivermectin, which is unjustified scientifically due to the persistent effect of this drug; see Table 3.2).

2. Strategic dosing
   The use of anthelmintics at specific times of year to disrupt the seasonal cycle of transmission has been widely and effectively employed in farm animal practice. The seasonality of horse strongyles is well established, so strategic dosing at turn-out, in the middle of the grazing season and again in the autumn is a rational approach to parasite control. Problems can arise with such a system in years with abnormal weather patterns, leading to early or late peak pasture larval burdens. Such a system is susceptible to breakdown if heavily parasitized horses are added to the population. Also, the fact that horses do not develop a significant degree of protective immunity to some intestinal helminths, and the fact that they graze in mixed age groups, make this method more difficult to institute than in farm animal practice. The seasonality of tapeworm infection is not very strong, so anticestode treatments can be included at any time of year.

3. Targeted strategic dosing
   This is a modification of the strategic dosing system. Strategic dosing is employed to suppress pasture contamination at critical times of the year, but all horses have fecal egg counts performed prior to dosing. Treatment is then targeted at animals with significant (>200 eggs per gram) adult parasite burdens. Diagnostic limitations mean that mucosal larval parasites can not be detected by fecal egg counts, so such a regimen must include larvicidal dosing of young, susceptible horses. Most anthelmintics currently available lack efficacy against mucosal-stage larvae in a state of arrested development. Therefore, it is important that these stages are not allowed to build up in large numbers in the colon wall of young, susceptible horses. Mass activation and re-emergence of these arrested stages results in clinical larval cyathostomosis. Anticestode treatments can be targeted by identification of significantly infected animals using the tapeworm antibody ELISA.[10]

- Whatever the strategy employed, owners should be aware of the recommended minimum dosing interval for each anthelmintic and should not dose more frequently.

A RATIONAL APPROACH TO PARASITE CONTROL

Given the limitations of parasite control and the problems discussed above, how can veterinary surgeons best advise their clients in order to minimize parasite-associated disease? The present authors recommend a combined approach that utilizes the strengths of both management and chemotherapeutic strategies. A key element of this approach is to monitor parasite burdens periodically, either coprologically for strongyles or serologically for tapeworms. This has three benefits:

1. It allows the efficacy of the control program to be monitored constantly.
2. It allows the targeting of expensive anthelmintic drugs at those animals with significant parasite burdens.
3. It reduces selection pressure for anthelmintic resistance.

It is important to realize that blanket recommendations, applicable to every managemental situation, can not be made. Recommendations for a stud with limited grazing and a high turnover of horses are going to be very different from those for three middle-aged horses in private ownership with extensive pasture and limited contact with other horses. Several features of a horse population, and its recent history, will help to indicate the likely extent of intestinal parasitism and the parasites involved:

- Are the horses managed by one person (e.g. single owner, trainer) or are they in multiple ownership?
  ❏ To be most effective, all horses in the population should be included in the control program.
- What is the age profile of the horse population?
  ❏ Young horses are more likely to develop high worm burdens that cause clinical disease and more likely to contaminate pasture with infective stages of intestinal parasites.
- Is there any history of parasite-associated disease? If so, which parasite?
  ❏ Larval cyathostomosis (springtime diarrhea) or weight loss may indicate a cyathostome problem. Both cyathostomes and tapeworms have been associated with colic.
- What is the previous worming history of the horses?
- Is there any indication of anthelmintic resistance?

- What are the pastures like?
  - ❑ Over-stocked, heavily grazed pastures where feces are never removed are far more likely to result in high parasite burdens.

The flow diagram in Fig. 3.7 gives an indication of how a rational control program for intestinal parasites can be instituted, monitored and maintained. At the initiation of such a strategy it is advisable to monitor strongyle egg count at least every 3 months. As a picture of the herd's parasite status emerges it is often possible to decrease the frequency of sampling. Regular re-evaluation of the herd's parasite status will allow fine-tuning of the control program. This often takes the form of much reduced anthelmintic use, thus saving the client money and reducing the pressure towards anthelmintic resistance. Clients are often surprised how effective their efforts at pasture hygiene are and this tends to encourage them in their efforts. The essential strategies involved in reducing the spread of infection are summarized in Fig. 3.8.

Should a veterinary surgeon decide to recommend an interval-dosing regimen, it is useful to establish the nature of the parasite burden at the start of the control program. Fecal and serological assessment of parasite burdens can indicate the parasites that need treating and the infection intensity. Periodic re-assessment of parasite status is recommended to monitor for anthelmintic resistance.

Whatever the strategy for anthelmintic use (interval dosing, strategic dosing, targeted strategic dosing), care should be taken to recommend a combination of anthelmintics that will control both roundworms and tapeworms (see Table 3.2). A number of reports exist of horse populations that have received ivermectin exclusively for periods of several years. Although this effectively suppressed strongyle infection, it also allowed tapeworm infection intensity to increase

unchecked. In some reports this led to tapeworm-related intestinal disease.

The use of a serological assay to estimate tapeworm infection intensity is a recent advance in equine parasitology. The results of this assay indicate the parasite burden in an individual animal. It is suggested that as many horses as possible are tested at the start of a targeted strategic parasite control program. Because an infected horse is likely to become re-infected, anticestode treatment should be concentrated on those animals with moderate or high tapeworm burdens. Re-testing needs only to be done infrequently (e.g. every 1–2 years).

SUMMARY

Veterinary surgeons undertaking equine practice should be aware of the problems of intestinal parasite control in horses. Knowledge of scientifically proven control strategies and the anthelmintic drugs currently available will allow practitioners to recommend the

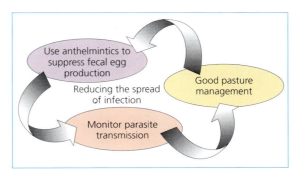

Fig. 3.8 Essential strategies to reduce the spread of infection.

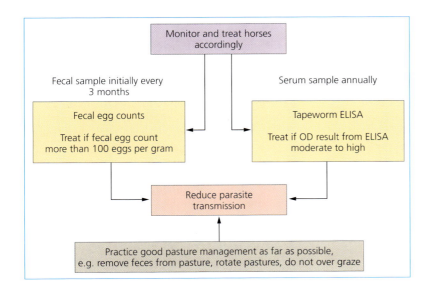

Fig. 3.7 A rational approach to parasite control. OD, optical density.

most appropriate control strategy for each circumstance. Interval dosing alone increases the risk of anthelmintic resistance developing and can not be guaranteed to control intestinal parasitism. Periodic evaluation of each horse's parasite status is recommended.

- Dung removal is a highly effective method of parasite control if done properly (i.e. twice a week in summer and once a week in winter). If no clean grazing is available, regular removal of feces in concert with strategic worming treatments will dramatically reduce larval challenge to grazing horses. From the management point of view, removal of feces will improve both quality and quantity of the grazing available. Disposal of feces should be such that pasture contamination is avoided. Middens must be used and feces from stables and yards must never be spread on pastures to be used for horses. The top layer of middens must be turned weekly.

Note:
- Harrowing of pastures is not recommended; it merely spreads the parasites over a wider range and may upset the selective feeding habits of the horses.
- Horses prefer to graze in areas away from droppings, so creating 'lawns and roughs' on pastures.

- Mixed grazing can be practiced. Only *Trichostrongylus axei* is capable of infesting cattle, sheep, pigs and horses, and this parasite, which is a stomach dweller, has little pathogenic effect.
- Avoid grazing young animals on pastures in successive years, particularly for the control of *Parascaris equorum*. If this is impossible, rest the paddocks for at least 5 winter months (from January to June in the northern hemisphere) to reduce infection levels of strongyles and, in particular, cyathostome larvae that may have over-wintered.
- Routine anthelmintic usage is commonly used as an excuse to avoid pasture control, but this is bad policy on a stud farm. Dramatic outbreaks of heavy parasitism can develop where good pasture management is not practiced. There is a vast wastage of anthelmintic with unnecessary regimens or over-worming. Most drugs are very effective against adult worms but have varying efficacy against different developmental stages of cyathostomes. Furthermore, resistance to benzimidazole drugs (and fenbendazole in particular) is a significant and increasing problem with cyathostomes.
- New horses admitted to stud farms should be wormed on admission and kept in isolation for 3 days after worming to minimize contamination of pastures. Previous worming histories are often misleading.
- One month before foaling, the mare should receive a full single adulticidal dose of anthelmintic (assuming no resistance in the case of benzimidazoles). This eliminates the majority of adult worms in the gut.
- Ten days after foaling, a larvicidal dose of ivermectin or fenbendazole is administered to the mare. Thereafter routine worming every 6 weeks using either ivermectin or fenbendazole or pyrantel is carried out.
- The first worm to mature to egg-laying stages in foals is *Strongyloides westeri*. This parasite can produce large numbers of eggs in foals about 2–3 weeks of age. At around 8 weeks the first strongyle and ascarid eggs will usually be detectable. Foals can significantly contaminate a pasture by 6–8 weeks of age and they should therefore be wormed at 6 weeks of age using a full, calculated dose of fenbendazole or pyrantel. Thereafter, deworming should be repeated every 4 weeks until 6 months of age with each alternate dose being an avermectin compound. After 6 months the interval should be lengthened to 6 weeks.
- Tapeworms are not likely to affect foals in their first year but it is useful to administer a double dose of pyrantel in the autumn of the first year to be certain.
- Different stud farms may need different regimens, so the veterinary surgeon must be able to make a logical and economical program for the individual stud farm, taking into account the likely challenge, the efficiency of pasture management and the worm egg build-up.
- Continuous worm egg counts (taken from a significant sample of the population of horses) should always be performed on a horse farm under the strict guidance of the attending veterinary surgeon. This will establish the effects of the measures and early detection of resistance.
- Targeted strategic treatments are recommended. This allows monitoring of the spread of infection and reduces the likelihood of resistance to anthelmintics developing. Ideally, the fecal egg counts should be done on the day of worming.
  - ❏ The aim is to achieve a mean worm egg count of less than 200 eggs per gram of feces.
  - ❏ Horses with fecal egg counts of over 100 eggs per gram should be wormed.
  - ❏ Any adulticidal anthelmintic can be used in the summer and should be rotated annually if wormers are used regularly.
  - ❏ All animals should receive a cyathostome larvicidal dose of fenbendazole (i.e. 5-day course) in the autumn, to reduce as much as possible larvae that have built up in the

intestinal mucosa. This is especially important in weanlings and yearlings.

❑ A double dose of pyrantel to reduce tapeworms (*Anoplocephala perfoliata*) is included once in the annual worming program.

A clean pasture is defined as one that:

- Has never been grazed by horses.
- Has not been grazed by horses until mid-summer (1 June in the northern hemisphere) of that year.
- Has been grazed by other species (cattle or sheep) for two grazing periods (i.e. cattle and/or sheep have twice grazed the pasture down and then been moved on).

Additional aids to the creation of 'clean pastures' include:

- Ploughing.
- Pastures used for foals and yearlings MUST receive priority for clean pasture management. Mares are the chief source of infection for foals, and pasture contamination by them is almost unavoidable. Therefore, barren mares, maiden mares and geldings should never be run with young foals. They can, however, be used to graze paddocks after the young foals and mares have left them.

CONTRACEPTION

Contraception is not usually a major feature of horse stud management but there are circumstances when it is a useful technique. The matter has received little research but historically it has been limited to castration of the stallion or ovariectomy in the mare. The former is a standard procedure but the latter is a major surgical intervention (no matter how it is performed) and carries a significant risk. Control of populations of wild horses cannot of course be effected by these methods and so other systems need to be explored. Population control is usually directed at the female because the endocrinology is easier to manipulate and because the mare can only carry one foal, whereas the stallion can mate many mares in a season. Unless the whole male population is neutered (as is the current state with most male horses), the fecundity of the mares will likely remain high. A wild population of horses requires only that one or two fertile stallions are available for the population to continue to grow.

Stallions

Several methods of hormonal manipulation (either by regular injections or by implants) have been attempted.[11] However, no suitable oral drug has yet been found. In principle, therefore, contraception in the male horse is not yet feasible.

Vasectomy, however, is used to create teaser males for stud purposes but, again, free running teasers may mate a mare several times and this can introduce significant infection. For the most part vasectomy is probably not the best option. Surgical deviation of the penis can be used to prevent intromission, but the ethical considerations of this are very questionable.

Mares

Contraception in the mare offers a better opportunity of success, but again little success has been achieved. Naturally occurring steroids appear to be well tolerated by the mare, but large doses of prostagens and estrogens are required to inhibit ovulation and sexual activity. Implants of hormones have been tried with mixed success.[12]

Ovariectomy is a feasible option for mares that will not be required to breed again (although they may be used as surrogates for embryo transfer; see p. 222). The technique is described in standard texts but the advent of laparoscopy makes it more feasible and safer.

REFERENCES

1. National Research Council. Description of individual condition scores. In: Nutrient requirements of horses. 5th edn. Washington, DC: National Academy Press; 1989:5.
2. Baker G, Easley J. Equine dentistry. Philadelphia, PA: WB Saunders; 1999.
3. Koterba AM. Diagnosis and management of normal and abnormal foals: general considerations. In: Koterba AM, Drummond WM, Kosch PC, eds. Equine clinical neonatology. Philadelphia, PA: Lea & Febiger; 1990:5–6.
4. Liu IK, Brown SL, Kuo J, et al. Duration of maternally derived immunity to tetanus and response in newborn foals given tetanus antitoxin. American Journal of Veterinary Research 1982; 43:2019–2022.
5. McClure TJ, Lunn DP. Practical applications of equine vaccination. In: Colahan PT, Mayhew IG, Merritt AM, et al., eds. Equine medicine and surgery. 5th edn. Philadelphia, PA: Mosby; 1999:191–196.
6. Jacobs DE. Colour atlas of equine parasites. London: Baillière Tindall; 1986:5.8–5.11.
7. di Pietro JA. A review of *Strongyloides westeri* infection in foals. Equine Practice 1989; 11:35–37.
8. Georgi JR, Georgi ME. Parasitology for veterinarians. 5th edn. Philadelphia, PA: WB Saunders; 1990:158–160.
9. Green SL, Mayhew IG. Neurologic disorders. In: Koterba AM, Drummond WH, Kosch PC, eds. Equine clinical neonatology. Philadelphia, PA: Lea & Febiger; 1990:525–526.
10. Proudman CJ, French N, Trees A. Tapeworm infection is a significant risk factor for spasmodic colic and ileal impaction colic in horses. Equine Veterinary Journal 1998; 30:194–199.
11. Kirkpatrick JF, Turner JW. Contraception. In: McKinnon AO, Voss JL, eds. Equine reproduction. Philadelphia, PA: Lea & Febiger; 1992:353–356.
12. Plotka ED, Eagle TC, Vevea DN, et al. Effects of hormone implants on estrus and ovulation in feral mares. Journal of Wildlife Diseases 1988; 24:507–514.

Chapter 4
THE STALLION

Cheryl Lopate,
Michelle LeBlanc,
Derek Knottenbelt

ANATOMY

A complete understanding of the normal anatomy and physiology of the stallion is required in order to evaluate accurately and completely a stallion's ability to be a successful breeding animal.[1–4] The reproductive anatomy of the male horse includes:

- The testicles and associated ducts. There are two testicles, located in the scrotum. There are two epididymides and spermatic cords, two vas deferens and two ampullae, which empty into the pelvic urethra.
- The accessory sex glands. These include the prostate, the seminal vesicles and the bulbourethral glands.
- The external genitalia (Fig. 4.1), comprising the penis and the prepuce.

The testicles

The testicles are located in the scrotum between the hind legs. They lie in a horizontal plane with the long axis of the body and are oblong in shape (Fig. 4.2). They are quite resilient to palpation, resembling a new tennis ball in character. The testicles are the site of spermatogenesis and the production of the hormones testosterone and dihydrotestosterone. They are surrounded by two connective tissue tunics that are loosely apposed to each other (Fig. 4.3; see also Fig. 4.4):

- The tunica albuginea is directly associated with the testicles and is the thicker of the two structures.
- The tunica vaginalis is the thinner of the structures and lies outside the tunica albuginea.

The testicles comprise:

- The seminiferous tubules, which are lined with germ cells.
- Sertoli (or nurse or sustentacular) cells.[5,6] These cells have gap junctions between them, which provide a barrier, known as the blood–testes barrier, between the systemic immune system and the germ cells. The horse's immune system is never exposed to the developing spermatocytes or spermatids and would therefore see them as foreign cells and destroy them if it was not for the protection of the Sertoli cells. Disruption of this protective barrier may result in subfertility or infertility. The Sertoli cells produce proteins that facilitate sperm production and carry nutrients to the sperm cells.
- Muscle (myoid) cells and fibroblasts line the tubules, which facilitate movement of spermatozoa and fluids along the tubules.
- The interstitium and Leydig cells, which are in the area between the tubules.[7] The interstitial tissue is composed of connective tissue, blood and lymphatic vessels and nerves. Testosterone is

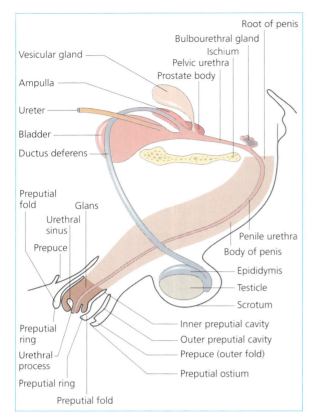

Fig. 4.1   The genitalia of the stallion.

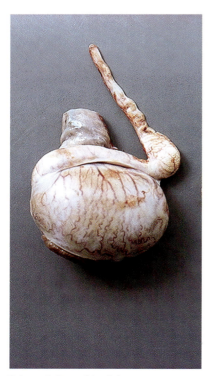

Fig. 4.2   External view of testicle.

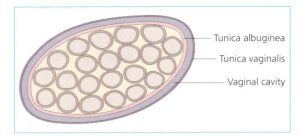

Fig. 4.3   The testicular tunics. The tunica vaginalis is an extension of the peritoneum which lines the scrotum. The tunica albuginea is a thick fibrous coat surrounding the testicle. A thin layer of fluid fills the vaginal cavity to allow the testicles to move smoothly in the scrotum.

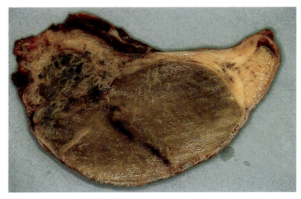

Fig. 4.4   Longitudinal section of testicle.

produced by the Leydig cells and is one of several hormones that facilitate sperm production, as well as supporting the male characteristics of libido, behavior, and masculine appearance.

- The seminiferous tubules empty into the straight tubules, which empty into the rete testis, which empties into the efferent ductules and on into the epididymis (Fig. 4.5). From the epididymis the sperm and associated fluids empty into the vas deferens.

The stallion is a seasonal breeder and thus the size and nature of the testicles change with the season.[8–10] There are also changes associated with age.

- During the breeding season, there are more Leydig cells, more Sertoli cells and more spermatozoa per gram of testis.
- As the stallion matures, the Leydig cells change from postpubertal to adult-type cells, which produce significantly more testosterone.
- The number of Sertoli cells per gram of testis decreases with increasing age. This change is thought to be associated with the decline in fertility associated with old age in stallions and is known as testicular degeneration.

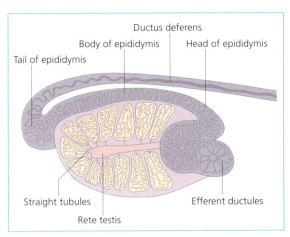

Fig. 4.5   The tubular system of the testicle. Spermatozoa leave the tubules, move through the straight tubules and empty into the rete testis, then to the efferent ductules which in turn empty into the head of the epididymis. The spermatozoa mature progressively as they pass through the epididymis and are finally stored in the epididymal tail until ejaculation.

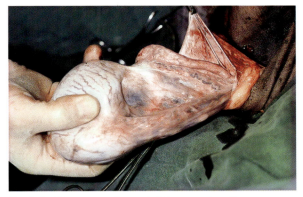

Fig. 4.6   The spermatic cord. This comprises the vas deferens and the pampiniform plexus. The pampiniform plexus contains the testicular vein surrounded by the tightly coiled testicular artery. This arrangement allows for heating and cooling of blood entering and leaving the testicle.

The scrotum

The scrotum is an outpouching of the skin from the inguinal region. There are two sacs, one surrounding each testicle, and they are separated by a septum. The scrotum has four layers:

- The skin. This has minimal underlying fat and has an abundant supply of sweat glands, which are important in the thermoregulation of the testicles.
- The tunica dartos. This comprises smooth muscle fibers and connective tissue. In warm weather, the muscle cells within the tunica dartos relax and allow the testicles to drop away from the body wall; in cold weather, the dartos muscle contracts, helping to pull the testicles closer to the body.
- The scrotal fascia. This allows the testicles to move freely within the scrotum.
- The common vaginal tunic. Two layers of connective tissue, called tunics, surround the testicles themselves. The outer tunic, the tunica vaginalis or common vaginal tunic, is considered by some to be part of the scrotum and by others to be part of the testicles themselves. The tunica vaginalis is an invagination of the peritoneal lining and passes through the inguinal rings when testicular descent occurs. The tunica albuginea closely adheres to the testicle whereas the tunica vaginalis is separated from the inner tunic by a very thin layer of fluid. This fluid facilitates the movement of the testes in the scrotum.

The spermatic cord

The spermatic cord runs from the internal inguinal ring to the base of the testicles in the scrotum (Fig. 4.6). It consists of:

- The testicular artery, vein and nerve. The testicular artery is a tightly coiled and convoluted structure, which is important in heating and cooling the blood both entering and leaving the testicles. The testicular vein is intimately associated with the testicular artery. The convoluted testicular artery and vein together are termed the pampiniform plexus.
- The vas deferens.
- The cremaster muscle, which is on the lateral aspect of the spermatic cord. It works to raise and lower the testicles during changes in temperature and provides a means of support for the testicles in the scrotum.

The testicles are maintained approximately 4–6°C cooler than body temperature for maximal sperm production. The ability to maintain this preferred temperature gradient is provided through the interworkings of several components, including the scrotal skin, the dartos muscle, the cremaster muscle and the pampiniform plexus.

- In warm weather, the many sweat glands in the scrotal skin provide for evaporative heat loss. The dartos and cremaster muscles relax to allow the testicles to hang further away from the body wall, moving them further from the higher core temperature of the abdominal cavity. This relaxation also allows the spermatic cord to stretch out, resulting in a longer time for blood to pass through the pampiniform plexus, thereby allowing more cooling of the blood to occur.
- In the winter, there is no sweating on the scrotal skin and the tunica dartos and cremaster muscles contract. This contraction pulls the testicles closer

to the body wall (exposing the testicles to a higher core body temperature). This action effectively shortens the spermatic cord and pampiniform plexus, thereby decreasing the transit time of the blood through the cord and so reduces the alterations in the temperature of the blood as it passes through the cord.

The epididymis

Maturation and storage of spermatozoa occur in the epididymis. The epididymis is divided into three sections (Fig. 4.7):

- The head (caput epididymis) is an extension of the efferent ductules of the testicle. The head is rather flat in shape and is closely adherent to the testicle itself. It takes a 180° turn as it courses caudally along the testicle and turns into the corpus epididymis.
- The body (corpus epididymis) is tubular and is loosely attached to the dorsal surface of the testicle.

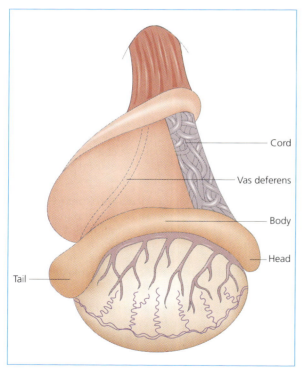

Fig. 4.7 The epididymis. This comprises three portions. The caput (head) is bound firmly to the testis, where spermatozoal maturation takes place. The corpus (body) is less closely attached to the testis and leaves a small pocket (the epididymal sinus). The cauda (tail) is attached to the caudal extremity of the testis by the proper ligament of the testis and continues as the vas deferens. Spermatozoa are stored in the cauda (tail) prior to ejaculation.

- The tail (cauda epididymis) is circular to ovoid in shape and is also loosely attached to the testicle. It terminates in the vas deferens, which takes a 120° turn dorsally as it courses up the spermatic cord.

The epididymis functions to resorb excess fluid (caput) associated with spermatogenesis, and produces secretions (corpus and cauda) that are important in the maturation of the spermatozoa. Sperm are stored in the terminal cauda epididymis until ejaculation occurs. It takes on average 8–11 days for sperm to traverse the length of the epididymis, although passage may occur as quickly as 3 days in cases of high breeding volume.

The vas deferens

The vas deferens leaves the tail of the epididymis and follows the spermatic cord up into the abdomen and empties in the pelvic urethra. It becomes markedly thicker as it approaches the urethra as a result of increased numbers of crypts and glands. This area of the vas deferens is termed the ampulla and is characterized by a thickening of the wall up to 18 mm in diameter (from 4–5 mm as it passes along the spermatic cord). The entire length of the vas deferens has a thick wall of smooth muscle tissue, which facilitates emptying of spermatozoa into the urethra during ejaculation.

The accessory sex glands

The accessory sex glands of the stallion include (Fig. 4.8):

- The prostate. This comprises two portions: a bi-lobed structure surrounding the urethra and a connecting structure, called the isthmus, between the two lobes. The prostatic lobes are approximately 7 × 4 × 1 cm in size; the isthmus is about 3 cm long.
- The seminal vesicles. These are a paired gland comprising vesicular sacs which are filled with the gelatinous fraction of the ejaculate. The seminal vesicles are approximately 15 cm long and 5 cm wide. They empty via a single duct at the seminal colliculus on the dorsal aspect of the pelvic urethra.
- The bulbourethral glands. This paired set of glands, at the level of the ischial arch, produce secretions for the maintenance of sperm longevity in the female tract.

The urethra

The urethra is a muscular tube extending from the bladder to the free end of the penis. The pelvic urethra is surrounded by a thick layer of skeletal muscle, which

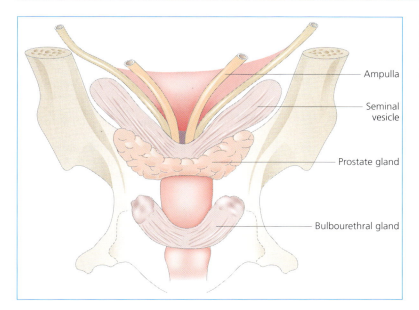

Fig. 4.8   Accessory glands of the stallion. They include paired ampullae, paired seminal vesicles, paired prostate lobes and an adjoining isthmus with paired bulbourethral glands.

Ampulla

Seminal vesicle

Prostate gland

Bulbourethral gland

contracts during ejaculation, resulting in the forceful expulsion of semen through the genitourinary tract. The corpus spongiosum penis, part of the erectile tissue of the penis, surrounds the urethra. The distal end of the urethra terminates in the urethral process.

- A diverticulum (fossa glandis) surrounds the urethra.
- Dirt, debris and secretions will often fill this groove (Fig. 4.9). This accumulation of debris (commonly known as the bean) may cause pain or difficulty in association with ejaculation.
- There is also a urethral sinus dorsal to the fossa glandis.
- This sinus may harbor infectious organisms, such as that causing contagious equine metritis.

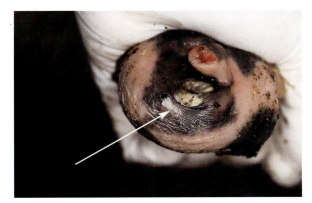

Fig. 4.9   Photograph of the end of a stallion's penis showing the urethral opening surrounded by the urethral fossa and the prominent dorsal urethral sinus. The fossa in this case has a large smegma bean inside it (arrow).

The penis

The penis of the stallion is musculocavernous in nature. It is composed of three general areas (Fig. 4.10):

- The base or root. This is attached to the ischium by the paired crural muscles, the paired ischiocavernosus muscles and a pair of suspensory ligaments. There are paired retractor penis muscles, which relax to allow the penis to be extended and contract to pull the penis back into the prepuce.
- The shaft.
- The glans (free end).

The urethra runs through the center of the penis and is surrounded by the corpus spongiosum penis.

- The corpus spongiosum penis contains some erectile tissue, which becomes engorged when sexual stimulation occurs.
- The corpus cavernosum penis surrounds the corpus spongiosum penis.
- The corpus spongiosum penis is not surrounded by any connective tissue and continues distally as the glans (free end) of the penis.
- The corpus cavernosum penis is an intricately sinusoidal structure, which becomes engorged with blood during sexual arousal. A connective tissue covering called the tunica albuginea surrounds the corpus cavernosum penis.
- The glans (free end) of the penis will increase 300–400% in size with engorgement and ejaculation. There are many nerve endings in the glans penis. There is a prominent rim of tissue on the glans (free end) of the penis called the corona glandis, which becomes firm and prominent with penile engorgement.

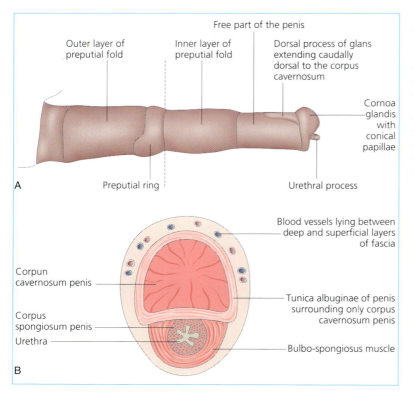

Fig. 4.10 The penis. (A) The glans free end of the penis comprises the corona radiata, the urethral process and the urethral diverticulum. (B) The corpus cavernosus penis (1) is the major component of the shaft of the penis and fills with blood during erection, resulting in penile engorgement; the corpus spongiosum penis (2) surrounds the urethra (3) and aids in muscular contraction of the urethra during emission. The base of the root of the penis attaches to the pelvis.

Labels in figure A:
- Free part of the penis
- Outer layer of preputial fold
- Inner layer of preputial fold
- Dorsal process of glans extending caudally dorsal to the corpus cavernosum
- Cornoa glandis with conical papillae
- Preputial ring
- Urethral process

Labels in figure B:
- Blood vessels lying between deep and superficial layers of fascia
- Corpun cavernosum penis
- Corpus spongiosum penis
- Urethra
- Tunica albuginae of penis surrounding only corpus cavernosum penis
- Bulbo-spongiosus muscle

Engorgement of the penis results in a significant (50%) increase in its length and diameter.

The prepuce (sheath)

The prepuce includes two portions (Fig. 4.11):

- A layer that covers the proximal portion of the penis.
- A layer that provides an external orifice into which the penis enters and exits.

The external prepuce in the stallion is significantly larger than the penile portion. There is a preputial fold that straightens and elongates as erection occurs.

DESCENT OF THE TESTICLES[11,12]

- The fetal testicle is suspended from the abdominal wall.
- The mesonephric duct, which will become the vas deferens and the epididymis, courses caudally towards the pelvic canal.
- The vaginal process invaginates to form the inguinal canal.
- At around day 150 of gestation, the epididymis is pulled towards the inguinal canal by the gubernaculum; however, due to the large size of the testicle, it cannot pass through the inguinal ring.
- The cauda epididymis continues to enlarge as the fetus grows and this stretches the inguinal ring and canal.

- At around day 300 of gestation, the testicle is able to enter the inguinal canal.
- Abdominal pressure from fluid and intestinal contents help push the testicle into and through the canal.
- The right testicle precedes the left testicle in most cases.

The testicles of the male equid are typically descended at birth or descend shortly after birth. However, in some cases, testicular descent may be delayed until 2–6 months after birth.

- Testicles that descend during this time period are considered to have descended within a normal time frame.
- Testicles may descend at 6–24 months of age, although these stallions would be considered to be cryptorchid (also known as false rigs or ridglings).
- In cases where descent is delayed, the testicle(s) are in the inguinal canal and it may take extra time for them to reach the external inguinal ring and/or scrotum.

Failure of normal testicular descent (cryptorchidism)

Failure of testicular descent (cryptorchidism) may be a result of:

- Inappropriate abdominal pressure.
- Stretching of the gubernaculum.

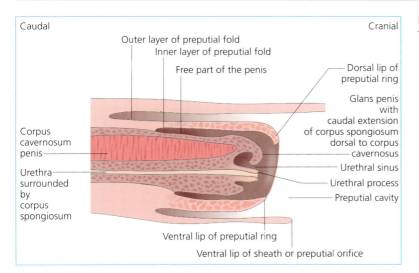

Fig. 4.11   Cross-sectional drawing of the penis and sheath of the male horse.

Caudal

Cranial

Outer layer of preputial fold
Inner layer of preputial fold
Free part of the penis

Dorsal lip of preputial ring

Glans penis with caudal extension of corpus spongiosum dorsal to corpus cavernosus

Corpus cavernosum penis

Urethral sinus

Urethra surrounded by corpus spongiosum

Urethral process
Preputial cavity

Ventral lip of preputial ring
Ventral lip of sheath or preputial orifice

- Inadequate growth of the gubernaculum and cauda epididymis resulting in insufficient stretching of the inguinal ring and canal.
- Displacement of the testicle to a position where it cannot be pulled/pushed into the inguinal canal by natural forces.

> Note:
> - Cryptorchidism is an important clinical and reproductive problem. The condition results in difficulties with diagnosis and with surgery.[13] Further, there appears to be some hereditary component to retention of the testicles (cryptorchidism) as it is most common in Quarter Horses and there has been a high incidence along some familial lines.
> - **It is recommended that cryptorchid horses are not used for breeding animals; they should be castrated.**

When atypical male behavior develops in a supposed gelding, a diagnosis of cryptorchidism can sometimes be made by a combination of:

- Deep palpation and/or ultrasound of the external inguinal canal.
- Rectal palpation and ultrasound examination following the vas deferens from its exit in the pelvic urethra forward either into the internal inguinal ring or into the abdominal cavity.
- Hormone testing. If there is uncertainty about the presence or absence of an abdominal or inguinal testicle, hormonal testing can provide strong evidence for the presence or absence of testicular tissue[14] (see p. 94).

PUBERTY

Puberty is defined as the commencement of successful reproductive function in a young animal. In the colt, puberty is usually attained by the age of 18 months, although in some individuals it may be reached earlier (12 months). The pubertal stallion will begin to show male characteristics, including increased muscle mass and increased jowl size, and will begin to display typical male behavior, including vocalization in the presence of females, erection, masturbation and copulation. Libido typically continues to improve with age after the onset of puberty.

> - At birth, the testes contain very few Leydig cells, stem cells and primordial Sertoli cells.
> - At 6 months of age, the colt will enter a prepubertal stage of development during which the cell types common to the testicle begin to develop and increase in number.
> - At around 9 months of age, concentrations of luteinizing hormone and follicle-stimulating hormone begin to increase in the systemic circulation.
> - At 12 months of age, the testes begin to increase in size. Total scrotal width increases approximately 1 mm per week from 12 months through to 18 months of age.[15]

Physiologically at puberty, spermatogenesis begins as a result of increased testosterone production. Leydig cells produce increasing amounts of dihydrotestosterone, which is converted to testosterone, providing a very high local concentration of testosterone surrounding the germ cells and their nurturing Sertoli cells. Dihydrotestosterone also stimulates the transformation of the stem cells (spermatogonia) into spermatozoa.

Surges of luteinizing hormone occur with greater frequency and amplitude, thereby increasing testosterone concentrations. Prolonged stimulation of the Leydig cells is believed to be required for their maturation.[16]

It has been suggested that, in the prepubertal stallion, production of estradiol results in a negative feedback on the hypothalamus and its production of gonadotropin-releasing hormone.[17,18] When production of gonadotropin-releasing hormone increases in frequency and amplitude at puberty, there is also an increased concentration of estradiol receptors, which results in a change from negative to positive feedback. This results in increased amounts of gonadotropin-releasing hormone, which in turn results in increased luteinizing hormone production. Sustained increases in concentrations of the gonadotropic and steroid hormones result in increased testicular growth and development of spermatogenesis.

PHYSIOLOGY OF SPERM PRODUCTION

Hormonal control

Spermatogenesis is a complicated process involving communication between the testicles and two parts of the brain: the hypothalamus and the pituitary. Several hormones are involved in the production and maturation of spermatozoa, the male sex drive and copulation (Fig. 4.12).[19,20]

- Hormones produced in the hypothalamus flow through the portal vessels to the pituitary gland, specifically the pars distalis.
- The hypothalamus produces short pulses of gonadotropin-releasing hormone, which is the driving force for the rest of the hormonal cycle.
- Gonadotropin-releasing hormone exerts its effect on the anterior pituitary gland and stimulates the release of two hormones: follicle-stimulating hormone and luteinizing hormone.
- Both luteinizing hormone and follicle-stimulating hormone are released in a pulsatile fashion, although, during the breeding season, pulses of luteinizing hormone may occur so close together that they are physiologically indistinguishable.
  - ❑ Follicle-stimulating hormone exerts positive feedback on the testicles by acting on the Sertoli cells and induces release of androgen-binding protein, inhibin and activin.[21]
  - ❑ Follicle-stimulating hormone is not completely dependent on gonadotropin-releasing hormone secretion in the male. Inhibin and activin are released into the general circulation and feed back on the hypothalamus and pituitary to inhibit and

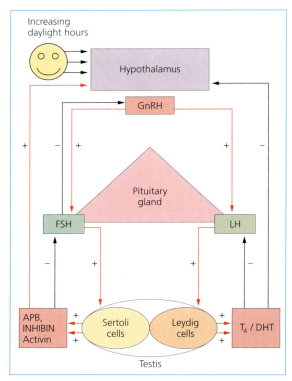

Fig. 4.12 Hormone production and control in the male horse. GnRH, gonadotropin-releasing hormone; FSH, follicle-stimulating hormone; LH, luteinizing hormone; APB, androgen-binding protein; T_4, testosterone; DHT, dihydrotestosterone.

promote, respectively, the release of follicle-stimulating hormone.
  - ❑ Androgen-binding protein binds to both dihydrotestosterone and testosterone and provides a high concentration of both of these hormones locally around the germ cells.

The Leydig cells produce the steroid hormones in the testicle:[22]

- Luteinizing hormone acts on the Leydig cells to produce testosterone, which is delivered to both the local testicular environment and the systemic circulation.
- Testosterone feeds back negatively on the hypothalamus and pituitary gland to curtail their production when its concentrations are elevated and positively when its concentration is low.
- Some of the testosterone is converted to estrogen by the Leydig cells and some by the hypothalamus and pituitary.
- The Leydig cells probably also produce oxytocin, which stimulates contraction of the seminiferous tubules and promotes transport of the germ cells through the tubules.

Note:
- The stallion's testicles produce significant proportions of estrogens.[23]
- The source of these estrogens is not completely understood.
- The Sertoli cells, the Leydig cells or other testicular cells may be involved in the complex production of estrogens (conversion from testosterone may be involved in this).

Spermatogenesis

Spermatogenesis is the process of maturation of the testicular germ cells from stem cells to spermatozoa.[24] The maturation process requires both mitotic and meiotic division of the germ cells. Spermatozoa are produced by the progression of germ cells.

- The primordial germ cells line the prepubertal testicle (with the Sertoli cells) along the outside of the spermatogenetic tubule.
- These primordial germ cells are termed spermatogonia. They are few in number until puberty, when the hormonal axis begins to result in a local increase in testosterone concentration.
- At this time the number of spermatogonia increases and the first spermatogenetic wave begins.

Spermatogenesis occurs in cycles, or waves. Depending on the location in the seminiferous tubule one may find a different stage of the cycle. In a cross-section of a tubule, 4–5 generations are arranged in definitive cellular associations. There are eight stages of the cycle of the seminiferous epithelium (Fig. 4.13):[25]

- Stage 1: from the disappearance of mature spermatids lining the tubular lumen to the beginning of spermatid nuclei elongation.
- Stage 2: from the beginning to the end of spermatid nucleus elongation.
- Stage 3: from the end of spermatid nuclei elongation to the start of the first meiotic division.
- Stage 4: from the start of the first meiotic division to the end of the second meiotic division.
- Stage 5: from the end of the second meiotic division to the first appearance of type B-2 spermatogonia.
- Stage 6: from the first appearance of type B-2 spermatogonia to the onset of migration of elongated spermatids towards the tubular lumen.
- Stage 7: from the onset of migration of elongate spermatids towards the lumen to the conclusion of their migration and disappearance of all B-2 spermatogonia.
- Stage 8: from elongate spermatids all residing at the tubular lumen and the appearance of preleptotene primary spermatocytes until all spermatids have disappeared from the lumen.

A single cycle of the seminiferous epithelium takes 12.2 days in the stallion. Different stages of the cycle can be detected along the length of the tubule. This change in the stages is termed 'a wave of the epithelium'. It takes around 57 days for spermatogenesis to be completed from the stage of spermatogonia until a mature spermatozoon is formed.

There are three phases of spermatogenesis:

1. Spermatocytogenesis: 19.4 days of spermatocytogenesis (mitosis and differentiation of the spermatogonia).
2. Meiosis: 19.4 days of meiosis (first of primary spermatocytes, followed by two divisions of meiosis which produce spermatids).
3. Spermiogenesis: 18.6 days of spermiogenesis (differentiation into fully differentiated spermatids). These spermatids are called spermatozoa once they are released from the seminiferous epithelium into the tubular lumen.

Spermatogenesis changes with the season of the year.[26,27]

- Daily sperm production increases during the breeding season. There is a 20% decrease in the efficiency of sperm production in mature stallions during the nonbreeding season.[28]

Spermatogenesis is also influenced by the age of the stallion.[29,30]

- As the stallion matures from a postpubertal to a mature stallion, daily sperm production increases along with testicular size.
- In aged stallions (over 13 years of age), efficiency of sperm production decreases by around 35%.

Spermatozoa are continuously produced after the onset of puberty.[31] There is continuous production of differentiated and committed spermatogonia, which go on to become spermatocytes and then on to spermatids and eventually spermatozoa. Uncommitted spermatogonia are replaced so that the germinal epithelium always has a supply of stem cells from which spermatozoa can be produced.

Thermoregulation

Thermoregulation of the testicles is an important function of the scrotum and spermatic cord.[32]

- Normal thermoregulation is required for spermatogenesis to proceed in an ordinary fashion.
- The scrotum regulates temperature by altering the position of the testicles, either closer to or further away from the body wall, depending on the environmental temperature. The dartos and

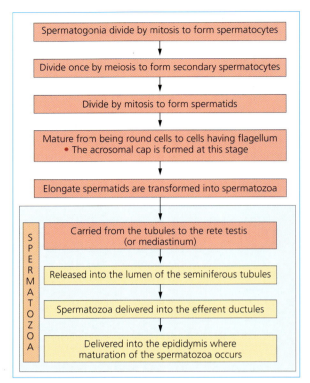

Fig. 4.13 Spermatogenesis.

cremaster muscles contract in cool temperatures and relax in warm temperatures to bring the testicles closer or further from the body wall, respectively.
- The scrotum and the pampiniform plexus control testicular temperature through vascular exchange.

Note:
- Elevation in testicular temperature above 40.5°C for 2 hours or more will result in alterations of spermatogenesis.[33,34]
- Pachytene primary spermatocytes, B spermatogonia and round spermatids are the most sensitive to overheating.
- Decreased semen concentration and alterations in sperm morphology will be noted approximately 40 days after overheating and will remain evident for up to 70 days.
- If insulation of the testes is prolonged, epididymal sperm may be affected as early as 4 days after insult. This would be first evidenced as an increase in detached heads, followed by other morphologic abnormalities.
- It will take up to 3 months before spermatogenesis returns to normal.

Erection and ejaculation

Erection, emission and ejaculation are complex neurological and physical processes.[35,36]

Erection

Erection results from penile engorgement; the penis lengthens and increases in diameter as a result of venous distension of the corpus cavernosus penis and the corpus spongiosum penis.

- Sensory stimulus of the glans penis and psychological stimulation of the cerebral cortex initiate erection.
- Parasympathetic impulses from segments S2–S4 pass to the penis resulting in dilation of the penile arterioles.
- There is an increase in the amount of blood entering the corpus cavernosus penis and the corpus spongiosum penis.
- The muscles of the penile root simultaneously contract and compress the veins of the penis against the ischial arch; this blocks the venous return from the penis, leading to penile engorgement. Cardiac output also increases, resulting in increased blood flow and pressure in the caudal aorta.
- Erection is lost when sympathetic impulses dominate again, resulting in arteriolar contraction, and the penile root muscles relax, resulting in the restoration of normal venous outflow.

Emission

This is the movement of fluids and spermatozoa through the ductal system and fluids from the accessory sex glands into the pelvic urethra.

- Emission is mediated and controlled by the sympathetic nervous system.

Ejaculation

Ejaculation is the forcible expulsion of fluids and spermatozoa through the urethra.

- It is controlled by parasympathetic impulses.
- During emission and ejaculation the urethralis and bulbospongiosus muscles contract strongly, resulting in pulsation and deposition of semen into the female tract.
- Prostatic fluid is emitted first (pre-ejaculatory fluid).
- Then the sperm-rich fraction is produced in 3–6 jets. The sperm-rich fraction also contains prostatic, bulbourethral and epididymal fluids.
- The last portion of the ejaculate comes from the vesicular glands and is gelatinous in nature (the so-called gel fraction).

Daily sperm output

- Daily sperm output can be determined by collecting the stallion daily for 5–7 days. At this time, the extragonadal sperm reserves are stabilized. When the stallion is collected on day 8, an accurate assessment of daily sperm output can be made. It can also be estimated by using testicular dimension measurement (see below).

- When stallions are collected daily, the daily sperm output will vary from 3.2 to 6.6 billion spermatozoa.
- The number of spermatozoa per milliliter of semen differs between first and second ejaculates, collected 1 hour apart, by approximately 55%.[37] There is a minimal reduction in gel-free semen volume for the second ejaculate.
- In stallions collected once versus twice daily, the sperm output is similar, regardless of the frequency of ejaculation. Therefore, a defined number of sperm is available on a daily basis for ejaculation and once the daily sperm output is reached there is no benefit of collecting twice daily for artificial insemination programs.
- In stallions being utilized in natural service programs, adequate time between services must be provided such that extragonadal sperm reserves are replenished.

The daily sperm output (DSO) can be calculated using the following formulae:[38]

$$DSO = (3.36 \times 10^9) + (0.066 \times 10^9 X)$$

where X is the scrotal width in mm

or

$$DSO = 0.024Y - 0.76$$

where Y is testicular volume in milliliters (see p. 52)

Factors affecting sperm production/output

The primary factors that influence daily sperm output include:

- Season of the year.
- Age of stallion.
- Frequency of ejaculation.
- Testicular size and consistency.

- Each of these factors may affect sperm output individually or in concert with other factors.

Other, secondary, factors that may affect sperm output include:

- Environmental conditions.
- Nutrition.
- Medication administration.
- Hormonal status.

Season of the year

There is a significant effect of season on daily sperm production.[39]

- The normal breeding season in the northern hemisphere is May–August. In the southern hemisphere the season extends from September to December.
- Semen volume is approximately 40% higher during the breeding season than during winter. The average number of spermatozoa per ejaculate is about 50% higher during the breeding season than during the nonbreeding season.
- If stallions are exposed to decreasing day length in autumn and then stimulated by an artificial photoperiod (16 light hours, 8 dark hours), the seasonal increase in sperm production can be stimulated earlier in the breeding season such that maximal sperm production in the northern hemisphere will occur in April rather than in June.[40] However, in these stallions, sexual recrudescence will occur earlier in the breeding season. Therefore, if the majority of mares are to breed in February–May, placing stallions under artificial lighting will be of benefit. However, if the majority of mares will be bred during May–July, artificial lighting is not recommended.

Age of the stallion

Age is an important factor to consider when determining the potential daily sperm output and the book of mares to a particular stallion.

- The more mature a stallion is, the larger his epididymal sperm reserves will be.[41]
- However, an aged stallion may have fibrosis of the epididymis resulting in decreased epididymal sperm reserves.
- Younger stallions produce less total semen volume, less gel-free volume and less total spermatozoa per ejaculate than do mature stallions (>6 years).
- There is no difference between 6-year-old stallions and 16-year-old stallions. It is evident, therefore, that maturation of the stallion is complete by 6 years of age.

Testicular volume (TV) can be calculated from the following formulae:

$$TV = A \times C$$

where A is the cross-sectional area through the widest portion of the testicle and C is (testicular length)/2

or

$$TV = a \times b \times c$$

where a is (testicular height)/2, b is (testicular width)/2 and c is (testicular length)/2

Frequency of ejaculation

Frequency of ejaculation will affect total volume and number of spermatozoa per ejaculate until the daily sperm output is reached (Table 4.1).[42–44]

- The more frequently an individual stallion is collected the lower will be his semen volume. Once the daily sperm output is attained, a similar frequency of ejaculation will not result in further decreases in semen volume.
- In stallions that are collected at least every other day, the number of spermatozoa per ejaculate decreases as the frequency of ejaculation increases.
- When stallions are collected every other day, all the spermatozoa being produced are being ejaculated.
- Therefore collecting any more often than every other day will result in decreased semen concentration per ejaculate.
- Young stallions that are collected twice daily may have inadequate sperm production for normal fertility (especially when used for natural service).

Sperm stored in the ampulla, vas deferens and cauda epididymis can be released during ejaculation.

- Sperm located in the caput and corpus of the epididymis are not available for ejaculation until maturation and transit of the sperm are completed.
- The number of sperm available for ejaculation depends on the size of the epididymal sperm reserves and the frequency of and interval between ejaculations.[45,46]
- Approximately 62% of the sperm available for ejaculation is stored in the tail of the epididymis.

Testicular size and consistency

Testicular size affects daily sperm production since daily sperm output depends on the number of spermatozoa produced per gram of testicular tissue.

- The larger the testicles, the greater the potential for increased sperm production.
- Although testicular size is an important factor, it is also important that the testicular tissue that is present is normal and completely functional for sperm output to be maximal.
- There are pathological reasons for enlargement of testicles and in this circumstance the output will be significantly impaired.

Testicular measurements can be made using calipers (Fig. 4.14) or by using an ultrasonographic measurement system.

- When measuring the testicles, they should be pressed downwards fully into the scrotum with one hand, while the other hand performs the measurements.
- Measurement of testicular depth, width and length should be repeated at least three times to be sure that an accurate overall measurement is made.
- If total scrotal width is used as an indicator of daily sperm output, again at least three measurements should be made to reduce the degree of error.

Table 4.1 Effect of frequency of ejaculation on total semen volume and number of spermatozoa per ejaculate (estimated for a mature stallion)

	Frequency of ejaculation		
	One per day	Four per week	One per week
Semen volume (ml)	50	55	55
Sperm per ejaculate	5.0×10^9	10.0×10^9	10.0×10^9

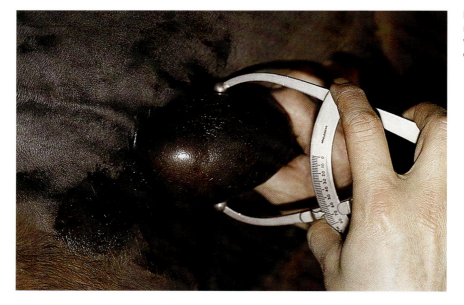

Fig. 4.14 Testicular measurements being taken with the help of a calibrated caliper.

Testicular size, daily sperm production and extragonadal sperm reserves continue to increase for several years following puberty.

- Testicular size is highly heritable in other species and is likely heritable also in the stallion.
- Stallions with a total scrotal width of less than 80 mm should not be used in breeding programs as they may pass on the genetic characteristics of hypoplasia. Additionally, stallions with low total scrotal width are poor sperm producers and will likely suffer fertility problems.
- Forty percent of the variation in testicular size is accounted for by difference in age.
- For the young stallion, collection or service once daily throughout the breeding season should be possible if all physical parameters are normal.
- In the older stallion, collection or service is possible up to three times daily, if libido will allow it.

Testicular consistency should resemble a new tennis ball. The epididymis should be compliant to compression.

- Any abnormality resulting in firmness, decrease in size or wrinkling of the tunics should be noted and should be considered a potential cause for a decrease in sperm output.
- These changes often occur as a result of fibrosis or degeneration.

BREEDING SOUNDNESS EXAMINATION

There are many factors that affect the inherent ability of an individual stallion to reproduce successfully. This may include the stallion's age and genetic make-up, his current and past health status, his body condition, the season of the year, and the environment in which he is housed. Assessment of the stallion's ability to breed successfully includes:

- Evaluation of the physical status of the entire animal.
- Specific examination of the reproductive tract.
- Determination of the normality of the spermiogram.
- Calculation of the number of mares that can successfully be bred during the ensuing breeding season, which includes determination of daily sperm output via evaluation of testicular function.

Evaluation may need to be performed:

- As part of a pre- or postpurchase examination.
- Prior to the breeding season.
- If fertility should decline.
- If breeding behavior changes.
- If infectious disease is suspected.

The evaluation should at a minimum consist of two semen collections taken 1 hour apart. For more in-depth evaluations, semen may be collected daily for 7–10 days in order to determine the daily sperm output.

The Society of Theriogenology has established guidelines for evaluating fertility potential of stallions.[47] The results of the breeding soundness examination should be recorded carefully, preferably using a standardized form.[48] These results are often required for legal and medical reasons and errors and omissions should be avoided. The breeding soundness examination is used to make recommendations on the number of mares that a stallion may mate successfully each season.

A stallion can be rated as:

- An unsatisfactory prospective breeder.
- A questionable prospective breeder.
- A satisfactory prospective breeder.

Prospective purchasers, mare owners and stud managers need to understand the implications of this classification. Stallions that are considered satisfactory and given reasonably good management and mares of good fertility are expected to render at least 75% of 40 or more mares pregnant when bred naturally, or 120 mares pregnant when bred artificially in one breeding season.

However, even poor breeders can be useful stallions and some that are classified as satisfactory have problems in other areas and so may be less effective breeders than the other classes. The whole status of the stallion should be considered carefully at the start of a breeding program. The role of the veterinarian in enhancing breeding potential of a stallion cannot be over-emphasized.

- For example, timing of service or insemination or the selection of highly fertile mares may enhance fertility in a poor breeder.

The breeding soundness examination represents a single assessment of the animal's breeding status at the time of the examination. Events and physiological status may change with age, management and medical manipulations.

- Significant fluctuations occur in the health status of a horse.
- Many causes of infertility in stallions are temporary (e.g. illness, injury, and reduced libido) so a breeding soundness examination performed when the stallion is not in his normal state could easily lead to his being condemned unjustifiably.

The breeding soundness examination identifies (and eliminates) *most* stallions with genetic defects and also alerts owners to potential problems.

The standard examination comprises the following:

1. The stallion should always be positively identified from documents provided. The identification should include:
   - Name.
   - Age.
   - Breed.
   - Registration number.
   - Microchip number.
   - Identifying marks: lip tattoo, hide brands (hot and freeze brands), color markings and hair whorls.

   It is helpful, especially when the sale of the horse is involved, that a photograph is taken for permanent identification. Most stallions will have an official document of identification and many now have microchip implants, so mistaken identity should be rare.

2. A complete history that details medical problems, injuries, drug therapy the stallion has been receiving over the past 6 months, and vaccination status needs to be taken. It should also include:
   - The dates of the athletic performance career (beginning and end).
   - The present use of the stallion (if used other than for breeding).
   - Previous breeding performance, including first cycle conception rates.
   - The pregnancy rate for the previous seasons and the current year.
   - Libido, mating behavior record.
   - Abnormalities encountered during breeding.
   - Results of previous fertility examinations and past breeding management should be evaluated and compared with the present findings, especially if the stallion has decreased fertility.
   - Any positive or negative experiences should be noted, especially if the stallion has a behavioral problem.
   - Mismanagement, inadequate nutrition, or a concurrent medical disorder may lead secondarily to deterioration in semen quality.

3. Physical examination of the whole horse to assess general health, including blood and serological testing for infectious or other disorders that may be directly involved in breeding (e.g. dourine, equine viral arteritis):
   - The examination must be thorough and the results properly recorded: reports and results are often required for sale purposes, for obtaining fertility insurance or for making recommendations on breeding management.
   - Particular attention should be directed to auscultation of the heart, evaluation of the eyes and the ability of the stallion to move freely.
   - Observation of the stallion moving in a small paddock may help to identify any musculoskeletal problems such as lameness due to chronic degenerative joint disease, laminitis or back disorders.
   - Potentially heritable traits such as cryptorchidism, brachygnathia, or cervical vertebral instability ('Wobbler') syndrome need to be recorded.
   - Rectal examinations are not routinely performed due to the inherent risks involved to both the examiner and the stallion.

4. Detailed evaluation of external genitalia (and possibly the accessory sex glands):
   - Examination of the reproductive tract of the stallion is conducted primarily to evaluate fertility potential and to diagnose gross abnormalities of the external genitalia.
   - The scrotum and its contents should be evaluated for symmetry and size:
     - Total scrotal width or testicular volumes are measured using calipers or testicular ultrasonography, respectively.
     - The size of the testicles is directly related to the male's daily sperm output and the number of mares he is able to breed during one breeding season (see p. 52).
     - Testicular consistency is assessed. The testicles and epididymides are palpated for tone, symmetry, and the presence of any abnormally firm or soft areas (see p. 55).
     - Both testicles should be present in the scrotum.

   - Cryptorchid stallions should not be used as breeding animals as there is a hereditary component to this congenital defect.

     - The spermatic cords are palpated for the presence of the vas deferens, sperm granuloma, varicocele (dilation of the blood vessels), excessive fat or masses in the cord.

5. Evaluation of libido and sexual behavior requires observation of mating behavior when presented with an estrus mare.

6. Evaluation of mating ability requires direct observation of mating.

7. Semen quality requires collection of a truly representative semen sample:
   - Spermatozoal and semen characteristics and the microbial flora of semen.
   - Ejaculated semen is composed of heterogeneous subpopulations of sperm cells, making an accurate diagnosis of dysfunctional sperm very challenging.
   - Some stallions, under good breeding management systems, that have normal to moderately low numbers of morphologically

normal, motile sperm in their ejaculates, either fail to have normal conception rates or have decreased conception rates.

- If pus, bacteria or blood are present in the ejaculate, or abnormalities such as azoospermia or cryptorchidism are noted, a rectal examination should be performed to assess the internal genitalia and inguinal rings.

Many of these parameters are relatively well correlated to fertility, but not all subfertile stallions will be identified by the examination.

- Supporting diagnostic tests (such as radiography, endoscopy, and blood sample analysis) should be performed if there is any doubt about the findings of the physical examination.
- Additional methods for identifying possible causes of the subfertility are currently available in specialized laboratories.

- Unfortunately, control values used for these tests are frequently of human origin and differences between the two species have not been completely identified, making interpretation of test results difficult.

Technological advances in semen preservation have changed breeding management strategies.

- Breeding soundness examinations may be performed on stallions that are to breed only 10–20 mares, but semen collected from that particular stallion must be cooled and shipped.
- Semen may be collected for cryopreservation.

Traditional breeding practices have also changed.

- Very few popular Thoroughbred stallions breed only 40 mares in a season.
- These changes make interpretation of the breeding soundness examination difficult, as stallions to be examined may not fit the classical defined criteria for fertility recommendations.

The breeding soundness examination provides valuable information on the health of the stallion and the daily sperm output, both of which are important prerequisites for breeding management decisions.

SPECIFIC EXAMINATION OF EXTERNAL GENITALIA

External genitalia are examined to rule out anatomic or pathologic conditions that will interfere with fertility.

- The scrotum, testicles, epididymis, penis and prepuce are examined routinely by manual palpation.
- Ultrasonography or endoscopy can be used to complement the examination.

Note:
- Considerable care must always be taken to avoid personal injury during examination as the stallion can kick in any direction.
- Not every stallion will allow the examination to be performed and some form of restraint may be needed.
- The examiner and the handler should stand on the same side.
- During the examination the examiner should keep in close contact with the horse's body and all movements should be slow and gentle.
- It is most common to examine the scrotum and spermatic cords after semen collection since most stallions are more manageable after collection, rather than before.

Suitable restraint can be obtained by:

- Placing the stallion in a stock/chute with the sidebars placed at a level above the ventral abdominal wall of the stallion. This allows the examiner to grasp the scrotum below the bar while either standing or bending down next to the horse's flank.
- Backing the stallion into a corner so that the animal's hindquarters and one side are against a wall.
- A twitch over the nose or chain over the stallion's upper gum is useful in diverting attention during examination.

The examiner needs to move slowly and keep his body close to the stallion when the scrotum and its contents are palpated. A preferred technique when the horse is not restrained in a stock is:

- To approach the horse from the left just behind his shoulder.
- Grasp the mane on the withers with the left hand, and while keeping close contact with the stallion's body slide the right hand medially along the ventral abdominal wall until the scrotum is grasped.

Many stallions will squeal, flinch, and withdraw the scrotum up close to the body. However, by remaining in contact with the horse's body, and by moving the hand slowly, most stallions tolerate the examination reasonably well. Once the stallion has relaxed, both hands can be used for manual palpation of the scrotal contents. Experienced well-handled stallions are usually more tolerant but safety should always be considered.

The scrotum

- The scrotum in the stallion is pendulous, smooth, thin, elastic, and hairless.
- During manual palpation or extremely cold temperatures, the scrotum may be withdrawn towards the body because of contractions of the cremaster muscles.
- Each testis and attached epididymis should be freely movable within the scrotal pouch.
- There should be no obvious free fluid within the scrotum (hydrocele) nor should there be any tissue within the sac other than the testis, epididymis or spermatic cord (scrotal hernia).
- The scrotal skin should be free of scars and granulomatous lesions, tumors or other thickenings.

The testes

- The testes should be palpated carefully to determine their general shape, size, orientation, and texture.
- Normal testes are oval and turgid, of similar size with a smooth surface.
- Testicular parenchyma should bulge slightly beneath the fingers when compressed, having the consistency of dense rubber.
- The testes lie horizontally, with the head of the epididymis closely apposed in an anterior position.
- The body of the epididymis is loosely apposed on the dorsolateral surface of the testis, with the tail located on the caudal pole of the testicle.
  - ❏ The epididymis should be palpable in its entirety; the prominent tail and the remnant of the gubernaculum (caudal ligament of the epididymis) serve as landmarks for orientation of the testis. The caudal ligament of the epididymis remains palpable during adult life as a small (1–2 cm) fibrous nodule adjacent to the epididymal tail, which itself is attached to the caudal pole of the testis.[49]
  - ❏ The epididymis should have a soft, spongy texture. There should not be any firm nodules, heat or pain on palpation.
  - ❏ It is not uncommon for some stallions to have one of the testes rotated 180° without the animal showing any pain or it having a negative effect on fertility (Fig. 4.15).

Testicular size correlates highly with daily sperm output and can be used to predict a stallion's breeding potential.[50] Therefore, if a stallion is being examined for fertility potential the testes may be measured either with calipers (scrotal width) or with ultrasonography (testicular volume):

- Scrotal width is measured by grasping the neck of the scrotum with one hand above the testes and pushing the testes down into the scrotum.

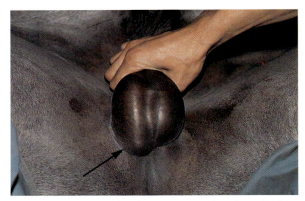

Fig. 4.15 Rotation of (left) testis. Note that the tail of the rotated (left) testicle is lying cranially and not obvious to view. Normal (right testis) epididymis is lying caudally in the correct position and visually obvious (arrow).

- The ends of the calipers are placed on the widest part of the testes and closed so that there is slight pressure on the scrotum.
- The measurement is read in millimeters from the base of the calipers. The width between the two ends of the calipers is measured with a measuring tape.
- Total scrotal width of mature stallions with normal fertility ranges from 95 to 120 mm.[51]

Ultrasonographic examination can easily be performed and provides an accurate measure of testicular volume.

- Each testis should be approximately the same size and consistency and should be free of abnormal echodensities.
- It is also possible to measure the testicular size accurately using ultrasonography.

The spermatic cord

- A small portion of the spermatic cord can be palpated through the neck of the scrotum, though its specific contents are not always definable.
- The two cords should be of equal size and of uniform diameter (2–3 cm).
- Acute pain in this area is usually associated with inguinal herniation or torsion of the spermatic cord.

The penis and prepuce

The penis, prepuce and sheath should be examined during the breeding soundness examination (Fig. 4.16):

- It is important to fully extend the penis during this examination so that the preputial reflection can be examined.
- The nonerect penis should have a uniform slightly turgid texture.

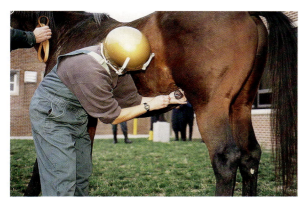

Fig. 4.16 Breeding soundness examination of penis and prepuce.

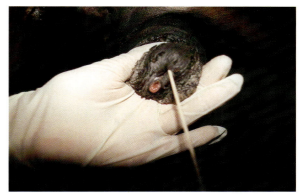

Fig. 4.17 A smegma bean being removed from the urethral fossa with a cotton swab. The same technique is used to obtain bacterial cultures from the fossa.

- Any evidence of past trauma, infections or deviations from normal is noted.
- The ability to obtain a normal erection along with the stallion's libido and serving capacity should be noted.
- The penis and prepuce are best examined by presenting the stallion to a mare in estrus. This procedure also permits assessment of sexual behavior, including erection capability.
- The penis can also be examined while the horse urinates.
- Tranquilization may be used to relax the penile supportive musculature, making the penis accessible.

> Note:
> - **Tranquilizers, especially phenothiazine derivatives, can result in penile paralysis or priapism (irresolvable erection) and should therefore not be used indiscriminately.**
> - Acepromazine should never be used in stallions (whether used for breeding or not).

- The penis should be washed to remove accumulated smegma on the body of the penis.
- The penis can then be grasped gently just behind the glans, rinsed with warm water and dried prior to inspection.
- The bean (smegma aggregation and inspissation) that may be present within the urethral fossa needs to be removed (Fig. 4.17), then the urethral process, glans penis and diverticulum carefully cleaned and examined. A bacteriological swab may be taken at the same time.
- Lesions commonly found on the penis include:
  - ❑ Nodules or cutaneous pustules associated with coital exanthema (see p. 192).
  - ❑ Habronema granuloma.
  - ❑ Papilloma.
  - ❑ Sarcoid (usually type A or type B nodules) (see p. 102).
  - ❑ Squamous cell carcinoma (of the shaft of the penis, the glans or the preputial skin/reflections or rings) or precarcinomatous changes (see p. 100).
  - ❑ Scarring, abrasions, or the presence of a hematoma or bruising are indicative of trauma.
- The skin of the prepuce and the internal lining should be free of distortions and thickenings. There should be no ulcerative lesions and the diameter of the preputial rings (internal and external) should allow free movement of the penis. It is usually possible to easily insert a lubricated gloved hand into the prepuce of a normal Thoroughbred stallion.

EXAMINATION OF INTERNAL GENITALIA

> - Examination of the pelvic area per rectum of a highly excitable or aggressive stallion is not without risk both to the operator and to the stallion.
> - Because of the risks, examination of the internal genitalia is not always performed at each breeding soundness examination.
> - If there is suggestive evidence of a problem such as pus, bacteria or inflammatory cells in the ejaculated semen or there is no semen in the ejaculate, evaluation of the accessory glands is warranted.

Stallions that are to be evaluated should be tranquilized properly to avoid injury to themselves and to the examiner:

- Phenothiazine and its derivatives have been associated with penile paralysis and so should not be used on stallions.

- α_2-Adrenoceptor agonists such as xylazine, romifidine and detomidine have been associated with hypersensitivity through the hindquarters. Therefore, they should be combined with another drug, such as butorphanol, to decrease the horse's tendency to kick.

- The doses and contraindications of the various drugs should be carefully checked prior to use.

A rectal examination should include:

- The prostate, seminal vesicles, ampulla, vas deferens and inguinal rings are examined by palpation and ultrasound examination.
- The bulbourethral glands are not palpable due to the heavy muscular coating and caudal location in the pelvis; however, they can be visualized on the ultrasound examination.
- There are differences in the appearance and size of the accessory sex glands, depending on whether the examination is performed prior to or following semen collection.

ACCESSORY SEX GLANDS

The stallion has four distinct accessory sex glands:

1. The paired ampullae, which surround the terminal segment of each deferent duct.
2. The paired vesicular glands (seminal vesicles).
3. The bi-lobed prostate.
4. The paired bulbourethral glands.
   - The glands change in shape and size according to the extent of sexual stimulus.
   - All four glands contribute to the watery fluids that are secreted at ejaculation.

Although they are readily accessible by rectal palpation it is difficult to locate all four glands accurately due to their indistinct texture. Therefore, if pathology is suspected, it is best to examine the glands with ultrasound per rectum using a linear 7.5-MHz probe and culture the seminal fluids after the stallion has been exposed to a mare in estrus.

- There is great variability in ultrasonographic findings of the accessory sex glands within the normal stallion population, making it sometimes difficult to identify pathology solely on the ultrasonographic findings.

The ampullae

These are paired, tubular, glandular thickenings of the distal ductus deferens located dorsal to the bladder. They are easily located by rectal palpation by moving the hand forward along the pelvic urethra until the two ductus deferens are palpated near the neck of the bladder.

- The ampullae are identifiable as 20–25-cm long pencil-like widening of the ductus deferens, located 2–4 cm cranial to the bifurcation of the ductus deferens.
- Anatomically, the ampullae have a central fluid-filled lumen surrounded by an inner glandular layer and an outer muscular layer.
- Ultrasonographically, the lumen appears dark (echolucent), the glandular parenchyma appears gray and the muscular layer appears bright (echogenic).[52] Within the wall there may be echolucent areas.[53]
- The diameter of the ampulla averages 13-mm but varies between horses and within individuals. The lumenal diameter of the ampulla doubles in size following teasing and decreases to resting values following ejaculation.
- The prominent size of the ampullae and the large cross-sectional area of the glandular tissue create potential for excessive accumulation of sperm and glandular secretions. This may result in distension of the glandular portion and possible blockage of the duct and azoospermia.

The prostate gland

The prostate gland is located above the intersection of the pelvic urethra and the bladder neck. It is entirely external to the urethra and is divided into a narrow central isthmus and two lobular portions that follow the lateral edges of the pelvic urethra. It is not usually palpable per rectum, but is easily visualized on ultrasonography.

- The interior of the prostate usually contains gray glandular parenchyma and narrow bands of dark fluid.
- The prostate gland increases in size and fluid content following teasing and decreases to sexually rested values following ejaculation.

The bulbourethral glands

The bulbourethral glands are ovoid organs located dorsolateral to the pelvic urethra in the vicinity of the ischial arch. They are difficult to identify by rectal palpation because of their thick muscular covering.

- Ultrasonographically, the bulbourethral gland contains homogeneous gray parenchyma and small (1–2 mm) pockets of dark fluid. The border is highly echogenic due to the muscular covering.
- The average size of the glands is 28 mm long and 19 mm wide. They do not change significantly in size or shape with teasing and ejaculation.

The vesicular glands

The gel portion of the seminal fluid originates from the vesicular glands, which are elongated, pyriform sacs with a central lumen located on either side of the bladder neck. They are usually located within the pelvic cavity, dorsomedial to the ampullae. They often extend beyond the pelvic cavity, hanging over the pelvic brim. Their shape appears to depend on their position, surrounding structures and contents. Their long axes radiate cranially and laterally from the origin at the proximal pelvic urethra. They can be difficult to palpate per rectum unless they are filled with fluid or are inflamed.

- To locate them via the rectum one locates the urethra on the floor of the pelvis and moves the hand cranially until the bifurcation of the ductus deferens is palpated. The examiner then rotates the wrist laterally, opens the hand and gently gropes along the lateral wall of the pelvic inlet. If the vesicular gland is filled with fluid, a soft, spongy, long structure is palpable.
- Inflamed vesicular glands may be enlarged and firm, and occasionally have a lobulated texture and irregular borders.
- They are rarely painful except in acute stages of disease.
- Semen of stallions with seminal vesiculitis has varying numbers of neutrophils with clumps of purulent material. Bacteria may be seen on microscopic examination.
- Ultrasonographically, vesicular glands are irregular in shape with thin, bright walls and a dark central lumen.
  - ❑ The vesicular glands of sexually rested stallions are dorsoventrally flattened pouches with gray muscular walls and a dark central lumen.
  - ❑ The lumen increases in diameter following teasing, and decreases or disappears following ejaculation.

The inguinal rings

The inguinal rings are most commonly explored by rectal palpation to determine the location of a retained testis and to evaluate the contents of the inguinal canal in horses experiencing inguinal or scrotal hernia. The arrangement of the inguinal rings and the problems associated with them have been well described.[54]

- To permit an accurate evaluation, the stallion must be adequately restrained during this procedure.
- To identify the location of a retained testis, both the superficial inguinal ring and the deep inguinal ring on the side of the retained testis need to be palpated.
  - ❑ The superficial inguinal ring can be located by palpating the ventral abdominal wall between the penis and the medial aspect of the thigh. If the examiner has difficulty identifying the ring on the side of an undescended testis, the spermatic cord of the descended testicle can be palpated and followed up to the superficial inguinal ring to estimate the other ring's location in relation to the thigh and penis. The opening of the superficial inguinal ring is 2–3 cm in diameter and the canal is 10–12 cm long.[55] The ring is directed laterally, cranially and slightly ventrally from the edge of the prepubic tendon.
  - ❑ The deep inguinal ring (also referred to as vaginal ring) is identified on rectal palpation as a slit-like opening on each side, ventrolateral to the pelvic brim. To locate them, the examiner clears all feces out of the rectum as far forward as can be safely reached. The examiner then passes a well-lubricated hand just cranial to the pelvic brim and moves the hand ventrally and laterally until contact is made with the abdominal wall. The examiner then sweeps the hand medially and laterally while slowly retracting the hand caudally. During the procedure the hand will come into contact either with vessels entering the inguinal ring or with the ring itself.

ULTRASONOGRAPHIC EXAMINATION OF STALLION GENITALIA

Ultrasonography is helpful in assessing:

- The accessory sex glands[56] (see p. 47).
- The scrotal contents (see p. 45).
- Testicular volume to determine daily sperm output (see p. 52).
- The location of an undescended testis.

- A 5-MHz transducer is most commonly used to measure testicular volume and to locate an undescended testis (see Fig. 4.48, p. 93).
- The 7.5-MHz transducer is used for scanning the accessory sex glands.[57]
- Each accessory sex gland has a standard approach for examination using a transrectal linear 7.5-MHz scanner.

The testes and scrotum

Ultrasonographically, normal testes have a homogeneous, echogenic appearance. In the center of the testes is a small (2–3 mm) circular nonechogenic area that corresponds to the central vein. The epididymis has a mottled appearance ultrasonographically as it contains many echogenic and nonechogenic areas due to fluid within the convoluted seminiferous tubules.

The accessory sex glands

The normal ultrasonographic appearance of the accessory gland varies with the breeding state of the stallion and the timing of the examination relative to ejaculation. Specialist interpretations can be useful but there is little information on the range of normal and abnormal ultrasonographic features of the stallion.

SEMEN COLLECTION

Collection of semen from stallions has become standard practice in stud farm management and is used both to evaluate semen quality and for artificial insemination. Although there are strict prohibitions on its use in some breeds and in some countries, it is likely that it will become a more common practice. Stallions that cannot mate naturally for other reasons, such as orthopedic pain or disability, can be used effectively in a breeding program in spite of the limitations on their physical function. Artificial insemination has been instrumental in improving other species of animals and could be used in horses to this end also. Although frozen semen is still not as reliable as it is in other species, it does widen the scope of breeding programs across the world. More usually, however, chilled fresh semen is used in equine breeding establishments so that mares do not have to travel and stallions are not subjected to the same risks as natural breeding.

Semen collection in the stallion can be performed by several methods:

- Artificial vagina.
- Condom.
- Ground (standing) collection (manual stimulation or chemical stimulation).

Technique for collection of semen

i. A mare in estrus or an ovariectomized, hormone-treated mare is used as a mount animal (Fig. 4.18); alternatively, the stallion is allowed to mount a phantom or dummy mare (Fig. 4.19).
  - If a mare in estrus is used as a mount mare, she should be in a good 'standing' estrus (heat) and willing to let the stallion mount, without any resentment or aggression.
  - She should be twitched and sedated or hobbled (Fig. 4.20).
  - The mare's tail should be wrapped and preferably tied to the right side.
ii. The mare's perineum should be washed thoroughly, any soap residues rinsed completely off and then dried with a clean paper towel.
iii. The person handling the stallion should be comfortable in the breeding shed.

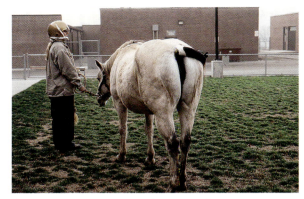

Fig. 4.18   Estrous mare used as mount for semen collection.

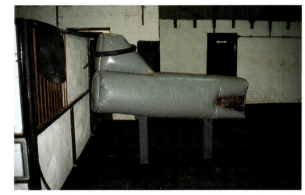

Fig. 4.19   Phantom/dummy mare.

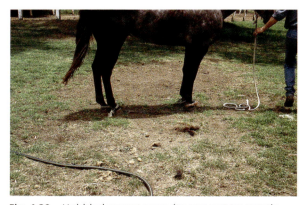

Fig. 4.20   Hobbled mount mare (to prevent traumatic injuries to the stallion).

- He/she should be able to alter the handling techniques based on the behavior of the stallion.
- Some stallions will require little more than vocal commands, while other stallions will require the use of a chain shank through the mouth or under the lip in order to maintain control and provide a safe environment for mare, stallion, handler and semen collector.

Collection using the artificial vagina

Several different artificial vaginas for semen collection are commercially available. Each of these has its attributes and peculiarities.[58] Basically, all the artificial vaginas have an outer rigid tube and an inner, soft, liner with the space between the two filled with warm water. The collecting system is arranged so that semen contacts the latex liner for the shortest time possible. The Missouri artificial vagina (Nasco, Ft. Atkinson, WI, USA) is widely used in the USA and has fairly good heat retention.

i. The artificial vagina should be prepared immediately before attempting semen collection.
ii. It needs to be filled with warm water (48–50°C) to provide an internal artificial vagina temperature of 44–48°C.[59] Because the glans penis should extend beyond the water jacket at the time of ejaculation, the internal temperature of the artificial vagina may exceed the 45–48°C spermatozoal tolerance thresholds without causing heat-related injury to ejaculated sperm.[60] An artificial vagina temperature of 6–8°C above that of the body seems to stimulate copulation without damaging sperm. The artificial vagina and semen receptacle should be kept insulated in cold weather.
iii. Before collection, the inner surface of the artificial vagina needs to be well lubricated with a nonspermicidal lubricant.
iv. The lumenal pressure of the artificial vagina should be adjusted so that the penis fits snugly within it but not to the extent that it is difficult for the stallion to penetrate the artificial vagina with his penis and to remove it after ejaculation.
v. A semen filter is placed in the receptacle to filter out the gel portion of the ejaculate, which emanates from the seminal vesicles.
vi. It is important that everyone involved is completely aware of the procedure, particularly with respect to personal safety issues.
   - All individuals in the breeding shed should wear helmets.
   - The person collecting the stallion should stand on the same side as the stallion handler (left).
   - If the stallion is difficult to handle or has never been collected it is recommended that a fourth person be present to assist the collector. This person should stand to the right of the collector facing the stallion's hip and if needed should place pressure on the stallion's hip to keep the horse up on the mount. This person will also monitor the behavior of the stallion and mare and if a problem occurs will pull the collector out of harm.

vii. Prior to collection, the stallion should be teased with a mare in behavioral estrus to stimulate erection.
   - Once erect, the penis and associated external genitalia need to be inspected for lesions and the penis cleansed to minimize contamination of the ejaculate with bacteria, dirt and epithelial debris from the surface of the penis.
   - The 'bean', or debris, should be cleaned out of the urethral fossa (see p. 58).
   - The penis is routinely rinsed with warm water only because repeated cleansings with soap scrubs removes the normal bacterial flora and may allow overgrowth of potentially pathogenic organisms (Fig. 4.21).
   - After washing, the penis should be dried with paper towels, as water may be spermicidal.
   - The washing procedure can be performed in the center of the breeding shed or, if the stallion is fractious, it can be done with the stallion backed into a corner of a loose box.
viii. Semen collection
   - For a general breeding soundness examination, semen is collected twice, with an hour between collections.
   - The stallion is teased to the mare until an erection is obtained and he is allowed to mount.

   - If a mare is used, she should have good footing and should be twitched.
   - If an artificial (phantom) mount is used, this must be capable of withstanding the weight and force of the stallion's activity.

   - Once the stallion has settled onto the mare (or phantom), his penis should be deflected to the left and introduced into the artificial

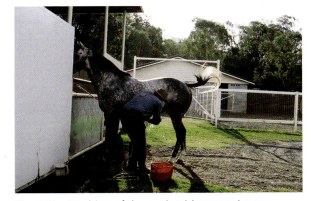

Fig. 4.21 Washing of the penis with soap prior to collection is not advisable. Rinsing with warm water is usually all that is needed and avoids harmful alterations in the bacterial flora of the penile skin.

vagina (Fig. 4.22). The stallion will thrust forward to 'couple' with the mare/dummy.

- The penis needs to be inserted into the artificial vagina at the first thrust so that 50% or more of the shaft of the penis is inserted into and maintained within the artificial vagina. If this does not occur, the glans penis may 'bell' (dilate) near the opening of the artificial vagina and will then be too large to permit full penile penetration into the artificial vagina, resulting in ejaculatory failure from inadequate penile stimulation.
- Once the penis is in the artificial vagina, the collection receptacle needs to be kept level with the ground. The artificial vagina should be held at an angle that is appropriate for the stallion (usually with the opening slightly downward) and the semen receptacle slightly upward (Fig. 4.23).
- The left hand is used to hold the artificial vagina (the collector can lean into the mare to put pressure on the artificial vagina if

necessary) and the right hand is placed with the thumb dorsally and four fingers ventrally on the base of the penis (Fig. 4.24).

- Ejaculation usually occurs after 4–6 thrusts.
- There are usually 3–5 ejaculatory jets, which can be felt on the ventral surface of the penis with the right hand. Many stallions 'flag' their tails during ejaculation, which appears as a pumping action of the tail.
- As the stallion ejaculates, the end of the artificial vagina should be lowered so that the ejaculate can flow freely into the receptacle and none is lost onto the ground (Fig. 4.25).
- As the penis relaxes, the right hand is used to strip the penis/urethra of the remaining semen.
- Water is immediately allowed to flow out of the artificial vagina to reduce the internal pressure and so that all the semen flows into the receptacle.
- If the stallion is reluctant to thrust, it may be necessary for the semen collector to change

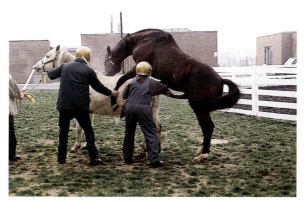

Fig. 4.22 The penis is deviated to the left and directed into the artificial vagina.

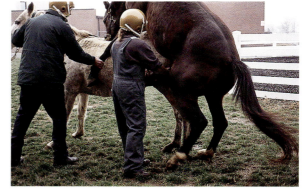

Fig. 4.24 The right hand can be used to check for the characteristic pulsations in the urethra that are a sign of effective ejaculation.

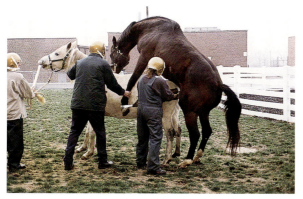

Fig. 4.23 The semen receptacle is maintained level with the ground or slightly downwards to ensure free flow of the ejaculate into the receptacle.

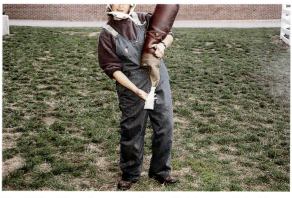

Fig. 4.25 After dismount, the artificial vagina is held up to allow all the semen to flow into the receptacle.

the pressure or temperature of the water in the water jacket. Warm wet compresses or pressure with one's hands on the base of the penis may help stimulate ejaculation.

- It should not take more than a few attempts at collection for ejaculation to occur.
- Difficulties or abnormalities should be noted as part of the evaluation.

Condom collection technique

i. If a condom is used to collect the stallion, he is washed as described above.
ii. A small amount of nonspermicidal lubricant is placed on the rim of the prerolled condom, and the condom is placed over the penis.
iii. Nonspermicidal lubricant is applied to the vulvar lips of the jump mare.
iv. The stallion should not be allowed to lose his erection in case the condom falls off.
v. The stallion is allowed to breed the mare, assisting with intromission if necessary.
vi. After ejaculation occurs, the stallion dismounts and the condom is removed before the erection is completely lost.
vii. The semen is filtered and poured into a semen container and handled as above.

Ground (standing) collection techniques

i. Stallions that have musculoskeletal injuries and or physical reasons that prevent them from mounting a mare may be trained to ejaculate while standing on the ground using manual stimulation techniques.[61,62]
ii. These stallions can also be ejaculated using chemical stimulation.[63,64]

Collection by chemical ejaculation

i. Chemical ejaculation using xylazine and/or imipramine and manual stimulation leading to ejaculation usually results in a very concentrated sample of low volume.
ii. Collection is sometimes problematical.

> Note:
> - There is no effective, humane and safe electro-ejaculatory method for horses.

SEMEN EXAMINATION

- Two semen samples are collected 1 hour apart after the stallion has had a week of sexual rest.
- If the two samples are representative, the total number of live, progressively motile, morphologically normal sperm in the second ejaculate is a fairly accurate assessment of daily sperm output.

> - The term 'representative' refers to the ability to produce and collect two complete ejaculates.
> - A sample is representative if the second ejaculate contains between 30% and 70% of the total sperm numbers seen in the first ejaculate.

The number of live, progressively motile, morphologically normal sperm needed for a stallion to pass the breeding soundness examination varies according to the month of the breeding season. Typical values are presented in Table 4.2 for the northern hemisphere.

The minimum number of live, progressively motile sperm needed to impregnate a mare has not been established. Minimum accepted sperm doses are:

- Mare to be inseminated with fresh semen: 250 million, live progressively motile sperm.
- Mare to be inseminated with cooled semen: 500 million, live progressively motile sperm.
- Mare to be inseminated with frozen semen: 200 million, live progressively motile sperm.

> Note:
> - Conception may be achieved with lower doses of live progressively motile sperm.
> - Breeding must be timed with ovulation to achieve maximal pregnancy rates.
> - Mares bred with fresh semen should ovulate within 48 hours of the last insemination.
> - Mares bred with cooled semen should ovulate within 24–36 hours of insemination.
> - Mares bred with frozen semen should ovulate within 8–12 hours of insemination.

Semen should be evaluated following every collection. The quantity and quality of sperm produced are influenced by many factors, including:

Table 4.2 Numbers of sperm required for a stallion to pass the breeding soundness examination in the northern hemisphere

For a stallion in the northern hemisphere with a book of 40 mares, the product

[sperm concentration] × [gel-free volume] × [% progressive motile sperm] × [% morphologically normal sperm] should exceed:

September–January	1100×10^6
February–April	1700×10^6
May	2000×10^6
June	2200×10^6
July–August	1700×10^6

- Season of year.
- Frequency of ejaculation.
- Age.
- Thermal shock.
- Drug administration.
- Stress of performance.

In general, stallions produce more sperm in the summer than in the winter, with intermediate numbers found in the spring and autumn. Unlike cattle and small ruminants, there is no definite link between semen quality and fertility, most probably because most stallions standing at stud are generally not chosen for their reproductive capability but on past athletic performance.

Equipment

The equipment required for semen evaluation does not need to be elaborate and should be assembled before collection. The following items are required:

- A binocular phase-contrast microscope, preferably with a heated stage.
- A hemocytometer (improved Neubauer ruling) or densitometer.
- Slides, coverslips, calibrated pipettes (such as those used for blood cell counting).
- Buffered formal–saline.
- Receptacle for measuring volume.
- Stains for assessing morphology (e.g. nigrosin–eosin).
- Semen extenders.
- Some means to keep the semen sample at 37°C. A thermostatically controlled water bath, slide warmer or incubator is usually used.

Note:
- All materials that come into contact with the semen, including slides, coverslips, semen extenders, also need to be maintained at 37°C.
- This can be accomplished by placing them in an incubator or on a slide warmer prior to use.

Parameters

Semen parameters (see Table 4.3) that are routinely evaluated in an ejaculate are:

- Color: normal semen is pale white or skimmed milk-like in color.
- Volume: mean volume is 60–70 ml (range 30–300 ml) per ejaculate. The volume will depend to some extent on the volume of the gel fraction.
- Motility (total and progressive): at least 50% of the sperm should be progressively motile (i.e. able to swim in a forward direction).

Table 4.3 Semen parameters for a mature stallion (at daily sperm output)

	Acceptable	Average
Volume (ml)[a]	30	50
Motility (total/progressive) (%)	60/50	70/60
Velocity (on a scale of 4)	2	3
Concentration (10^6/ml)[b]	>50	100–200
Concentration per ejaculate ($\times 10^9$)	>2.0	4.0–6.0
Morphology (% normal)	>60	>80

[a]Varies with concentration and level of excitement.
[b]Depends in part on volume.

- Morphology: at least 50% should be morphologically normal.
- Concentration: this will be in the range $75–800 \times 10^6$ per ml, with a total sperm output of 1–20 billion sperm in each ejaculate.

Additional procedures include measuring the pH, staining semen samples to identify bacteria or inflammatory cells and longevity studies.

All findings should be recorded using a breeding soundness certificate.

Semen handling

i. During semen collection and transport to a laboratory, the receptacle should be kept at body temperature to prevent cold shock of the sperm. All semen should be maintained at 37°C until evaluation and all equipment that comes into contact with the semen should be warmed to 37°C.
ii. The collection vessel should be detached from the artificial vagina; the filter with its contained gel should be removed immediately upon collection of the semen to prevent seepage of gel into the gel-free portion of the ejaculate.
   - Separating the gel from the gel-free fractions maximizes the number of spermatozoa in the collection.
   - Nylon micromesh filters are superior to polyester matte for separating gel from gel-free fractions because they are nonabsorptive and do not trap as many sperm.
iii. Air, UV light, water, blood and urine are spermicidal and contact with these should be avoided. The air should be squeezed out of the collection container.
iv. Ideally, the semen needs to be at the laboratory and placed in an extender within 3 minutes of collection.
   - The semen is poured in a gentle manner into a warm graduated cylinder to measure its volume.

- Alternatively, it may be poured or gently aspirated into a warmed, nonspermicidal syringe, which has no rubber stoppers.
- The semen is immediately placed in an incubator at 37°C.
- Warmed microscope slides, coverslips and pipettes should always be used to prevent cold shock.

v. Three to five milliliters of raw semen should be reserved for immediate evaluation of its sperm concentration and motility (see below).

vi. Immediately after the initial examination of the raw semen has been performed, a small aliquot is extended using an appropriate extender (see below) and allowed to remain at 37°C for further examination.
- Semen is usually extended 1:20 to maximize motility evaluation.
- Semen should be evaluated at a magnification of ×10 (or ×40).

vii. The remaining (bulk) specimen is extended in a prewarmed (37°C) milk-based extender at a ratio of 1:2 to 1:4 semen to extender and placed in an incubator set at 37°C. The greater the dilution ratio of semen, the better the spermatozoal survival rate.[65]

Semen extenders

Semen extenders are used to provide the spermatozoa with nutrients that prolong their lifespan, especially if the environmental conditions are unfavorable for sperm survival in its raw form. Semen extenders will also increase the viability of semen from subfertile stallions and will increase the volume of the inseminate in artificial insemination programs where only a few milliliters of raw semen are required for a proper insemination dose. Extenders are used to deliver antibiotics and therefore prevent transmission of certain bacterial diseases.

The qualities of a good extender:

- It provides a favorable environment for the spermatozoa.
- It is easy to prepare and store.
- It allows for accurate semen evaluation.
- It is inexpensive.

Most equine semen extenders are based on either skim milk or egg yolk.[66,67] Those most commonly used are based on nonfat, dried, skim milk (see Table 4.4). Some contain buffers that regulate osmolarity and/or pH. Antibiotics, including polymyxin B, amikacin, amikacin and penicillin, and ticarcillin, are commonly added to the extender. Several commercially prepared extenders are available.

Plasma or colostrum (both having high concentrations of immunoglobulin) have been used instead of semen extenders but they are less satisfactory from handling and use perspectives.

Table 4.4 Preparation of a semen extender

Instant dried, low fat skimmed milk powder	2.5 g
Gelatin	0.5 g
Glucose	5.0 g
Penicillin (crystalline, sodium benzathine)	300 mg
Streptomycin (crystalline)	300 mg
Water	100 ml

The choice of which semen extender to use is based on the semen characteristics of an individual stallion because semen from a particular stallion will perform better in certain extenders than in others. This may be due to differences in specific constituents and their concentrations in each stallion's semen or to differences in the make-up of the extender.

- Semen extenders should always be warmed to 37°C before semen is added.
- Once the semen is extended it should be kept at 37°C until insemination, if the insemination is to be performed within 1 hour of collection. Semen can also be maintained at room temperature (25°C) for up to 12 hours in a suitable extender without significant decrease in fertility.[68]
- Typical dilution rates are 1:2 to 1:4, although some stallions with high-volume, low-concentration ejaculates need only be extended 1:1. Alternatively, semen from these stallions can be centrifuged at 500 g for 10 minutes and then re-suspended to improve concentration.[69]
- Some subfertile stallions will also benefit from this centrifugation/re-suspension process as it removes the association of semen with the seminal fluid, which is sometimes detrimental to safe semen storage.

DETAILED SEMEN EVALUATION

In addition to the direct examination described above, a complete evaluation of semen quality includes:

- Motility and percentage of live sperm.
- Morphology.
- Longevity studies (see p. 70).

Motility assessment

Motility needs to be evaluated within 5 minutes of collection. Both initial motility and longevity of sperm motility (see below) of undiluted and extended semen should be assessed and recorded. Assessment of motility is subjective, but the same observer can become very consistent. Phase-contrast microscopy is ideal for motility evaluation, although bright-field microscopy is acceptable. Use of a warmed microscope stage is recommended to prevent cold shock to the spermatozoa and consequent errors in motility evaluation.

Technique

i. A drop of raw semen is placed directly onto a warmed slide (37°C).

ii. A coverslip is carefully placed so as to avoid air bubbles.

iii. The motility of at least 50 sperm is assessed under ×40 magnification.
- *Individual motility* is estimated by counting 10 or more fields for progressive, forward motility of the cells (described as a percentage).
- Five sperm are chosen per microscope field and the number moving is counted. This number represents *total motility*.
- The fields chosen should be towards the center of the slide.
- The proportion of the five sperm swimming across the slide represents the *progressive motility*.

iv. The procedure is repeated for 10 or more fields to determine the percentage of total motile and progressively motile sperm in the sample.

v. The procedure is then repeated using the semen samples diluted in extender.

The total motility and the progressive motility should be estimated and recorded for each ejaculate evaluated.

> - Motility evaluation can also be performed using a computer-assisted semen analysis (CASA) machine.

Morphological examination

Sperm can be evaluated as stained smears using standard bright-field microscopy or as wet mounts using either phase-contrast microscopy or differential interference-contrast microscopy. Semen morphology is evaluated by mixing a small drop of semen with a stain; eosin–nigrosin is usually used. This is a vital stain that is mixed with the fresh specimen; sperm that are alive when the stain is applied will not take up the stain and will appear white or clear, whereas sperm that are dead will take up the stain and appear pink when viewed under the microscope (Fig. 4.26).

Microscopy

Technique

i. One drop of semen is mixed with one to two drops of stain at one end of a glass slide.

ii. A second glass slide is laid on this slide at an angle of 45° and pushed slowly into the mixture of semen and stain.

iii. When the stain and semen mixture has flowed under the edge of the top slide, the top slide is pulled slowly over the bottom glass slide as if

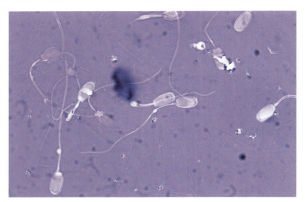

Fig. 4.26 Photomicrograph of semen stained with eosin–nigrosin stain.

making a blood smear. Gentle pushing of the stained semen is required to prevent damage to the sperm, resulting in abnormalities during the evaluation.

iv. The slide is allowed to air dry then examined under the microscope.

v. If a vital stain is not available, one of the following stains can be used:
- Indian ink.
- Eosin–aniline blue.
- Giemsa or (modified) Wright–Giemsa.
- New methylene blue.
- Spermac.

vi. When these stains are used, a smear of semen is made in similar fashion to the preparation of a blood smear, dried, fixed and then stained before being viewed under oil immersion (×100) for evaluation.

Wet mounts

This enhances visualization of the structural detail of sperm.

Technique

i. Fix a few drops of sperm in 3–5 ml of buffered formal–saline or buffered 4% glutaraldehyde solution.

ii. A few drops of the fixed sample are placed on a slide and a coverslip is carefully placed to ensure minimal air bubbles.

iii. The slide is then examined at ×1000 magnification (high-power, oil immersion). It is also examined for the presence of:
- Leukocytes (white blood cells).
- Erythrocytes (red blood cells).
- Spheroids (immature germ cells). Since the exact nature of the spheroid cells cannot be determined with eosin–nigrosin stain, when these are present another slide should be prepared using a nonvital stain such as modified Wright–Giemsa or Wright's stain.
- Bacteria.

- Some CASA machines can also perform morphologic analysis.

Interpretation

  i. A minimum of 200 cells should be counted to assess their staining characteristics.
 ii. Normal sperm cells as well as those with acrosomal, head, mid-piece, droplets and tail defects should to be carefully recorded.
iii. Artifactual changes are negligible using wet mounts. It may be difficult, however, to evaluate sperm heads due to the three-dimensional field and the tendency of the cells to roll or float in the wet mount preparation.

Traditionally, abnormal sperm are categorized as having:[70]

1. Primary abnormalities.
   - These defects reflect defects in spermatogenesis and are therefore testicular in origin.
   - They include head and acrosomal defects, diadem defects, bent/coiled mid-pieces, distal mid-piece reflexes, proximal cytoplasmic droplets and tail stump defects.
2. Secondary abnormalities.
   - These abnormalities are believed to occur after the sperm leave the testicles and pass through the rest of the ductal tract or occur during semen processing.
   - They arise in the excurrent duct system and include kinked tails and distal cytoplasmic droplets.
3. Tertiary abnormalities.
   - These develop in vitro as a result of improper semen collection or handling procedures and include detached heads and kinked tails (see below).

Other classifications of abnormal sperm morphology include:

1. Major and minor defects.
   - Major defects are believed to interfere with fertility.
   - Minor defects are abnormalities that do not affect the spermatozoa's fertility.
2. Compatible and incompatible defects.
   - Compatible defects are those that are compatible with fertilization.
   - Incompatible defects are not compatible with normal fertilization.

Errors and problems

Poor collection technique and specimen handling results in artifactual changes, primarily:

- Increased numbers of detached heads.
- Kinked tails.
- Head shape abnormalities.
- Clumping of sperm.

Certain antibiotics, either in normal or high concentrations, can cause significant changes in sperm morphology, and the use of cold glass slides (as opposed to prewarmed ones) may produce acrosomal and mid-piece damage. If the technique is likely to be questionable, the raw semen should be fixed in buffered formal–saline prior to the preparation of the smear.

Estimation of semen concentration

Semen (sperm) concentration of gel-free semen can be measured by:

- Hemocytometer.
- Densitometer.
- Spectrophotometer.
- Computer-assisted sperm analysis (CASA) machines.

Method for counting sperm numbers with a hemocytometer

  i. Using a standard white cell counting Unopette®, 50 µl of raw semen are diluted with 5 ml of buffered formal–saline and mixed well by turning (not shaking).
 ii. The coverslip is placed over the counting grid and the diluted semen is slowly added along the outer edge of the coverslip until the entire counting area is covered with liquid. Care should be taken that no air bubbles exist under the coverslip and that the fluid does not overflow the edges of the counting chamber.
iii. The fluid is allowed to settle for 3–5 minutes.
 iv. The heads of sperm in 5 small squares in the large central square of the hemocytometer (Neubauer chamber), or all 25 squares, are counted.
   - Both sides of the grid should be counted and the average taken.
   - The number of squares counted and the dilution needed differ with the semen concentration in the sample.
   - Five large squares in the center square are counted; or, if fewer than 100 cells are counted, 10 squares are counted.
   - If 5 squares are counted, the number is multiplied by 5.
   - If 10 squares are counted the figure is multiplied by 2.5.
   - This number is then multiplied by 10,000 and by any dilution factor that was used in the preparation of the sample prior to counting.

This then provides the number of sperm per milliliter of semen:

- If only 5 squares are counted, the number of sperm per milliliter of ejaculate is the number of sperm counted multiplied by 5 million.
- If all 25 squares are counted, the number of sperm per milliliter is the number counted multiplied by 1 million.

Measurement by densitometer/spectrophotometer

- Use of a densitometer requires dilution in a formalin solution to kill the sperm.
- The densitometer measures concentration by comparing the density of the formalin solution with semen added to the density of the formalin solution alone.
- A light beam is first passed through the formalin solution and again after the semen has been added. The concentration can then be calculated by the difference in the two measurements based on a known density curve.
- A spectrophotometer functions in a similar manner. Semen must first be diluted; then the value obtained is compared with a plot on a known curve to determine the concentration.

- Accurate measurement of the sperm concentration is critical because multiplying sperm concentration by semen volume provides the total number of sperm in an ejaculate.

Semen longevity/survival estimation

Longevity analysis should be performed on any stallion whose semen is to be transported in a chilled state or is to be frozen.

Technique

i. Longevity of spermatozoal motility is determined on raw semen samples and on samples diluted in various extenders stored in a refrigerator at 4–5°C.

ii. Evaluations using raw semen should be done as quickly as possible following collection because the semen tends to agglutinate, making evaluation difficult.

iii. The semen is extended with skim milk extender plus antibiotics and is maintained at room temperature (25–27°C) and at 5°C.

iv. For longevity studies semen is diluted at either:
   - 4 parts extender to 1 part of semen (or 25–50 million sperm per milliliter).
   - 5 parts extender to 3 parts of semen.

v. It is then evaluated for motility at 2, 12, 24, 48, and 72 hours post collection.
   - This analysis is useful to help determine the type of extender best used for each stallion and the dilution rate for the extender chosen.
   - Motility evaluation should be performed using both raw and extended semen (as described above).
   - Motility evaluations should be made immediately after rewarming for 5 minutes at 37°C, by placing a small drop of semen on a warmed microscope slide and applying a coverslip.
   - The semen drop should be large enough to have fluid extend to all corners of the coverslip, but should not be so big as to have semen extending beyond the coverslip edges.

Interpretation

- Motility is evaluated until progressive motility drops below 25–30%.
- The time post collection at which the motility drops to 25–30% is the maximum time the cooled semen should be stored.
- Insemination should definitely occur before the calculated time.

pH and osmolarity determination

Determination of the pH of the semen is beneficial, especially if fertility problems exist. The following factors may influence the pH of normal stallion semen:

- Time of the year (season).
- Frequency of ejaculation.
- Spermatozoal concentration.

Technique

- For the most accurate assessment the pH of gel-free semen should be determined using a properly calibrated pH meter, although pH paper may be used if a pH meter is unavailable.

Interpretation

- The normal pH of equine semen in the sperm-rich fraction is 7.2–7.7.[71]
- Osmolarity of stallion semen ranges between 290 and 310 mOsm. Values greater than 350 mOsm can be indicative of urospermia, whereas values less than 200 mOsm will affect morphology of the sperm observed as coiling of the tails.
- With infections of the accessory sex glands, the pH may be altered.
- Abnormally high semen pH can be associated with:
   - ❑ Contamination of the ejaculate by urine or soap.
   - ❑ Inflammatory lesions of the genital tract.

Bacteriological culture and sensitivity

Bacteriological cultures may be performed on an elective basis during a Breeding Soundness Examination or as a diagnostic tool if any leukocytes (white blood cells) are seen in the ejaculate or there is a history of infectious disease or sub/infertility.

Cultures may be taken from:

- Pre-ejaculate urethra (fluid).
- Prepuce.
- Sheath.
- Urethral diverticulum.
- Postejaculate urethra.
- Semen.

Normal equine semen contains a variety of bacteria.[72] The majority are nonpathogenic, whereas others are capable of causing infection in mares. Bacteria currently considered to be pathogenic are:[73]

- *Taylorella equigenitalis*.
- *Klebsiella pneumoniae* (capsule types 1, 2 and 5).
- *Pseudomonas aeruginosa* (some strains).

Technique

Cultures of swabs taken from the urethra prior to and after semen collection, and culture of the semen itself are routinely performed during a Breeding Soundness Examination.

i. Prior to collection of samples for bacterial isolation, the penis is rinsed thoroughly with warm water and dried.
ii. Debris from the glans penis and fossa glandis should be removed.
iii. Brisk rubbing of the glans penis during the washing process usually stimulates secretion of clear fluid out of the urethra. A cotton swab is then inserted 3–5 cm into the urethral orifice.
iv. The procedure is repeated post ejaculation.
v. A sterile swab is inserted into the semen specimen and placed in transport medium.
vi. All swabs are carefully placed into a suitable transport medium and delivered as quickly as possible to the laboratory.

Interpretation

- The results from the three cultures (semen, pre- and postejaculation urethral fluid swabs) are compared to identify the quantity and the predominance of an individual organism.
- If there is heavy growth of a pathogenic bacterium such as a *Pseudomonas aeruginosa* or *Klebsiella pneumoniae*, the stallion may be harboring the bacteria in the accessory sex glands and a thorough examination of the internal genitalia should then be performed.

SEMEN HANDLING AND STORAGE

SEMEN CHILLING

Chilled, transported semen can be used in an artificial insemination program where the mare and stallion are not on the same farm.

The benefits of using liquid, chilled semen include:

- It eliminates the need to transport the mare (and possibly her foal) to the stallion and is therefore safer.
- It increases the opportunities for the owner of a mare to breed her to a stallion at distant sites or where there are inadequate facilities for mare housing or management. The speed and efficiency of modern postal transportation make the process very effective worldwide.
- It reduces the use of genetically inferior stock and increases the use of genetically superior stallions by wider dissemination of the semen.
  ❑ Owners can be more selective and the costs are reduced; therefore financial savings can be made or a better stallion can be selected.
- It reduces disease transmission between farms by eliminating the possibility of spread of venereal and other infectious disease.
- It significantly reduces the costs for mare housing and management.

If insemination is to be postponed for longer than 12 hours then the semen should be chilled.

- Cooling of semen will prolong longevity by decreasing the metabolic rate of the spermatozoa thereby reducing their energy and nutrient requirements.
- When the semen is re-warmed, the metabolic rate of the sperm will return to normal and motility and fertility will return towards normal.
- The rate of cooling determines the active lifespan of the sperm once rewarming has occurred.
- To maximize sperm viability and motility:
  ❑ Cooling should be performed at a controlled rate (see below). Cooling at too fast a rate will result in damage to the spermatozoa.[74,75] The damage is to the membrane, with subsequent loss of lipids, ions and other substances, and resulting in diminished motility and depressed cellular metabolism. These changes are irreversible and are commonly known as cold shock.
  ❑ Rewarming should also be performed slowly.

Technique

Equine semen can be chilled rapidly (0.5–0.3°C/ minute) from 37°C to 20°C, and then cooled slowly (<0.1°C/minute) from 20°C to 5°C (Fig. 4.27).[76] There are several methods that can be used to cool semen safely at a slow, methodical, stepwise rate.[77]

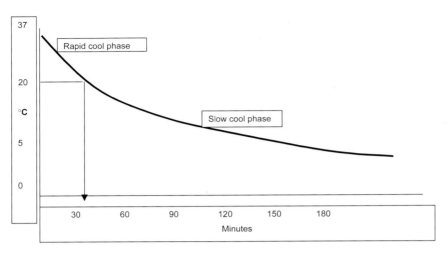

Fig. 4.27 Optimal chilling curve for liquid chilled semen.

1. A specially designed shipping container (Equitainer®), provides the most controlled incremental cooling process.
   - If the lid is not opened, it will cool the semen over 6 hours and maintain the semen at 5°C for 48 hours without decay or significant rises in the temperature.
   - This is the recommended method and has been proven reliable.
   - Instructions for its use are delivered with the container.
2. Styrofoam shipping boxes (Fig. 4.28).
   - The styrofoam shipper boxes contain an ice coolant pack, which is responsible for the cooling process.
   - Semen is cooled at a more rapid rate in these shipping containers than in the Equitainer®.
   - If the semen is to be transported in a styrofoam shipper and is not to be picked up for several hours, the entire box can be placed in the refrigerator to slow the thawing of the ice pack inside.
   - In winter months and during air transit, the freight storage area temperatures are sometimes not controlled and temperatures may reach well below freezing. Styrofoam shipper boxes may not then maintain 4°C. If the semen is held at less than 4°C for more than a short period the spermatozoa may be seriously damaged.
3. Direct refrigeration in a refrigerator.
   - If the semen is placed in the refrigerator directly, it is advisable to use a water buffer (at 25–28°C) to retard and control the cooling process.

SEMEN FREEZING

Factors that affect successful semen cryopreservation include:

- The stallion's inherent fertility.

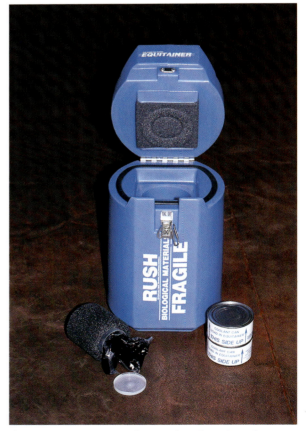

Fig. 4.28 A purpose-made container for safe and effective transport of fresh (chilled) equine semen.

- The use of an adequate centrifugation and cryopreservation medium.
- The correct cooling/freezing rate.
- Consistent storage temperature.
- The use of an appropriate thawing/warming protocol.
- Insemination into the mare in a timely fashion.

Table 4.5 Centrifugation and cryopreservation media[78]

	Centrifugation	
	Citrate–EDTA	Glucose–EDTA
Glucose (g)	1.5	59.98
Sodium citrate (g)	25.95	3.7
Disodium EDTA (g)	3.69	3.69
Sodium bicarbonate (g)	1.2	1.2
Polymyxin B sulfate (IU) (dilute to 1 liter with deionized sterile water)		10^6
	Cryopreservation	
Lactose solution (11%, w/v) (ml)	50	
Glucose–EDTA solution (ml) (see above)	25	
Egg yolk (ml)	20	
Glycerol (ml)	5	
Equex-STM (ml)	0.5	

In spite of the increasing availability of artificial insemination using frozen semen, the use of chilled or fresh semen still carries improved results. The latter is often used even over long distances as transportation and communication facilities have improved. Nevertheless, chilled or fresh semen inseminations have limitations in time and insemination doses.

Technique

- Cryopreservation involves cooling of the semen and extender plus cryoprotectant.
- This is a complex process, which begins with centrifugation and then involves combination of the spermatozoa with cryopreservation medium (Table 4.5).[78]
- This is cooled slowly to 4°C and then cooling process proceeds rapidly to –196°C.
- Some spermatozoa will experience cold shock.[79] Slow cooling followed by rapid cooling minimizes cold shock.
  - ❑ Cold shock occurs as a result of increased membrane permeability and subsequent loss of intracellular ions.
  - ❑ Energy production decreases and the acrosome swells.
  - ❑ Cold shock changes are irreversible and result in decreased fertility.
  - ❑ Continued freezing and subsequent thawing typically aggravates cooling-induced changes in spermatozoa.
  - ❑ Determination of the appropriate cooling and warming rates will depend on the media used, the semen concentration and the size/type of packaging system used.
- In order for stallion semen to maintain adequate fertility after freezing, the spermatozoa must have:
  - ❑ Adequate post-thaw motility.
  - ❑ Normal acrosomal enzymes.
  - ❑ Proteins on their surface that allow attachment to the oviduct.
  - ❑ Adequate energy to get to the oviduct and to fertilize the oocyte.

Advantages and disadvantages of frozen semen

The advantages of frozen semen include:

- Ability to breed the mare at any time of the day or year, regardless of the availability of the stallion.
- Ability to breed to stallions at distant locations or on different continents without shipping the mare.
- Cost-effectiveness of shipping semen and nitrogen tank compared with transporting the mare (with the associated boarding fees).
- The stallion can be used for breeding while his performance career still continues.
- Semen can be stockpiled before the stallion ages or has health problems, allowing continued use of the stallion beyond his normal reproductive career.
- Ejaculate can be divided to provide several insemination doses so that: the number of mares can be increased without the need to overwork the stallion, and the number of mares can be maintained using a lower number of ejaculates.
- Prevention/control of venereal disease and the transmission of exotic disease while at the same time allowing the genetic material to be used.

The disadvantages of frozen semen include:

- Reproductive monitoring of the mare and ovulation timing require more expertise and time.
- Fertility of frozen semen is typically lower than that of fresh semen or chilled semen.
- The cost of processing semen is significantly higher.
- A specialized laboratory and equipment are required for successful semen cryopreservation.

The principles of cryopreservation

This involves several concepts and processes.[80–82]

- As the media is cooled, freezing does not begin until the media is a few degrees below the freezing point. This is termed supercooling and the process occurs around –6°C to –15°C.
- Extracellular ice crystals begin to form from the freezing of water in the extender.
- As the water freezes, there is a relative increase in the concentration of salt, protein and sugar in the media surrounding the spermatozoa.
- This increased concentration of solutes causes water to move, by osmosis, from inside the spermatozoa to the extracellular environment resulting in dehydration of the sperm (see Fig. 4.29).

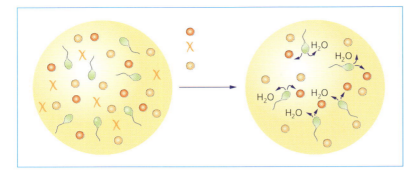

Fig. 4.29 The process of semen freezing. Formation of extracellular ice crystals begins at −15°C. This causes a relative increase in the other ions in the cytoplasm due to the decreased fluid volume component. Water moves out of the sperm cells by osmosis, resulting in cellular dehydration. Glycerol moves into the cells from outside and the combination of glycerol and dehydration protects the cells from intracellular ice formation.

- Since water moves out of the spermatozoa, there is less available to form ice crystals and the ice crystals that do form are smaller. This results in less cellular damage.
- The rate at which semen and extender is cooled depends on the concentration of spermatozoa and the type (constituents) of extender used.

In order to partially protect the spermatozoa from these cellular changes, the semen is frozen with a cryoprotectant in the media (see Table 4.5).

- Cryoprotectants may either be absorbed into the spermatozoa or may remain in the extracellular environment.
- Glycerol, dimethylsulfoxide and propylene glycol are termed penetrating cryoprotectants.
- Glycerol is the most commonly used.
  - ❏ The freezing point of glycerol is significantly lower than that of water. Therefore, as it is absorbed into the cell, it takes longer for intracellular ice to form, thereby decreasing cellular damage.
  - ❏ Glycerol increases the proportion of unfrozen solvent at a given point in time, and decreases the solute concentrations in the media.
  - ❏ Increased amounts of glycerol in the extracellular environment and increased solute concentrations result in more areas of unfrozen solvent where the sperm can survive between ice formations.
- Nonpenetrating cryoprotectants include polyvinylpyrrolidone, egg yolk lipoprotein, and lactose.
  - ❏ These act by drawing water osmotically out of the spermatozoa as the temperature drops.
  - ❏ This dehydrates the cells and reduces the chances that large ice crystals form in the cells.

Note:
- Cryoprotectants are toxic to spermatozoa.[83,84]
- There is damage to subcellular components of the spermatozoa and there is osmotic injury.
- The acrosome and plasma membrane are most sensitive to injury.

- During thawing, the movement of glycerol out of the cell will result in significant membrane injury.
- The addition of glycerol either in a stepwise fashion, or following slow cooling (once the media reach 4°C), will decrease the amount of membrane damage that will occur.
- The optimal concentration of cryoprotectant is designed to maximize its beneficial effects (extracellular) and to minimize its detrimental effects (intracellular).

Freezing of semen requires several steps:[85,86]

1. The semen is extended and centrifuged.
   - Centrifugation is an important step in that it separates the spermatozoa from the seminal plasma and it provides a highly concentrated spermatozoal pellet, allowing for optimal packaging.
   - Most centrifugation extenders use either skim milk or egg yolk as the base solution. Sodium citrate/EDTA media are also commonly used.
   - The semen is then centrifuged for 10–15 minutes at <400 g.
2. The spermatozoa are then found in a loose pellet at the bottom of the centrifuge container.
   - The fluid layer above the sperm (the supernatant) is poured off, and the semen pellet re-suspended.
   - This second suspension may be in a different centrifugation extender and centrifuged again, or it may be a freezing medium.
3. The freezing medium is typically lactose-based and contains EDTA, sodium bicarbonate, egg yolk, detergent and glycerol (as the cryoprotectant).
   - Sometimes the spermatozoa are added to the cryoprotectant media without the glycerol and cooled to 4°C before the glycerol is added.
4. After the sperm have been placed in the cryoprotectant medium (or after the glycerol is added), the straws are filled and sealed.
   - Straws of 0.25 ml, 0.5 ml or 5 ml capacity are typically used.[87]

5. A small air bubble is left at the top of each straw, so that when thawing is performed the straw does not burst.
6. The straws are placed on a horizontal surface.
   - If 0.25- or 0.5-ml straws are used they are placed 3 cm above nitrogen vapor on a wire rack for 10 minutes and then plunged into liquid nitrogen.
   - If 5-ml straws are used they are placed in the refrigerator, horizontally, for 15 minutes, at 4–5°C.
   - Then they are placed 3 cm above nitrogen vapor for 15 minutes and then plunged into liquid nitrogen.
   - The straws are then stored in liquid nitrogen tanks at −196°C.
   - Freezing rates of 0.05°C/minute from 18°C to 4°C and then at −10 to −25°C/minute from 4°C to −100°C are used.[78]
   - Thawing rates depend on the freezing rate used and the size of the packaging system.

- Fast freezes require fast thaws (75°C for <10 seconds), whereas slow freezes require slow thaws (38°C for 30 seconds).
- The type and thickness of straw used will also dictate the required thawing times.
- The specific instructions for the semen being used must be understood prior to thawing. Mistakes are disastrous! All frozen semen received by the mare owner for insemination should be accompanied by specific thawing and inseminating (dose) instructions.

Assessment of freezability of semen samples

Frozen semen, stored properly, is believed to be viable for several years, but the actual duration of 'normal' fertility has yet to be determined.

Evaluation of pregnancy rates obtained with frozen semen is difficult to make because of differences in:

- Semen packaging.
- Freezing methods.
- Cryoprotectants.
- Timing of insemination.
- Number of inseminations per cycle.
- Breeding dose used.
- The number of mares bred to a particular stallion.

On average, with insemination doses of 200 million progressively motile cells, the 'per-cycle pregnancy rate' for quality semen and fertile mares is around 50% with a range between <10% and >90% depending on the stallion and mares selected.

Assessment of the freezability of stallion semen can be performed by several methods.[88] The most commonly used method involves:

- Evaluation of post-thaw motility.
- Determination of the percentage of intact acrosomes.

Another common method of evaluating frozen semen is to determine first- and/or second-service conception rates.

Factors involved in determining the fertility of frozen semen

1. Individual characteristics.
   - Differences in motility and fertility vary from stallion to stallion and between different ejaculates from the same stallion.[89]
   - Semen from individual stallions will freeze well, with good post-thaw motility and good fertility, whereas the semen from some others freeze well, with good post-thaw motility but with poor fertility.
   - Alternatively, sometimes a stallion's semen will freeze poorly, show poor post-thaw motility but still have good fertility.
   - It is not known why there is such a difference in the freeze-ability of different stallions but it may be dependent on differences in the seminal plasma and its molecular constituents.[69]
   - Use of different freezing media, cryoprotectants, centrifugation protocols, straw sizes or freeze times and rates will sometimes provide more acceptable results with an individual stallion.
   - The variability and unpredictability of these factors has resulted in less use of frozen semen in equine artificial insemination.

- It is critical that practitioners who are freezing semen realize that each stallion must be treated as an individual and that alterations in freezing protocols are frequent and necessary.
- Advice is usually available from the supplier on the special requirements for particular semen doses.

---

2. Seasonality.
   - There is apparently little or no effect of season on freezability of stallion semen, although there may be a very small decrease in fertility in semen frozen during the nonbreeding season.[90,91]
   - Differences in fertility are likely due to differences in the seminal plasma during the different times of the year.
   - There is a significant difference in post-thaw motility between first and second collections (1 hour apart), with the second ejaculate having lower post-thaw motility.

- It is recommended that semen be collected once every 3–4 days for freezing. Collection every 3–4 days allows for accumulation of extragonadal sperm reserves and therefore maximizes the total spermatozoa/ejaculate for each freezing session.

3. Age.
   - There is no evidence that age affects fertility rates with frozen semen, providing that motility and morphology are normal prior to freezing.
   - Therefore, as soon as it is determined that a stallion is a candidate for freezing, it is recommended that semen is frozen, thereby reducing the chance that an injury or illness will prevent his sperm being available in the future.

4. Timing of insemination.
   - Time of insemination itself has a considerable impact on fertility.[92,93]
   - It is desirable to use as small a breeding dose as is necessary, and to breed as few times per cycle as is required for several reasons.
   - The breeder pays for each breeding dose, so the minimal number used means economic savings for the producer.
   - The fewer the number of straws per insemination means the more breeding doses that will be produced from each collection, thereby increasing the number of mares that can be bred per stallion.
   - In order to utilize the minimum amount of semen per cycle, careful breeding assessment of the mare must be performed around the time of ovulation, such that inseminations can be performed within 4 hours of ovulation (either pre- or postovulation) (Fig. 4.30).

- Inseminations occurring more than 6 hours after ovulation or more than 24 (–36) hours before ovulation are associated with decreased fertility.
- There are some stallions whose semen freezes so well, that insemination up to 48 hours prior to ovulation will result in comparable pregnancy rates to those inseminated within 6 hours of ovulation.

   - Use of a lower volume of frozen semen placed in a mare's uterus will reduce the postbreeding endometritis commonly associated with frozen semen. Acute postmating-induced endometritis reactions occur more with frozen semen than with fresh or chilled semen, possibly because more damage to the spermatozoa occurs during the freezing process, resulting in either more dead or more abnormal spermatozoa in the uterine lumen at the time of breeding.

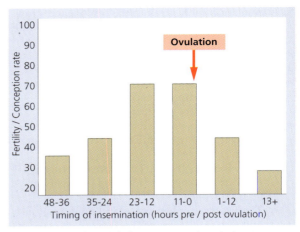

Fig. 4.30 Fertility with frozen semen in relation to insemination time.

5. Semen type.
   - Early embryonic death occurs at a 1.5 times higher rate in mares bred with frozen semen than in mares bred with fresh semen. This may be due to:
     - ❑ Altered sperm function.
     - ❑ Damage to the spermatozoal nucleus during freezing resulting in abnormal embryonic development.
     - ❑ Inseminating mares in such close proximity to ovulation.
   - Around 25% of stallions whose semen is frozen, will have an acceptable pregnancy rate.[94]
     - ❑ Selecting stallions with above average fertility of frozen semen and selecting against stallions with poor fertility of frozen semen, may increase the number of stallions with acceptable freezability.
     - ❑ This may be the case, if as occurs in cattle, the ability to freeze and thaw semen for a particular stallion is slightly heritable.
     - ❑ This will not likely occur in the majority of the horse industry, however, since the selection to use a horse in frozen semen program is generally determined by his own athletic performance and that of his progeny.

THE STALLION BOOK

The stallion book[95–97] (the number of mares he can be expected to serve in a breeding season) is compiled from the stallion's:

- Age.
- Fertility.
- Libido.

Most mature stallions with good libido can breed a mare twice a day for 6 days a week throughout the breeding season. If the mares are of normal fertility, it can be assumed that two covers per mare will result in conception (one cover for each of two cycles). If this is the case, approximately 80–90 mares can be bred in one season. Some stallions will have the libido to cover three mares in a day. The book for these stallions will be higher, whereas for stallions with poor libido the book may have to be less, as they may only be bred every other day.

A semen sample should be obtained from each stallion prior to the start of the breeding season and his fertility assessed (see p. 65). If the fertility begins to decline during the breeding season, semen should be collected again and reassessed. The book may need to be re-organized as a result of these changes. If more than 50% of the mares return for breeding for more than two cycles, the stallion's fertility should be reassessed. As the breeding season progresses, there is usually a higher proportion of infertile mares to be covered (mares returning over two cycles or more). These mares should be managed carefully, using procedures to maximize their chances of conceiving. It is easy to blame the stallion for a declining fertility when in reality his mares are the most likely source of the problem.

Libido and serving capacity should always be evaluated using natural service or artificial vagina collection techniques (see p. 62). Some stallions are very vocal, whereas others may not make many sounds when approaching a mare. A stallion that has been used in a natural service situation for an extended period of time may approach the mare from the side and mount from the side. This is considered normal behavior and is often used to prevent an injury from a kick from an unwilling or nervous mare. The stallion should approach the mare, obtain an erection and be willing and capable of copulating in a timely fashion.

TEASING THE STALLION

Teasing is defined as the presentation of a mare to a stallion (or vice versa) to evaluate the mare's response to that stallion, indicating her receptivity and facilitating the determination of the stage of her cycle.[98]

Depending on the farm management and layout, the mare can be brought to the stallion or the stallion can be brought to the mare.

Signs of estrus in the mare include:

- Squatting and urination.
- 'Winking' (repeated clitoral eversion).
- 'Nickering' (gentle vocalization).
- Turning the haunches to the stallion.
- Backing up to the stallion.
- Standing willingly for the stallion.

Signs of diestrus in the mare include:

- Pinning of the ears.
- Baring the teeth.
- Biting.
- Striking.
- Kicking.
- Moving away from the stallion.
- Clamping the tail.
- Squealing.

The teaser male

An entire stallion is the best method of teasing. Although some mares will exhibit signs of heat in response to geldings or even other mares, these signs are often unreliable and may be misleading. On some large breeding farms it is common practice to have a 'teaser' stallion with excellent libido that will not be used for breeding, or teaser ponies are used (Fig. 4.31). On smaller farms, the breeding stallion may also be used for teasing. Pony stallions usually make excellent teasers. They have excellent libido, are easy to handle, require less space to house, and the chances of accidental breeding are lessened due to their small size.

Management of the teaser depends on the type and number of teasers available on the farm. If the breeding stallion is used, he may become less interested in teasing a large number of mares, unless he is allowed to breed occasionally. Even if the semen is not to be used for breeding, it is best to use the collection to maintain a normal degree of libido. In situations where teasers are used for heat detection it is best to separate the teaser from the mares for some period of time during the day. Ideally, the teaser will be presented to the mares twice daily for at least 30–60 minutes at a time.

If possible, the teaser should be left across a wall or semi-solid fence which is either open for nasal and visual contact or arranged so that the teaser can get his

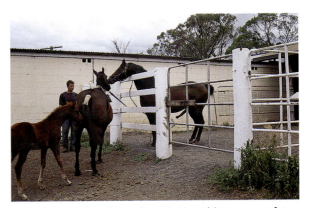

Fig. 4.31 Teasing the stallion. During this process safety for both operators and horses must be paramount. The foal is in obvious jeopardy here if the mare kicks backwards.

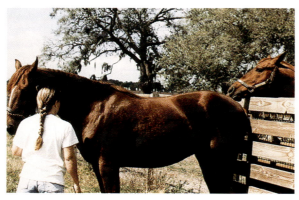

Fig. 4.32 A teaser restrained behind a solid or semi-solid barrier so that his head can gain access to the mare but he cannot climb over.

head over, but cannot climb over (Fig. 4.32). The more vocal the teaser is, the more mares will respond to him. In this situation, the more aggressive mares will go up to the teaser to display signs of heat, while the more timid mares will need to be brought up individually to the teaser for the best detection of heat. Teasers that do not have to perform breeding, especially ponies, will often maintain higher degrees of libido than will breeding stallions, who are less tolerant of teasing that is not followed by coitus. Teaser ponies that have never bred may perform their role with great enthusiasm without any subsequent mating.

> • It is possible to allow the teaser to mount the mare to help determine whether she is receptive or not. If the teaser is allowed to mount, some means of preventing penetration of the mare, such as a penile shield, must be used.

VENEREAL (SEXUALLY TRANSMITTED) DISEASES

Transmission of disease through breeding can occur with bacterial, viral or protozoal organisms (Table 4.6). These diseases might result in:

• Decreased fertility by causing early embryonic death.

• Endometritis.
• Placentitis.
• Abortion.
• Systemic illness in the mare with generalized clinical signs attributable to one or more body systems.
• The birth of an infected, weak foal.

Depending on the infectious agent involved, the signs of infection may be noted in the mare, the stallion, or both, or may not be apparent in carrier animals. These diseases are most commonly transmitted during natural service, but can also be transmitted through artificial insemination if strict hygiene and management are not adhered to. The use of sterile techniques and semen extenders with antibiotics will make the chances of transmission of venereal diseases quite unlikely.

There are three important venereal diseases in horses:

• Coital exanthema: this is a self-limiting disease caused by equine herpesvirus 3 (see p. 192).
• Contagious equine metritis (*Taylorella equigenitalis*) (see p. 193).
• Equine viral arteritis (an RNA pestivirus of the Togaviridae family) (see p. 259).
• In some parts of the world dourine is an important venereal infection of horses (see p. 196).

Stallions typically do not display clinical signs of infection from these bacteria (carriers), although if signs are present they typically involve aberrations of the spermiogram. Infection of the accessory sex glands, testis or epididymis will result in one or more of the following:

• Inflammatory cells in the ejaculate.
• Pain upon ejaculation.
• Decreased fertility.
• Signs of inflammation in the mares to which the stallion is bred.

Apart from *Taylorella equigenitalis* infection (see p. 193), the other bacteria mentioned below are transmitted during coitus, either directly from the penile surface or through infected seminal fluids.

• *Pseudomonas aeruginosa* and *Klebsiella pneumoniae* are both considered to be venereally transmitted organisms.

Table 4.6 Sexually transmitted diseases

Viral	Bacterial	Protozoal
• Equine viral arteritis • Coital exanthema (equine herpesvirus 3)	• Contagious equine metritis (*Taylorella equigenitalis*) • *Pseudomonas aeruginosa* • *Klebsiella pneumoniae* • *Escherichia coli* • *Streptococcus zooepidemicus*	• Dourine (*Trypanosoma equiperdum*)

These diseases are described in detail on pp. 192–195.

- Although *Streptococcus zooepidemicus* and *Escherichia coli* may be transmitted from stallion to mare, no direct evidence of their venereal transmission has been proven.
- Although some mares may be resistant to infection and others susceptible, the transmission of *Streptococcus zooepidemicus* and *Escherichia coli* does not occur in every mare bred to a stallion with these organisms in his seminal fluid.
- Only certain strains of *Klebsiella pneumoniae* are associated with venereal disease after transmission from stallion to mare (capsule types K1, K2 and K5).[99]
- The natural immune function of the mare and her ability to clear fluid and debris from the reproductive tract following coitus may be significantly more important than the fact that the stallion is infected.

The presence of pathological bacteria in sufficient numbers to cause disease is important in the transmission of disease to the mare. Some of these bacteria will exist as normal flora of the skin or as contaminants, either from the environment or from feces. This normal flora is concentrated in the stallion's smegma and in the debris (bean) of the urethral fossa/diverticulum (see p. 47).

- Pathologic infection of the stallion's accessory sex glands, testicles or epididymis will usually result in decreased fertility.

Diagnosis of venereal infection requires culture of swabs taken (both pre- and postejaculation) from:

- The urethra.
- The urethral fossa.
- The penile shaft.
- The prepuce.
- Semen.

Note:
- Use of an individual sterile artificial vagina for each stallion, disposable liners, disposable sleeves, sterile lubricants, antibiotic-containing semen extenders and minimum contamination techniques should be used for artificial insemination or natural service.
- The stallion's penis should not be cleaned with disinfectants such as chlorhexidine or povidone iodine as this destroys the normal flora and allows for overgrowth of more pathogenic and resistant strains of bacteria.
- The penis should be washed with a mild nonscented soap intermittently during the breeding season and rinsed with water only on a daily basis.[100,101]
- Additionally, washing should be done gently, as scrubbing may remove the complete resident population of normal flora.

Infection/inflammation of the testicles (orchitis)

Etiology
Orchitis involves infection and inflammation of the testicles and is rare in the stallion. Possible causes include:

- Infectious organisms which may enter via the bloodstream.
- Penetrating wounds.
- Ascending infections.

The most common infective bacteria are:

- *Streptococcus zooepidemicus.*
- *Klebsiella pneumoniae.*
- *Salmonella abortus equi.*

Common viruses causing infectious orchitis are:

- Equine herpesvirus 1.
- Equine viral arteritis.
- Equine infectious anemia.

Noninfectious causes of orchitis include:

- Testicular torsion with infarction of the testicle.
- Testicular trauma.

- Testicular trauma is the most common cause of orchitis in the stallion, with secondary bacterial infection from the scrotal skin inwards being the causative factor. If there is no penetrating wound, the inflammation is probably noninfectious in origin.

- Larval migrations (*Strongylus edentatus*).
- Autoimmune orchitis may result from a breakdown of the blood–testes barrier, thereby allowing the systemic immune system to contact the seminiferous epithelium. Antigen–antibody complexes form as the immune system sees the spermatozoa as foreign cells.

Clinical signs
- Testicular swelling, pain and heat in the early stages of the disease (Fig. 4.33).
- Epididymitis is often associated with orchitis. Scrotal and preputial edema are common sequelae (Fig. 4.34).
- Often there is pain associated with ejaculation and the stallion is unwilling to mate.
- Prolonged orchitis will lead to testicular degeneration if it is left untreated.

Diagnosis
- If semen can be obtained, its quality is generally decreased, with many neutrophils ± bacteria and germ cells present.

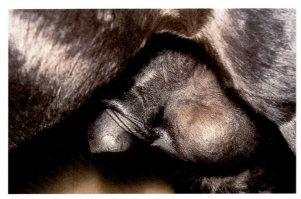

Fig. 4.33 Swollen and painful testicles typical of orchitis.

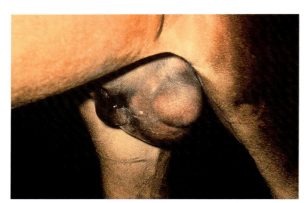

Fig. 4.34 Scrotal and preputial edema arising secondarily to orchitis.

- There is usually a decrease in concentration, motility and normal morphology.
- Primary spermatozoal defects are common (head, acrosome, mid-piece lesions).

Treatment

The mainstays of treatment include:

- Cold water hydrotherapy for 15 minutes every 2–4 hours; this is beneficial in restoring normal testicular thermoregulation by reducing edema and thereby scrotal temperature.
- High levels of systemic antibiotics to prevent or treat bacterial infection.
- Nonsteroidal anti-inflammatory drugs to reduce inflammation.

If the orchitis is unilateral and response to treatment is not rapid, hemicastration may be the best option.

- Hemicastration should be considered early in the condition and may prevent spread to the other testicle either by ascending infection or local inflammation and will help prevent derangement of spermatogenesis due to overheating in the normal testicle.
- The stallion must be given complete reproductive rest until the condition resolves.

Prognosis

- Sperm granuloma may result from extravasation of sperm from the tubules, and testicular degeneration and fibrosis are common sequelae.
- The prognosis for a compromised testicle is very poor. Any reduction in size or softening indicates chronic (probably irreversible) changes that are unlikely ever to return to normal.
- The biggest risk in unilateral cases is the involvement (either by infectious process or by thermal changes) in the other (normal) testicle. The future fertility of the stallion may be significantly improved by early intervention.

Infectious disease of the accessory sex glands

Etiology

- Seminal vesiculitis and ampullitis are very uncommon.[102]
- Prostatitis and bulbourethritis are even rarer.
- Infections from *Streptococcus zooepidemicus*, *Pseudomonas aeruginosa*, *Klebsiella pneumoniae* and *Staphylococcus* spp. are the most common etiology.
- Infection may result from ascending infection, descending infection, hematogenous infection or by infiltration/extension from adjacent infected tissues.

Clinical signs

- Affected glands are enlarged and lobulated but may be difficult to palpate.
- Pain is not usually a prominent sign although acute inflammation may be painful.
- There is usually no outward clinical signs of inflammation, such as pain on urination or ejaculation.
- Typically, the semen is light pink in color with or without clumps of purulent material.
- In chronic infections, the glands may be small, firm and fibrosed.

Diagnosis

- Diagnosis is made by culturing from various aspects of the penis, prepuce, urethra, and ejaculatory secretions.[103] Heavy growth of a single organism from the semen and postejaculatory urethra are indicative of infection of the accessory sex glands (testicles or epididymides).
- Localization of the source of infection involves physical examination, rectal examination, ultrasonography and differential staining of semen to determine the type of round cells present in the ejaculate and cultures.
- Ultrasonography is a good diagnostic aid.[104,105]
- White blood cells are often seen in the ejaculate along with varying degrees of hemospermia.

- Red blood cells (erythrocytes) may indicate hemospermia but there are other sources of this.
- The spermiogram is usually normal (unless the proximal reproductive tract is also affected), although longevity is often diminished.

- Collection of vesicular fluid is possible by teasing the stallion for 10 minutes, and thoroughly washing and drying the penis. A sterile catheter can be passed along the urethra to the base of the seminal vesicles (using palpation per rectum or via endoscopy of the seminal colliculus). The seminal vesicles can be manually expressed and their fluid contents aspirated and evaluated by cytology and culture. Alternatively, a small flexible endoscope may be passed directly into the seminal vesicle and fluid aspirated following visual examination of the lumen of the gland.

Treatment

Long-term systemic antibiotics and sexual rest are required for the resolution of signs.

- The choice of antibiotics should be based on sensitivity analysis from bacteriological cultures of semen.
- Additionally, the selected antibiotic should be lipid-soluble, have low binding affinity to plasma protein, have a high pK_a, and be of sufficiently small molecular size to maximize penetration of the glandular tissue.

- Trimethoprim has been shown to be absorbed into the vesicular glands of several species and therefore may be a good choice for treatment.

- Alternatively, antibiotic may be infused directly into the glands via endoscopically guided catheter placement. In this case the affected glands should be flushed with saline prior to antibiotic infusion.

- This may be the best method of treating vesiculitis.

- Vesiculectomy (removal of the affected gland in cases of seminal vesiculitis) may be necessary if the disease becomes chronic and fails to respond to conservative medical treatment. Vesiculectomy usually does not affect fertility.[106] This specialized procedure can be performed in standing stallions under epidural anesthesia.
- Where vesiculitis cannot be treated effectively, the use of an appropriate antibiotic-containing semen extender or minimum contamination breeding technique may be used to minimize spread of the infection to the mare, and to maximize spermatozoal longevity.[107]
- If possible, semen should be allowed to remain in the antibiotic-containing extender for 15–30 minutes prior to insemination to destroy all bacteria.

Infectious disease of the penis and prepuce

These diseases include the important venereal diseases of the horse:

- Coital exanthema (see p. 192).
- Dourine (see p. 196).

CONGENITAL AND ACQUIRED DISORDERS OF THE REPRODUCTIVE ORGANS

INTERSEX AND HERMAPHRODITISM

Intersex conditions are where the external genitalia and the internal reproductive organs are from opposite sexes, or a combination of both male and female reproductive organs is present.

True hermaphrodites have both ovarian and testicular tissue. Pseudohermaphrodites have only one or the other (testis or ovary). Thus, a male pseudohermaphrodite has only testes and a female pseudohermaphrodite has only ovaries. Other than the gonads, the reproductive tract of hermaphrodites is usually intermediate between male and female.[108]

Surgical removal of the gonadal tissue is desirable if the horse is to have any use, but this is extremely difficult in many cases. Laparoscopy holds out the best chance of removing small but hormonally significant gonadal tissue from both male and female pseudohermaphrodites.

Male pseudohermaphroditism

- This is the most common intersex condition in the horse.
- The external genitalia consist of a vulva with an enlarged clitoris (similar in appearance to the glans penis) (Fig. 4.35).
- The external genitalia are smaller than normal; the vagina is shortened and is often a blind-ended sac. The vagina is incomplete, and the urethra may lie on the floor of this structure.
- In some cases there is a deformed penis-like structure in the inguinal region.
- Hypoplastic testicles are retained either inguinally or, more commonly, abdominally.
- The tubular reproductive tract is infantile or absent.
- Genetically, the animal is female.

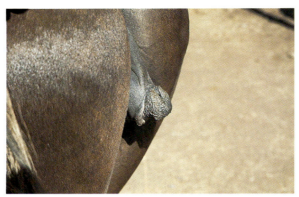

Fig. 4.35   A grossly enlarged clitoris with a penile-like appearance typical of a male pseudohermaphrodite.

- The horse exhibits either stallion-like behavior or nymphomania (persistent aggressive estrous behavior).
- Testicular feminization is a specific inherited type of male pseudohermaphroditism with a female appearance (phenotype) but with an XY (male) genotype.[109] The testes are normally formed but are invariably retained in the abdomen and the animals show masculine sex behavior. However, the rest of the male tract is not developed; thus there is an apparent vulva and clitoris but no vagina and uterus.
- All affected animals are sterile.

Female pseudohermaphroditism

- The external genitalia are male or ambiguous and small, and the internal reproductive organs include ovaries (Fig. 4.36).
- Genetically, the animal is male.
- The X–Y sex reversal syndrome occurs in which the genetic make-up is that of a stallion but the physical appearance is that of a mare.[110] The ovaries are infantile and the tubular tract is very poorly developed.
- These horses are best regarded as sterile.

True hermaphroditism

- This is very rare in horses.
- The external genitalia may reveal both a small penis between the back legs and an enlarged clitoris and small vulva.
- Internally both ovaries and testicles or ovotestes are present.
- Sexual behavior is very unpredictable because the ratio and dominance of ovary or testis are unpredictable.
- These animals are all sterile.

THE PENIS AND PREPUCE

Congenitally small or short penis
(Fig. 3.37)

- With this condition, the breeding stallion is unable to achieve intromission. Selection of small mares or the use of artificial insemination will allow these stallions to be used in a breeding program.
- The condition may be inherited and so the ethics of breeding from such stallions is questionable.

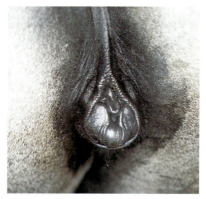

Fig. 4.36   A female pseudohermaphrodite showing the typical poorly developed external genitalia. Typically there are infantile ovaries associated with a small, poorly developed tubular tract.

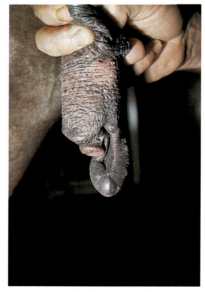

Fig. 4.37   A congenitally short penis that prevented this stallion from breeding naturally. The condition was detected during routine breeding soundness examination and he was not used for breeding.

Congenital stenosis or stricture of the preputial orifice (phimosis)

- This may preclude extension of either a part of, or the entire, penis out of the preputial orifice and thereby make erection impossible.
- Surgical correction or widening of this type of narrowing is possible.

Varicosities of the preputial veins

- A varicosity is the enlargement and distension of veins on the prepuce.
- They are detected as soft, fluctuant swellings on either side of the prepuce.
- They are sometimes noted in young colts or stallions.
- This condition usually does not interfere with breeding but may occasionally rupture and bleed.
- Surgical ligation may be required if simple pressure alone does not stop the bleeding.

Balanitis/balanoposthitis (inflammation of the penis and prepuce)

This condition is termed balanitis if only the penis is involved or balanoposthitis if the penis and prepuce are involved. It may be caused by noninfectious inflammation or irritation (usually from the application of strong chemicals) or by infective organisms, including:

1. Viruses.
   - Coital exanthema (equine herpesvirus 3) (see p. 192).
2. Bacteria.
   - Bacterial balanitis usually occurs following trauma (or viral infection).
   - *Streptococcus* spp., *Klebsiella pneumoniae* and *Pseudomonas aeruginosa* are the most common species of bacteria involved in these infections[111].
   - Contagious equine metritis (*Taylorella equigenitalis*) (see p. 193).
3. Protozoa.
   - Dourine (*Trypanosoma equiperdum*) is the most serious protozoal cause of balanitis/balanoposthitis (see p. 196).
4. Parasites.
   - Habronemiasis (*Habronema musca*).
   - Myiasis (fly strike/maggots).

Noninfectious balanoposthitis

This is usually the result of direct trauma (see below) or of application of strong irritant washes. The latter circumstance is a relatively frequent event when a stallion is known to have served an infected mare. The penile skin and the preputial lining are delicate and strong chemicals may be harbored in the semi-closed prepuce.

Treatment

Inflammation of the penis and preputial lining is not specific and so treatment should be directed at the cause. One of the most difficult conditions to treat is the chronic irritative balanoposthitis that occurs in older stallions and much more frequently in older geldings. A detailed history and careful clinical examination should establish the cause and then specific measures can be undertaken to restore the normal state.

As a general rule, no antiseptics or strong chemicals should ever be applied to the penile skin. Long-term disturbances in the normal bacterial population may cause serious chronic inflammation that is difficult to treat.

Penile trauma

Profile

Injury to a stallion's penis, prepuce or scrotum may occur from a variety of causes:

- Kick injuries during breeding (Fig. 4.38).
- Fighting with other animals.
- Puncture wounds.
- Poor fitting or inappropriate use of stallion rings or brushes.
- Frostbite.
- Photosensitization.
- Application of irritant/caustic chemicals (Fig. 4.39).
- Complications of castration.
- Congenital defects.

Clinical signs

- Trauma usually results in acute swelling of the penis and prepuce.
- Excoriation of the penile and preputial epithelium may allow secondary bacterial infection of the tissue.

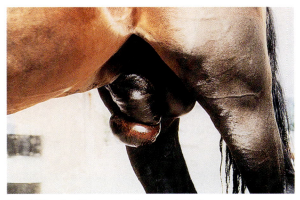

Fig. 4.38   Penile trauma due to a kick from an unrestrained mare.

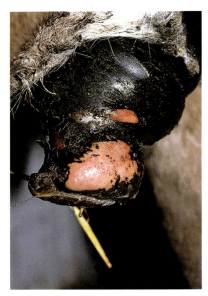

Fig. 4.39   Inflammation and swelling of the penis due to irritant chemical contact during ill-advised washing of the penis.

- Treatment of these lesions/injuries involves several general principles:
  - ❏ Reduction of edema and inflammation.
  - ❏ Support for the normal circulation.
  - ❏ Maintenance of normal urination.
  - ❏ Protection from drying and further trauma.
  - ❏ Maintenance of good hygiene.
  - ❏ Return of the reproductive system to normal function.

Treatment

- Penile support is essential if continued deterioration is to be avoided (Fig. 4.40).
- Hydrotherapy by running cold water from a hose pipe over the area at frequent intervals is a useful measure if it can be tolerated.
- Some irritation and excoriation can follow from this approach.
- The skin should be protected by petroleum jelly or udder creams, etc.
- Systemic and/or topical antibiotics may be required.
- Steroid creams and systemic nonsteroidal anti-inflammatory drugs may help reduce inflammation.
- Sexual rest is essential.

Penile hematoma

Etiology

Penile hematoma occurs as a result of traumatic rupture of subcutaneous vessels on the penis, leading to the accumulation of blood between the tunica albuginea and the skin. It can occur if:

- The stallion is kicked by the mare during copulation (Fig. 4.41).
- The penis is bent during a forceful thrust on intromission.

> Note:
> - Kicks that occur during the mating ritual usually involve the penis rather than the prepuce.

Other causes include:

- Mating a mare with a Caslick suture in place.
- Attempting to achieve erection with tight stallion ring in place.
- Improper handling of the artificial vagina during collection of semen.
- Becoming entangled in fencing.
- Traumatic laceration of the tunica albuginea or corpus cavernosum penis.

Clinical signs

- The appearance of a penile hematoma changes as the injury progresses from acute to chronic.
- Immediately after injury, bleeding results in enlargement on the dorsal surface of the penis, usually just below the preputial reflection, which may act as a cuff on the penis. The penis and the prepuce then rapidly enlarge due to inflammatory edema.[112,113]
- In the early stages the stallion will experience pain.
- As the injury becomes more chronic, the pain response is lost due to peripheral nerve damage.
- The penis hangs downwards and is usually curved, with the glans penis pointing posteriorly.
  - ❏ The edema is worsened by the effects of gravity on the penis.
  - ❏ Edema will progress caudally from the prepuce to the scrotum and inguinal region.
- The penis cannot be retracted into the prepuce due to its enlarged size from the blood and edema.

> - The inability to retract the penis into the prepuce is termed paraphimosis.

- The exposed penile tissue will dry out and become necrotic. Balanoposthitis will ensue. As the injury becomes more chronic, the penile skin will crack and thicken and the infection will worsen (Fig. 4.42).
- Eventually, contraction of the hematoma will occur. **However, because the penile nerves and muscles have usually been chronically stretched, the stallion is unable to retract the penis back into the prepuce and a permanent state of penile prolapse ensues.**

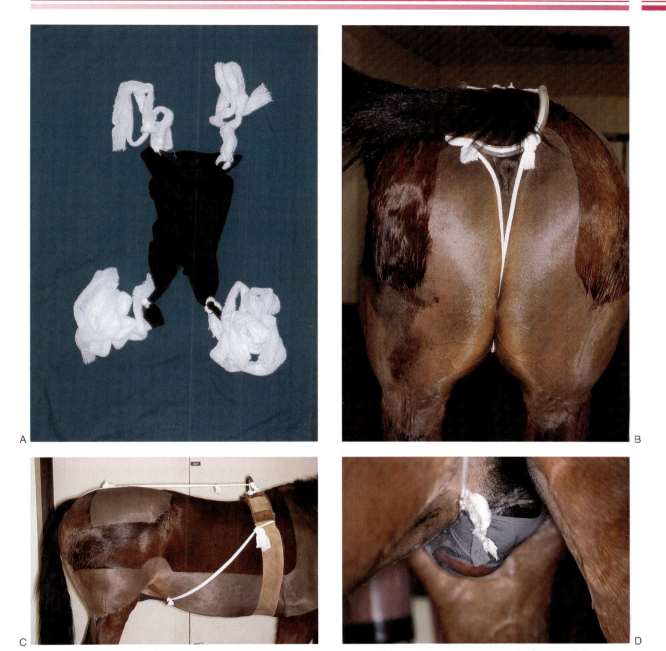

Fig. 4.40   A supportive sling can be made from a pair of nylon tights. This apparatus supplies good support while not restricting urination

Treatment

> • **Failure to manage this condition as an emergency can be catastrophic for a breeding stallion.**

Management requires several immediate and important steps, including:

• Reduction of the amount of edema.

• Prevention of secondary thrombosis of the penile veins.
• Prevention of (further) excoriation and trauma to the penile skin.
• Return of the penis to the prepuce.

1. Immediate treatment
   i. The penis should be supported with a sling close to the abdominal wall until it can be replaced in the prepuce (Fig. 4.43).
   ii. This can be constructed from nylon stocking

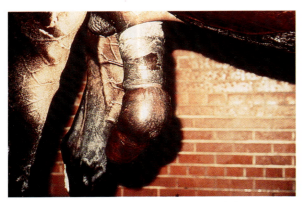

Fig. 4.41   Penile hematoma caused by a kick from a poorly restrained mare immediately prior to service.

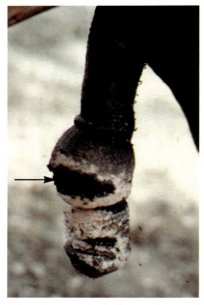

Fig. 4.42   A chronic, extensively damaged penis that had been neglected in the early stages following injury.

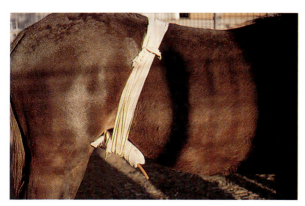

Fig. 4.43   A penile sling used to provide support for the penis in an attempt to reduce the gravitational accumulation of edema and blood.

and lengths of bandage. This has the added advantages of being easily replaced and allowing urination without any resistance.

iii. This sling may be needed for some days and the stallion will usually accept it.

iv. Cold water hydrotherapy, 3–4 times daily for 15 minutes, and compression bandages. Care should be taken to avoid excessive pressure as this may crack the skin and damage compromised blood vessels.

v. Because water will tend to dry and crack the delicate skin, oil-based antibiotic ointments or petroleum jelly are applied following hydrotherapy.

vi. If urination is not possible due to edema and inflammation, a urethral catheter should be passed and maintained until some of the edema decreases and urination is possible.

2. After the first 48 hours
  i. Hydrotherapy may be changed to cold water for 15 minutes followed by 2–3 minutes of warm water at the end of the hydrotherapy session.

  ii. The sling is maintained.

  iii. As soon as the penis is supple enough to be replaced in the prepuce, a purse-string suture of umbilical tape can be placed in the preputial ring to retain it.

   - Either local or general anesthesia is typically required depending on the nature of the stallion.
   - The purse-string suture should be tied sufficiently tightly to prevent prolapse and sufficiently loosely to allow urination to occur.
   - The purse-string should be opened daily for evaluation and cleansing of the penis.
   - Once the penis is back in the prepuce, application of topical ointment is not required unless local inflammation or infection is present.
   - The purse-string is left in place for 10–14 days or until the stallion can maintain retraction on his own. The retention suture should not be left in place for too long because it results in further edema, inflammation and fibrosis of the prepuce.

  iv. Systemic nonsteroidal anti-inflammatory drugs are maintained to minimize inflammation and control pain.

  v. If balanoposthitis is present, systemic broad-spectrum antibiotics are also indicated.

Note:
  - Sedation is contraindicated as it results in further relaxation of the penis.
  - If thrombosis of the corpus cavernosus penis occurs, flushing may be performed under general anesthesia.

- In certain cases, this may result in a return of the ability to obtain an erection.
- If this procedure fails, a shunt may be created to divert blood flow from the corpus cavernosus penis to the corpus spongiosus penis so that erection may be obtained.

vi. Sexual stimulation must be avoided until at least 2–3 months after recovery.
  - A slow and careful return to supervised service is recommended.
  - The stallion is usually first presented to an estrus mare, allowed to drop his penis, and then is immediately removed from the mare to determine if he can retract the penis normally.
  - If this is adequate and normal, the stallion may be teased to a partial erection, and then stopped. If this is normal, then the stallion is teased to a full erection, and again stopped.
  - If this is normal, the stallion is allowed to breed a mare; intromission should be guided to minimize the seeking thrusts required by the stallion.
  - Obviously, further traumatic events must be prevented because a second episode usually carries a bad prognosis.

Note:
- This entire testing process should occur over several days, so that any fresh hemorrhage that may occur as a result of sexual stimulation is noted early on.

Prognosis

- The prognosis must be guarded and the outcome is sometimes unsatisfactory even if the best possible care is provided.
- Stallions that have had this type of penile trauma will be more likely to sustain similar injury in the future due to the weakness of the scar tissue in the penis.
- Complications of penile hematoma include:
  - ❑ (Total) (permanent) penile paralysis (a flaccid paralysis of the penis) (Fig. 4.44).
  - ❑ The inability to retract the penis due to injury to dorsal nerves of the penis.
  - ❑ Stretching of the retractor penis muscles and nerves.
  - ❑ Thrombosis (blood clotting) of the cavernosum penis, resulting in the inability to obtain an erection.
  - ❑ Fibrosis of the cavernosum penis and tunica albuginea, resulting in the inability to obtain a hard erection.

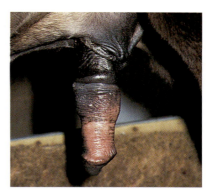

Fig. 4.44 Penile paralysis. There is a flaccid relaxation of the retractor muscles of the penis without any direct penile trauma. The penis may, however, become secondarily traumatized and this may complicate the condition.

Penile paralysis[114]

Etiology

This condition is defined as the flaccid extension of the penis from the prepuce (Fig. 4.44). The causes of penile paralysis include:

- Trauma.
  - ❑ To the third and fourth sacral nerves or their branches.
  - ❑ To the penis or pelvis.
  - ❑ To the penis during castration.
- Spinal neurological disease.
- Equine herpesvirus 1 infection.
- Rabies.
- Equine protozoal myeloencephalopathy.
- Exhaustion.
- Starvation/debility (particularly associated with low serum albumin).
- Phenothiazine tranquilizers.
- Idiopathic penile paralysis without any apparent cause.

Clinical signs

- Inability to retract the flaccid penis.
- The stallion maintains good libido but no erection is possible.
- There may or may not be sensation to the glans penis (free end of the penis) depending on the cause of the paralysis.
- Dependent edema and excoriation of skin will develop with continued penile exposure.
- There is often edematous cuffing at preputial reflection, which develops over time.

Diagnosis and differential diagnosis

- Penile hematoma.
- Penile trauma.
- Debility.

Treatment

The primary disease should be treated if possible. The treatment is similar to that for penile hematoma, including:

- Continued penile support using a sling is essential.
  - ❑ A suitable sling can be constructed from nylon stockings/tights (Fig. 4.40).
- Hydrotherapy (pressure water applied 3–4 times daily for 15 minutes).
- Topical soothing, oily ointments.
- Systemic nonsteroidal anti-inflammatory drugs to control inflammatory responses that might aggravate the condition, although the condition is seldom painful.
- Antibiotics may be indicated.
- Return of the penis to the prepuce as soon as possible to prevent further damage and drying.
  - ❑ Application and management of a purse-string suture.
- Penile amputation or retraction procedures may be required for refractory cases.[115]
  - ❑ This outcome is clearly catastrophic for a breeding stallion.

> Note:
> - If penile paralysis occurs following phenothiazine tranquilization, 8 mg of benztropine mesylate may be administered within the first few hours. This has limited success; however, the condition is potentially catastrophic so this treatment should be attempted.
> - **In general, phenothiazine tranquilizers should not be administered to male horses at any time.**

Prognosis

- The prognosis for recovery is poor in most cases.
- The prognosis may depend heavily on the initial cause.

Priapism

Etiology

- This condition is defined as a persistent erection followed later by penile paralysis.
- There is inability of the sympathetic and parasympathetic nervous systems to communicate and promote, then diminish, the blood flow to the corpus cavernosus penis.
- It occurs in stallions much more commonly than in geldings.
- Causes of this condition include:
  - ❑ Systemic debilitating disease.
  - ❑ Inflammation of the spinal cord.
  - ❑ Trauma or surgery in the pelvic region.
  - ❑ Phenothiazine tranquilizers.
  - ❑ Use of antihypertensive agents during surgery due to parasympathetic dominance.
  - ❑ Inflammatory reaction to urethritis or urethral stricture.[116]

Clinical signs

- Penile engorgement and persistent erection followed by penile paralysis.
- Dependent edema.
- Excoriation of the penile skin.
- Cuffing of the preputial reflection.
- Thrombosis of the corpus cavernosum penis blood vessels followed by fibrosis may occur over time.

The complications of this disorder have been described in the section on penile paralysis.

Treatment

Treatment is the same as described for penile paralysis (p. 87).

Habronemiasis

Profile

- *Habronema muscae or microstoma* (larval forms of stomach parasite) and *Draschia megastoma* are common causes of parasitic lesions on the penis and less commonly on the prepuce.[117]
- Transmission is by flies (*Musca* spp.).
- The larvae are deposited by the intermediate host (the fly), which feeds in moist areas on the horse.
- The larval invasion stimulates rapid formation of granulomatous lesions containing numerous small, yellow caseous (pus-like) granules. These necrotic foci contain encysted larvae, the remnants of dead larva and many eosinophils.
- The parasite also causes cutaneous habronemiasis or 'summer sores' and conjunctival habronemiasis.
- The lesions usually occur in the late summer or autumn. They disappear in winter months in cold climates.

Clinical signs

- The lesions are seen most commonly at the preputial ring or urethral process (Fig. 4.45).
- The lesions are some 1–3 cm in diameter and will bleed freely if traumatized. The ejaculate may contain blood (hemospermia) and a lowered fertility is usual.
- A characteristic of these lesions is that they are severely pruritic (itchy).
- Lesions on the urethral process may interfere with normal urination.
- The penis is generally reddened and swollen.
- Often a fetid odor is noted from the prepuce or smegma.

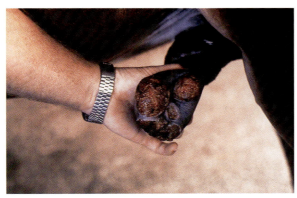

Fig. 4.45 Habronemiasis of the glans penis (and urethral fossa in particular). The stallion consistently showed pain during service and hemospermia resulted in loss of fertility.

- Lesions may occur on face and legs.
- The stallion may have difficulty copulating.
- The stallion may be unwilling to mate due to pain on intromission.

Diagnosis and differential diagnosis

- The larvae can usually be seen easily by scrapings and washings from affected sores.
- Sometimes there is extensive inflammation and few larvae can be found.
- Diagnosis can be confirmed by response to specific treatment.
- The lesions must be differentiated from neoplastic conditions that occur on the penis and prepuce.

Treatment

- Healing of the lesions results in scar tissue formation, which may affect extension and retraction of the penis in severe cases.
- Treatment involves the use of anthelmintics:
  - ❏ Ivermectin orally (at 0.2 mg/kg) once is effective for smaller lesions.[118] This treatment may be repeated in a month for larger lesions.
  - ❏ A diluted ivermectin solution in saline may be used to wash the sheath. This is usually effective from one treatment.
  - ❏ Organophosphate cream (trichlorfon) may be applied topically at a dose of 4.5 g/100 g (where this is available); nitrofurazone cream can be used in cases with refractory or large lesions.
  - ❏ Use of systemic trichlorfon is not recommended since adverse reactions have been noted and may result in mortality.
  - ❏ Surgical excision or cryosurgery may be required to remove mineralized and granulomatous lesions on the urethral process if hemospermia persists.[119]

Hemospermia

Etiology

There are several causes of blood in the ejaculate.[120] It often affects stallions under heavy breeding use more than others.

1. Viral urethritis/coital exanthema (equine herpesvirus 3) or other viruses.
2. Bacterial urethritis, or infection of the urinary tract.
   - Primary infections:
     - ❏ *Streptococcus* spp.
     - ❏ *Escherichia coli*.
     - ❏ *Pseudomonas aeruginosa*.
     - ❏ Contagious equine metritis (*Taylorella equigenitalis*).
   - Secondary infection following trauma to the urethra.[121]
   - Infections are most commonly seen in the pelvic urethra near the seminal colliculus.
   - Infection and/or inflammation of any of the accessory sex glands.
     - ❏ Seminal vesiculitis is the most common infection of the accessory sex glands.
3. Dilation and trauma to the urethral epithelium and blood vessels during the muscular contraction that occurs during ejaculation.
   - Affected animals are reluctant to breed and are painful on ejaculation.
4. Rupture of the corpus spongiosum penis.
   - At the level of the ischial arch or rupture of the urethra.
   - More often fresh bleeding is associated purely with erection or the end of urination.
   - This may also occur as a result of breeding trauma or long-term urethral inflammation.
5. Ulcers or prolapsed subepithelial vessels in the urethra or secondary sex glands.
6. Parasitic infections of the glans penis.
   - Habronemiasis of the urethral process may result in hemorrhage (see p. 88).
   - Larval migration of the parasite results in inflammation and ulceration of the urethral process.
7. Urethral strictures or diverticulum forming as a consequence of healing.
8. Trauma.
   - Use of stallion rings to prevent masturbation can result in scarring and fibrosis of the urethra and the associated vessels. With ensuing erections there may be tearing of this scar tissue resulting in hemorrhage.
   - Small lacerations or puncture wounds to the glans penis or urethral process can result in hemospermia.
   - Lacerations may occur if the glans penis becomes entangled in the mare's tail hairs during service. These lesions typically bleed

during erection. There will be frank blood in the ejaculate.

- Direct trauma to the glans penis or to the penile shaft during unsupervised/unattended mating can also cause serious penile bleeding.

9. Neoplasia of the genitourinary tract (see p. 100).
   - Tumor invading epithelial tissue resulting in ulceration or prolapse of subepithelial vessels.
   - Squamous cell carcinoma is very rare in working stallions but can be highly erosive. Mating also easily traumatizes the proliferative forms.
   - Viral papilloma is a benign disorder that can bleed when traumatized by coitus.
   - Sarcoid is an unusual cause of penile bleeding during mating.
   - Rarely melanomas also ulcerate within the sheath and bleeding can contaminate the ejaculate.

10. Uncommonly, cystic calculi in the bladder may result in discharge of blood and urine into the ejaculate.

The presence of blood in the ejaculate can result in either diminished fertility or infertility, depending on the amount of blood present (Fig. 4.46).[122] The cause of the infertility is difficult to determine as motility, morphology and concentration are typically normal in ejaculates with blood in them. The erythrocytes (red blood cells) seem to be the cause of the problem. They may release enzymes that are detrimental to the sperm's ability to penetrate or fertilize the oocyte. Alternatively, the erythrocytes

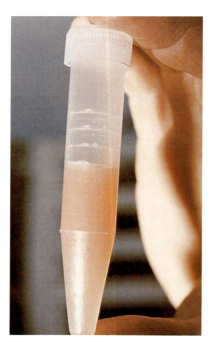

Fig. 4.46 Hemospermia. This semen sample was taken from a stallion with injury to the urethral process which bled during service, contaminating the semen.

may affect the sperm's ability to capacitate, to attach to the oviductal wall, or to become hyperactive in the presence of the oocyte.

> Note:
> - Vaginal injury can cause misleading blood on the stallion's penis.
> - Blood may be seen dripping from the stallion's penis following natural service. This may be the result of damage within the mares reproductive tract including:
> - Rupture of a persistent hymen.
> - Rupture of vaginal varicosities.
> - Rupture of the anterior vagina.
> - This occurs when small mares are bred to stallions with a long penis but does sometimes occur with comparable-sized horses.
> - Use of a breeding roll will help prevent this situation.
> - Mares should be checked by vaginoscopy followed by manual examination when a stallions dismounts with blood on his penis, or blood is noted dripping from the vulva following breeding if an immediate cause from the stallion cannot be identified.
> - Peritonitis (sperm or septic) may occur following vaginal rupture and ejaculation into the abdomen.

Clinical signs

- Depending on the amount of blood, a difference in the color will be noted. Frank and significant hemorrhage will result in a deep red color; seepage from capillaries or smaller bleeding sites will result in a light pink ejaculate.
- Depending on the cause of the bleeding, it may be associated with pain on ejaculation. In cases with disease of the accessory sex glands in particular, the stallion rarely shows any clinical signs of disease and there is rarely pain with ejaculation.
- In coital exanthema (equine herpesvirus 3) vesicles along the urethral epithelium can be seen. Rupture of these vesicles may result in mild hemorrhage.
- Habronemiasis is typically seen in the warm summer months. Nodules filled with caseous material which rupture and bleed easily with erection and physical contact with the mare (or artificial vagina) are typical. The lesions are commonly mildly pruritic (see p. 88).

Diagnosis

- Diagnosis can be difficult. There are no characteristic features of hemospermia that provide diagnostic information apart from the character and amount of the blood. Micro-hemorrhage can be impossible to detect without laboratory assistance. A specimen of semen can

be diluted with water and a urine dipstick inserted. The blood detection portion is extremely sensitive.
- Careful examination of the external and internal reproductive organs is essential.
- Bleeding can be derived from any part of the tract.
- Diagnosis of seminal vesiculitis is based on rectal palpation, ultrasonography and culture of the third fraction of the ejaculate, the gel portion, which originates from the seminal vesicles.
- Bacterial culture of the urethra, semen and urine or direct culture of the inflamed areas identified during (sterile) endoscopy.

> Note:
> - Endoscopy can be used to determine the location of abnormal bleeding sites and the severity of the lesions.

Differential diagnosis
- Other causes of stallion infertility.
- Bleeding into the urinary tract from:
  - ❏ Kidneys.
  - ❏ Ureters.
  - ❏ Bladder.
  - ❏ Pelvic urethra.
- Bleeding on the skin of the penis or prepuce.
- Blood-clotting disorders.
- Cystitis.

Treatment
- Identification of the cause is almost essential.
- Treatment involves long-term systemic antibiotics or short-term topical antibiotic therapy where practicable. Delivery of antibiotics to nondefined infections can be very problematic and unrewarding.
- Nonsteroidal anti-inflammatory drugs may help reduce swelling and relieve some discomfort associated with the inflammatory disorders.
- External wounds should be kept clean and topical antibiotics may be applied if necessary.
- Sexual rest for a minimum of 2 weeks[123] until healing has occurred, depending on the cause.
- Cases of urethral bleeding may require up to 12 weeks of sexual rest.
- Animals that do not respond to therapy may benefit from subischial urethrotomy. This procedure has been thought to benefit these stallions by temporarily diverting urine away from the inflamed tissues.
- Vesiculectomy can be performed in refractory cases of seminal vesiculitis without material effect on fertility.
- Neoplastic lesions may be amenable to surgical excision. If the tumor has invaded significant areas of tissue, complete resection may not be possible, meaning that bleeding may only be temporarily controlled.

- Surgery to remove cystic calculi will often result in resolution of signs.

Prognosis
- Urethral strictures or diverticulum may form during the healing process.

Urospermia

Etiology
The cause of urospermia is unknown, since affected stallions typically show no other signs of systemic or organic disease. Potential causes include:

- Neurological dysfunction.
  - ❏ Bladder sphincter closure and emission are controlled by α-adrenergic fibers of the sympathetic nervous system. Any disease affecting these pathways may affect the ability to keep the sphincter closed during ejaculation.
  - ❏ Urinary incontinence due to cauda equina syndrome or equine herpesvirus 1 infection.
- Urinary incontinence.
  - ❏ Urination during ejaculation will result in contamination of the ejaculate and decreased fertility of the semen from that ejaculate. The presence of even a small amount of urine is detrimental to spermatozoal motility.
  - ❏ Urospermia occurs in only 30–40% of the ejaculates obtained from stallions with this tendency.

Clinical signs
- Affected stallions typically have normal libido and behavior.[124]
- There are no characteristic signs apart from infertility.

Diagnosis
- Examination of ejaculate that has:
  - ❏ A yellow color
  - ❏ Odor of ammonia.
  - ❏ Calcium carbonate crystals evident with microscopic examination.
- Determination of urea nitrogen and creatinine concentrations will confirm the diagnosis.

> - A laboratory reagent test strip may be dipped in the semen and held for only 10 seconds (rather than the typical 60 seconds for blood, to prevent false positives from occurring) prior to determination of urea nitrogen level.
> - If a multiple urine type dipstick is used instead, the sample should be evaluated for nitrate level 3.5 minutes after exposure to the semen.
> - Use of an open-ended artificial vagina will allow fractionation of the ejaculate.

Treatment

- This is very difficult at best, since there is no way to determine whether or not urine contamination will occur for any given ejaculate.
- Collection of semen immediately following urination is the best way to minimize urine contamination.
- Urination may be stimulated by the use of a chemical diuretic, by presenting the stallion to the fecal pile of another stallion or from cycling mares.
- Catheterization should not be routinely performed since the chances of an ascending infection are high following routine catheterization.
- Variable results have been obtained with bethanecol chloride and oxytocin.

THE SCROTUM

Scrotal trauma

Etiology

- Trauma usually occurs as a result of a kick to the scrotum and causes a hematocele (hemorrhage with blood collecting between the two testicular tunics or hematoma).
- Blood between the tunics will cause derangement of the thermoregulatory mechanism of the scrotum and will result in abnormal spermatogenesis.

Clinical signs

- Initially, the scrotum is warm, fluctuant, enlarged and painful.
- As the hematoma organizes it becomes firm and painless.
- Adhesions may develop between the two tunics or between the testicle and the tunica albuginea, reducing the natural ability of the testicle to slide smoothly within the scrotum.
- Thermoregulatory mechanisms are impaired.[125]
- Scrotal trauma may result in orchitis and subsequent testicular degeneration.

Treatment

- Immediate cold water hydrotherapy or ice packing should be used at least 3–4 times daily until the swelling subsides.
- Lacerations should be surgically debrided and closed. If the lacerations penetrate the testicular tunics, broad-spectrum systemic antibiotics are also indicated.
- Topical antibiotic ointments and systemic antibiotics are necessary.
- Nonsteroidal anti-inflammatory drugs should be used to decrease inflammation.

- Spermatogenesis will inevitably be affected for up to 60 days after all clinical signs have resolved.
- Unilateral castration may be indicated in some cases, to allow for normal thermoregulation of the uninjured testicle.

Prognosis

- Semen should be evaluated every 30 days to determine when to return to breeding.
- If semen quality is still poor 3 months after resolution, the effects on fertility may be permanent.

Scrotal dermatitis/edema

Etiology

- This may occur in association with systemic diseases that cause peripheral fluid accumulation, such as equine infectious anemia, equine viral arteritis or a result of varicosities.
- Dermatitis may be caused by irritating chemicals, soaps or ointments.
- Nettles and thistle awns, etc. can also cause serious scrotal inflammation and swelling.
- Scrotal edema is also seen when movement is restricted (e.g. with orthopedic disease).

Clinical signs

- Dermatitis and edema cause the scrotal skin to be thickened, resulting in derangement of thermoregulation (Fig. 4.47).
- If it is persistent, it may result in infertility.

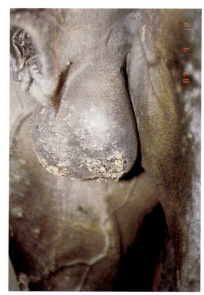

Fig. 4.47 Scrotal dermatitis and thickening sufficient to cause a reduction in fertility from thermal injury.

Treatment

- Treatment of the primary disorder or etiology is required.
- Exercise is essential for resolution of most scrotal edema conditions.
- Cold water hydrotherapy is helpful.
- Diuretics and topical emollient/antibiotic ointments may be indicated.

THE TESTICLES

Testicular hypoplasia/degeneration

Etiology

Testicular hypoplasia is typically a congenital disorder and is probably hereditary. There is usually a history of a young stallion with poor conception rates after breeding multiple mares. It may be unilateral or (more commonly) bilateral.

Testicular degeneration is a condition of older stallions with a history of normal fertility that has declined.[126,127] Degeneration may be unilateral or bilateral. Causes of testicular degeneration include:

- Age.
- Testicular torsion.
- Hydrocele.
- Hematocele.
- Scrotal edema.
- Orchitis.
- Autoimmune disease (sperm granuloma).[128]
- Varicocele.
- Inappropriate use of anabolic steroids.
- Systemic disease.
- Neoplasia.
- Cryptorchidism.
- Injury or traumatic damage to testis, spermatic cord, epididymides or deferent ducts, or vasculature/nerve supply to the testicle(s).
- Malnutrition or toxin ingestion.
- Exposure to damaging chemicals, heavy metals, or radiation.

Clinical signs

- Testicular hypoplasia is characterized by small testes, poor semen quality and infertility/sterility.
  - ❑ Hypoplastic testicles are prone to testicular degeneration with time.
  - ❑ Early in the course of the disease the testicles are smaller and softer than normal.
- Adhesions between the tunics and the testicle will restrict free movement of the testicle in the scrotum.
- Discrepancy between estimation of daily sperm output and actual daily sperm output early in the disease process.
- The testicles may become progressively firmer as a result of scar tissue replacing the testicular tissue in end-stage disease.

- A wrinkled texture may be felt as the testicular tissue decreases in volume and the tunics become less tightly stretched.
- The epididymis will become more prominent as testicle size decreases.

> Note:
> - Occasionally there may be localized degeneration due to a previous injury or hemorrhage in the testicle from trauma, which resolves with fibrosis and calcification.

Diagnosis

Diagnosis of hypoplasia or degeneration is based on age, history, physical examination, ultrasonography (Fig. 4.48), evaluation of the spermiogram, testicular biopsy (Fig. 4.48, see also below), and hormonal analysis.[129]

- If the condition is bilateral, azoospermia or oligospermia is usually noted; if it is unilateral there may be a normal to azoospermic spermiogram.
- Teratospermia (dead sperm) and necrospermia (abnormal forms) are common findings. Germ cells may be noted in the ejaculate.

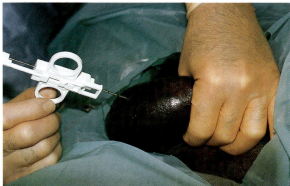

A

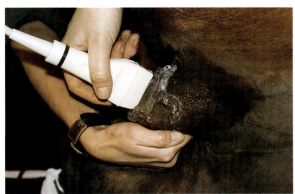

B

Fig. 4.48 (A) Testicular biopsy. (B) Testicular ultrasound.

- Testicular biopsy can be used to define the extent and type of change.[130,131]
  - ❑ Focal lesions identified by ultrasonography or diffuse lesions involving a single testis are candidates for biopsy.
  - ❑ Diffuse diseases or obviously different types and locations of lesions of both testicles may warrant multiple biopsies but in principle the fewer biopsies the better.
  - ❑ Local anesthesia of the skin at the site is essential (and some sedation may be wise).
  - ❑ Antibiotics should not be required if performed as a sterile procedure but may be used prophylactically.

Interpretation

Biopsy may reveal:

- Decreased thickness of the germinal epithelium.
- Germ cell hypoplasia.
- Maturation arrest.
- Decreased tubular diameter.
- Increased giant cell formation, mineralization of the tubules and fibrosis with seeming Leydig cell hyperplasia due to decreased tubular mass.[132]
- After the disease becomes more chronic, tubular hyalinization and Sertoli cell only syndrome may be diagnosed.

Hormonal evaluation from blood samples may reveal:

- Normal, high or low gonadotropin concentrations.
- Normal to low circulating testosterone concentrations.
- Normal or diminished response to stimulation of the testicles with human chorionic gonadotropin or gonadotropin-releasing hormone.[133]

Treatment

The specific cause of the disorder must be treated.

- If fever is present, antipyretics should be administered.
- Injury to the testicles or edematous conditions should be treated to restore the thermoregulation of the testicles and scrotum as quickly as possible.
- If only one testicle is affected, the contralateral testicle may respond by hypertrophy, resulting in some return to normal spermiogram values, although they usually do not return to pre-injury levels.
- In animals with hypogonadotropic hypogonadism, where circulating gonadotropin concentrations are low, treatment with gonadotropin-releasing hormone may be of benefit to either slow the course of the disease or to provide some return to a more normal spermiogram.[134,135]
  - ❑ In order for gonadotropin-releasing hormone to be effective, the pituitary must be functional and the testes must be able to respond normally to gonadotropin stimulus.
  - ❑ Pulsatile administration of gonadotropin-releasing hormone is ideal; the hormone is provided by a pump system, which releases low doses every 30 minutes.
- Hemicastration may be indicated if this procedure will result in return to a normal scrotal environment (e.g. testicular torsion), or prevent production of excessive amounts of anti-sperm antibodies and breakdown of the blood–testes barrier.
  - ❑ If hemicastration is considered, closed castration should be carried out using sterile technique with closure of the scrotal incision to minimize the inflammation associated with the surgical procedure.

Prognosis

- Treatment is frequently unsuccessful, unless the cause of the insult is resolved or can be treated quickly.
- Degeneration or hypoplasia of the testicles will result in diminished fertility.
- The severity of the lesions will determine the degree of subfertility.
- Late spermatogonia, spermatocytes and spermatids are the most susceptible germ cells. If the cause of the degeneration is temporary (e.g. fever), regeneration may occur and spermatogenesis will return to normal in due course.
- Stallions with hypoplastic testicles may have adequate libido to be used as teaser stallions.
  - ❑ Otherwise, they are usually castrated because their fertility is too low to be acceptable even as a subfertile stallion.
  - ❑ In stallions with early stages of degeneration, use of hormonal therapy may prolong their reproductive lifespan, although the disease is progressive and eventually will lead to unacceptable levels of fertility.
- In stallions that have diminished spermatogenic function, maximal fertility can be achieved by:
  - ❑ Use of excellent management techniques.
  - ❑ Limiting the book of mares.
  - ❑ Selection of only highly fertile mares.
  - ❑ Breeding as close to ovulation as possible.
  - ❑ Using fresh, extended semen rather than chilling and shipping.
  - ❑ Using the proper semen extenders.

Testicular biopsy

- **Testicular biopsy is a surgical procedure and requires aseptic methods.**

Technique

Incisional biopsy

i. Following a small skin incision a single incision (no longer than 0.5 cm) is made into the tunica propria of the testis.
ii. The testicular tissue will normally bulge out from the incision.
iii. This is cut parallel to the surface of the testis and placed in a suitable fixative.
iv. The tunica is closed with fine sutures of absorbable material and the skin is closed with subcuticular sutures of fine absorbable material such as polyglactin.
v. This method carries extra risks of adhesions so the incisions should be as small as possible.

Split-needle biopsy

Testicular biopsy with a spring-loaded split-needle biopsy instrument is a simple procedure (see Fig. 4.48).

i. The instruments are available in a variety of sizes giving a biopsy specimen of 1–1.5 mm in diameter and 0.2–2 cm long.
ii. A small stab incision is made in the skin to allow unrestricted movement of the needle during the cutting stage.
iii. The biopsy instrument is passed through the skin incision and into the testis (under ultrasound guidance if a specific site is to be sampled).
iv. The biopsy is obtained by advancing the central needle and then releasing the cutting mechanism.
v. The needle is withdrawn and the biopsy placed in fixative.
vi. There is usually no need to suture the skin incision.

Fine-needle aspirate

This technique is not well established in horses.

i. A 20-g 2.5–3.5-cm needle attached to a 20-ml syringe is introduced into the testicle.
ii. Cells are aspirated into the needle and the syringe by vacuum applied to the plunger.
iii. The cells are ejected directly onto a glass slide or into fixative for examination.

Hydrocele

Etiology

- This is a condition in which fluid accumulates between the vaginal tunic and the tunica albuginea.
- The fluid may emanate from the abdominal cavity, result from parasite migration (*Strongylus edentatus* or *Fasciola hepatica*), or result from exposure to high environmental temperatures for an extended period of time.
- The condition results in abnormal thermoregulation of the scrotum.

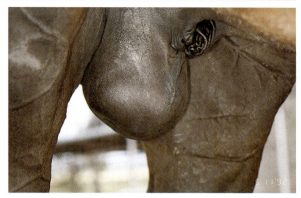

Fig. 4.49 Hydrocele. Fluid has accumulated between the vaginal tunic and the tunica albuginea.

Clinical signs

- Fluid accumulation between the tunica vaginalis and the tunica albuginea (Fig. 4.49).

Diagnosis

- Diagnosis is by palpation and ultrasonography.
- Aspiration of fluid from the vaginal cavity can be performed to confirm the nature of the fluid as a transudate.
- Centesis will allow differentiation from hematocele.

Treatment

- Hemicastration using closed technique, with removal of the entire vaginal cavity, is recommended to return the thermoregulation of the unaffected testicle as quickly as possible.

Cryptorchidism/rig

Etiology

Cryptorchidism is the retention of one or both testicles in the abdominal cavity or in the inguinal canal. As the testicles grow, they slowly descend into the scrotum, usually by 3 years of age. Failure of the normal descent mechanism is thought to cause the condition (see p. 48), the retained testicles more commonly being located in the inguinal rings than in the abdomen.

The condition probably has some hereditary component which is believed to be an autosomal recessive gene.[136] There are certain cryptorchid stallions that throw a much higher incidence of cryptorchid foals than the average population; and there is a breed predilection in the Quarter Horse and Paint Horse populations. Other cases are sporadic.

Temporary inguinal retention

- Occurs primarily but not exclusively in ponies with small testicles (<40 g).

- Over 75% of temporary inguinally retained testicles are on the right side.
- If inguinally retained testicles are not removed they can descend into the scrotum up to 3 years of age.
- The retained testicle is macroscopically normal but, as it is small, the epididymis may appear to be over large, especially in the older horse.[137]
- Microscopically the testis appears immature with prominence of the tubular structures and few interstitial cells. The nearer the testis gets to the scrotum the more normal will be its microscopic features.

Permanent inguinal retention

- Affects all types of horses. Affected animals are commonly called high flankers, false rigs, or ridglings.
- Affected testes are larger than 40 g and may be misshapen.
- The testis is retained in the inguinal canal and usually has a very short vaginal tunic and therefore can only be exteriorized with difficulty.
- Usually unilateral, with equal frequency between left and right.
- Occasionally the contralateral testis is abdominally retained.
- The retained testis is often not palpable in the standing horse and only with difficulty in most anesthetized horses.
- Microscopically the testis is immature with prominent tubular structures and few interstitial cells.

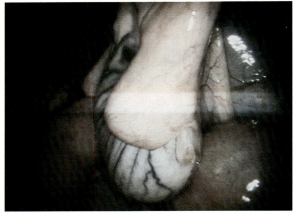

Fig. 4.50 A laparoscopic view of a cryptorchid testicle in a pony stallion that had a good breeding history in his first year of use (aged 2 years) (slide courtesy of J Walmsley).

Complete abdominal retention

- Abdominal retention of both testis and epididymis on the affected side.
- The testis is suspended in the abdominal cavity from the sublumbar region (Fig. 4.50).
- The retained testis is relatively mobile within the abdomen, but usually lies close to the deep/internal inguinal ring. However, it can be found in coils of intestine, dorsal to the rectum or lateral to the bladder.
- Abdominally retained testicles are usually small, weighing between 10 and 50 g, and are characteristically soft and flabby in texture (Fig. 4.51).

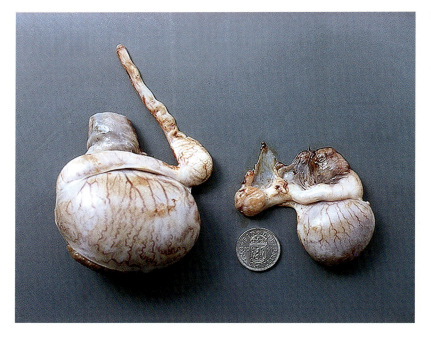

Fig. 4.51 The two testicles of a unilateral cryptorchid stallion. The retained testicle (right) was abnormally small and had an elongated epididymis.

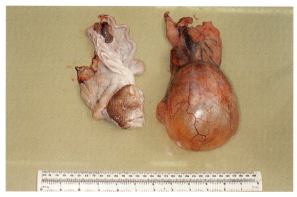

Fig. 4.52 Testicular teratoma (two types). Left: teratoma containing cartilage and bone. Right: large fluid-filled cystic teratoma.

- Sometimes the retained testicle is grossly enlarged, being either cystic or teratomatous (Fig. 4.52).
- The histological appearance is remarkably similar to that of the fetal testis; there are isolated islands of tubules with very sparse interstitial cells surrounded by extensive loose connective tissue. Fibrous tissue increases with age.

Incomplete abdominal retention
- The vaginal process is well developed, has an attached well-developed cremaster muscle and contains the tail of the epididymis.
- The vaginal tunic can sometimes be palpated in the inguinal region in the standing horse and can be mistaken for a small testis in the anesthetized horse in dorsal recumbency.
- Incomplete retention occurs in about half of the cases of unilateral, right-sided abdominal retention but only in about 15% of unilateral left-sided cases.
- Bilateral cases usually have the same distribution, being either both complete or both incomplete.
- In Thoroughbreds and other larger horses (as opposed to ponies), left-sided retention is more common than right-sided retention.
- The testis is usually located at the deep inguinal ring but is relatively immobile due to the firm location of the vaginal tunic in the scrotum.

Note:
- In the foal, palpation of the scrotum can be confusing.
- The gubernaculum and the attached epididymal tail may be larger than the testis itself.
- This may give the impression of normal testicular descent when both testes are still abdominal.

Significance of cryptorchidism
- A cryptorchid testis is infertile.
- Cryptorchid testes cannot be removed using normal castration techniques; special approaches need to be taken to ensure effective castration even when the retention is within the inguinal canal.
- A retained testis will continue to produce androgens such as testosterone and so the animal will retain its masculine characteristics and behavior.[138]
- Cryptorchidism is an inherited disorder in some lines of horse.
- It is an unfortunate fact that some horses are castrated on the one side and then sold. These animals are a persistent problem and a diagnosis is essential if behavior is to be controlled. Unilateral castration should not be performed. The retained testicle should be removed first to ensure that an animal that is designated as a gelding is not subsequently found to be a cryptorchid.

Clinical signs
- The testis is not palpable in the scrotum.
- If one or both testes cannot be palpated in an animal that has not been castrated, cryptorchidism should be suspected.

Note:
- Palpation may result in withdrawal of the testis.

- In some cases the testicle(s) may be temporarily retained between the inguinal rings.
- In a quiet or sedated animal an inguinally retained testicle may be palpable in the inguinal canal and can usually be palpated when the horse is under general anesthesia in dorsal recumbency.

Diagnosis
- Palpation of the scrotum fails to reveal one (or both) testes in an animal that is known not to have been castrated.
- Palpation of the scrotum under sedation or even general anesthesia fails to reveal the testis.
- Rectal palpation and transrectal or transabdominal ultrasonographic examination are commonly used to locate the retained testis.
- Laparoscopic examination of the inguinal region is very useful and can be followed immediately by removal of the retained structures.
- Blood samples are highly diagnostic.

In horses less than 2 years old and donkeys of any age, clotted blood sample is obtained immediately prior to administration of 6000 iu human chorionic gonadorophin (IV).

A second sample is obtained 30–120 min later.

In horses 3 years old or older, a single sample of clotted blood is submitted for oestrone sulphate analysis.

Samples submitted for testosterone analysis. Expected values:

	Testosterone		Oestrone sulphate
	(nmol/l)		(ng/l)
	Before	*After*	
Entire male	–	–	10–50
Cryptorchid	0.3–4.3	**1.0–12.9**	0.1–10
Gelding	0.03–0.15	**0.05–0.19**	< 0.02

Treatment

- The only effective treatment is complete castration.
- Laparoscopic castration is an effective way of avoiding surgical laparotomy for abdominally retained testicles.

Prognosis

- If the condition is unilateral the stallion is either fertile or subfertile.
- If the condition is bilateral the stallion either has very poor fertility or is sterile.
- Testicles that remain at elevated temperatures for extended periods of time (i.e. years) are more prone to neoplastic transformation.
- Affected stallions should never be used for breeding purposes because of the possible hereditary component. By far the best approach is to castrate all stallions with a retained testicle to ensure that they do not breed.

Anorchidism/monorchidism/polyorchidism

1. Anorchidism.
   - This is very rare.
   - Neither testicle develops and there is no gonadal tissue present, yet the animal is genetically male.
2. Monorchidism.
   - This is also rare,[139] but less so than anorchidism.
   - This is a condition in which only one testicle develops.
   - The structures associated with the testicle are usually present; it is just the gonad itself that is missing.
3. Polyorchidism.
   - This a condition in which more than two testicles are found.[140]
   - True polyorchid horses are extremely rare; indeed, it is unlikely that it has ever occurred. They may be confused with animals whose epididymis is in the inguinal canal and the testicle is in the abdomen, or animals with a cystic structure on the spermatic cord that is mistaken for a third testicle.

Testicular torsion

Etiology

Testicular torsion is rotation of the testicle on the spermatic cord. Possible causes that have been suggested include a strong and abnormal cremaster reflex, a long gubernaculum, presence of a large scrotum with small testicles, presence of a long spermatic cord and neoplasia. Rotation may be partial or complete.

Partial torsion

- This is defined as a rotation through 90° and retraction close to the abdominal wall.
- It is believed to be due to the improper attachment of the cremaster muscle to the vaginal tunic.
- The torsion is common in young stallions and usually is not detrimental to future fertility.
- Partial torsion may be up to 180°, so that the tail of the epididymis is located cranially (Fig. 4.53). It may be a developmental defect in testicular descent and usually does not affect fertility.

Complete torsion

- This involves rotation beyond 180° and up to 360° or more (Fig. 4.54).
- It is more common in trotting Standardbreds and Thoroughbreds, which implies there may be a breed predilection, hereditary component or an association with heavy exercise.
- There is usually a history of a sudden onset of abdominal pain, which often begins following mating or exercise.

Clinical signs

- Colic is often the presenting sign.

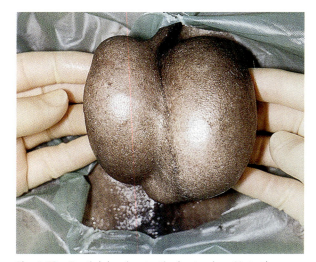

Fig. 4.53 Partial, benign testicular torsion. Note the anteriorly facing tail of the epididymis in the torsed testicle. This is a benign condition without significant effects on fertility.

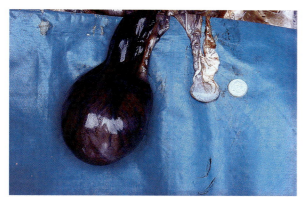

Fig. 4.54 Complete torsion of the testicle resulting in massive local edema and severe unremitting pain. There is invariably severe and irreversible compromise to the testicular tissue.

- Trotters will often break stride or begin to pace and Thoroughbreds will assume a hopping gait with a hitch in stride on the affected side.

> - The scrotum and testicles (and the inguinal rings) of a stallion should always be examined during an examination for colic.

- The affected testicle swells quickly due to inability to drain blood from the testicle.
- Torsion beyond 360° results in ischemia, thrombosis and variable degrees of degeneration depending on the severity and duration of the torsion.

Diagnosis

- Torsion needs to be differentiated from scrotal hernias. This differentiation is made through palpation and ultrasound of the testicles and inguinal rings.
- Differential diagnoses:
  - ❑ Testicular trauma (traumatic orchitis/hematoma/hematocele).
  - ❑ Infectious orchitis.

Treatment

- Treatment of torsion consists of emergency hemicastration to prevent changes in thermoregulation in the normal testicle.
- If the disease process is caught in the very early stages, attempts at resolving the torsion followed by tacking the testicle in the scrotum have been made with varying success.

> - Tacking of the testicle may result in the inability to lower the testicles completely during hot weather and abnormal thermoregulation with subsequent infertility.

Prognosis

- The prognosis for a testicle that has suffered serious or prolonged torsion is poor.
- Testicular size will usually reduce and may never approach normality again.
- Fertility is invariably impaired to some extent, if not totally.

THE EPIDIDYMIS

- Abnormalities of the epididymis are uncommon in the stallion.

Epididymitis

- Epididymitis is usually secondary to orchitis, with the same causative agents or processes.
- Occlusion of the duct system with purulent exudate or sperm granuloma formation is common following or during orchitis/epididymitis.
- Treatment of epididymitis is the same as for orchitis.

Congenital hypoplasia or aplasia of the tubular ductal system

- This is very rare and may occur unilaterally or bilaterally.
- The associated testicle is usually smaller than normal due to pressure necrosis from backup of spermatozoa and the associated tubular fluids.
- The daily sperm output is diminished if unilateral abnormalities occur; azoospermia exists if the condition is bilateral.
- There is no treatment for these conditions at this time.
- A more common cause of apparent hypoplasia is retention of the testicle (cryptorchidism) in which all the testicular structures are altered significantly (see p. 95).

THE SPERMATIC CORD

Varicocele

- This is a rare, apparently congenital condition and is usually unilateral.
- It causes dilation of the spermatic vein and significant enlargement of the vessel (Fig. 4.55). The pathological enlargement of the vein is detectable by careful ultrasonographic examination.
- Varicocele results in the inability of the pampiniform plexus to cool the blood effectively before it enters the testicle.

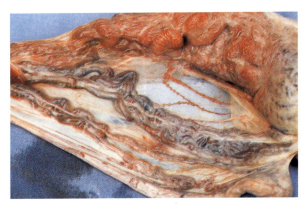

Fig. 4.55 Varicosity of the spermatic cord showing obvious enlargement of the vessels. Under these conditions it may be difficult for normal thermoregulation to take place.

- Testicular swelling and scrotal edema may result in more severe cases.
- Testicular degeneration may ensue.
- There is no pain associated with palpation.
- Hemicastration is usually curative.

Verminous granulomas

- Granulomas may result from parasitic migrations and cause testicular degeneration by altering the blood flow to the testicle.
- The consequent abnormal thermoregulation causes testicular degeneration.
- Hemicastration with removal of the entire spermatic cord may result in some return of fertility in the remaining testicle if the degenerative changes are not too severe.

NEOPLASMS OF THE REPRODUCTIVE ORGANS

PENIS AND PREPUCE[141]

The penis and prepuce should be examined carefully in detail in the extended position and then the prepuce is examined again following retraction of the penis. Diagnosis of neoplasia of the penis and prepuce is made by palpation of these structures in their entirety. The scrotum should be evaluated at the same time, because dermatological neoplasia (such as sarcoid) may extend to this structure as well. Excisional biopsy will usually establish a definitive diagnosis.

Note:
- Inguinal (both superficial and deep) and pelvic lymph nodes should be examined for enlargement prior to aggressive surgical or medical therapy being instituted.

Treatment for the various neoplastic lesions will vary of course, depending on the extent, character and location of the tumor. The therapeutic options include:

- Surgical excision.
- Cryotherapy/cryonecrosis.
- Chemotherapeutic agents (topical and/or systemic).
- Laser resection.[142]
- Radiation.

For cases in which the disease has spread extensively, penile amputation or reefing may be required.[143]

Squamous cell carcinoma

Etiology

- This is the most common neoplasia of the penis.[144]
- Smegma (sebaceous secretion of the penile epithelium and epithelial cells shed from the prepuce) is suggested as being the most likely carcinogen.[145]
- Nonpigmented skin surfaces of the prepuce and penis are more susceptible.
- Geldings are far more often affected than stallions, possibly because geldings produce more smegma than do stallions and the penis of geldings is less likely to be cleaned.
- The severity ranges from a mild (but sometimes extensive) precancerous, mildly ulcerative, dermatitis-like condition to highly aggressive malignant tumors (Fig. 4.56).
- The condition has a lower malignancy in older horses.

- Young horses that are affected generally carry a much poorer prognosis.

- The tumor commonly has either a proliferative or a destructive nature.
  - Proliferative tumors produce cauliflower-like lesions; sometimes these are ulcerated also. There may be extensive proliferation over wide areas of the penile skin and the glans.
  - The destructive form results in extensive distortion of the penis/glans.
  - Involvement of the preputial rings and surrounding skin is a serious complication and this can occur in its own right.

Clinical signs

- Squamous cell carcinoma is typically found on the urethral orifice, the glans penis or the internal prepuce.
- Common clinical signs include blood observed in the ejaculate or in the urine.

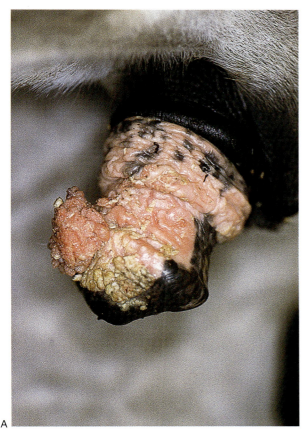

A

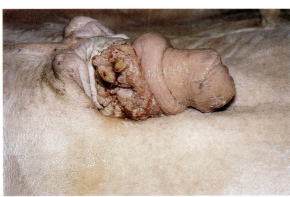

B

Fig. 4.56 (A) Precarcinomatous changes characterized by thickening and depigmentation. There may be slight hemorrhage. (B) An invasive, destructive squamous cell carcinoma of the penile shaft.

- Sometimes a bloody, fetid preputial discharge will be noted.
- Pain may be associated with the penis.
  Early lesions appear as small, heavily keratinized plaques (<5 mm).
- The tumor infiltrates the surrounding tissue and forms crusted, ulcerative lesions that bleed freely.
- The lesions may take on a cauliflower-like appearance and have a necrotic center.

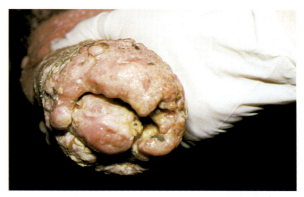

Fig. 4.57 Extensive ulcerative and proliferative squamous cell carcinoma of the penis. The iliac lymph nodes were grossly enlarged, suggesting that the tumor was malignant.

- This tumor will spread by local infiltration over the entire penis and prepuce if left unchecked (Fig. 4.57).
- The aggressive (often malignant) forms cause a wooden feel to the shaft of the penis (this is more common in younger horses).
- Secondary metastases in the pelvic organs, lumbar vertebrae and other major organs may cause signs apparently unrelated to the tumor.
- Extensively ulcerated tumors usually have a fetid odor, a heavy, hemorrhagic preputial discharge and can become infested with fly maggots.

Treatment

- Early treatment of the precancerous stage is based upon removal of all possible carcinogens and ensuring that the penis, penile skin and preputial lining are healthy and clean.
- Surgical treatment of squamous cell carcinoma includes any of the following alone or in combination:
  ❏ Cryosurgery.
  ❏ Radical excision.
  ❏ Reefing procedures (stripping of the penile and preputial skin).
  ❏ Penile amputation.
- Medical treatment may include:
  ❏ Local infiltration with chemotherapeutic agents, such as 5-fluorouracil or cisplatin, either alone if the lesions are small, or following surgical debulking therapy.
  ❏ Some chemotherapeutic creams are also now available for topical application.
  ❏ Radiation treatment using interstitial gamma brachytherapy or teletherapy.

Prognosis

- Fortunately, penile or preputial squamous cell carcinoma is very rare in working stallions.
- Metastasis to local lymph nodes may occur. However, spread to other organs is uncommon.

Melanoma

- Melanoma is most commonly seen on the penis or prepuce (Fig. 4.58) in older gray horses (stallions or geldings).
- Melanomas will commonly be noted on other areas of the body such as the anus, the face, the neck, the limbs, within the guttural pouches and parotid salivary and lymph nodes, or along the body wall. Perineal melanomas are particularly common.
- In cases where melanoma is diagnosed on a nongray horse, spread to other organs is more common.
- If the external genitalia are involved, masses are usually seen on the prepuce, but may occur on the penis as well. The masses are round, smooth, hairless and generally small (<2 cm).
- This tumor is slow to spread to other sites or organs and treatment is usually not required unless the tumor interferes with mating or urination. Some melanomas can be aggressive, so biopsy of the tumor and microscopic assessment is recommended.

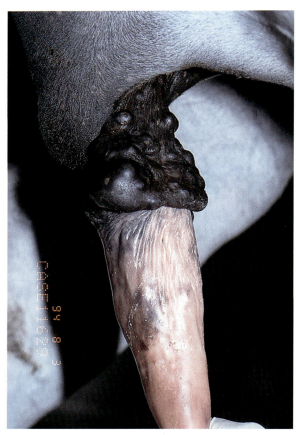

Fig. 4.58 Extensive melanoma in the penile skin of a gray stallion. There was no apparent effect on his fertility but the tumors were inclined to ulcerate and bled from time to time, causing delays in breeding.

- If the tumor is found to be aggressive on microscopic examination of a biopsy specimen, surgical removal is recommended. In these cases, surgical excision or cryotherapy is generally effective.
- If the tumor is not aggressive, but growing actively, or in cases where the number of tumors is excessive, cimetidine administration may sometimes result in a decrease in the size of the tumor(s).[146]

> Note:
> - Cimetidine is administered orally (2.5 mg/kg once a day) until no further decrease in size is noted (usually within 3–4 months).
> - Therapy can be resumed if growth recurs at a later date.

- Autogenous vaccine prepared by a commercial laboratory from X-irradiated autogenous cell cultures is a new method being developed.
  - ❑ The tumor is resected and sent to the laboratory. An autogenous vaccine is made from irradiated cells grown from the tumor.
  - ❑ This vaccine stimulates the immune system of the animal to recognize tumor cells as foreign and to attack them. This results in tumor regression.

Viral (squamous) papillomas (warts)

- Squamous papillomas (warts) are benign tumors found on the penis and prepuce.
- They typically occur in young stallions (or geldings).
- A papilloma virus is responsible.
- The virus usually induces seroconversion, so the papillomas are usually self-limiting.
- Typically there are small (1–2 mm) cauliflower-like growths of epithelial tissue. Similar lesions on the nares, muzzle or lips may be noted. They may grow in multiple sites. They rarely become large.
- Spontaneous resolution generally takes 1–3 months depending on the size and number.
- There is little chance of recurrence but a few lesions will persist.
- Treatment is usually unsuccessful in getting the lesions to resolve more quickly.

Scrotal/preputial/penile sarcoid

Etiology

- These are fibroblastic skin tumors.
- Sarcoids are the most common tumor of the horse (all locations included).
- The tumors are more common in younger horses (under 6 years of age).

- The fibroblastic form often arises from the site of an old wound. Most commonly they are encountered on the head, limbs and ventral midline.
- Metastasis has not been reported with this neoplasm.
- The tumors tend to grow quickly.
- Sarcoids are commonly regarded as a virus disease affecting the skin, but they may best be regarded as a neoplastic disorder affecting both the dermis and epidermis or the subcutaneous tissue (or both).
- Scrotal sarcoids commonly develop in horses that have sarcoids at other sites.

Clinical signs

Individual lesions can be small or large and multiple lesions are common (Fig. 4.59). Sarcoid tumors are more common on the prepuce (Fig. 4.60) than on the penis. They can also occur on the scrotal skin. Scrotal sarcoids take one of the six recognized forms of sarcoid tumor.[147]

1. Most are nodular in nature.
   - Some are spherical type A nodules (without cutaneous involvement).
   - Others have variable dermal and epidermal involvement (type B nodules) and are usually less spherical in nature.

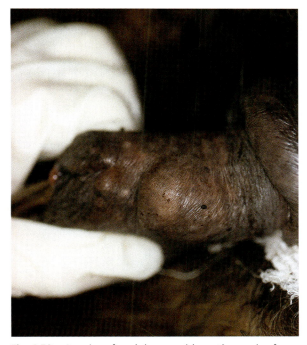

Fig. 4.59 A series of nodular sarcoids on the penis of a stallion. The stallion had not been used for breeding for some 12 years and these were discovered during prebreeding examination.

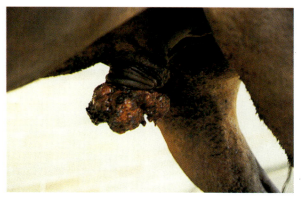

Fig. 4.60 Extensive fibroblastic sarcoids involving the prepuce.

- There may be few or several hundred lesions.
2. Fibroblastic and malignant sarcoid can be found on the penile skin or the preputial rings and occasionally in the skin of the prepuce and scrotum.
3. Superficial involvement of the scrotal and preputial epidermis and dermis alone results in verrucose lesions that have a wart-like rough, hyperkeratotic appearance.
4. Occasionally the occult form is found on the skin, but seldom on the penis. These are very superficial in character and often present with a gray, slightly scaly circular lesion.
5. Mixed lesions are common on the skin of the prepuce and scrotum (Fig. 4.61).
6. Each of the former lesions can develop into true fibroblastic lesions with a fleshy, ulcerated character. These are rare on the scrotal skin.

Diagnosis

- The clinical appearance is easily recognized.
- Biopsy is probably the only definitive way of identifying the lesions, but is regarded as potentially dangerous.

Treatment

- Surgical excision is the attractive option and the results can be satisfying.
- Cytotoxic treatments can be dangerous for both fertility and scarring (which in itself can cause adhesions and loss of fertility).
- Interstitial radiation brachytherapy has a high success rate but has serious implications for operator safety and for the possibility of mutation of spermatogonia.

Prognosis

- The prognosis is always guarded.
- There is a high rate of recurrence with most therapies and recurrences are likely to be more aggressive and infiltrative.

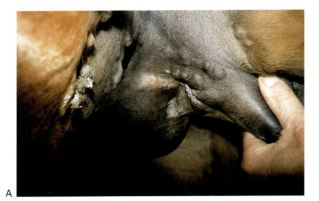

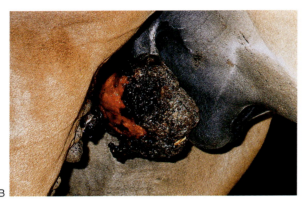

Fig. 4.61 (A) Mixed sarcoids in the scrotal skin of a stallion. (B) Fibroblastic sarcoid on the scrotum.

THE TESTICLES[148,149]

Profile

Tumors of the testicle are uncommon and are usually unilateral. Testicular tumors are divided for descriptive purposes as follows:

1. Germ cell tumors
   - Seminoma.
     - ❑ This is the most common tumor of the equine testicle.[150]
     - ❑ Aged stallions are most often affected (Fig. 4.62).
   - Teratoma and teratocarcinoma.
     - ❑ They arise directly from the cells of the seminiferous epithelium and therefore can transform into endoderm, mesoderm or ectoderm.
     - ❑ For this reason, on cut surface, these tumors will have many different types of tissue, including differentiated hair, fat, teeth, and bone.
     - ❑ Malignancy is rare.
     - ❑ The tumors are usually round or oval in shape, with irregular surfaces.
     - ❑ They are most common in abdominal testicles.

2. Nongerminal tumors
   - Interstitial cell tumors.
     - ❑ These are rare in the horse.[151]
     - ❑ They are usually small, may be multiple in number and are usually found incidentally at necropsy or after castration.
   - Sertoli cell tumors
     - ❑ These are rare.[152]
     - ❑ They result in increased estrogen secretion and feminization in the dog but whether this so in the horse is unknown due to their rarity.

- Germ cell tumors are more common than stromal/interstitial tumors.
- Cryptorchid testicles may be more predisposed to neoplastic transformation due to their constant exposure to increased temperature and the resultant alterations in cell types and structures, alterations in blood supply and local hormonal milieu.
- Retained testicles tend to have a higher incidence of transformation into teratomas.

Clinical signs

- Some stallions with cryptorchid testicular tumors may present for weight loss or colic.
- Stallions with a scrotal testis affected by neoplasia usually present because of the noticeable increase in size of the affected testicle.
- These stallions do not usually experience pain on ejaculation or palpation.
- The presence of neoplasm in one testicle may affect the thermoregulation of the other testicle, resulting in a decrease in fertility; this may therefore be the presenting complaint.
- In most cases, the spermiogram is normal. On very rare occasions, abnormal germ cells may be shed into the ejaculate.

Seminoma

- Usually there are no clinical signs; the seminoma is found on routine palpation or ultrasound examination of the testicles.
- The affected testicle has lobulated soft to firm masses that are gray-white in color on cut surface.
- Seminomas may be small to large and occasionally become aggressive and metastasize to other organs.[153]

Diagnosis

- Tumors must be differentiated from other causes of scrotal/testicular enlargement such as:
  - ❑ Orchitis (traumatic or infectious).
  - ❑ Testicular torsion.
  - ❑ Hematocele/varicocele/hydrocele.
  - ❑ Hematoma.
  - ❑ Sperm granuloma.
  - ❑ Hernia.

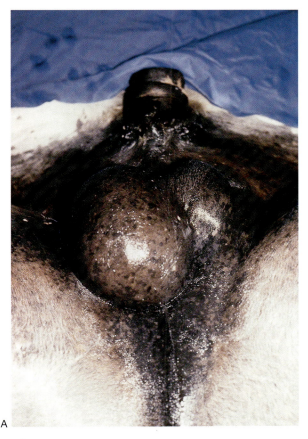

A

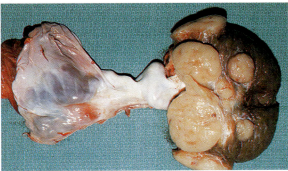

B

Fig. 4.62 Testicular seminoma in an aged Welsh stallion that had developed a slow enlargement of one testicle.

- Physical examination and history will assist in ruling out these other conditions.
- History of recent trauma, acute onset of swelling, pain associated with mating or palpation will make neoplasia a less likely diagnosis.
- Additional diagnostic aids include:
  - ❏ Ultrasonography. This will help identify discrete masses and characterize their density.[154]
  - ❏ Fine-needle aspiration.
  - ❏ Cytology.
  - ❏ Biopsy.

- Biopsy of tumors in man has an increased incidence of neoplastic re-occurrence. For this reason, if, based on palpation and ultrasound examination a tumor is suspected in a stallion, immediate hemicastration should be considered.

Treatment
- Hemicastration should be performed using closed techniques. The skin incision should be closed to minimize swelling and alterations in thermoregulation of the remaining testicle.[155]
- The testicle and as much spermatic cord as possible should be removed.
- Hyperplasia of the remaining testicle often occurs, resulting in partial return to the previous level of spermatogenesis (up to two-thirds of normal).

Prognosis
- Growth of testicular tumors is usually slow, but on occasion a tumor may grow quickly enough to result in pain due to pressure on the tunics.
- Metastasis of all tumors is uncommon but, when it occurs, local spread to the inguinal or iliac lymph nodes, posterior abdomen and pelvic canal is common.

OTHER CONDITIONS THAT LIMIT FERTILITY

Impotence and abnormal sexual behavior

Impotence is defined as the consistent inability to achieve or sustain an erection of sufficient rigidity for sexual intercourse.[156] It can be divided into disorders involving:

- Poor libido.
- Organic disease.
- Psychogenic dysfunction (a relatively common cause[157]).

Abnormal sexual behavior includes, but is not limited to:

- Failure to attain or maintain an erection.
- Incomplete intromission or lack of pelvic thrust.
- Dismounting at onset of ejaculation.
- Failure to ejaculate despite multiple mounts, required repeated intromission.
- Diminished libido or aggressive sexual behavior.

Management and training

Many aspects of sexual behavior are learned. Thus appropriate sexual behavior depends to a large extent on management and training. Stallions with good libido are easier to train than stallions with poor libido.

- Overbearing management or excessive discipline in the training barn and show-ring to prevent performance animals from displaying normal sexual behavior often leads to aggressive or abnormal behavior or poor libido when they are asked to perform in the breeding shed.
- Improper management of equipment for artificial insemination will quickly lead to abnormal mating behavior and willingness to breed.

> - For example, caustic/irritating soaps, incorrect artificial vagina temperature, inadequate lubrication inside the artificial vagina and improper placement of the artificial vagina onto the penis are all factors that might induce either resentment or impotence.

- Overuse (especially in young stallions) can lead to decreased libido and impotence due to exhaustion.
- Some stallions will show mare or color preference.

> - For example, some Thoroughbred stallions will not breed gray mares because they are unaccustomed to the color. These stallions should not be forced to breed these mares, but should be gradually introduced over time to similar types of mares until they become acceptable.

- Excessive use as a teaser without positive reinforcement in the breeding shed can lead to decreased libido.

> - On the other hand, use of a stallion with poor libido for teasing multiple mares just prior to breeding may improve his reaction time when it comes time to actually collecting the semen or breed the mares.
> - Allowing slow teasing stallions access to a harem of estrous mares or access to a tease chute or stall prior to collection can increase libido.

- Previous injury from a kick or accident during natural service may result in unwillingness to breed.

> - Slowly reintroducing these stallions to calm, quiet mares in good standing heat will facilitate their reintroduction into the breeding shed.
> - The use of valium in nervous or timid stallions will often increase their libido and willingness to breed.

- The presence of a more dominant stallion within view of a subordinate, or younger, stallion breeding a mare may lead to intimidation and refusal to breed.

> - On the other hand, allowing a young, timid stallion to watch more experienced stallions breed mares, may help improve the young stallion's willingness to breed.

Organic causes of sexual dysfunction

- Orthopedic disease (e.g. painful hind limb joints or musculoskeletal back pain).
- Systemic disease.
- Chronic debilitating diseases.
- Parasitism.
- Neurological disease.
- Vascular disease.
- Endocrine imbalance.
  - ❑ Impotent stallions may have low blood concentrations of chorionic gonadotropin and 17β-estradiol.

> Note:
> - It is important to be patient when training or retraining stallions.
> - Short sessions with positive reinforcement are imperative.
> - When a problem arises efforts should be made to establish if the problem is physical or psychological.
>   - ❑ Physical problems should be treated promptly and the stallion returned to breeding as soon as practicable.
>   - ❑ Psychological problems also must be dealt with in a timely manner before negative behavior is reinforced and retraining is more difficult.
> - Abnormal behavior in the breeding shed is often due to a combination of factors.
> - The abnormal behavior may start with a physical or hormonal cause and then be reinforced with psychological ones.
> - Each problem must be addressed before normal breeding behavior will return.

Masturbation

- Masturbation is *not* a vice; it is best regarded as normal sexual behavior and should not be discouraged.
- Stallions rarely ejaculate when masturbating, so the myth that semen is wasted by allowing masturbation to occur is not true.
- Masturbation may increase in stallions that are bored, so all breeding stallions should get adequate exercise and turn-out time.
- Providing a companion (e.g. a goat, pregnant mare in next stall) to a stallion that cannot receive adequate exercise will reduce boredom.

Self-mutilation

- Stallions in the breeding shed that can smell the semen of other stallions may begin to self-mutilate.[158]
- Affected stallions will bite and chew at the flanks (or any other part of their anatomy) either persistently or intermittently.
- The skin damage is often mistaken for pruritus (itchiness).
- The horse can usually be distracted from self-mutilating by minimal interference until it becomes a neurosis.
- Neuroses or habits can be difficult to manage. Prevention of boredom and sufficient exercise are helpful.
- Regular breeding will also help.
- 'Toys' such as a ball or rubber tire in the stable can help.

Effects of pharmacological agents on spermatogenesis and behavior[159]

- Medications administered may adversely affect spermatogenesis or sexual behavior.
- The changes noted in the spermiogram may be characteristic for a specific drug.
- In some cases, the effects of a drug are well known for the male species while other medications have unknown or uncertain effects.
- Some individuals are more sensitive to the effects of certain drugs than are others.
- In many cases, the side-effects of a certain drug are extrapolated from other species. Whether the same types of changes will be seen in the stallion may be unknown.

- Alterations in spermatogenesis may be seen as sub- or infertility, or may not be noted at all if they are not severe.
- Changes in testicular size, shape or tone may be noted.

- Alterations in behavior may range from increased aggressiveness to lack of libido.
- Circulating hormone concentrations may also be affected.

Drugs that affect the rapidly dividing germ cells include:

- Chemotherapeutic agents such as cyclophosphamide and doxorubicin.
- Cytotoxic and antimitotic agents such as cisplatin may harm sperm production.
- Alkylating agents and colchicine.
- Radiation may also affect the germ cells.[160]

Alterations are seen as a decrease in total sperm per ejaculate. Some changes in morphology may also be noted. The reserve spermatogonia are usually spared since they do not divide actively and may replenish the tubules once the treatment is concluded.

Medications that affect the Sertoli cells include:

- Chemicals such as dinitrobenzene and diphthalate. These drugs affect the function of the Sertoli cells and therefore indirectly will affect spermatogenesis since they are the support cells of the germinal epithelium.

The Leydig cells may have diminished steroid production following the administration of steroids or anabolic agents. This can result in decreased circulating testosterone and abnormal sexual interest.

Effects of testosterone

- Administration of exogenous steroids containing testosterone will result in high concentrations of testosterone in the circulation.[161,162] This results in negative feedback on the hypothalamus and pituitary.
- Decreases in gonadotropin-releasing hormone and subsequently follicle-stimulating hormone and luteinizing hormone will result in a lack of secretion of testosterone from the Leydig cells.
- Since the Leydig cells do not secrete testosterone the intratesticular testosterone secretion is significantly lowered, resulting in derangement (to cessation) of spermatogenesis.
- Estrogen production by the testicle will be similarly affected.
- Changes in spermatogenesis may be noted within 75 days of the start of treatment.

- **These changes are reversible in nature, taking from 3 months to years for complete recovery depending on the length of treatment, the dose used and the type of drug administered.**

Effects of anabolic steroids

- Administration of anabolic steroids such as boldenone undecylenate (Equipoise), stanozolol (Winstrol-V) and nandrolone decanoate (Deca-Durabolin) will result in:
  - ❏ Decreased total scrotal width.
  - ❏ Decreased semen concentration and sperm motility.
  - ❏ Changes in sperm morphology.[163]
- These changes are usually reversible with adequate time.
- Decreases in circulating testosterone concentrations will result in diminished libido.

- For these reasons, the use of exogenous steroids and anabolic agents is contraindicated in breeding stallions, or in those stallions that may have future reproductive use.

REFERENCES

1. Dyce KM, Sack WO, Wensing CJG. Textbook of veterinary anatomy. Philadelphia, PA: WB Saunders; 1987.
2. Sack WO, Habel RE. Guide to the dissection of the horse. Ithaca, NY: Veterinary Textbooks, 1982.
3. Dellman HD, Brown EM. Textbook of veterinary histology. Philadelphia, PA: Lea & Febiger; 1987.
4. Little TV, Holyoak GR. Reproductive anatomy and physiology of the stallion. Veterinary Clinics of North America: Equine Practice 1992; 8(1):1–30.
5. Setchell BP. The mammalian testis. Ithaca, NY: Cornell University Press; 1978.
6. Russell LD, Griswold MD, eds. The Sertoli cell. Clearwater, FL: Cache River Press; 1993.
7. Payne AH, Hardy MP, Russell LD. The Leydig cell. Vienna, IL: Cache River Press; 1996.
8. Berndtson WE, Squires EL, Thompson DL. Spermatogenesis, testicular composition and the concentration of testosterone in the equine testis as influenced by season. Theriogenology 1983; 20:449–457.
9. Johnson L, Tatum ME. Sequence of seasonal changes in numbers of Sertoli, Leydig, and germ cells in adult stallions. Proceedings of the Eleventh International Congress on Animal Reproduction and Artificial Insemination, Dublin 1988:373.
10. Clay CM, Squires EL, Amann RP, et al. Influences of season and artificial photoperiod on stallions: testicular size, seminal characteristics and sexual behavior. Journal of Animal Science 1987; 64:517–525.
11. Stickle RL, Fessler JF. Retrospective study of 350 cases of equine cryptorchidism. Journal of the American Veterinary Medical Association 1978; 172:343–346.
12. Bergin WC, Gier HT, Marion GB, et al. A developmental concept of equine cryptorchidism. Biology of Reproduction 1970; 3:82–92.
13. Cox JE, Edwards GB, Neal P. An analysis of 500 cases

of equine cryptorchidism. Equine Veterinary Journal 1979; 11:113–116.
14. Cox JE. Cryptorchid castration. In: McKinnon AE, Voss JL, eds. Equine reproduction. Philadelphia, PA: Lea & Febiger; 1993.
15. Naden J, Amann RP, Squires EL. Testicular growth, hormone concentrations, seminal characteristics and sexual behavior in stallions. Journal of Reproduction and Fertility Supplement 1990; 88:167–176.
16. Naden J, Amann RP, Squires EL. Testicular growth, hormone concentrations, seminal characteristics and sexual behavior in stallions. Journal of Reproduction and Fertility Supplement 1990; 88:167–176.
17. Amann RP. Endocrine changes associated with the onset of spermatogenesis in Holstein bulls. Journal of Dairy Science 1983; 66:2606–2622.
18. Amann RP. Physiology and endocrinology. In: McKinnon AE, Voss JL, eds. Equine reproduction. Philadelphia, PA: Lea & Febiger; 1993.
19. Purvis K, Hansson V. Hormonal regulation of spermatogenesis. International Journal of Andrology Supplement 1981; 3:81–143.
20. Bedrak E, Samuels LT. Steroid biosynthesis by the equine testis. Endocrinology 1969; 85:1186–1195.
21. Russell LD, Griswold MD, eds. The Sertoli cell. Clearwater, FL: Cache River Press; 1993.
22. Payne AH, Hardy MP, Russell LD. The Leydig cell. Vienna, IL: Cache River Press, 1996.
23. Raeside JI. Seasonal changes in the concentration of estrogens and testosterone in the plasma of the stallion. Animal Reproductive Science 1979; 1:205–212.
24. Johnson L. Spermatogenesis. In: Cupps PT, ed. Reproduction in domestic animals. 4th edn. New York: Academic Press; 1990:173–219.
25. Swiestra EE, Pickett BW, Gebauer MR. Spermatogenesis and duration of transit of spermatozoa through the excurrent ducts of stallions. Journal of Reproduction and Fertility Supplement 1975; 23:53–57.
26. Berndtson WE, Squires EL, Thompson DL. Spermatogenesis, testicular composition and the concentration of testosterone in the equine testis as influenced by season. Theriogenology 1983; 20:449–457.
27. Johnson L, Tatum ME. Sequence of seasonal changes in numbers of Sertoli, Leydig and germ cells in adult stallions. Proceedings of the 11th International Congress on Animal Reproduction and Artificial Insemination Dublin 1988:373–374.
28. Johnson L, Thompson DL. Age-related and seasonal variation in the Sertoli cell population, daily sperm production and serum concentrations of follicle-stimulating hormone, luteinizing hormone and testosterone in stallions. Biology of Reproduction 1983; 29:777–789.
29. Johnson L, Neaves WB. Age-related changes in the Leydig cell population, seminiferous tubules and sperm production in stallions. Biology of Reproduction 1981; 24:703–712.
30. Johnson L, Varner DD, Thompson DL. Effect of age and season on the establishment of spermatogenesis in the horse. Journal of Reproduction and Fertility Supplement 1991; 44:87–97.
31. Johnson L. Spermatogenesis. In: Cupps PT, ed.

Reproduction in domestic animals. 4th edn. New York: Academic Press; 1990:173–219.

32. Harrison RG. Effect of temperature on the mammalian testis. In: Hamilton DW, Greep RO, eds. Handbook of physiology, Vol 5. Washington, DC: American Physiology Society; 1975:219–233.

33. Harrison RG. Effect of temperature on the mammalian testis. In: Hamilton DW, Greep RO, eds. Handbook of physiology, Vol 5. Washington, DC: American Physiology Society; 1975:219–233.

34. Austin JW, Hupp EW, Murphree RL. Effect of scrotal insulation on semen of Hereford bulls. Journal of Animal Science 1961; 20:307–310.

35. Tischner M, Kosiniak K, Bielanski W. Analysis of the pattern of ejaculation in stallions. Journal of Reproduction and Fertility Supplement 1974; 41:329–335.

36. McDonnell SM. Ejaculation: physiology and dysfunction. Veterinary Clinics of North America: Equine Practice 1992; 8:57–70.

37. Pickett BW, Faulkener LC, Seidel GE, et al. Reproductive physiology of the stallion. VI. Seminal and behavioral characteristics. Journal of Animal Science 1976; 43:617–625.

38. Varner DD, Schumacher J, Blanchard TL, et al. In: Diseases and management of breeding stallions. Goleta, CA: American Veterinary Publications; 1991.

39. Clay CM, Squires EL, Amann RP, et al. Influences of season and artificial photoperiod on stallions: testicular size, seminal characteristics and sexual behavior. Journal of Animal Science 1987; 64:517–525.

40. Burns PJ, Jawad MJ, Weld JM, et al. Effects of season, age and increased photoperiod on reproductive hormone concentrations and testicular diameters in Thoroughbred stallions. Journal of Equine Veterinary Science 1984; 4:202–208.

41. Gebauer MR, Pickett BW, Swierstra EE. Reproductive physiology of the stallion. III. Extra-gonadal transit time and sperm reserves. Journal of Animal Science 1974; 39:737–742.

42. Amann RP, Thompson DL Jr, Squires EL, et al. Effect of age and frequency of ejaculation on sperm production and extragonadal sperm reserves in stallions. Journal of Reproduction and Fertility Supplement 1979; 27:1–6.

43. Squires EL, Pickett BW, Amann RP. Effect of successive ejaculation on stallion seminal characteristics. Journal of Reproduction and Fertility Supplement 1979; 27:7–12

44. Pickett BW, Neil JR, Squires EL. The effect of ejaculation frequency on stallion sperm output. Proceedings of the Ninth Equine Nutrition and Physiology Society Symposium 1985:290–295.

45. Squires EL, Pickett BW, Amann RP. Effect of successive ejaculation on stallion seminal characteristics. Journal of Reproduction and Fertility Supplement 1979; 27:7–12.

46. Amann RP, Thompson DL Jr, Squires EL, et al. Effect of age and frequency of ejaculation on sperm production and extragonadal sperm reserves in stallions. Journal of Reproduction and Fertility Supplement 1979; 27:1–6.

47. Kenney RM, Hurtgen J, Pierson R. Manual for clinical fertility evaluation of the stallion. Manual of the Society for Theriogenology 1983:97–100.

48. Hurtgen JP. Breeding soundness evaluation of the stallion. Proceedings of the Nineteenth Bain-Fallon Memorial Lectures. New South Wales: Australian Equine Veterinary Association; 1997:1–8.

49. Amann RP. A review of anatomy and physiology of the stallion. Equine Veterinary Science 1983; May/June: 83–105.

50. Picket BW. Factors affecting sperm production and output. In: McKinnon AO, Voss JL, eds. Equine reproduction. Philadelphia, PA: Lea & Febiger; 1993:689–704.

51. Varner DD, Shumacher J, Blanchard TL, et al. Diseases and management of breeding stallions. Goleta, CA: American Veterinary Publications; 1991.

52. Little TW, Woods GL. Ultrasonography of accessory sex glands in the stallion. Journal of Reproduction and Fertility Supplement 1987; 35:87–94.

53. Pozor MA, McDonnell SM. Ultrasound evaluation of stallion accessory sex glands. Proceedings of the Annual Meeting of the Society for Theriogenology 1996:294–297.

54. Cox JE. Surgery of the reproductive tract in large animals. Liverpool: University of Liverpool Press.

55. Sack O, Habel RE. Rooney's guide to the dissection of the horse. Ithaca, NY: Veterinary Textbooks; 1982:65–70.

56. Weber JA, Woods GL. Transrectal ultrasonography for the evaluation of the stallion accessory sex glands. Veterinary Clinics of North America: Equine Practice 1992; 8:183–190.

57. Love CC. Ultrasonographic evaluation of the testes, epididymis and spermatic cord of the stallion. Veterinary Clinics of North America: Equine Practice 1992; 8:167–182.

58. Samper JC. Diseases of the male system. In: Kobluk CN, Ames TR, Geor RJ, eds. The horse. Philadelphia, PA: WB Saunders; 1995:947–955.

59. Hillman RB, Olar TT, Squires EL, et al. Temperature of the artificial vagina and its effect on seminal quality and behavioral characteristics of stallions. Journal of the American Veterinary Association 1980; 177:720–722.

60. Cooper WC. The effect of rapid temperature changes on oxygen uptake by and motility of stallion spermatozoa. Proceedings of the Society of Theriogenology 1979:10–13.

61. McDonnell SM, Love CC. Manual stimulation collection of semen from stallions: training time, sexual behavior and semen. Theriogenology 1990; 33:1201–1210.

62. Crump J Jr, Crump J. Stallion ejaculation induced by manual stimulation of the penis. Theriogenology 1989; 31:341–346.

63. McDonnell SM, Love CC. Xylazine-induced ex copula ejaculation in stallions. Theriogenology 1991; 36:73–76.

64. McDonnell SM, Garcia MC, Kenney RM, et al. Imipramine-induced erection, masturbation, and ejaculation in male horses. Pharmacology and Biochemistry of Behavior 1987; 27:187–191.

65. Varner DD, Schumacher J, Blanchard TL, et al. In: Diseases and management of breeding stallions. Goleta, CA: American Veterinary Publications; 1991.

66. Douglas-Hamilton DH, Osol R, Osol G. A field study of the fertility of transported equine semen. Theriogenology 1984; 22:291–304.

67. Householder DD, Pickett BW, Voss JL, et al. Effect of extender, number of spermatozoa and HCG on equine fertility. Journal of Equine Veterinary Science 1981; 1:9–13.

68. Province CA, Squires EL, Pickett BW, et al. Cooling rates, storage temperatures and fertility of extended equine spermatozoa. Theriogenology 1985; 23:925–934.

69. Pickett BW, Sullivan JJ, Byer WW, et al. Effect of centrifugation and seminal plasma on motility and fertility of stallion and bull spermatozoa. Fertility and Sterility 1975; 26:167–174.

70. Jasko DJ. Evaluation of stallion semen. Veterinary Clinics of North America: Equine Practice 1992; 8:129–148.

71. Varner DD, Schumacher J, Blanchard TL, et al. In: Diseases and management of breeding stallions. Goleta, CA: American Veterinary Publications; 1991.

72. Kenney RM. Clinical fertility evaluation of the stallion. Proceedings of the American Association of Equine Practitioners 1975:336–355.

73. Codes of practice on infectious diseases. London: Horserace Betting Levy Board; 2000:1–17.

74. White IG, Wales RG. The susceptibility of spermatozoa to cold shock. International Journal of Fertility 1960; 5:195–201.

75. Watson PF. The effects of cold shock on sperm cell membranes. In: Morris GJ, Clark A, eds. Effects of low temperature on biological membranes. New York: Academic Press; 1981:189–218.

76. Squires EL, Amann RP, McKinnon AO, et al. Fertility of equine spermatozoa cooled to 5 or 20°C. Proceedings of the International Congress of Animal Reproduction and Artificial Insemination 1988; 3:297–299.

77. Katila T, Combes GB, Varner DD, et al. Comparison of three containers used for the transport of cooled stallion semen. Theriogenology 1997; 48:1085–1092.

78. Cochran JP, Amann RP, Froman DP, et al. Effects of centrifugation, glycerol level, cooling to 5°C, freezing rate and thawing rate on post thaw motility of equine spermatozoa. Theriogenology 1984; 22:25–38.

79. Watson PF. The effects of cold shock on sperm cell membranes. In: Morris GJ, Clark A, eds. Effects of low temperature on biological membranes. New York: Academic Press; 1981:189–218.

80. Amann RP, Pickett BW. Principles of cryopreservation and a review of cryopreservation of stallion spermatozoa. Journal of Equine Veterinary Science 1987; 7:145–173.

81. Blach EL, Amann RP, Bowen RA, et al. Changes in quality of stallion spermatozoa during cryopreservation: plasma membrane integrity and motion characteristics. Theriogenology 1989; 31:283–298.

82. Hammerstedt RH, Crichton EG, Watson PF. Comparative approach to sperm cryopreservation: Does cell shape and size influence cryosurvival? Proceedings of the Society of Theriogenology San Diego 1991:8–11.

83. Demick DS, Voss JL, Pickett BW. Effect of cooling, storage, glycerolization and spermatozoal number on equine fertility. Journal of Animal Science 1975; 43:633–637.

84. Hammerstedt RH, Crichton EG, Watson PF. Comparative approach to sperm cryopreservation: Does cell shape and size influence cryosurvival? Proceedings of the Society of Theriogenology San Diego 1991:8–11.

85. Sullivan JJ. Characteristics and cryopreservation of stallion spermatozoa. Cryobiology 1978; 15:355–357.

86. Pace MM. Sullivan JJ. Effect of timing of insemination, numbers of spermatozoa and extender components on the pregnancy rate in mares inseminated with frozen stallion semen. Journal of Reproduction and Fertility Supplement 1975; 23:115–121.

87. Volkmann DH, Van Zyl D. Fertility of stallion semen frozen in 0.5 ml straws. Journal of Reproduction and Fertility Supplement 1987; 35:143–148.

88. Tischner M. Evaluation of deep-frozen semen in stallions. Journal of Reproduction and Fertility Supplement 1979; 27:53–59.

89. Klug E, Treu H, Hillmann H, et al. Results of insemination of mares with fresh and frozen stallion semen. Journal of Reproduction and Fertility Supplement 1975; 23:107–110.

90. Nishikawa Y, Shinomiya S. Freezability of horse semen collected during the nonbreeding season. Proceedings of the International Congress on Animal Reproduction and Artificial Insemination 1972:1539–1543.

91. Magistrini M, Chanteloube P, Palmer E. Influence of season and frequency of ejaculation on production of stallion semen for freezing. Journal of Reproduction and Fertility Supplement 1987; 35:127–133.

92. Kloppe LH, Varner DD, Elmore RG, et al. Effect of insemination timing on the fertilizing capacity of frozen/thawed equine spermatozoa. Theriogenology 1988; 29:429–439.

93. Woods J, Bergfelt DR, Ginther OJ. Effects of time of insemination relative to ovulation on pregnancy rate and embryonic loss rate in mares. Equine Veterinary Journal 1990; 22:410–415.

94. Pickett BW, Amann RP. Cryopreservation of semen. In: McKinnon AE, Voss JL, eds. Equine reproduction. Philadelphia, PA: Lea & Febiger; 1993:769–789.

95. Ley WB. Method of predicting stallion to mare ratio for natural and artificial insemination programs. Journal of Equine Veterinary Science 1985; 5:143–146.

96. Amann RP, Thompson DL, Squires EL, et al. Effect of age and frequency of ejaculation on sperm production and extragonadal sperm reserves in stallions. Journal of Reproduction and Fertility Supplement 1979; 27:1–6.

97. Pickett BW, Anderson EW, Roberts AD, et al. Management of the stallion for maximum reproductive efficiency, II. Fort Collins, CO: Colorado State University Animal Reproduction Laboratory Bulletin 05; 1989.

98. Rossdale PD, Ricketts SW. Equine stud farm medicine. 2nd edn. London: Baillière Tindall; 1980:33.

99. Kikuchi N, Iguchi I, Hiramune T. Capsule types of *Klebsiella pneumoniae* isolated from the genital tract of mares with metritis, extra-genital sites of healthy mares and the genital tract of stallions. Veterinary Microbiology 1987; 15:219–228.

100. Bowen JM, Tobin N, Simpson RB, et al. Effects of

washing on the bacterial flora of the stallion's penis. Journal of Reproduction and Fertility Supplement 1982; 32:41–45.

101. Jones RL. The effect of washing on the aerobic bacterial flora of the stallion's penis. Proceedings of the American Association of Equine Practitioners 1984:9–16.

102. Blanchard TL, Verner DD, Hurtgen JP, et al. Bilateral seminal vesiculitis and ampullitis in a stallion. Journal of the American Veterinary Medical Association 1988; 192:525–526.

103. Cooper WC. Methods of determining the site of bacterial infections in the stallion reproductive tract. Proceedings of the Society for Theriogenology 1979:1–4.

104. Little TV, Woods GL. Ultrasonography of accessory sex glands in the stallion. Journal of Reproduction and Fertility Supplement 1987; 35:87–94.

105. Weber JA, Woods GL. Ultrasonographic studies of accessory sex glands in sexually rested stallions and bulls, sexually active stallions, and a diseased bull. Proceedings of the Society for Theriogenology 1989:157–165.

106. Klug E, Deegan E, Liesk R, et al. The effect of vesiculectomy on seminal characteristics in the stallion. Journal of Reproduction and Fertility Supplement 1979; 27:61–66.

107. Blanchard TL, Varner DD, Love CC, et al. Use of a semen extender containing antibiotic to improve the fertility of a stallion with seminal vesiculitis due to *Pseudomonas aeruginosa*. Theriogenology 1987; 28:541–546.

108. Varner DD, Schumacher J. Diseases of the scrotum. In: Colahan PT, Merritt AM, Moore JN, et al., eds. Equine medicine and surgery. 5th edn. Mosby, Philadelphia, PA: Mosby; 1999:1034–1035.

109. Kieffer NM. Male pseudohermaphroditism of the testicular feminizing type in a horse. Equine Veterinary Journal 1976; 8:38–41.

110. Kent MG, Shoffner RN, Buoen L, et al. XY sex-reversal syndrome in the domestic horse. Cytogenetics and Cell Genetics 1986; 42:8–18.

111. Hughes JP, Asbury AC, Loy RG, et al. The occurrence of *Pseudomonas* in the genital tract of stallions and its effect on fertility. Cornell Veterinarian 1967; 57:53–59.

112. Clem MF, DeBowes RM. Paraphimosis in horses – Part I. Compendium of Continuing Education for the Practicing Veterinarian 1989; 11:72–75.

113. Clem MF, DeBowes RM. Paraphimosis in horses – Part II. Compendium of Continuing Education for the Practicing Veterinarian 1989; 11:184–187.

114. Carr JP, Hughes JP. Penile paralysis in a Quarter horse stallion. California Veterinarian 1984; 13:16–18.

115. Walker DF, Vaughan JT. Bovine and equine urogenital surgery. Philadelphia, PA: Lea & Febiger, 1980.

116. Pearson H, Weaver BM. Priapism after sedation, neuroleptanalgesia and anaesthesia in the horse. Equine Veterinary Journal 1978; 10:85–90.

117. Larsen RE. The stallion. In: Mansmann RA, McAllister ES, eds. Equine medicine and surgery. 3rd edn. Santa Barbara, CA: American Veterinary Publications; 1982.

118. Bridges ER. The use of ivermectin to treat genital cutaneous habronemiasis in a stallion. Compendium of Continuing Education for the Practicing Veterinarian 1985; 7:S94–S97.

119. Stick JA. Amputation of the equine urethral process affected with habronemiasis. Veterinary Medicine for the Small Animal Clinician 1979; 74:1453–1457.

120. Voss JL, Pickett BW. Diagnosis and treatment of haemospermia in the stallion. Journal of Reproduction and Fertility Supplement 1975; 23:151–154.

121. Sullins KE, Bertone JJ, Voss JL, et al. Treatment of haemospermia in stallions: a discussion of 18 cases. Compendium of Continuing Education for the Practicing Veterinarian 1988; 10:1396–1403.

122. Voss JL, Pickett BW, Shideler RK. The effect of haemospermia on fertility in horses. Proceedings of the Eighth International Congress of Animal Reproduction, Vol. 4. Krakow; 1976:1093–1095.

123. Voss JL, Pickett BW. Diagnosis and treatment of hemospermia in the stallion. Journal of Reproduction and Fertility Supplement 1975; 23:151–154.

124. Nash JG, Voss JL, Squires EL. Urination during ejaculation in a stallion. Journal of the American Veterinary Medical Association 1980; 176:224–227.

125. Friedman R, Scott M, Heath SE, et al. The effects of increased testicular temperature on spermatogenesis in the stallion. Journal of Reproduction and Fertility Supplement 1991; 44:127–134.

126. McEntee K. The male genital system. In: Jubb KVF, Kennedy PC, eds. Pathology of domestic animals. 3rd edn. New York: Academic Press; 1970.

127. Zhang J, Ricketts SJ, Tanner SJ. Antisperm antibodies in the semen of a stallion following testicular trauma. Equine Veterinary Journal 1990; 22:138–141.

128. Squires EL, Todter, GE, Berndtson WE, et al. Effect of anabolic steroids on reproductive function of young stallions. Journal of Animal Science 1982; 54:576–582.

129. Miskin M, Bain J. Use of diagnostic ultrasound in the evaluation of testicular disorders. Progress in Reproductive Biology 1978; 3:117–130.

130. Finco DR. Biopsy of the testicle. Veterinary Clinics of North America 1974; 4:377–381.

131. Threlfall WR, Lopate C. Testicular biopsy. In: McKinnon AO, Voss JL. Equine reproduction. Philadelphia, PA: Lea & Febiger; 1993:943–949.

132. McEntee K. The male genital system. In: Jubb KVF, Kennedy PC, eds. Pathology of domestic animals. 3rd edn. New York: Academic Press; 1970.

133. Burns PJ, Douglas RH. Reproductive hormone concentrations in stallions with breeding problems: case studies. Equine Veterinary Science 1985; 5:40–42.

134. Roser JF, Hughes JP. Prolonged pulsatile administration of gonadotrophin-releasing hormone (GnRH) to fertile stallions. Journal of Reproduction and Fertility Supplement 1991; 44:155–168.

135. Blue BG, Pickett BW, Squires EL, et al. Effect of pulsatile or continuous administration of GnRH on reproductive function of stallions. Journal of Reproduction and Fertility Supplement 1991; 44:145–154.

136. Leipold HW. Cryptorchidism in the horse: genetic implications. Proceedings of the American Association of Equine Practitioners 1986; 31:579–590.

137. Bishop MWH, David JSE, Merservey A. Some observations on cryptorchidism in the horse. Veterinary Record 1964; 76:1041–1048.

138. Cox JE, Williams JH, Rowe PH, et al. Testosterone in normal, cryptorchid and castrated horses. Equine Veterinary Journal 1973; 5:85–90.

139. Parks AH, Scott EA, Cox JE, et al. Monorchidism in the horse. Equine Veterinary Journal 1989; 21:215–217.

140. Foster AEC. Polyorchidism. Veterinary Record 1952; 64:158.

141. McEntee, K. The male genital system. In: Jubb KVF, Kennedy PC. Pathology of domestic animals. 3rd edn. New York: Academic Press; 1970.

142. Vaughan JT. Surgery of the penis and prepuce. In: Bovine and equine urogenital surgery. Philadelphia, PA: Lea & Febiger; 1980.

143. Schumacher J, Vaughan JT. Surgery of the penis and prepuce. Veterinary Clinics of North America: Equine Practice 1988; 4:473–493.

144. Strafuss AC. Squamous cell carcinoma in horses. Journal of the American Veterinary Medical Association 1976; 168:61–62.

145. Plaut A, Kohn-Speyer AC. The carcinogenic action of smegma. Science 1947; 105:391–392.

146. Goetz TE, Ogilvie GK, Keegan KG, et al. Cimetidine for treatment of melanomas in three horses. Journal of the American Veterinary Medical Association 1990; 196:449–452.

147. Pascoe RR, Knottenbelt DC. Manual of equine dermatology. London: WB Saunders; 1998.

148. McEntee, K. The male genital system. In: Pathology of domestic animals. 3rd edn. New York: Academic Press; 1970.

149. Caron JP, Barber SM, Bailey JV. Equine testicular neoplasia. Compendium of Continuing Education for the Practicing Veterinarian 1985; 7:53–59.

150. Vaillancout D, Fretz P, Orr JP. Seminoma in the horse: report of two cases. Journal of Equine Medicine and Surgery 1979; 3:213–218.

151. Smith HA. Interstitial cell tumor of the equine testis. Journal of the American Veterinary Medical Association 1954; 124:356–357.

152. Rahaley RS, Gordon BJ, Leiopold HW, et al. Sertoli cell tumor in a horse. Equine Veterinary Journal 1983; 15:68–69.

153. Trigo FJ, Miller RA, Torbeck RL. Metastatic equine seminoma: report of two cases. Veterinary Pathology 1984; 21:259–300.

154. Nachtsheim DA, Scheible FW, Nachtsheim D, et al. High resolution ultrasonography of scrotal pathology. Radiology 1979; 131:719–722.

155. Hoagland TA. Effects of unilateral castration on morphological characteristics of the testis in one-, two-, and three-year old stallions. Theriogenology 1986; 26:397–405.

156. Krane RJ, Goldstein I, Tejada IS. Impotence. New England Journal of Medicine 1989; 321:1648–1659.

157. Pickett BW. Sexual behavior. In: McKinnon AO, Voss JL, eds. Equine reproduction. Philadelphia, PA: Lea & Febiger; 1992:812–813.

158. Mayhew IG. Large animal neurology. Philadelphia, PA: Lea & Febiger; 1980.

159. Mattison DR, Thomford PJ. Mechanism of action of reproductive toxicants. In: Working PK, ed. Toxicity of the male and female reproductive systems. New York: Hemisphere Publishing; 1989:101–129.

160. Oakberg EF. Irradiation damage to animals and its effect on their reproductive capacity. Journal of Dairy Science Supplement 1960; 43:54–64.

161. Berndtson WE, Hoyer JH, Squires IL, et al. Influence of exogenous testosterone on sperm production, seminal quality and libido of stallions. Journal of Reproduction and Fertility Supplement 1979; 27:19–23.

162. Squires EL, Berndtson WE, Hoyer JH, et al. Restoration of reproductive capacity in stallions after suppression with exogenous testosterone. Journal of Animal Science 1981; 53:1351–1359.

163. Blanchard TL et al. The effects of stanozolol and boldenone undecylenate on scrotal width, testis weight, and sperm production in pony stallions. Theriogenology 1983; 20:121–131.

Chapter 5
THE MARE

Michelle LeBlanc,
Cheryl Lopate,
Derek Knottenbelt,
Reg Pascoe

REPRODUCTIVE ANATOMY OF THE FEMALE GENITAL TRACT

A thorough understanding of the mare's reproductive anatomy is needed to differentiate normal from abnormal, and to identify structures during reproductive examinations. In this section important anatomical considerations are reviewed. The main structures of the breeding organs of the mare are shown in Fig. 5.1.

The perineum is the area that includes the anus, vulva and the adjacent skin (usually hairless) under the tail. The normal conformation of the perineum prevents the ingress of air and bacteria into the genital tract. This area is very important because of its protective role for the genital tract and its implications in some forms of infertility in particular. It is also a common site for injury at parturition. The anatomic arrangement of the perineum, including its length relative to the pelvic bones and its angle relative to the vertical plane, are important features for the fertility of the mare; for example, mares that experience bouts of infertility frequently have a flat-topped croup with a tail setting that is level with the sacral iliac joint and a sunken anus (Fig. 5.2). Alterations of angle and length have been used to determine a Caslick score[1] (see p. 185) which is used to provide an index of the need to perform a vulvoplasty operation (Caslick's operation, see p. 184). The normal/ideal anatomic arrangement is that the vulva should be vertical (or at least less than 10% from the vertical) and that more than 80% of its length (from dorsal commissure top ventral commissure) should lie below the level of the ischial tuberosities (Figs 5.3, 5.4). Variations in either the relative length below the ischium or an increase in the angle of declination (or both) results in a tendency for the vulva to be drawn forwards into the perineum below the anus, especially during later pregnancy (Fig. 5.5). This combination results in an increased chance of aspiration of air into the vagina and a higher Caslick score.

Three seals protect the genital tract:

- The vulvar seal (created by close contact between the vulvar lips or labiae and the skin and muscles of the perineum).
- The vestibulovaginal seal (formed by the posterior vagina, the pillars of the hymen and the floor of the pelvic girdle).
- The cervix, which acts as a final barrier for the uterus.

Any deficiency in one or more of these 'seals' has implications for the reproductive efficiency of the mare. During a normal reproductive examination these seals are broken and air allowed into the vagina. The presence of air in the vagina allows bacteria to be carried into the anterior reproductive

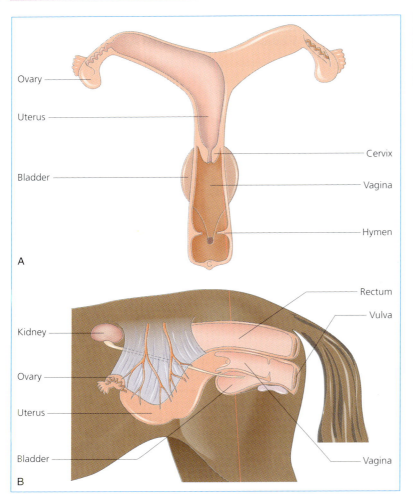

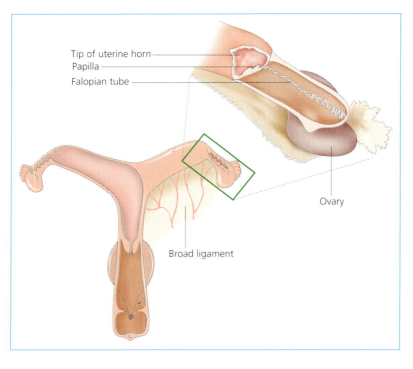

Fig. 5.1 Reproductive organs of the mare: (A) left lateral view; (B) viewed from above; (C) detail of the falopian tube region and the relationship of the horn of the uterus to the broad ligament.

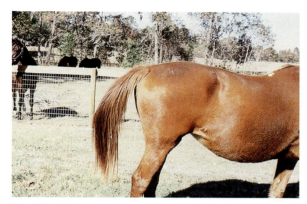

Fig. 5.2   Flat-crouped mare.

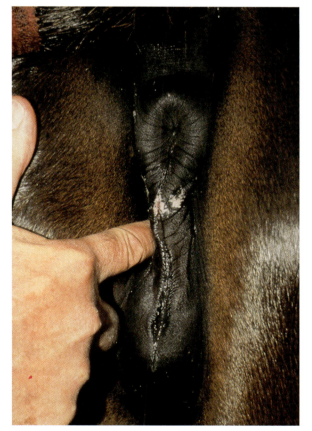

Fig. 5.3   Evaluating perineal conformation in a normal mare.

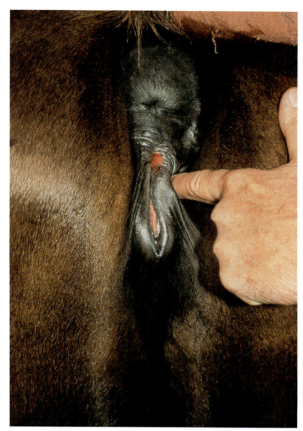

Fig. 5.4   Evaluating perineal conformation in a mare with poor conformation.

and vestibulovaginal seals usually restrict the ingress of clinically significant bacteria. The vagina and uterus should be free of significant infection although some incidental bacteria are commonly found.[2]

- Simply gently parting the lips of the vulva and listening for aspiration of air into the vagina can test the integrity of the vestibulovaginal seal.
- Normally the vestibulovaginal seal will maintain an airtight seal when the lips of vulva are parted in this way. In-rushing air suggests poor vestibulovaginal seal efficiency.

tract. The presence of the air itself is responsible for a typical inflammatory response with blood vessel engorgement. When any of the three seals are disrupted (either through trauma, faulty acquired or congenitally poor perineal conformation, or poor body condition) air may be intermittently or consistently aspirated into the vagina and the resulting contamination and infection can be a serious cause of infertility. The vulvar

Vulva and vestibule

The vulva comprises the two vulvar lips (labiae) (and the clitoris) and is one region of the reproductive tract that is in common with the urinary system. The two vulvar lips meet dorsally at the tightly angled dorsal commissure and ventrally at the more

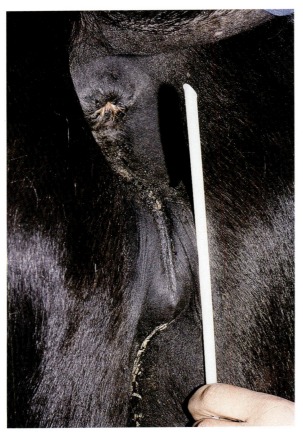

Fig. 5.5 An example of very poor vulvar conformation. The upper half of the vulva slopes forward and is almost horizontal. The anus is drawn forward.

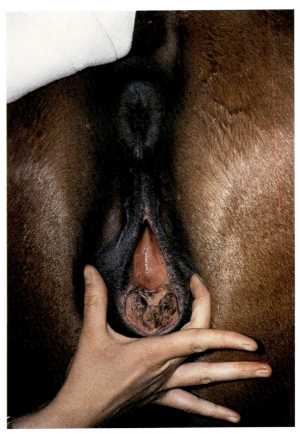

Fig. 5.6 The clitoris is visible in the ventral vulvar commissure.

rounded ventral commissure. Just inside the lips themselves lies the junction between the highly glandular skin and the nonglandular mucous membrane of the vestibule (the area of the reproductive tract that lies outside the level of the vestibulovaginal seal/hymen). The mucocutaneous junction is continuous with the clitoral prepuce or fold. The vulvar constrictor muscle continues into the external anal sphincter dorsally. The clitoral retractor muscle lies over the vulvar constrictor muscle ventrally. These muscles are variously responsible for the protective function of the vulva and the winking of the clitoris that occurs at the end of urination and during estrus, and the arrangement allows considerable expansion during delivery of the foal.

The vestibule is the tubular portion of the tract between the lips of the vulva and the vestibulovaginal seal. The lateral and ventral walls contain the strong vestibular constrictor muscles. The vestibular wall and the muscles of the anus create the roof. The external urethral orifice lies on the ventral floor of the mid-vestibular region.

- The vulvar lips should be vertically orientated and approximately two-thirds of the vulvar cleft should lie below the level of the ischial arch.
- The anus should not be located anterior to the dorsal commissure of the vulva.
- There should be no aspiration of air into the vagina (vaginal wind-sucking) during normal exercise. If this occurs it suggests a poor vulvar seal and an inefficient vestibulovaginal seal.

Clitoris

The erectile clitoris of the mare is held in a protective pouch (the clitoral prepuce) just inside the ventral commissure of the vulva. It can readily be everted by gentle manual pressure applied across the ventral commissure of the vulva (Fig. 5.6). This process reveals the clitoral glans itself, which has a wrinkled appearance in most mares. The clitoris lies in the clitoral fossa created by the clitoral prepuce and it is common to encounter an accumulation of moist smegma in this area. On the crown of the clitoris are three depressions (the clitoral sinuses) with a deep central sinus and two smaller, shallower lateral sinuses. All of these commonly harbor a variable amount of smegma derived from the clitoral sebaceous glands.

The clitoral sinuses and fossa have considerable importance in the investigation of venereal disease. Bacteriological swabs are routinely taken from the clitoral sinuses and from the clitoral fossa (see p. 152).

Vagina

The vagina is the portion of the reproductive tract between the vestibulovaginal seal and the cervix. The cervix projects into the vagina at its anterior aspect. The vaginal walls need to be able to dilate sufficiently to allow delivery of the foal, so any scarring or distortion may be significant. Accumulation of air (pneumovagina), urine (urovagina), or both, in the anterior vagina is a common cause of infertility and results from some abnormality of the anatomical arrangement of the more caudal structures. Normally the vaginal walls are closely applied and there is little or no bacterial or other contamination. Examination of the vagina by manual palpation or by vaginal speculum results in a rapid (usually transient) inflammation of the vaginal walls.

Cervix

The cervix is a muscular structure 5–7.5 cm long and about 2–5 cm in diameter. It is a very important structure for reproductive efficiency. It projects some 2.5–4.0 cm into the anterior vagina. It forms the final barrier to the ingress of contamination and infection. During estrus it dilates to allow the passage of semen into the uterus and at this time it is easily dilated manually. An operator should easily be able to pass one or two fingers through its entirety during estrus. During diestrus and pregnancy the cervix is firm and tightly closed and it is difficult to dilate manually. During parturition it has to dilate very considerably; failure to dilate sufficiently during delivery of the foal at parturition can result in traumatic laceration (see p. 303). The surface of the cervix is a delicate mucous membrane that is easily traumatized by strong chemicals.

Adhesions and damage are important causes of infertility (see p. 174). Examination of the cervix usually involves manual palpation per vaginum and visualization using a speculum or endoscope (see p. 136).

Uterus and broad ligaments

The uterus is a T-shaped structure. The two uterine horns and body are located entirely within the caudal part of the abdominal cavity. Distension and movement of the intestines and bladder as well as pregnancy influence the position of the reproductive tract.[3] The uterine horns range from 20 to 25 cm in length. The uterine body averages 18–20 cm in length.

The uterus is suspended within the abdomen by two large broad ligaments that extend along the lateral sublumbar and lateral pelvic walls from the third or fourth lumbar vertebra to the level of the fourth sacral vertebra. These ligaments serve as attachments to the body wall and support blood vessels, lymphatic vessels, and nerves. The broad ligaments also contain a large amount of smooth muscle that is continuous with the outer longitudinal muscular layer of the uterus and oviducts. Although the broad ligaments are a continuous sheet they are commonly divided into three nondemarcated areas:

- The mesometrium, attaching to the uterus.
- The mesosalpinx, attaching to the oviducts.
- The mesovarium, attaching to the ovaries.

Cystic remnants of mesonephric tubules and ducts (epoöphoron and paraoöphoron) occur commonly in the mesovarium and mesosalpinx.

The ovaries

The ovaries are kidney-shaped with a very prominent depression (the ovulation fossa) on the free or ventral border. The ovary has two surfaces (lateral and medial), two borders (dorsal or attached and ventral or free), and two poles (cranial and caudal). These are used in the description of normal and pathological changes.

The mare's ovaries are larger than those of other domestic species and vary considerably in size during the year depending on the number and size of follicles on their surface. During reproductive quiescence, the ovaries may be the size of walnuts. During the cyclic season when there is a 50-mm follicle on the ovary, it may be the size of a large orange. On cut section, there may be follicles in different stages of development and atresia. There may be a developing or regressing corpus luteum along with remnants of corpora lutea of previous cycles; 10–12 days later, the appearance of the same ovary will have completely changed.

- It is extremely important, therefore, to record all palpable and ultrasonographic findings during reproductive examinations (see p. 134).

The ovaries can move freely within the abdomen, thus their orientation and location are variable, making it difficult to identify poles and surfaces. The mesovarium attaches at the dorsal aspect of the ovary and extends for a considerable distance over the medial and lateral surfaces. Blood vessels and nerves reach the ovaries through the broad ligaments and enter each ovary at the dorsal convex border and spread over the lateral and medial surfaces.

The equine ovary is unique in its internal structure. Unlike other organs that have the cortical area as the outer portion or external layer and the medulla in the center, the adult equine ovary has the opposite arrangement. The medullary (vascular) zone is superficial and the cortical zone that contains the oocytes and follicles is partially within the interior of the gland. The cortex reaches the surface only at the depression (ovulation fossa) on the free border, which is the only area from which normal ovulation occurs. The corpus luteum does not project from the greater surface of the ovary as in other species and is therefore not palpable during rectal examination.

Oviduct

The oviducts are tortuous tubes within the meso-salpinx, with a total length of some 20–30 cm.

The oviduct is divided into:

- Infundibulum.
- Ampulla.
- Isthmus.

At ovulation, ova drop into the expansive funnel-shaped infundibulum that covers the ovulation fossa. They travel quickly through the infundibulum to the ampulla where fertilization and early development of an ovum occurs. The fertilized ovum then travels through the narrow isthmus and enters the uterine horn at the uterotubal junction. Unfertilized ova normally are retained for a considerable time in the oviduct before degeneration occurs.[4] Unfertilized ova rarely enter the uterus.

PHYSIOLOGY

PUBERTY

Puberty is the onset of reproductive activity. There are considerable changes that are associated with this event, relating to the physical stature and the behavior of both mares and stallions. Little is understood about the mechanisms for the onset of puberty but maturation and onset of activity in the hypothalamus, pituitary and ovarian (or testicular) tissues may control its onset. A late foal (May–June, northern hemisphere) may reach puberty at an earlier age than an early foal (January–February, northern hemisphere). In any case, the onset of reproductive activity is timed to ensure that parturition occurs at a favorable time of the year for survival of the offspring. However, there are physiological and pathological causes of delay or total inhibition of the onset of puberty.

The onset of puberty usually occurs, and is currently presumed to result, from a combination of endocrinological events within the hypothalamus, the pituitary gland, and the gonads (Fig. 5.7). The onset of puberty is well recognized as a primary reproductive event and occurs at around 12–24 months of age,[5] but this can be significantly affected by several factors, including:

- Age (and timing of birth within the breeding season).
- Photoperiod (daylight hours). This is likely to be a significant event in the onset of puberty in horses, but this area has been poorly researched. Prolonged daylight hours result in a delayed onset of puberty; the best stimulus to puberty is the natural fluctuations in daylight hours.[6] This

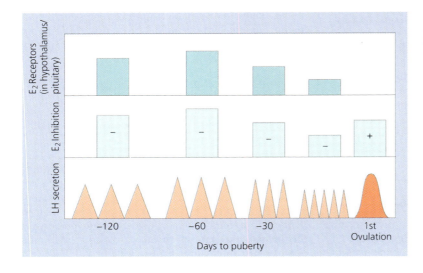

Fig. 5.7 Model for endocrine control of puberty. A minus sign (–) indicates inhibitory effects of estradiol; a plus sign (+) signifies a positive effect. E_2, estradiol; LH, luteinizing hormone.

contrasts with the effect of photoperiod in mares and stallions of mature breeding age (see p. 156).

- Nutritional status (body condition score) and growth rate. Although there are no data relating to the effects of nutritional status on the onset of puberty, this does occur in other species and there is no reason to suppose that it would not be similar in the horse. In ruminants, nutritional deprivation usually results in delayed onset of puberty. Whether precocious puberty occurs in response to high energy and rapid growth and weight gain in horses is uncertain. Most breeders are not driven to encourage early onset of puberty in mares in particular and prefer to rely on natural events.[7]
- Contact with other horses of breeding age (pheromone-governed). Typically, the effects of pheromones may be altered by the endocrine status of the animal and it may be that these factors have little overall influence on the onset of puberty itself.

THE NORMAL ESTROUS CYCLE AND SEASONALITY

The estrous cycle is a synchronized interplay of anatomic, endocrine, and behavioral events resulting in ovulation. Despite the high level of stud farm management and veterinary attention they receive, horses have an inherently low reproductive efficiency. A few highly significant factors contribute to this problem. They include:

- A disparity between the breeding season arbitrarily imposed by racing and performance industries and the physiologic breeding season of mares.
- Failure to select for fertility, including retention of breeding stock with heritable defects that reduce fertility (e.g. bad vulvar confirmation, cryptorchidism).
- Breeding geriatric animals.
- Prohibition of artificial insemination (in some breeds only and in particular the thoroughbred).

It is essential to understand basic equine reproductive physiology to manage normal mares for maximum fertility and to treat abnormal mares. There are wide variations in events within the cycle, particularly related to season of the year. These must be put in perspective and, if possible, used to best advantage.

Mares are regarded as 'long-day, seasonally polyestrous breeders', meaning that they exhibit a distinct breeding season characteristically during the spring, summer, and early autumn months. During this period, normal nonpregnant mares show repeated estrous cycles lasting about 21 days. Estrus

lasts for between 4 and 6 days. During this time one or more follicles mature and the mare is receptive to the stallion. Estrus is followed by 16–17 days of diestrus, when a corpus luteum is functional and the mare rejects the stallion.

During winter, most mares pass through a period of anestrus or sexual inactivity, when neither follicles nor corpora lutea are present. The response to the stallion is neutral (being neither receptive nor rejective). Day length is the primary factor controlling this seasonal ovarian activity.[8,9] Long day length (15–16 hours), such as occurs during the summer, stimulates ovarian activity. The effects of day length are mediated negatively by melatonin secretion from the pineal gland within the brain. Prolonged periods of high melatonin secretion during the short winter days suppress gonadotropin-releasing hormone release from the hypothalamus. Increasing day length in spring causes shorter periods of high melatonin production, allowing an increase in the frequency and amplitude of pulsatile gonadotropin-releasing hormone release.

Seasonal effects on ovarian cycles can be divided into three phases:

1. The ovulatory phase: the period from first ovulation in the spring until the last ovulation in the autumn.
2. Anestrus: the period of ovarian inactivity during the winter months.
3. Transition: the period of irregular or prolonged estrus receptivity that occurs in early spring or late autumn.

During the spring transition period, the ovaries develop numerous follicles of varying sizes which grow and regress until finally one follicle progresses to ovulation.

In both northern and southern hemispheres, 75–80% of mares demonstrate seasonally polyestrous behavior, whereas 20–25% have estrous cycles all year. The percentage of mares that cycle throughout the year increases nearer the equator and year-round cyclicity is more common in Arabian mares.[10]

Anestrus

In response to the diminished photoperiod of winter and other related factors governing seasonality, the anestrus mare is best described as sexually dormant.

- The ovaries are small, smooth, and firm, with no palpable follicular activity or functional luteal tissue.

Without the stimulus of estrogens and progesterone that accompany cyclicity, the uterus becomes atonic and thin-walled.

- Uterine changes that can be seen microscopically include glandular atrophy and compaction of the stroma resulting from the absence of edema.

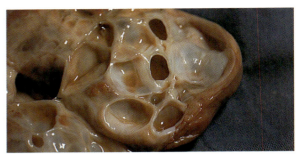

Fig. 5.8 Normal ovary (spring transition ovary). Note the numerous small atretic follicles with a few medium-sized follicles developing.

The cervix is similarly flaccid and difficult to palpate. The cervix, seen through a speculum, is pale, dry, and often relaxed, sometimes to the point of appearing open. The vaginal tract also is quite pale and devoid of obvious secretions.

- Distension of the vagina with air (such as follows manual examination of the vagina or the use of a vaginal speculum) produces little hyperemia or engorgement of superficial blood vessels.

During anestrus, the endocrinological functions that govern cycles essentially are shut down. As a result of a shortened photoperiod, small and infrequent pulses of gonadotropin-releasing hormone from the hypothalamus lead to baseline levels of plasma luteinizing hormone concentrations. Baseline concentrations of plasma follicle-stimulating hormone remain relatively high but fluctuate randomly during anestrus, presumably as a result of the lack of any negative feedback effect from ovarian inhibin and estrogen.[11]

- Plasma progesterone concentrations are less than 1 ng/ml because there are no corpora lutea in the ovaries.

The behavior patterns of seasonal anestrus are less specific and less predictable than endocrine function. Most mares are passive to mildly resistant in the presence of a stallion. It is not unusual, however, for a mare in deep anestrus to be sexually receptive to the point where she accepts the stallion at any time. In the absence of follicular development, this behavior seems paradoxical. It is possible that minute amounts of steroid hormones produced by the adrenal glands could be responsible for this. In addition, the cervix is partially to completely relaxed in mares in anestrus.

Anestrous mares behave similarly to ovariectomized mares because they are under similar endocrine control. Very small doses of exogenous estrogens cause sexual receptivity in both. For this reason, spayed (ovariectomized) mares make excellent teasers for semen collection because they can be predictably induced into estrous behavior with small doses of estrogenic hormones.

Transition

The transition phase frequently coincides with the time when owners are eager to breed mares for early foals. Managing transitional mares is a major concern for practitioners and stud managers during the spring months.

In most mares, the changeover from anestrus to a fully functional ovulatory phase is gradual. This transition is characterized by the re-establishment of endocrine function, erratic sexual behavior, and follicle development without accompanying ovulation. Increasing follicular activity causes the ovaries to enlarge considerably in comparison to their size during anestrus. There is a noticeable change in consistency as multiple small follicles begin to grow (Fig. 5.8). A springy resilience is evident on deep palpation, in contrast to the dense, firm consistency noted during the anovulatory phase.

A large variability is noted in transitional mares in the number of the various types of follicles palpated. Commonly, many small (10–15 mm) follicles are clustered on the ovarian surface, suggesting bunches of grapes. These small structures remain firm and are barely distinguishable in consistency from the ovarian stroma. As the season progresses, most mares develop one to two follicles that slowly progress to 25–30 mm but remain firm and then slowly regress. Mares in transition eventually develop follicles greater than 35 mm in diameter. Although these follicles can grow to a large size, initially they regress without ovulating.

- Lack of estrogen synthesis appears to be the underlying defect in these anovulatory follicles.

In pony mares, three to four follicles greater than 30 mm develop sequentially during transition over a period of several weeks. The first and second follicles usually regress, whereas the third or fourth follicle will undergo the first ovulation of the season. Estrogen production is the hallmark of the follicles that successfully ovulate.[12] Most of the time, the first follicle of the year that ovulates is accompanied by uterine edema visualized on ultrasonography (see p. 217).

When follicles begin to develop on the ovaries early in spring, little physical change is detectable in the tubular reproductive tract. The uterus stays thin-walled and flaccid, lacking stimulation because of relatively low levels of ovarian hormones. As follicular activity increases, the uterus becomes more edematous, probably as a result of increasing estrogen concentrations.

The increase in day length during spring leads to an increase in both the amplitude and the frequency of pulses of gonadotropin-releasing hormone from the hypothalamus.[11]

Baseline plasma follicle-stimulating hormone concentrations rise during the early stage of the transition period but then fall steadily during the 15–20 days before the first ovulation of the breeding season, presumably because of an increasing production of inhibin by developing follicles. Plasma luteinizing hormone concentrations increase slowly and steadily throughout the transition phase, with minor pulses that coincide with the pulses of gonadotropin-releasing hormone. Concentrations rise more steeply during the few days immediately preceding the first estrus, eventually reaching a typical peak at or soon after ovulation.

Plasma progesterone concentrations are less than 1 ng/ml until after ovulation, when they rise sharply. Plasma estrogen concentrations also remain low during anestrus but then rise coincidentally with the wave of follicular growth that precedes the onset of the first ovulation.[13]

- Behavior patterns during transition are erratic.
- Mares may show either no signs of estrus behavior, or constant to erratic estrous behavior.
- Mares should not be bred during the transition phase as excessive breeding during this period may result in endometritis, especially in older, pluriparous mares.

Prolonged periods of full sexual receptivity are usual as follicular development progresses. It is particularly helpful to managers to determine the difference between transitional mares showing strong estrous behavior without ovulation and normally cycling mares. Unnecessary breeding during the early season can be avoided by careful reproductive tract palpation and ultrasonography. The benefits of conserving the stallion and avoiding contamination of mares during this unproductive stage of the cycle are obvious. Some transitional mares remain passive, whereas others respond to the teaser with no correlation to ovarian status, showing receptivity and resistance in no definable pattern.

The fall transition period after the ovulatory phase of the cycle receives little attention from owners or clinicians, because the breeding season does not correspond with this period of waning reproductive function. The decreasing photoperiod in the autumn has the reverse effect on the mare to the increasing photoperiod in the spring. Behavior and ovulation become more erratic as the ovulatory season nears its end.

After the last ovulation, it is not uncommon for a follicle to develop to a large size and then fail to ovulate or regress. These so-called autumn follicles have been mistakenly referred to as 'cystic follicles'. They are not pathologic and disappear spontaneously, often weeks to months later.

The ovulatory phase

During the ovulatory phase, mares establish cycles which, compared with those in females of other domestic species, are models of inconsistency. Acceptance of these inconsistencies as variations of the normal limits is the only reasonable way to approach broodmare management.

- Examples of these inconsistencies include mares 'normally' ovulating without showing estrous behavior, showing signs of estrus without ovulating, undergoing prolongation of the lifespan of the corpus luteum for a couple of months, or splitting heats with 8–10-day inter-ovulatory intervals.

The estrous cycle of the mare is defined as the interval from one ovulation to the subsequent ovulation when ovulation is accompanied by behavioral estrus and/or plasma progesterone concentrations below 1 ng/ml. Progesterone concentrations are included in the definition because ovulation may occur during the middle of the cycle (diestrus ovulation) when progesterone concentrations are high. Estrus is the period of sexual receptivity. Diestrus is the period from the end of one estrus to the beginning of the next estrus, characterized by the formation of a functional corpus luteum.

The duration of the individual components and the length of the total estrous cycle vary greatly (Table 5.1). The greatest variability is at the beginning and end of the ovulatory phase. Therefore the duration of estrus is shortest during the peak of the ovulatory season and corresponds with the peak of fertility. Breeding mares at the optimal time early in the imposed breeding season require closer management than breeding mares at the peak of the physiologic breeding season. For example, it can be assumed that ovulation occurs 24 hours before the end of estrus and

Table 5.1 Mean length of components of the estrous cycle

	Mean (days)	Range of means (days)
Estrus	6.5	4.5–8.9
Diestrus	14.9	12.1–16.3
Estrous cycle	21.7	19.1–23.7

that sperm is viable for 48 hours within the mare's reproductive tract. Without palpation for follicular development, if breeding commences on the second day of estrus, three breedings are necessary to adequately expose mares with an 8–9-day estrus. Mares with a 4-day estrus need only be bred once. Due to this variability, if palpation is not or cannot be used, mares are covered on the second day and then every other day until estrus has ended. This illustrates the value of accurate palpation in avoiding unnecessary stallion services.

CYCLIC EVENTS OF THE OVULATORY PHASE

Three main groups of hormones are involved in control of the estrous cycle. The 'brain hormones' (melatonin and gonadotropin-releasing hormone) convert external stimuli into direct stimulation of the pituitary gland. The 'pituitary hormones' [the gonadotropins (follicle-stimulating hormone, luteinizing hormone), prolactin, and oxytocin] exert a direct trophic action on the ovaries, uterus, and other parts of the genital tract. The 'genital or sex hormones' [estrogen, progesterone, inhibin, and prostaglandin $F_{2\alpha}$ ($PGF_{2\alpha}$)] are secreted in response to stimulation by pituitary hormones and control functional changes in the genital tract and behavioral changes in the animal. They feed back positively and negatively on hypothalamic and pituitary hormone secretion rates (Fig. 5.9).[14]

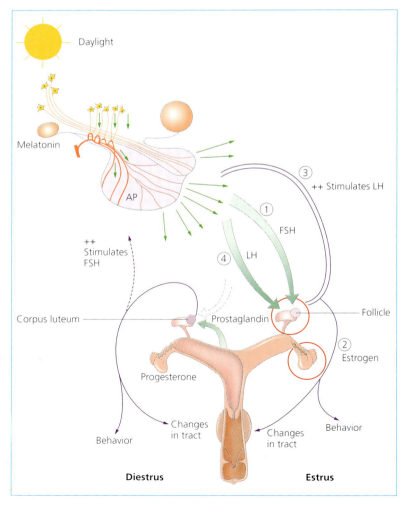

Fig. 5.9 Hormonal control of the estrous cycle in the mare. AP, anterior pituitary; LH, luteinizing hormone; FSH, follicle-stimulating hormone; GnRH, gonadotropin-releasing hormone.

Hypothalamic control

Gonadotropin-releasing hormone is secreted by cells in the hypothalamus and is released in brief pulses. After gonadotropin-releasing hormone reaches the pituitary gland via a portal venous system, it stimulates the secretion and release of both follicle-stimulating hormone and luteinizing hormone. The frequency of the gonadotropin-releasing hormone pulses is mediated by melatonin release. A low frequency occurs during anestrus when melatonin release is high because of the shortened day length. The frequency of gonadotropin-releasing hormone release is also reduced during diestrus as a result of negative feedback effects exerted by progesterone. The frequency of the pulses of gonadotropin-releasing hormone controls which gonadotropin is released from the anterior pituitary gland.

- High-frequency pulses of gonadotropin-releasing hormone stimulate luteinizing hormone release.
- Low-frequency pulses of gonadotropin-releasing hormone cause follicle-stimulating hormone release.[15]

Pituitary function

The pituitary hormones (follicle-stimulating hormone and luteinizing hormone) are responsible for the control of follicular growth and ovulation in mares:

- Follicle-stimulating hormone stimulates the initial growth of follicles in the ovaries during diestrus.
- Luteinizing hormone stimulates maturation of the follicles, maturation of the oocytes within the follicles, and ovulation during estrus.

Follicle-stimulating hormone

During the physiologic breeding season of mares, follicle-stimulating hormone concentrations peak twice during each cycle at about 10–11-day intervals (Fig. 5.10). Follicle-stimulating hormone secretion is stimulated by increased day length and suppressed by inhibin secreted by developing follicles. The first peak of follicle-stimulating hormone concentrations occurs near the end of estrus. This peak coincides with the luteinizing hormone peak at or soon after ovulation. The second follicle-stimulating hormone surge is seen in mid-diestrus, when follicular activity is at its lowest. It is theorized that this surge is responsible for initiating the wave of follicular growth that provides the ovulatory follicle during the ensuing estrus. Follicles stimulated after the first surge of follicle-stimulating hormone reach the luteinizing-hormone-dependent stage between days 5 and 7 of the estrous cycle and become atretic if luteinizing hormone is not available.[16]

Luteinizing hormone

Plasma concentrations of luteinizing hormone are low between days 6 and 15 (Fig. 5.10) after ovulation because of the negative feedback action of progesterone on the hypothalamus, causing the sup-

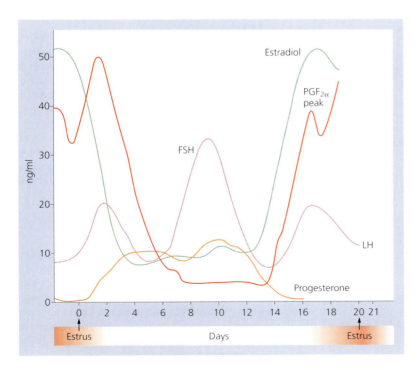

Fig. 5.10 Hormone changes occurring during the normal 21-day estrous cycle in the mare (the arrows depict ovulation). LH, luteinizing hormone; FSH, follicle-stimulating hormone; $PGF_{2\alpha}$, prostaglandin $F_{2\alpha}$.

pression of gonadotropin-releasing hormone. Blood concentrations start to rise near the beginning of estrus (day 17) as the suppressive effects of progesterone are removed and probably as a consequence of the positive stimulatory action of estrogen on gonadotropin-releasing hormone pulse frequency. Concentrations of luteinizing hormone peak about 2 days after ovulation and then decline slowly. Because of its prolonged half-life, luteinizing hormone reaches baseline concentrations at about day 5 or day 6 after ovulation.[3]

Ovarian function

Estrogen induces the major structural changes throughout the genital tract that are associated with estrus, including:

- Softening and relaxation of the cervix.
- Increased fluidity and volume of uterine and vaginal secretions.
- Uterine edema.
- Growth of the primary follicle.

It also acts on the brain, stimulating behavioral changes of estrus and having both positive and negative feedback on gonadotropin-releasing hormone (see Fig. 5.9). Shortly before the luteinizing hormone surge, plasma and urinary estrogens rise, reaching a peak 24–36 hours before ovulation. Estrogens are secreted mainly as estrone and 17β-estradiol. In the absence of concurrent high progesterone concentrations, high concentrations of estrogen cause estrous behavior.

Progesterone is secreted by the corpus luteum during days 1–17 after ovulation. Progesterone causes contraction of the cervix and increased viscosity of vaginal secretions. It stimulates proliferative changes in the uterine luminal epithelium and endometrial glands and acts on the brain to induce the rejection-type behavioral response shown by mares in diestrus. Plasma progesterone concentrations are low (less than 1 ng/ml) throughout estrus but rise sharply after ovulation, reaching values of 1.5–2.5 ng/ml by 24 hours and 2–5 ng/ml by 48 hours post ovulation (day 0). Peak concentrations of 8–20 ng/ml are attained by days 5–8 after ovulation, and these values remain high until luteolysis commences at days 14–15 after ovulation (Fig. 5.10).

> - The rapid rise in plasma progesterone concentrations after ovulation makes progesterone assay a useful clinical tool for confirming ovulation.

Oxytocin is released from the posterior pituitary by the estrous mare in response to sexual arousal, particularly if the arousal is a stallion call. During teasing, breeding, and artificial insemination, peaks in oxytocin levels are detected in pituitary venous blood. Exogenous oxytocin, now frequently administered as a postbreeding treatment, may stimulate luteinizing hormone secretion slightly, possibly advancing ovulation.

> - Oxytocin also stimulates oviductal and uterine contractions, facilitating the union of ovum and sperm in the oviduct, and assisting uterine clearance after breeding.

Graafian (mature) follicles secrete inhibin during their maturation. This hormone exerts a direct, negative feedback effect on follicle-stimulating hormone release, presumably by altering the sensitivity of follicle-stimulating hormone gonadotropins in the pituitary to stimulation by gonadotropin-releasing hormone.

Early estrus

The mid-cycle release of follicle-stimulating hormone (Fig. 5.11) stimulates follicular development. Around days 16–18 after ovulation, near the beginning of estrus, a few follicles (greater than 25 mm in diameter) are present, and one follicle is associated with the luteinizing hormone surge beginning on day 16 or 17 after ovulation, when levels of follicle-stimulating hormone are lowest. Resulting estrogen production from these growing follicles initiates the physical and behavioral changes of early estrus.

Late estrus

As the dominant follicle approaches maturation, a large preovulatory surge of estrogens produces a positive feedback on the pituitary, continuing the rise in luteinizing hormone concentrations. In contrast to females of other species, mares have a prolonged surge in luteinizing hormone levels that often lasts for 7–8 days and usually peaks after ovulation (Fig. 5.11). Because it is common for multiple follicles to develop during estrus, this long exposure to luteinizing hormone may account for the large number of multiple ovulations that occurs.

Ovulation

In its embryonic development, the cortex of the equine ovary folds at its hilus and becomes surrounded by medullary tissue. Mechanically, this only allows ovulation through the hilar area or ovulation fossa. Follicles are palpated on the general ovarian surface, but the follicle collapses at ovulation and forces the ovum through its tract to the ovulation fossa. Follicles usually increase rapidly in size (about 5 mm in

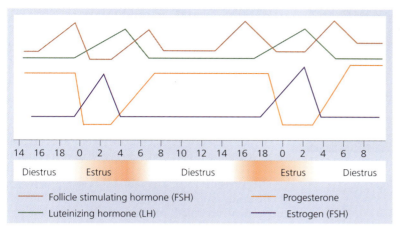

Fig. 5.11 Cyclical variations in circulating hormones during the normal estrous cycle of the mare.

diameter per day) before ovulation. Mares weighing 400–550 kg often ovulate from follicles 45–65 mm in diameter, whereas smaller mares weighing 225–350 kg may ovulate from follicles 35–45 mm in diameter.[17]

At ovulation, as detected by rectal palpation, there may be a perceptible softening of the follicle before rupture, but this is not a consistent finding. Mares frequently exhibit signs of mild pain at the site of a recently collapsed follicle, probably associated with the sudden change in tension of the visceral peritoneum that surrounds all but the ovulation fossa of the ovary.

The time of ovulation in relationship to estrus varies. It is virtually impossible to predict ovulation time based solely on the duration of estrus. One report indicated that only 46% of the mares studied ovulated on the day before the end of estrus and nearly 12% ovulated 3 days before the end of heat. Very few mares (1.4%) ovulated after sexual receptivity had ceased.

Ovulation usually occurs during evening or night hours, with approximately 75% of mares ovulating between 4:00 p.m. and 8:00 a.m. The incidence of multiple ovulation reportedly varies from 14.5% to 42.8%.[18]

Endocrine changes after ovulation are quite rapid in most mares, and physical and behavioral changes follow very shortly (Table 5.2; see also Fig. 5.7). Some luteinization probably occurs before ovulation; however, estrogen concentrations drop drastically when the follicle collapses and the corpus luteum develops quickly. The resulting reversal in circulating estrogen:progesterone ratio causes the rapid cessation of estrous behavior. At this point, progesterone rather than estrogen dominates behavior and the physical character of the tubular genitalia.

Diestrus

The corpus hemorrhagicum is palpable per rectum during the first 2–3 days after ovulation as a soft, spongy structure on the surface of the ovary. As it matures into a corpus luteum and the blood within the corpus hemorrhagicum clots, the consistency changes to that of a rubbery, firm structure that is difficult to distinguish from a firm follicle (Fig. 5.12). The ultrasonographic appearance of the corpus luteum

Table 5.2 Endocrine and physical characteristics of the estrous cycle of the mare (FSH, follicle-stimulating hormone; LH, luteinizing hormone)

| Estrus phase | Endocrine events | | Physical events | | |
	Pituitary	Ovary	Ovary	Genital tract	Behavior
Estrus					
Early	FSH increases	Estrogen increases	Follicle developing	Poor tone	Some receptivity
Late	LH rises	Estrogen peaks and begins to fall	Follicle maturation	Uterine edema Cervical relaxation	Strong receptivity
Ovulation	LH peaks	Estrogen falls Progesterone increases	Follicle collapse	Uterine contraction	Receptive
Diestrus					
Early	LH reducing	Progesterone increases	Corpus hemorrhagicum	Firm uterine tone	
Mid	FSH rises	Progesterone peaks	Corpus luteum	Maximal uterine tone	Rejection of stallion
Late	FSH peaks	Progesterone falls	Follicular activity	Uterine softening	

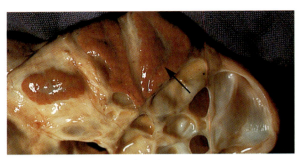

Fig. 5.12 Normal ovary, showing mature corpus luteum (brownish/yellow tissue; arrowed), smaller corpus luteum and atretic follicles. Note the thickened walls of atretic follicles.

is characteristic and is easily identified throughout its lifespan.

The corpus luteum is considered to be mature 5 days after ovulation. Until that time, the corpus luteum is refractory to luteolysis by prostaglandin. The mature corpus luteum induces high blood concentrations of progesterone (8–10 ng/ml) until about days 14–15 of the estrous cycle. At this time, the corpus luteum undergoes luteolysis in response to $PGF_{2\alpha}$, which is released from the endometrium. $PGF_{2\alpha}$ enters the systemic circulation and reaches the corpus luteum via arteriovenous transfer and/or in the lymphatics, where it precipitates luteolysis and so instigates the next estrous cycle.

RECOGNITION OF ESTRUS IN THE MARE

The correct and early recognition of estrous behavior in mares is an important part of stud farm management. Failure to detect estrus and the consequent failure to breed mares is a common (and largely unnecessary) cause of poor conception rates.

> • Early recognition results in better synchronization of mating with ovulation and reduces the number of rectal examinations that may be required.

Mares that fail to show overt estrous behavior may be more difficult to assess. Where visual inspection and obvious behavioral changes do not detect estrus, teasing (testing with a teaser pony, testosterone-implanted gelding or stallion) is standard practice in stud farm management. Although this procedure may seem to be tedious and time-consuming, it is clearly vital for the success of the breeding program. The best stud farms with the best results are expert at the process of teasing and take particular care to try and detect early signs of estrus in the mares, often when the behavioral and physiological changes are subtle.

Detailed breeding records may be very helpful in predicting when the mare is likely to come into estrus, although there may be variations in cycle length during the season and variations may also arise from early embryo loss, etc. (see p. 163).

Repeated examinations of the reproductive tract are also helpful in determining when the mare is in estrus, especially if there is no stallion available or she does not exhibit estrous behavior.

By far the most efficient method for estrus detection is to tease each mare individually with a stallion, but mares can also be teased by teasers, or on occasion by geldings (see p. 153). The interrelationship between a mare and stallion during estrus is probably more dependent on smell and taste rather than on sight. However, teasing is usually restricted to one or two 5–10-minute periods each day and this is clearly an artificial circumstance. While most mares will either show signs of estrus or diestrus (rejection behavior and absence of clinical evidence of estrus), some mares may not respond normally to this narrow time scale and often appear to be in diestrus throughout the cycle. The extent of estrus 'showing' is variable. Some respond quickly to contact with the stallion (often even on initial approach), but other mares may take considerable time to settle to the behavior pattern.

Managerial factors may influence the extent to which estrus is shown by behavioral signs alone. Management that involves separation of the mares from the stallions for the greater part of the time means that teasing (testing) must be performed more effectively.

- Maiden mares may also be difficult, especially those that are nervous and excitable; they may be reluctant to show estrus and may then not respond well even when teased individually.
- Mares do not show any overt sexual behavior (e.g. mounting each other) when grouped with other mares and overt changes in the physical characteristics (mucous secretions) of the vulva are not usually obvious.
- Mares with a high androgen concentration (resulting from administration of male hormones or anabolic steroids or certain ovarian tumors) may show masculine behavior rather than estrus.[19]
- Estrus signs may be much stronger in the presence of an active stallion. Estrus in paddock or free-bred mares will be detected quickly by the attending stallion(s).
- Mares with foals at foot may not show strong signs of estrus, either if the foal is separated from her at the time of teasing or if the foal is physically beside the mare during teasing. This is caused either by separation anxiety or by protectiveness, respectively.

Estrous behavior is defined as the pattern that results in acceptance of the approach of, and mating by, a stallion. Usually a mare is considered to have been in estrus if she shows 4–6 days of estrous behavior followed by a period of 10–14 days of diestrus during which she should show no receptivity to the stallion and no overt clinical signs of estrus[20] (see below). Individual mares may habitually show strong or weak estrous signs. In the latter cases, supportive testing (see alternative methods below), dates and records can be helpful.

Behavioral changes typical of estrus include:

- Docility (although behavior can be unpredictable).
- Ears relaxed either forward or in neutral position.
- Vocalization in the form of squealing often occurs with laid back ears when the mare is first approached by the stallion.
- Tail raising and swishing with adoption of a stance similar to urination but maintained for longer periods and without evidence of straining. The tail is usually held slightly to one side.
- Fence pushing.
- Lengthening and eversion of the vulvar lips with clitoral eversion ('winking').
- Squatting and frequent squirts of urine (usually with a characteristic odor and yellowish cloudy appearance).

Alternative methods of estrus detection

These are useful if either a teaser is not available (often for cost or management reasons) or the stallion cannot be used to tease the mare (usually for safety reasons and because some stallions become frustrated and develop behavioral problems such as self-mutilation or indifference to breeding). In any case, a single method should not be relied upon because there are variations from mare to mare.

Vaginal examination

Vaginal examination of estrous mares often identifies a thin mucoid secretion. Attempts to measure the electrical conductivity of vaginal mucus have not been rewarding. Vaginal cytology has also not proven to be an effective mechanism for estrus detection.

Vaginoscopic examination (Fig. 5.13) can be used to detect estrus (and diestrus) with some accuracy but it is a semi-invasive method and can cause problems with vaginal inflammation.

The normal state of the cervix changes during estrus (and during pregnancy).[21] During estrus the cervix shows hyperemia (a red or dark pink color). The mucosa is edematous (moist-looking and thickened) and the cervix itself is relaxed and lies on the floor of the vagina. The mucus consistency correlates closely with the rise in blood estrogen and is recognized as an

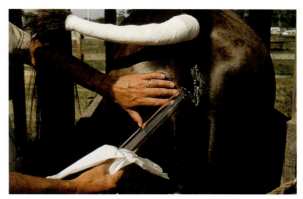

Fig. 5.13   Vaginoscope in use.

increased shininess of the mucosal surfaces. Introduction of the speculum is relatively easy due to increased mucous secretion during estrus but commonly causes a significant increase in blood vessel diameter and increased redness of the mucosal surfaces.

> Note:
> - An abnormal hyperemia and redness is associated with inflammation but this is noticeably different to the experienced examiner.

In diestrus under the influence of progesterone, the cervix is much more easily identifiable and changes to a paler almost gray color with a yellowish tinge, and appears dry and tightly closed and is elevated off the floor of the vagina. The surface blood vessels do not become more obvious when the speculum is introduced.

In anestrus, the vaginal and cervical mucosa is an almost white color with sparse vasculature. The cervix may be seen to be open and flaccid. It is usually found near the vaginal floor.

A classification system has been proposed for the description of the cervix during examination.[22] This has advantages because any repeat examinations can be considered with the previous ones.

> Thus:
> - In estrus, the cervix is relaxed, edematous and pink (i.e. **CR pink**).
> - In diestrus, the cervix is pale moist, located off the vaginal floor and has an obvious appearance (i.e. **CT pale**).
>
> [C is cervix, **R** is relaxed, **T** is tight]

This is just one classification scheme; many others have been created and can be used to describe the differences in cervical tone during estrus and diestrus.

As long as the examiner uses the same classification scheme consistently, it will be useful for comparison during repeated examination of the reproductive tract.

> Note:
> - During pregnancy the cervix is pale (almost white) and is tightly closed.
> - A sticky mucous plug covers its surface but the vaginal mucosa is dry.
> - In late pregnancy the cervix becomes less obvious and the vaginal surface is covered by thick sticky mucus that prevents the normal ballooning of the vagina during vaginoscopic examination.

Rectal and ultrasonographic examination

The value of an effective and thorough ultrasonographic examination cannot be overstated. With the use of a high-quality scanner the reproductive tract can be examined with sufficient detail to provide important information. The uterus of mares in estrus will have a 'cartwheel' appearance as visualized on ultrasonography (see Fig. 6.8), due to the increase in edema in the uterine wall. The 'cartwheel' breaks up approximately 24 hours prior to ovulation and can be used to identify mares in estrus and to time breeding. Mares in diestrus will have a homogeneous appearance to the uterus and a corpus luteum on one of their ovaries. Pathology, such as intrauterine fluid or lymphatic cysts, that can not be identified by rectal palpation can easily be visualized by ultrasonography.

Blood sampling

This is useful to obtain hormone profiles characteristic of estrus. Mares in estrus will have plasma progesterone concentrations of <1 ng/ml.

Body temperature

This is a very unreliable method of determining the presence of estrus.

Diestrus

The onset of diestrus in the mare is abrupt; usually by 2 days post ovulation she is totally nonreceptive to the stallion.

- The diestrus mare shows none of the features above.
- She will usually be more aggressive, often biting or kicking at the teaser and will certainly not permit mating.

EXAMINATION OF THE FEMALE GENITAL TRACT

BREEDING SOUNDNESS EXAMINATION

Breeding soundness examinations are performed to determine a mare's suitability as a broodmare and for identifying causes of infertility. Portions of the examination are performed routinely on normal mares during the breeding season to determine when they should be bred. Common use of new technologies, such as artificial insemination of mares with shipped, cooled semen or frozen semen and embryo transfer, require that the veterinarian excel in reproductive examination skills. A complete breeding soundness examination (see Fig. 5.14) is most commonly performed to identify a cause of infertility. Although in purely dictionary terms infertility can be defined as the failure to produce an offspring (whether or not that reflects failure to conceive), the stud farm definition is usually taken one stage further: that is, failure to produce a productive offspring that achieves its desired use and has the ability (if not the opportunity) to breed itself once it has reached breeding age.

When confronted with an infertility problem it is vital to collect and record a full history, including all aspects of management and as much detail about the mare as possible (including back-tracking to her own neonatal development).

1. Obtain a full reproductive and other history of the mare.
   - This should include as much detail as is practicable and should not be limited to the reproductive history.
   - There are many aspects of reproduction that are influenced by diseases and accidents/injuries involving other body systems.
   - Medications of all types can be responsible for difficulties with conception and maintenance of pregnancy.
   - A full history of the fertility rates and changes in these for the whole stud should be taken.
2. Perform a complete physical examination.
   - The examination of the infertile or problem mare should not be limited to the reproductive organs as there are many secondary reproductive effects from other diseases (e.g. equine Cushing's disease/pituitary adenoma, endotoxemia).
3. Perform a full reproductive examination in a logical order.
   - Inspect the external genitalia.
   - Rectal examination (see p. 133).
   - Ultrasound examination of the reproductive tract.
   - Collect clitoral swabs (clitoral sinus and fossa).
   - Speculum examination of vagina and collect cervical and endometrial swabs for culture and

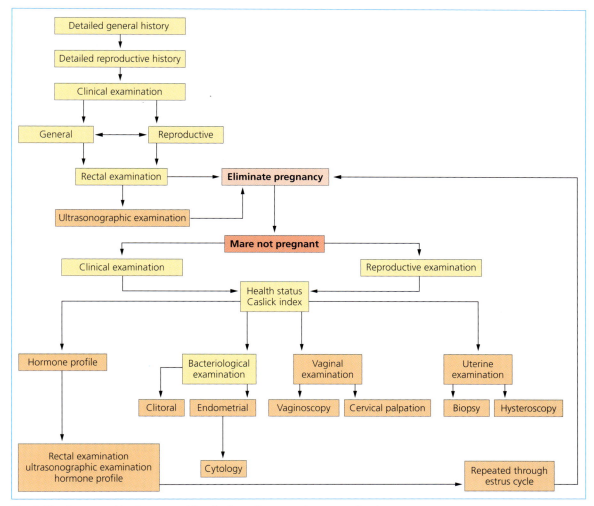

Fig. 5.14   Suggested basic protocol for the breeding soundness examination.

cytology (make smears immediately after collection).
- Manual examination of vagina, vestibule and cervix.
- Endometrial biopsy (see p. 144).
- Endoscopy of tract (record findings) (see p. 148).
4. Obtain peripheral blood samples for hormone analysis/chromosomal analysis.

There are many different ways of performing the breeding soundness examination of mares and no single method is universally accepted as being ideal. The clinician should establish a protocol that minimizes the risks of missing important aspects of the examination and needs to ensure that the mare has the best possible chance of conceiving quickly. Failure to carry out a full general clinical appraisal can easily lead to errors of diagnosis. An inadequate approach is likely to lead to problems of diagnosis.

An accurate record of the findings of a breeding soundness examination must be kept for each mare and for each breeding season. Reference to the previous history can be very useful in establishing the cause and likelihood of reproductive problems.

History

A complete history of the reproductive performance of the mare prior to examination is essential for:

- Making a diagnosis.
- Establishing a prognosis.
- Selecting appropriate treatments.

Because improper management is often the principal cause of infertility, a complete history is needed if no physical causes of infertility are found in the examination. Reviewing the history frequently reveals the cause of the problem. The ideal breeding history includes a sequential year-by-year account of the mare's entire racing, show or eventing and breeding career. Unfortunately, this is rarely obtained because mares frequently change owners and many owners keep incomplete records.

- The length of the performance (racing, showing, eventing, etc.) career, training, and age at which it began and finished, should be noted.
- Drugs, stress or injuries incurred during performance may adversely affect cyclic patterns, behavior, or general body condition.
- Behavioral attitudes developed in training may also compromise reproductive performance of the young mare for several months after arrival at the breeding farm.
- Performance mares that are to be bred may be housed at facilities that lack a stallion, making estrus detection difficult.

The age of the mare may have an influence on her ability to conceive. The young mare, at 2–3 years of age, may experience abnormal estrous cycles and have aberrant behavior. Older, pluriparous mares, more than 15 years of age, may have undergone anatomical changes leading to pneumovagina, refluxing of urine in the anterior vagina, or accumulating fluid within the uterine lumen after breeding.

Reproductive data should include when the mare was first bred, number of years bred, number of foals carried to term, difficulties incurred at foaling and whether the foal was born alive. The time of year that the mare was bred and whether she was subjected to artificial lighting needs to be noted. Abortions, placentitis, retained placenta and early embryonic death need to be recorded. A detailed reproductive history for the preceding 3 years, including teasing and breeding data, is invaluable because it may reveal cyclic patterns. Short cycles (suggesting uterine infection) and prolonged diestrual patterns (suggesting endocrine dysfunction) should be noted. Communication with the management personnel and other veterinarians who have previously attended the mare is helpful. They can supply information on estrous behavior such as ease with which estrus was detected, restraint needed to produce signs of estrus, and other 'personality' quirks.

Treatment history, ultrasonographic findings, cytology and culture results, drugs infused into the uterus and the schedule of drugs administered should be evaluated. These data will be invaluable when comparing them with results of a subsequent examination of the reproductive tract. Response to treatment, improvement, degeneration or failure to respond contributes to the prognosis as well as to evaluation of the efficacy of previous treatment. Evidence of, or recorded data relating to, previous surgery of the reproductive tract is indicative of a need to correct some abnormality that can compromise conception or maintenance of pregnancy.

Knowledge of the fertility of the stallion to which the mare has been previously bred and the method by which the mare was bred, natural service, artificial insemination with fresh, cooled or frozen semen, is needed. The contribution that the stallion may be making to the infertility can be assessed by consideration of:

- The number of estrous cycles per conception for the stallion's matings.
- The motility of the shipped, cooled semen or post-thaw motility of frozen/thawed semen.

If cooled or frozen semen is used, insemination must be timed properly if conception is to occur. First-cycle pregnancy rates are highest in mares bred with frozen/thawed semen when the mares are examined every 6–8 hours to determine ovulation. Such intensive management may be logistically impossible. In addition, some mares may experience an acute prolonged endometritis after being bred with frozen semen, resulting in early embryonic death.

Prior to examination of the reproductive tract, the general physical condition of the mare should be appraised. Any systemic problems that may interfere with fertility should be noted. Extremes in body condition from debilitation to obesity may affect fertility. Less than optimal feeding or management changes, dental care or parasite control can easily lower fertility.

External examination

- Examination of the external genitalia should include the entire perineal area as well as the tail and buttocks to detect signs of vulvar discharge.
- Perineal and pelvic conformation need to be examined thoroughly as the anatomical alignment of the mare's perineum is important for reproductive soundness (Fig. 5.15). The perineal body may be defective in older, pluriparous

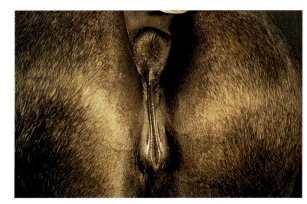

Fig. 5.15   Perineal conformation in a normal young mare. Note the vertical orientation of the vulva and the location of the tuber ischii, level with the lower third of the vulva.

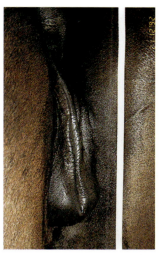

Fig. 5.16 Vulvar angulation (10%). Note the common (near-normal) conformational shape; requires vulvoplasty (Caslick's operation) for best fertility results.

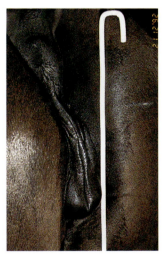

Fig. 5.17 Vulvar angulation (40%) Note the very poor conformation; always needs vulvoplasty (Caslick's operation). Surgery possible. Fertility is often significantly reduced.

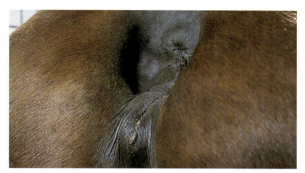

Fig. 5.18 Vulvar angulation (80%). Note that there is no prospect of conception without combined perineal construction (Pouret's operation) and vulvoplasty (Caslick's operation).

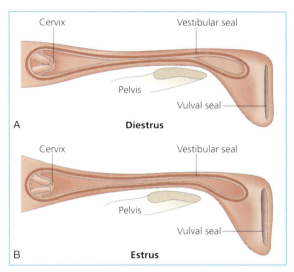

Fig. 5.19 Lateral view of the normal anatomical relationships between the posterior genitalia and the ischium, showing three functional seals between the uterus and the environment. (A) Diestrus: cervix closed, vulvar and vestibular seals effective. (B) Estrus: cervix and vulva relaxed, vestibular seal penetrated at coitus.

mares. The defect most likely occurs from repeated foalings and poor reproductive conformation and results in a sunken anus and lack of tissue between the rectum and the vagina.

- The pelvic conformation should be viewed laterally and caudally.
- Conformational characteristics that correlate with high fertility include a long sloping hip, a sacral iliac joint located dorsal to the tail setting and a vulva that is no more that 10° off the vertical. Various degrees of vulvar angulation and their relationship to fertility are illustrated in Figs 5.16–5.18.
- Mares that experience bouts of infertility frequently have a flat-topped croup with a tail

setting that is level with the sacro-iliac joint and a sunken anus (see Fig. 5.2). These conformational defects lead to pneumovagina, urovagina, and accumulation of intrauterine fluid.

- The vulva is best evaluated during estrus, when relaxation and elongation of the vulvar lips are greatest. The integrity of the vulvar lips, the angulation of the vulva and the location of the dorsal commissure of the vulva in relation to the pelvis need to be evaluated. The vulvar lips should meet evenly and appear full and firm. They function as a seal against external contamination of the uterus (see Figs 5.19, 5.20). The lips should lie vertically with a cranial to caudal slope of no more than 10° from the vertical. The dorsal commissure of the vulva

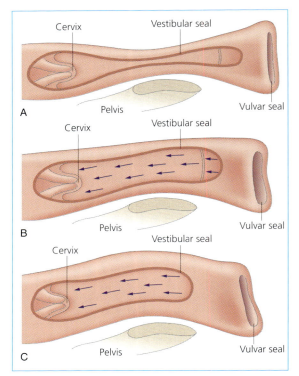

Fig. 5.20 As Fig. 5.19, but of a mare in diestrus with poor conformation. (A) Ischium is low in relation to vagina, so vestibular seal is ineffective, but in this case the vulva is competent so the cervix is not challenged. (B) As above, but with an incompetent vulva, so that pneumovagina occurs and the cervix is directly challenged by environmental microorganisms. (C) As above, but further aggravated by a sloping vulva which allows fecal contamination.

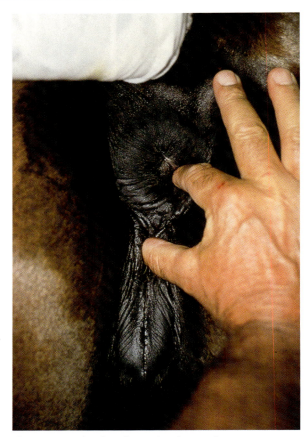

Fig. 5.22 Evaluating the perineal musculature.

should be no more than 4 cm dorsal to the pelvic floor.[23] If it is more than 4 cm, the vulva is predisposed to cranioventral rotation leading to pneumovagina and contamination[1] (Fig. 5.21).

- The lips of the vulva should be parted to determine the integrity of the vestibulovaginal sphincter. An intact sphincter is present in a mare when the labia can be spread slightly without air entering the cranial vagina. By parting the labia, the color and moisture of the vestibular walls can be assessed. Estrus produces a glistening pink to red mucosa. Anestrus generally is reflected by a pale, dry mucosa; a dark-red or muddy color suggests inflammation. A white, tacky mucosa indicates progesterone dominance.

- The integrity of the perineal body can be assessed by placing one finger into the rectum (usually the second finger) and the thumb into the vestibule. There should be at least 3 cm of muscular tissue between the two fingers (Fig. 5.22). Surgical correction of any defect may be possible.

Fig. 5.21 A lateral view of the anatomical relationship between the anus, vulva and ischium: (A) good conformation; (B) poor conformation, predisposing to (C) in which the labia are in the horizontal plane.

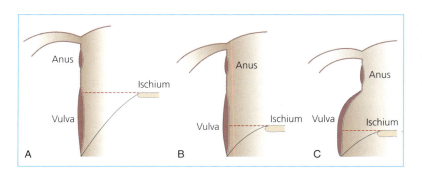

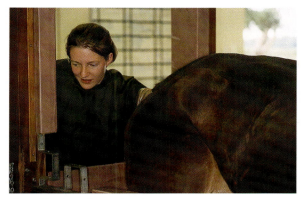

Fig. 5.23 Rectal examination.

DIAGNOSTIC METHODS

Rectal examination

Rectal examination is a routine procedure in stud medicine.[24] It is used to directly palpate the tubular genital tract and ovaries (Fig. 5.23). It is also an integral part of the transrectal ultrasonographic examination that has revolutionized reproductive medicine in mares.

The technique carries significant risks; no matter how careful the operator is there are serious accidents. Rough or careless examination can have a much higher rate of complications and the procedure should not therefore be taken lightly. Although it is tempting to expound the potential hazards to an owner, this is sometimes more alarming to them and may deter them from having the procedure performed. However, failure to warn of the potential dangers may equally cause acrimony in the event that a serious complication occurs.

The potential hazards are primarily related to rectal tears.

> - **Evidence of blood on the operator's sleeve following rectal examination should never be ignored** (Fig. 5.24).
> - Immediate measures should be taken to investigate the extent of the problem and to manage the consequences.
> - Management of rectal tears is described in standard surgical texts.

There are recognized classifications of rectal tears ranging from grade 1 (tearing of the superficial mucosa only) to grade 5 (total disruption of the rectal wall). The location of the tear also has serious implications for the prognosis. Tears in the retroperitoneal rectal wall are somewhat less serious than those involving peritoneal disruption because peritoneal contamination with fecal material is almost invariably fatal.

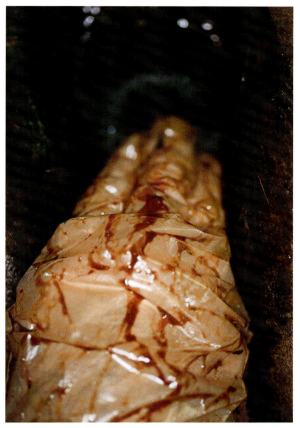

Fig. 5.24 Blood on rectal sleeve indicative of rectal damage. This can be an emergency situation and requires specialist assistance immediately if the mare is to be saved.

All veterinary surgeons should be familiar with the measures described in standard surgical and medical texts on the management of rectal tears.

> - Although owners are invariably inclined to blame the attending veterinary surgeon for the occurrence of a rectal tear, this is not justified in most cases.
> - Provided suitable care is taken and restraint is adequate (including sedation, if necessary), rectal examination should be safe.
> - In the event of a problem, the owners should be informed immediately and suitable emergency measures taken to maximize the chances of the horse's survival.
> - Even very experienced operators are occasionally faced with a rectal tear.
> - In the US and UK, the risk of the procedure is recognized legally and, provided due care has been taken and no negligence is involved, litigation is unlikely to succeed.

Technique

i. Adequate restraint is essential. Operator safety is paramount; problems (for both patient and operator) are far more common in mares (and stallions) that are poorly restrained. The use of protective walls and stable doors is not without risk and a proper chute/stocks (see p. 15) should be available on all stud farms. It is useful to apply a bridle or Chiffney to support the restraint. In any case, an assistant must be available to hold the head and another to lift the foreleg or to hold the tail.

- The procedure must never be performed without adequate help and restraint, no matter how docile the mare may appear to be.
- The increasing commercial value of mares and the high cost of ultrasound equipment make the provision of suitable stocks/chute a basic requirement for all reproductive examinations and procedures.
- Inappropriate restraint can result in serious personal injury and may also result in life-threatening or fatal injury to the mare.

---

ii. Sedation of fractious horses is a very wise precaution; problems are far more common in nervous animals that have not been subjected to repeated rectal examination.
- Sometimes a nose twitch and a lifted front leg are adequate, especially in older experienced horses.

iii. A protective overall and a thin plastic sleeve covered with copious lubricant should be used.

iv. An assistant holds the mare's tail to one side (away from the operator.)

v. The gloved, lubricated hand is introduced into the anus and any fecal matter in the rectum is evacuated. Each time the hand is re-introduced lubricant is re-applied.

vi. Individual veterinary surgeons will have a standard approach to ensure that all the required structures are examined carefully and adequately; it is far better to do one thorough examination than several inadequate ones.
- Usually the cervix is located initially with the hand inserted up to the wrist only.
- Thereafter the uterus can be followed and examined accordingly.
- As the operator reaches the apex of the uterine horn the ipsilateral ovary will be identified.

vii. As soon as the examination is completed the arm is withdrawn and the sleeve examined carefully for ANY evidence of blood.

viii. If the mare strains during the procedure the hand should be slowly withdrawn in response to the peristaltic wave in the rectum. The peristaltic wave should not be resisted.

ix. The whole pelvic and abdominal component of the genital tract of the mare (and the stallion) can be examined per rectum and with experience it can be a highly valuable procedure.

The results of the examination are recorded immediately. The rectal findings are often combined with those of the ultrasonographic examination and specific coded abbreviations are useful (see below).[25] The additional accuracy from ultrasonographic examination makes the procedure more meaningful, although experienced examiners are often very skilled at rectal examination. The combination of rectal examination and ultrasonography forms one of the foundations of reproductive medicine.

Example (after Asbury[25]):

DATE	LEFT OVARY	RIGHT OVARY
	Height × Width × Depth	Height × Width × Depth
7/07/2001: size:	$80 \times 50 \times 50$	$30 \times 40 \times 40$
characteristics:	FR/AP/40/#3	NSS

This example describes the results of a reproductive examination, performed on 7 July 2001, in which:
- The left ovary was $80 \times 50 \times 50$ mm in size, with a follicle of 40 mm diameter on the anterior pole, that is softening. (The code # is used to describe the extent of softening on a scale of 1 (firm) to 4 (fluctuant.)
- The right ovary is described as $30 \times 40 \times 40$ mm in size without any significant palpable structures (NSS).

If an ultrasound examination is to be conducted it is performed at this time. Otherwise the mare is prepared for vaginoscopy.

Vaginoscopic examination

The entire vagina and external cervical os can be inspected visually using a sterile instrument such as a plastic, cardboard or glass tubular speculum or a flexible endoscope.[26] The speculums are inexpensive, disposable and easily sterilized. Alternatively, the trivalve metal Caslick speculum may be used. It provides excellent visibility of the cervix and anterior vagina. It is used for evaluation of cervical tears, rectovaginal fistulas, and assessment of the integrity of urethral extensions. It is, however, cumbersome to sterilize and relatively expensive. A bright beam of light directed focally is needed to assess the vaginal walls and cervix. Light sources include penlights, halogen illuminators attached either to a long- or a short-handled transilluminator, and flashlights. An old endoscope with a functioning light source can be a very useful instrument. It takes up little space but provides a high-intensity light source that can be moved and manipulated easily.

In many examination procedures, the speculum examination is followed by collection of endometrial samples for:

- Culture.
- Cytological examination.
- Histopathological examination (see p. 145).

Aseptic preparation of the vulva is important in these procedures to prevent uterine contamination.

Note:
- Transient vaginal inflammation and bacterial flare can be detected after almost all procedures in which air is allowed to gain access to the vagina.

Features that have implications for the reproductive status of the mare include:

- The character and color of the mucosa.
- The shape, position and integrity of the cervix.
- The degree of cervical relaxation.
- The character of uterine, cervical and vaginal secretions.
- Anatomic abnormalities of the area and those caused by trauma also are easily detected.

Vaginoscopic examination is useful for:

- Detecting evidence of estrus or diestrus (or pregnancy, in conjunction with other methods).
- Detecting the presence of abnormal accumulations of fluid:
  - ❏ Urine in the vagina.
  - ❏ Fecal matter in perineal injuries such as rectovaginal fistula and perineal laceration.
  - ❏ Purulent material originating from the uterus or cervix.
- Detecting the origin of vaginal discharges seen at the vulvar lips.
- Detecting the presence of physical abnormalities of the vagina and cervix.

Technique (see Fig. 5.25)

Separate sterile instruments should be used for each successive mare if contagious disease is to be controlled. Disposable specula are available.

i. Apply suitable restraint to ensure safety of operator and mare, preferably in a chute or stocks in a darkened environment.
ii. Prepare the mare by application of a tail sleeve and tail bandage.

iii. Wash the perineal area with mild (nonscented) soap and rinse thoroughly with warm water. Dry with paper toweling and dry the inner margins of the vulva with a separate cotton gauze swab.
iv. The speculum is lubricated with a water-soluble, sterile, nonbactericidal, nonspermicidal obstetric lubricant.
v. The instrument is introduced in a slightly upward direction until the vaginal seal is broken and it is then directed more horizontally. As the seal is broken an obvious sucking sound will be heard.

- Repeated vaginoscopic examinations should be avoided if possible as each one induces a significant inflammation and risk of infection.
- Nevertheless the procedure is simple and requires little equipment to obtain much useful information.

Interpretation

Vaginoscopic examinations help determine the stage of the estrous cycle (Fig. 5.26) if used in conjunction with teasing and rectal palpation.

1. In estrus
   - The cervix progressively softens and drops toward the floor of the distended vagina.[26]
   - At the time of maximal relaxation, the cervix appears completely flattened on the vaginal floor, especially in pluriparous mares. The cervix in maiden and younger mares usually relaxes to a lesser degree.
   - Estrogen secretion by the developing follicle also produces edema, mucous secretion and hyperemia of both the cervical and vaginal mucosa.
   - Early in estrus, it is common for the external cervical os to have edematous folds of mucosa that resolve as ovulation approaches.
   - The degree of mucous secretion correlates with follicular development and is seen as increased shininess of the cervical and vaginal mucosal surfaces.
   - Judging the degree of hyperemia is important in evaluating the cervix and vagina for inflammatory and physiologic changes.
   - Artifactual reddening is produced quickly when air contacts the tissues, so evaluation of color must be made shortly after dilation of the vagina.

2. In diestrus
   - The cervical and vaginal surfaces become pale and dry.
   - The color of the mucous membrane is typically gray, with a yellowish cast.
   - The external cervical os projects into the

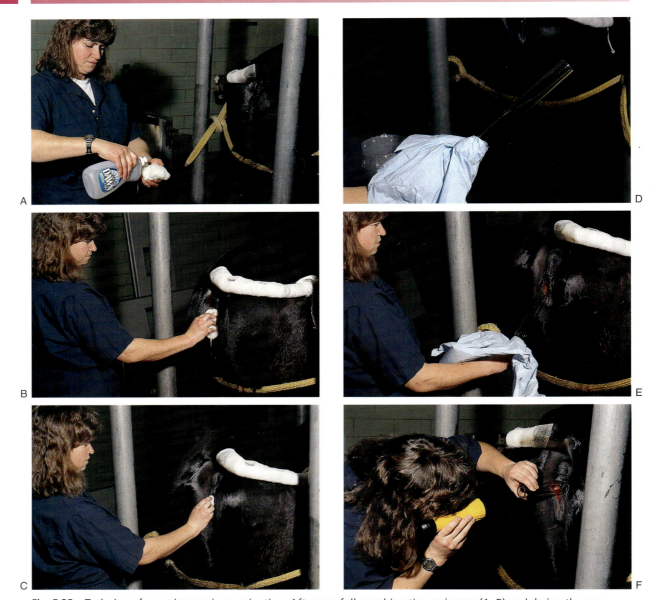

Fig. 5.25 Technique for vaginoscopic examination. After carefully washing the perineum (A, B) and drying the area, including the vulvar lips (C), the speculum (D) is introduced in a slightly upwards direction (E). Air will be heard to fill the vagina when the vestibular seal is broken. An illuminated speculum is helpful but not necessary to perform the procedure because a flashlight can be used (F).

cranial vagina from high on the wall and is tightly contracted, lending itself to the terms high, dry, and tight, or rosebud. The appearance of the cervix correlates well with its elongated shape and firm consistency on rectal examination.

3. In anestrus
   • Total lack of steroid production also results in a typical picture. Inactive ovaries are commonly found in winter anestrus and in conditions of gonadal dysgenesis.
   • Cervical and vaginal color is blanched, almost white.

   • The cervix becomes atonic and flaccid, and often gapes open to reveal the uterine lumen.
   • Blood vessels are sparse on the vaginal wall and little hyperemia occurs after exposure to air.
4. In pregnancy
   • The cervix may be intensely white and tightly closed.
   • In late pregnancy, the mucosa of the vaginal wall is covered by a thick, sticky exudate, which prevents the usual ballooning effect caused by introducing a speculum. It is sometimes difficult to visualize the cervical os

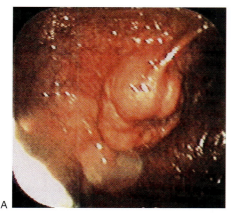
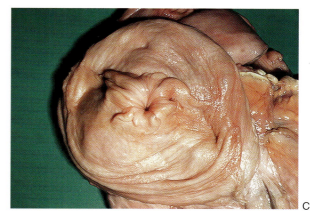
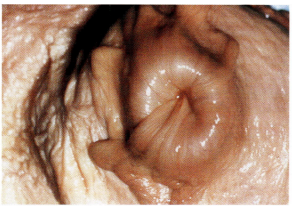
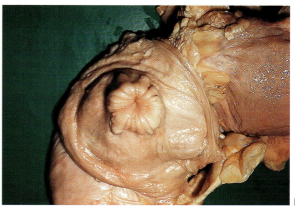

Fig. 5.26 Changes to the cervix during the estrous cycle and pregnancy. (A) Early estrus. (B) Estrous cervix. (C) Diestrous cervix. (D) Anestrous cervix. (Courtesy of Gary England.)

late in pregnancy because it is pulled cranioventrally.

5. Exudate and inflammation
   - Inflammatory changes, such as mucosal hyperemia and suppurative exudate, are often discovered by visual examination.
   - These changes are seen most frequently on the second or third day of estrus, after the perineum has relaxed under the influence of estrogens and prior to the flushing action of the increased uterine secretions.
   - On speculum examination, a grayish, watery to white, purulent exudate may be present on the vaginal floor.
   - Exudate may be seen passing out of the cervical os from the uterus and the vaginal mucosa may be hyperemic.
   - If pneumovagina is present, the mucus and exudate will often have a 'foamy' appearance because air has mixed with the mucus.

6. Urovagina (pooling of urine in the cranial fornix of the vagina)
   - This is encountered in older, multiparous mares that have developed problems associated with pneumovagina, such as a pelvic canal that slopes cranioventrally.
   - Urovagina might not be observed until the day before ovulation, when estrogen levels and perineal relaxation are greatest.
   - It may be seen during the first postpartum estrus when the vaginal structures are stretched, relaxed, and pulled forward by the weight of the involuting uterus.
   - Fluid in the vaginal fornix may be confirmed to be urine by visual inspection of color, by smell, or biochemically (osmolarity, urea content).
   - The urine may often be seen to cover at least a portion if not the entire cervix.
   - Inflammatory cells are often mixed with the urine and its salt sediment.
   - In severe cases, the urine flows into the uterus when the cervix is relaxed causing cervicitis and endometritis.

7. Physical abnormalities
   - Vaginal varicosities (Fig. 5.27).
     ❑ Usually occur in the region of the perforated hymen and are not uncommon.[27]
     ❑ May rupture late in pregnancy leading to blood dripping from the vulvar lips.
     ❑ If observed at breeding, the bleeding must be differentiated from vaginal rupture.

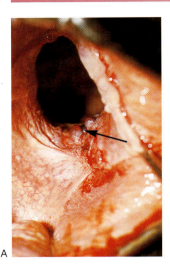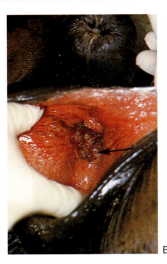

A B

Fig. 5.27 (A) Anterior vaginal varicosity. Note the varicose veins in the anterior vault of the vagina. Clots of blood overlie veins (arrow). The mare died 12 months later from a fatal hemorrhage, 1 month before foaling. (B) Posterior vaginal varicosity. Note the small hemorrhagic 'grape-like' varicose veins in the posterior vagina (arrow). The mare bled frequently after service and occasionally following urination.

❑ Varicose veins are detected by speculum examination. They are usually 1–2 mm in diameter and the color of venous blood inside a bluish translucent vascular wall.
- Rectovaginal fistula.
  ❑ A green watery exudate with fecal matter will be present on the vaginal floor in rectovaginal fistulas.
  ❑ Location of the fistula can be determined by examining the dorsum of the vagina and vestibulum as the speculum is extracted from the vagina. The fistula will appear as a small to large opening that contains feces.
- Persistent hymen.
  ❑ The hymen may persist in maiden mares.
  ❑ On vaginal speculum examination it will appear as a thin, bluish-white sheet of tissue covering the cranial aspect of the vestibulovaginal junction.
  ❑ If the hymen is complete, the speculum cannot be advanced into the vagina.
  ❑ The hymen may bulge out through the lips of the vulva in fillies that have reached puberty and are having estrous cycles. This results from uterine fluids produced during estrus accumulating in the anterior vagina.
- Necrotic/bacterial vaginitis may occur as a sequel to dystocia and can be life-threatening.
  ❑ On vaginal speculum examination, the vaginal walls will be black and necrotic or will be gray and granulomatous.
  ❑ There will be a foul odor when the speculum is passed into the vagina.
  ❑ After the delivery of a dead, necrotic fetus, severe vaginitis occurs if hair and necrotic tissue become embedded within the wall as a result of improper lubrication during delivery.
  ❑ Treatment of severe necrotic vaginitis consists of lavage with warm saline solution

and a nonirritating antimicrobial. This loosens necrotic vaginal tissue.
❑ Proper aseptic technique and ample sterile lubrication of the operator's gloved hand reduce further vaginal irritation.
❑ Mares should be given broad-spectrum antibiotics and metronidazole because many become systemically ill.

Manual vaginal examination

This is an almost obligatory part of the breeding soundness examination. Although it is tempting to use a vaginoscopic examination instead, there are several important conditions that are best detected by manual examination (e.g. cervical incompetence). The main purpose of this examination is to examine the cervix for integrity and character.

- Evaluation of the mare's genital tract is incomplete without manually exploring the vagina and the cervical integrity and character.

Technique

Aseptic technique is essential in these procedures, in preparation both of the mare and of the hand and arm of the examiner.

  i. Restraint and hygienic preparations are as above.
 ii. When the gloved hand is introduced into the mare's vagina, the vulvar labiae should be parted with the fingers of the other hand to reduce contamination.
- A well-lubricated gloved hand is inserted gently between the vulvar lips and directed gently upwards until the vaginal seal is broken.

- A sterile, shoulder-length latex glove is ideal, but a practical alternative is a clean plastic sleeve with a sterile surgeon's glove applied over it.
iii. Lubrication should be with a sterile, water-soluble product.
iv. It is possible to dilate the cervix of the estrous mare to permit uterine examination.

- A similar approach is made for introduction of an endometrial biopsy instrument, for uteroscopy with a fiberoptic or video endoscope (see below), or for harvesting a suitable specimen for endometrial culture and/or cytology.

Interpretation

i. The vestibulovaginal junction should be tight, making it difficult for the examiner to pass his or her hand. If the examiner's hand slips easily into the anterior vagina, the mare may be predisposed to pneumovagina. If the manual exam is performed after the speculum exam, pneumovagina, caused by the vaginoscopic exam, makes this assessment more difficult.
ii. The vestibulovaginal junction should be palpated in maiden mares to ensure the absence of tissue bands formed by hymen remnants. These bands could later contribute to a rectovaginal perforation at parturition.
iii. The cervix should always be palpated directly if a complete reproductive examination is performed.
   - By carefully dilating the external os of the cervix and then palpating the entire cervical canal, it is possible to locate lacerations and adhesions that are not evident simply by vaginoscopy. The cervical os may be torn or the cervical body may be ruptured such that it is permanently overstretched.
   - Because of the importance of the cervical seal during pregnancy, if a lesion is noted the cervix should be re-examined during diestrus to determine if it closes completely.
   - Evaluation of the cervix manually is extremely important in infertility evaluations, as tears are often very difficult to detect by speculum examination in older multiparous mares.

Technique

i. The operator may be confident in the use of only one hand. However, examination may be more accurate if the gloved thumb is introduced into the cervical canal and the index finger is used to palpate the cervix in a 180° clockwise sweep, starting at the dorsal rim.
ii. Particular note can be made of variation in thickness.

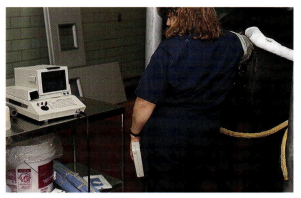

Fig. 5.28 Ultrasonographic examination of the reproductive tract.

iii. This procedure is then repeated from the dorsal rim in an anticlockwise sweep using the other hand.

Ultrasonography

Ultrasonographic examination of the reproductive tract of the mare (Fig 5.28) has revolutionized stud medicine. The procedure is nonhazardous (except for the accompanying risks of rectal examination; see p. 133). The accuracy and detail that can be provided by this technique have been instrumental in improving the breeding management of mares and stallions. The accuracy of the information is greatly increased when the findings are compared to the findings derived from rectal palpation.[28]

Usually the technique involves transrectal examination with a probe of 7.5 or 5.0 MHz with linear array configuration. A linear array 5-MHz transducer is most frequently used in routine equine reproductive work. Its enables the operator to detect a conceptus on day 11 or 12 (day 0 is day of ovulation), follicles as small as 3 mm in diameter, and the presence of a corpus luteum through most of diestrus.

A linear array 2.5- or 3-MHz transducer is used to evaluate fetal viability using a transabdominal approach (see p. 238).

Ultrasonography can be used to diagnose uterine disease, such as:

- Intrauterine fluid.
- Air.
- Cysts.
- Ovarian irregularities, such as anovulatory follicles.
- Neoplasia and hematomas.

Also, examination of the ovaries by ultrasonography may aid in determining the stage of the estrous cycle, status of preovulatory follicles, and development of the corpus luteum (see p. 142).

Excellent in-depth reviews of reproductive ultrasonography are available.[29,30]

Technique

Precautions:
- The procedure and precautions for transrectal ultrasound examinations are similar to those for rectal palpation.
- Feces must be thoroughly removed from the rectum before introducing the transducer.
- The transducer should be well lubricated, and care should be taken to avoid fecal material attaching to the transducer.
- Good contact must exist between the transducer and rectal wall.
- Air in the rectum or a gas- or fluid-filled loop of bowel will result in a distorted image.

i. The examination should be performed in a darkened environment so that greater detail can be appreciated and 'gain' can be reduced.
ii. The mare is prepared as for rectal examination (see above).
iii. The linear probe is held in the palm of the hand so that the working surface of the probe is directed downwards.
iv. The probe is guided onto the body of the uterus initially and then is gradually passed forwards along the body and up each horn of the uterus in turn. This part of the examination can provide very useful information about the uterine content. The ovary can be visualized easily and the various structures are highly characteristic.

Ultrasonographic diagnosis of pregnancy is a routine procedure and provides very useful information about the conceptus and its development.

Interpretation

A systematic scanning technique needs to be developed to eliminate the possibility of missing structures or an embryonic vesicle. One method of examination is to move the probe from uterine body to left uterine horn, left uterine horn to left ovary, re-examine the left uterine horn and uterine body, evaluate the right uterine horn and right ovary, return to the uterine body and then scan the cervix.

Normal anatomy

1. The uterus (Fig. 5.29)
   - The uterus is visualized as a cross-sectional image.
   - With the probe held in a sagittal plane, the cranial aspect of the uterus is seen on the right of the ultrasound screen and the caudal aspect on the left of the screen (this can be reversed by certain operators on the ultrasound machine by a probe-reversal function button).

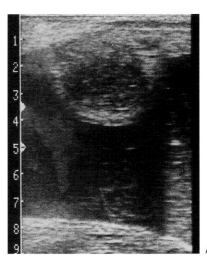

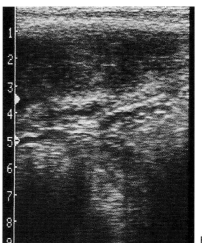

Fig. 5.29 (A) Normal uterine appearance on ultrasonography during diestrus. (B) Ultrasound appearance of normal uterine body.

- The uterus undergoes dynamic changes due to hormonal influences that can be visualized by ultrasonography.
   i. Estrus
      - The uterine horns are well rounded, and both horns and body have an interdigitated pattern of alternating echogenic and nonechogenic areas similar to the spokes on a wheel or slices of an orange.[31,32]
      - The areas of decreased echogenicity are the outer edematous portions of endometrial folds. The edema is caused by the influence of estrogen.
      - Endometrial folds generally parallel estrogen production and are visible at the end of diestrus, becoming quite prominent as estrus progresses and

decrease or disappear 12 hours before ovulation.

❑ A small amount of fluid may be present normally within the uterine lumen during estrus.

❑ These changes, in combination with loss of the endometrial folds and softening of the follicle, can be used to estimate time of ovulation.

❑ Endometrial folds are sometimes seen in early pregnancy (16–28 days of gestation), especially if large follicles are present on the ovaries.

ii. Diestrus

❑ The echo texture is more homogeneous, and the uterus is well circumscribed.

❑ A hyperechogenic white line in the area of apposing endometrial surfaces often identifies the uterine lumen.

iii. Anestrus

❑ The uterus is flat and irregular and may contour closely to surrounding abdominal organs.

iv. Pregnancy

❑ The uterus appears similar to that of diestrus during pregnancy except that endometrial folds may again appear after day 16 and a vesicle will be present.

2. The ovary (Fig. 5.30)

● Follicles are nonechogenic and appear as black, roughly circumscribed shaped images. They may appear irregular-shaped due to impending ovulation or due to compression by adjacent follicles or luteal structures.

● Within 24 hours of ovulation, the shape of the follicle changes from spherical to teardrop and the follicular wall becomes more hyperechoic.[33] Just prior to ovulation an increase in follicular fluid density may be evident.

● After the follicle ruptures, a corpus hemorrhagicum forms. It has one of two appearances on ultrasound:

i. It is either a uniformly echogenic circumscribed image or it contains a centrally nonechogenic center. Echogenic lines attributable to clotting and fibrinization in the central nonechogenic center may be present (Fig. 5.31).

ii. The corpus hemorrhagicum is highly echogenic on the day of ovulation. Echogenicity decreases and then plateaus during the first 6 days (now a mature corpus luteum) and then increases over days 12–16 (Fig. 5.32).

The characteristic ultrasonographic changes associated with pregnancy are described on p. 237.

Pathological changes visualized by ultrasonography

Uterine cysts, accumulation of intrauterine fluid, and air can be identified by ultrasonography (Fig. 5.33).[34,35]

1. Uterine cysts

Uterine cysts indicate an on-going degenerative process within the endometrium. Cysts will vary in size from <5 to >50 mm. There may be many small cysts that appear to be imbedded within the endometrium or just a single, large cyst that may contain many partitions. It is helpful to record the presence of intraluminal cysts visualized by ultrasonography because they may be confused with an embryo. Characteristics of the embryo that can be used to differentiate the two include:

● Early mobility of the embryo (days 10–16).

● The presence of specular reflection on the upper and lower surfaces of the embryonic vesicle.

● Spherical appearance without partitions.

● Growth rate.

2. Fluid

Fluid present within the uterus during diestrus and the early postovulatory period has been associated with early embryonic death, endometritis, and decreased conception rates (Fig. 5.34). A small amount of nonechogenic fluid in the uterine lumen during estrus does not appear to adversely affect fertility. Air within the uterus appears as multiple hyperechogenic reflections. If present in mares during estrus or directly after ovulation, the mare should be closely examined for pneumovagina.

3. Abnormalities

Ovarian abnormalities, such as anovulatory follicles, luteinized unruptured follicles, persistent corpus luteum, tumor, and hematoma can be identified by ultrasonography.[36] Anovulatory follicles result when preovulatory follicles grow to an unusual size (70–100 mm), fail to ovulate, fill with blood, and gradually recede. These follicles are distinctly echogenic, with criss-crossing fibrin-like strands without significant luteal tissue around the periphery (Fig. 5.35).

4. Tumors

The two most common ovarian tumors are:

● Granulosa theca cell (see p. 170).

● Teratoma (see p. 173).

Both of these characteristically have a 'honeycomb' appearance, with multiple small nonechogenic areas separated by echogenic trabeculae. However, the granulosa cell tumor can be highly variable in appearance. Some may contain one to two large cysts (Fig. 5.36); others may be homogeneously dense throughout. Measurement of plasma testosterone

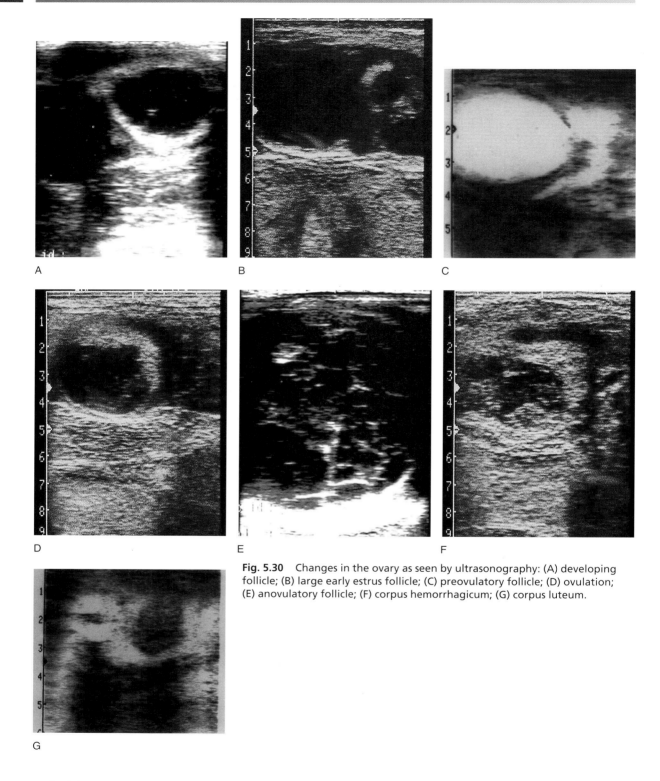

Fig. 5.30 Changes in the ovary as seen by ultrasonography: (A) developing follicle; (B) large early estrus follicle; (C) preovulatory follicle; (D) ovulation; (E) anovulatory follicle; (F) corpus hemorrhagicum; (G) corpus luteum.

and inhibin concentrations can be used to definitively diagnose these tumors (see p. 171).

Ovarian hematoma (see Fig. 5.37) can be confused with granulosa cell tumor because they appear similar on ultrasound examination, and some granulosa cell tumors have hematomas within their stroma. Frequently, ovarian hematoma appears uniformly echogenic. Some may appear as lucid areas separated by trabeculae, similar to those of a multi-cystic granulosa cell tumor (Fig. 5.37). It is likely that some

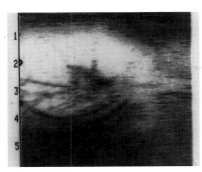

Fig. 5.31 Ultrasonographic image of a 48-hour-old corpus hemorrhagicum. The corpus hemorrhagicum is located centrally within the ovary and is surrounded by non-echogenic fluid.

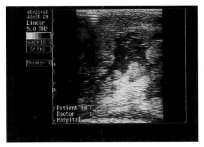

Fig. 5.34 Fluid in the uterine lumen is a significant finding in mares suffering from various forms of infertility. This fluid is free within the uterine lumen (arrow).

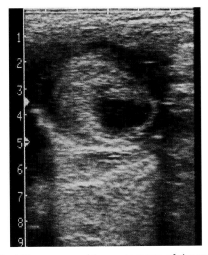

Fig. 5.32 Ultrasonographic appearance of the corpus luteum (arrow). Note the highly echogenic appearance which will gradually decline up to day 6 and then tends to enlarge slowly up to day 16 when it will again become less obvious and remain static for the rest of the cycle.

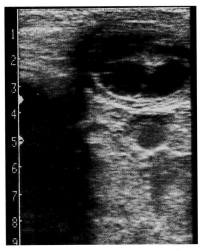

Fig. 5.35 Anovulatory follicles are a natural phenomenon in the mare but they can sometimes reach considerable size and have echogenic strands without significant luteal tissue.

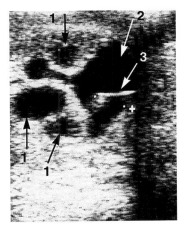

Fig. 5.33 Uterine/endometrial cyst (ultrasonographic appearance).

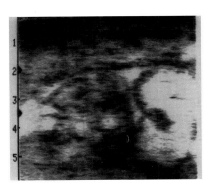

Fig. 5.36 Granulosa (thecal) cell tumor. Note the cystic multiloculated appearance.

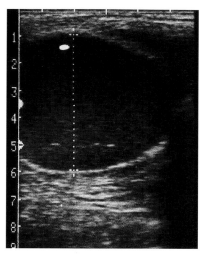

Fig. 5.37 Ultrasound image of an ovarian hematoma.

ovarian structures that were diagnosed as hematomas before the advent of ultrasonography were anovulatory follicles.

Diagnosis of granulosa cell (thecal) tumor and hematoma must be made on the basis of:

- Clinical signs and reproductive behavior.
- Rapidity of ovarian enlargement.
- The presence or absence of the ovulation fossa.
- The size of the contralateral ovary.
- The concentration of inhibin and testosterone in plasma.
- Response to prostaglandin administration.

Specific ultrasonographic features of the various reproductive structures are described in other sections.

Blood samples

Blood samples may be very useful for the assay of hormone profiles. Certain specific physiological changes are recognized in cycling, noncycling, and pregnant mares. Furthermore, there are significant changes in some pathological conditions, such as granulosa (thecal) cell tumor (see p. 170) and cryptorchidism in the male (see p. 95).

The specific types of blood sample (anticoagulant and volume) may vary for the various requirements and the laboratory should be consulted before sampling if there is any doubt about what is required.

Technique

Blood sampling technique is a routine matter for veterinary surgeons. Although complications are rare, localized infection (phlebitis) or thrombosis, or both (thrombophlebitis) can follow in certain conditions. The risks are probably similar to those of intravenous injection although the latter can involve irritant drugs that might add to the risks.

Uterine (endometrial) biopsy

Histological assessment of the endometrium is helpful in assessing the degree of inflammation, noting the presence or absence of fibrosis and lymphatic lacunae and evaluating glandular density (see Fig. 5.38, Table 5.3). The technique has been widely used for many years[37–39] and established standards for interpretation make this procedure an integral part of the reproductive examination.[40,41]

Endometrial biopsies may be obtained at any stage of the estrous cycle because the equine cervix is easily dilated. Endometrial architecture changes with the stage of the cycle and the season of the year. For this reason, the person evaluating the biopsy should be informed of the stage of the cycle and the physical findings at the time the sample was taken.

Suitable custom-made 70-cm alligator punch instruments with a basket size of $20 \times 4 \times 3$ mm are available for the purpose (Pilling, Fort Washington, PA; Arnolds Veterinary, UK) and make the procedure relatively safe and simple (see Fig. 5.39).

Candidates for endometrial biopsy include:

- Barren mares with clinical, endoscopic or ultrasonographic evidence of endometrial disease that fail to conceive after repeated breeding to a stallion of known fertility.
- Mares with a history of early embryonic death, or mares with a history of having abnormal estrous cycles.
- Nonpregnant mares presented for fertility evaluation as a part of a prepurchase examination should also have a uterine biopsy.
- Mares requiring genital surgery that may not be capable of supporting a pregnancy to term should be biopsied prior to surgical intervention.

- Clearly the mare must not be pregnant when a biopsy is taken!

Technique (Fig. 5.39)

i. The mare is restrained in stocks/chute as for rectal examination and the rectum is evacuated of fecal material.

ii. The perineum is washed and prepared as for vaginal examination.

iii. The closed biopsy instrument is inserted into the vagina in the cupped hand and is guided carefully into the uterus through the cervix with the index finger so as to avoid any risk of cervical trauma.

iv. The operator's arm is then withdrawn and introduced into the rectum. The instrument is located per rectum.
  - If a specific site is to be biopsied, the forceps is guided to that location.
  - If no specific site is identified, a single or multiple mid-horn biopsy is sufficient.

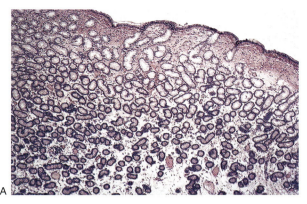

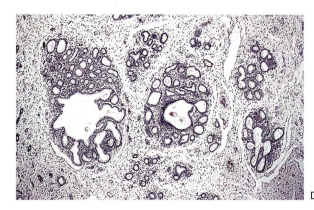

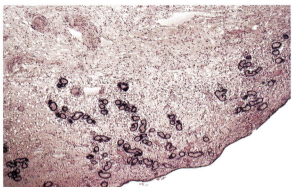

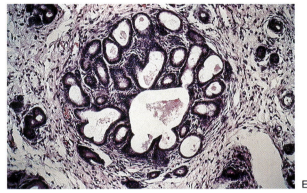

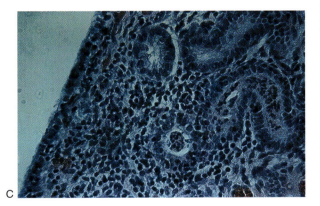

Fig. 5.38 Histological appearance of normal endometrium (A), non-glandular endometrium (B), diffuse, severe inflammation (C), fibrosis (D), lymphatic lacunae (E).

v. The instrument is turned onto its side and the jaws are opened. The endometrium is gently pushed between the open jaws, which are then closed firmly.

vi. A short, sharp tug may be needed to cut the tissue and the instrument is withdrawn.

vii. The specimen is carefully removed from the basket immediately (usually with a fine needle) and placed in a suitable fixative (Bouin's solution is usually recommended) or onto ice if bacterial culture is to be undertaken.

- In the event that the specimen is not to be processed for more than 3–4 days, it should be transferred to 70% ethanol to prevent deterioration.

- Formalin (10%) is also used but tends to create more tissue distortion on sectioning.
- Cryosections can be taken from the fresh biopsy if facilities exist for this.

viii. The fixed tissue is trimmed for embedding in paraffin so that sections are cut perpendicular to the endometrial surface.

- Paraffin-embedded sections are best stained with hematoxylin and eosin for routine examination.
- For proper interpretation, specimens need to have at least 1–2 cm of endometrium on histological sections.

ix. The histological significance of the findings is variable[42] but some are described in Table 5.3.

Table 5.3 Interpretive findings from endometrial biopsy in normal and abnormal horses

Stage	Endometrial epithelium	Glandular pattern	Comments
Normal horse			
Pre-estrus	Low columnar	Glands in clumps	
Estrus	Tall columnar	Edema and decreased glandular density	Neutrophil infiltration
Diestrus	Low cuboidal	Increased density; proliferation; reduced edema	
Anestrus	Cuboidal/atrophic	Glandular atrophy; low density	Possibly trapped amorphous inspissated secretions in mucosa
Abnormal horse			
Pyometra		Cystic glands distended with hyaline secretions; atrophy and fibrosis	Inflamed granulation tissue infiltration of endometrium
Acute endometritis			Diffuse acute inflammatory infiltrate
Chronic infiltrative endometritis			Mononuclear (histiocyte and plasma cell) infiltration of superficial stroma; eosinophils and mast cells; periglandular aggregations of cells ('lymphoid' follicles)
Chronic degenerative endometritis	Thin, low and inactive	Cysts and gland nests	Periglandular stromal fibrosis and edema (lymphatic lacuna)
Endometrial hypoplasia	Low cuboidal, inactive	Short, underdeveloped glands	No underlying inflammatory changes or degeneration
Endometrial atrophy	Cuboidal (in spite of cyclical ovary)	Atrophic and low in number	Chronic infiltrative inflammation and degenerative endometritis present

After Asbury AC. Endometrial biopsy. In: Colahan PT, Moore JN, Merritt AM, Mayhew IG, eds. Equine medicine and surgery. USA: Mosby, 1999:1088, 1097–1110.

Usually, however, interpretation is best left to specialist pathologists with experience of such specimens. Nevertheless, it is important to provide the pathologist with a detailed history of the mare and the results of any other tests that have been performed.

- Many endometrial disorders are diffuse and so the findings can usually be regarded as representative.[43]

x. Notwithstanding the need for a specialist pathological interpretation, it is possible for clinicians to develop interpretative skills. However, facilities for the preparation of sections are not usually available in normal practice so it seems sensible to rely on specialists.

Interpretation

i. The major pathologic changes in endometrial biopsies are:

- Inflammation.
- Fibrosis.
- Lymphatic stasis.

ii. To be of diagnostic and prognostic value, these changes must be characterized and quantified.

iii. Endometrial inflammation is characterized by increased numbers of inflammatory cells in foci or diffused in various areas of the lamina propria.

iv. The predominant cell type classifies the cellular infiltrate.

- Neutrophils are the predominant cell in acute endometritis.
- There is a mixture of neutrophils and lymphocytes in subacute endometritis.
- In chronic endometritis, there are lymphocytes, plasma cells, and macrophages.

v. Endometrial fibrosis occurs most commonly around the glands and appears in response to inflammation or glandular damage, or from other undefined causes.

- Periglandular fibrosis may interfere with gland

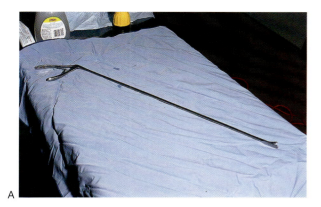

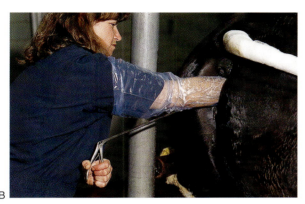

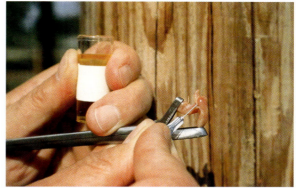

Fig. 5.39 Uterine alligator forceps (A) are used to obtain a biopsy from the endometrium. The instrument is introduced into the uterus through the cervix under manual guidance (B). The operator's arm is then introduced into the rectum to assist biopsy. The specimen is enclosed in the biopsy instrument cup and is then gently placed in fixative (C).

function to the extent that glandular support of the early conceptus is altered and causes early embryonic death between 35 and 70 days.

vi. Lymphatic stasis appears as large, fluid-filled spaces lined with endothelial cells.
  - When widespread and accompanied by a jelly-like consistency of the uterus on rectal palpation, this lesion is correlated with reduced fertility.
  - Because large areas of edema may be artificially produced during biopsy, care must be taken to identify the spaces as lymphatics.

When these basic pathologic changes are observed, they should be evaluated for severity and distribution. This allows mares to be categorized into three diagnostic and prognostic groups (categories):[40]

1. **Category I** includes mares with an endometrium compatible with conception and capable of supporting a foal to term. Pathologic changes are slight and widely scattered.
  - No endometrial atrophy or hypoplasia is seen on biopsies taken during the physiological breeding season. Mares in category I have a ≥70% chance of producing a live foal.
2. **Category II** includes mare with endometrial changes that reduce the chance of conception and pregnancy maintenance but which are reversible or only moderately severe. Endometrial changes

may include combinations of any of the following: slight to moderate, diffuse cellular infiltration of superficial layers; scattered but frequent inflammatory; fibrotic foci throughout the entire lamina propria. Other lesions include:
  - Scattered but frequent periglandular fibrosis of individual gland branches of any degree of severity.
  - ≤3 nests of gland branches per low-power field in five fields (fields 5 mm in diameter).
  - Mild to moderate lymphatic stasis.

Mares with glandular atrophy due to physiological seasonal changes are also placed in Category II. Pregnancy rates for mares in this category range from 30% to 70%, depending on the severity of the lesions.[41]

Frequently, category II is subdivided into:

- **Category IIa** where there is inflammation.
- **Category IIb** where fibrosis is detected and in cases where there is fibrosis and inflammation.

Since there is no treatment for fibrosis, mares in category IIb have a lower likelihood of carrying a foal until term.

3. **Category III** includes mares with endometrial changes that reduce the chances of conception and pregnancy maintenance, and which are essentially irreversible.
   - The endometrium may contain any of the following changes:
     - ❏ Widespread periglandular fibrosis of any degree of severity, with ≥5 nests in an average low-power field.
     - ❏ Widespread, diffuse, severe cellular infiltration of superficial layers.
     - ❏ Widespread lymphatic stasis accompanied by palpable changes in the uterus.
   - Additional findings include endometrial atrophy or hypoplasia with gonadal dysgenesis, and pyometra accompanied by rectally palpable endometrial atrophy or widespread, diffuse, severe inflammatory cell infiltration.
   - Mares in category III have less than a 10% chance of carrying a foal until term. Many of these mares may conceive but will not carry the full 11 months.

- Care should be taken before pronouncing a mare sterile on the basis of single or even multiple biopsies.
- The occasional exception can be embarrassing.

Hysteroscopy/uteroscopy

Uteroscopy has developed from vaginoscopy with the availability of suitable fiberoptic and video endoscopes.[44] The technique has significant benefits in providing visual information on the condition of the endometrium. Although it is tempting to take biopsies for histological examination, there are no instruments that will permit a suitable size of biopsy instrument for effective biopsy. Visual inspection can be used to guide an independently introduced instrument so that biopsy of specific locations can be undertaken with relative ease. Conditions such as endometrial cysts, polyps, adhesions, and hemorrhagic foci can be identified and treated directly, but endometrial biopsy is more effective in detecting pathological endometrial disease.[44]

A complete reproductive examination is essential before hysteroscopy because the procedure itself does cause pathological changes. Examination during diestrus is preferred.

Endoscopes used for hysteroscopy should be equipped with high-power insufflation, suction and effective washing facilities. Without these, the technique becomes frustrating and difficult to interpret. Insufflation invariably induces an acute inflammation, so maximal effort must be taken to obtain the full range of specimens at the initial occasion. Saline distension induces much less inflammation but can be difficult to control. Because it causes less straining and discomfort than air insufflation, saline distension is recommended.

Technique

i. The mare is restrained and if necessary sedated to allow safe examination.

ii. The perineum is cleaned and dried in the manner previously described.

iii. The endoscope is guided into the cervix with a gloved lubricated finger and the cervix can be gently held to retain the insufflation air or saline infusion under gravity feed (up to 1–2 liters is usually sufficient).

iv. The instrument can be guided up each uterine horn in turn and a recording taken of the findings for later detailed examination.

v. After the manipulations are complete the cervix can be released and suction used to remove as much air as possible from the distended uterus.
   - If the uterus has been distended with saline this is released and aspirated as far as possible.

vi. The instrument is removed.

Note:
The sterility of an endoscope is not always easy to maintain:
- Gas sterilization (using ethylene oxide) or glutaraldehyde washing should be used between each examination.
- The risk of transmission of infection is considerable if several mares are to be examined sequentially.
- It is virtually impossible to sterilize an endoscope by simply wiping it between mares.

Uterine cytology

Cytological examination of the uterus can also be helpful in establishing a diagnosis in chronic or low-grade endometritis, especially if the physical examination does not reveal signs of inflammation, such as hyperemia or exudate.

- The presence of neutrophils in a cytological specimen obtained from the uterine lumen indicates an active inflammatory process.[45,46]
- The number of neutrophils in the uterine lumen is probably representative of the presence of bacteria or foreign material of another type. Air, urine, feces, semen and bacteria will cause a uterine inflammatory response.
- The relationship between inflammatory cells and uterine inflammation is the basis for the use of cytological examination of cells obtained from the uterine lumen.

- Use of this technique provides early information on the breeding soundness of a mare in the face of an outbreak of infectious uterine disease.[47]

- There is no doubt that the results of combined cytology and bacteriological culture (and if necessary biopsy) provide the practitioner with a very helpful indication of uterine health.

Technique

Specimens may be obtained by:

- Aspiration.
- Lavage.
- Curettage.

Various methods for examining uterine lumenal cells are available (Fig. 5.40).[48] A guarded culture instrument (suitable instruments are made by: Kalayjian Industries Inc., Long Beach, CA; McCullough Cartwright, Barrington, IL; Haver Lockart, Kansas

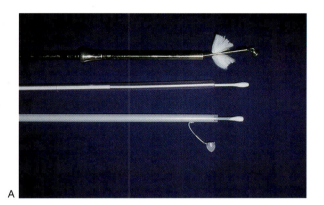

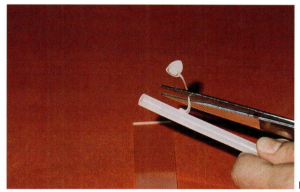

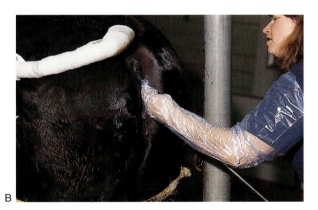

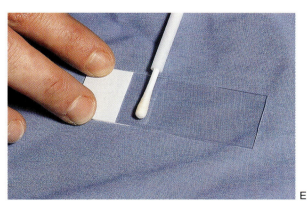

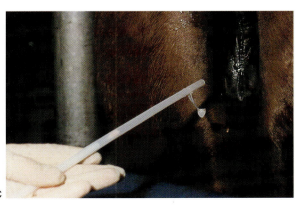

Fig. 5.40 A variety of methods are available for cytological collection, including brushes, simple cotton swabs and combined swab and fluid collection instruments (A). The procedure is carried out in a very clean (ideally aseptic) fashion (B) and the collection is performed according to the method used (C). If the fluid method of collection is used, the 'cup' is cut off and processed (D), whereas if a swab is used a direct smear is taken onto a glass slide (E).

City, KS) is usually used to obtain cells for cytological (and bacteriological) examination (see Fig. 5.40). To be diagnostically useful and practical under field conditions, examination of the slide must be rapid, simple and produce consistent results.

> * The use of unguarded culture rods carries risks of false results resulting from contamination from the vagina, vestibule and vulva, and also carries the risk of introducing infection into the uterus.

i. The mare should be in mid-estrus.
   * Most frequently the procedure is performed on day 2 or 3 of estrus.
   * If performed during diestrus, it is advisable to induce estrus after the procedure by administration of prostaglandin because iatrogenic infection can be introduced when the cervix is closed.
ii. The mare is restrained and hygienically prepared as above.
iii. A vaginal speculum is inserted into the vagina (see above) and the guarded culture instrument is passed through the cervix under direct visualization.
   * Alternatively, the culture instrument can be guided to the cervix using a sterile gloved arm.
   * A cap and the outer tube guard the swab in this instrument as it is passed through the cervix.
iv. Once in the uterus (Fig. 5.41), the inner sheath that contains the swab is pushed against the cap, which snaps open and exposes the swab.
   * The swab is rubbed along the endometrial surface.

* After the swab is saturated for the microbiological sample, it is retracted back into the tube and is withdrawn.

> Note:
> * For bacterial culture, the swab should be retained in the uterus for over 30 seconds to allow effective harvesting of bacteria (see Fig. 5.41).

* A direct smear from the swab is made immediately onto several glass slides; these are fixed immediately using an aerosol or alcohol fixative.
v. The cap remains attached to the tube by a flexible plastic stalk.
   * While the outer tube is still in the uterine lumen, the entire tube is rotated briskly several times.
   * This causes the cap to collect a sample of endometrial cells and fluid.
vi. As soon as the instrument is withdrawn from the mare, the cap is cut off and a slide prepared from the drop of fluid and cellular material it contains.
   * The open end of the cap is placed on a slide and tapped briskly with the index finger to transfer the sample to the slide.
   * The sample is spread gently onto the slide and allowed to air-dry.

> Note:
> * Air-drying and fixing can cause significant cell distortion.

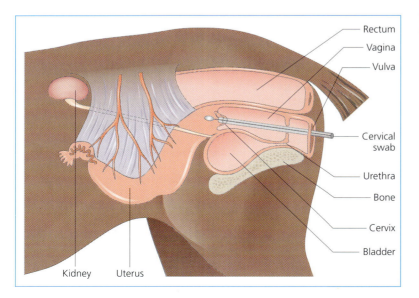

Kidney   Uterus

Rectum
Vagina
Vulva
Cervical swab
Urethra
Bone
Cervix
Bladder

Fig. 5.41 Diagram to show endometrial cytology swab in utero.

vii. The slides are stained with routine stains such as:
  - New methylene blue. This stain provides an excellent differentiation of cells but stained material cannot be stored permanently. A drop of stain is placed directly onto the slide and a coverslip applied.
  - Leishman.
  - Giemsa.
  - Modified Wright–Giemsa. A simple three-step Wright–Giemsa staining process has proved practical and effective for field use. Staining takes only a few minutes and slides may be examined wet or allowed to dry for later evaluation.
viii. Permanent mounting with a coverslip is recommended for long-term storage of slides.

Alternative method using endometrial lavage systems:

- A suitable flushing balloon catheter is introduced into the uterus as above and guided into the uterine horn.
- A small volume of warm saline is introduced and aspirated back.
- The specimen is subjected to cytospin separation and the cells transferred to a glass slide for routine staining and examination.

Interpretation

Interpretation of the specimens requires careful consideration and experience (see Fig. 5.42).

  i. A cytological specimen that has been collected and prepared properly will have sheets of epithelial cells throughout the slide (Fig. 5.42).
  ii. An effective sample will have a significant proportion of epithelial cells; if there are none, the sample is probably not cytologically useful.
  iii. If there is a high proportion of neutrophils with epithelial cells then the likelihood is that there is endometrial inflammation (a ratio of more than 1 neutrophil to 10 epithelial cells is significant).
  iv. If no epithelial cells are seen, there is no assurance that the uterine lining was scraped sufficiently. This problem tends to occur in older pluriparous mares whose uterus is located ventral to the pelvis.
  v. If many neutrophils are seen (>5 cells/high-power field, ×40), inflammation is present (Fig. 5.42).

- Interpretation of the vast majority of samples processed in this manner provides a straightforward positive or negative result.[47] Occasional samples show few neutrophils. In these cases, a ratio of neutrophils to epithelial cells should be calculated. If this ratio is more than 1 neutrophil to 10 epithelial cells, inflammation may be judged to be significant.

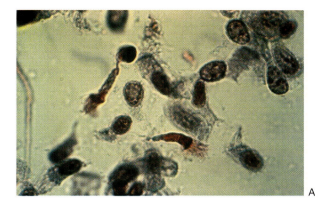

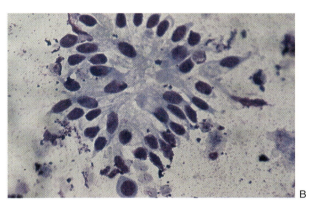

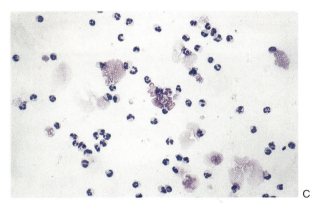

Fig. 5.42 (A, B) A properly prepared cytological specimen containing sheets of epithelial cells. (C) Cytology smear with numerous neutrophils present.

Microbiological swabbing

The significance of bacteriological cultures taken from uterine swabs has caused much debate.[48] Although most early work supported the hypothesis that all infection was significant, this opinion is now moderating and more regard is taken of the type of infectious organism and the consequences on the endometrium. It is likely that there are commensal organisms within the genital tract of mares and that a totally sterile tract is probably not achievable. It is fair to say also that there are many more bacterial organisms in the more caudal parts of the tract than in the uterus itself.[2,49]

Anestrus sampling appears to be the least reliable because there is an increased chance of not culturing the bacteria associated with chronic endometritis.[50] Probably the best time to recover uterine organisms is the first or second day of standing estrus, even if the cervix is not fully relaxed. At this time, uterine secretions are increasing, making a moist swab easier to obtain, and the full flushing action of estrus has not yet occurred. Late diestrus or early estrus specimens have been used but most opinion supports the use of mid-estrus samples as being the best indicators of the uterine status. At this time there is less risk of false results (either negative or positive) and less risk of introducing infection during the procedure. During diestrus, the endometrium is often dry, making bacterial recovery more difficult. Also, infection may be transferred into the uterus with bacteria carried in on the hand from the vestibulum and the absence of subsequent estrus may allow the development of this infection.

If an ultrasound examination is conducted to confirm pregnancy and the uterus contains a large amount of free fluid and no embryo, culture and cytology of the uterine fluid are frequently diagnostic.

Technique

Culture of microorganisms from the reproductive tract is accomplished in several ways.[51] The most

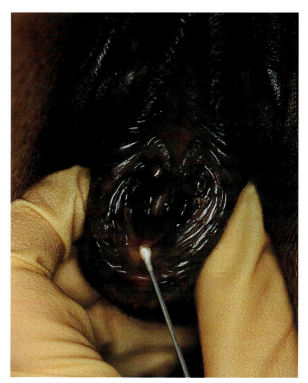

Fig. 5.43 Microbiological swabbing from the clitoris.

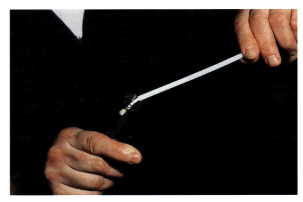

Fig. 5.44 Microbiological swabbing taken from the uterine lumen using a simple sterile guarded swab. Various forms of swabs can be used, ranging from the fine cotton swabs used for clitoral swabbing to the sophisticated guarded double-sheathed intrauterine swabs. These also have the facility to take endometrial cytology specimens.

relevant microbiological cultures are obtained from the clitoris fossa/sinuses and the endometrium (Fig. 5.43).

The logistics of the two types are quite different and the target organisms are likewise different:

- For clitoral swabs a fine cotton swab is usually used and the specimen is placed immediately in a bacterial transport medium to avoid desiccation. This technique is relatively straightforward (see Fig. 5.43).
- Instrumentation for uterine swabs varies from the traditional wire loop to various types of guarded swabs. Cultures are made either through a speculum or by manual insertion to the desired location. Care should be taken when procuring a sample to avoid contaminating the uterus with bacteria during the process.
    i. The mare is restrained appropriately.
    ii. To eliminate the risks of environmental, vulvar and vaginal contamination, the procedure must be carried out in a clean area and the mare should be prepared for aseptic examination.
    iii. An instrument that can obtain reliable uterine samples without risk of contamination should be used. Such instruments are commercially available and are the same as those used for cytological examination. (Suitable instruments are made by: Kalayjian Industries Inc., Long Beach, CA; McCullough Cartwright, Barrington, IL; Haver Lockart, Kansas City, KS.) Furthermore, the two investigative techniques can be performed at the same time and the results are then more reliable.
    iv. Immediately after collection, uterine swabs should be placed directly on the final medium

for culture or can be placed in a suitable transport medium for delivery to the laboratory. Immediate culture gives a positive correlation between numbers of organisms on the swab and numbers of colonies on the plate.

- Bacteria are invariably lost as the swab dries; therefore, any method that delays drying, such as refrigeration, addition of sterile saline to the swab or placement in a culture transport medium, extends bacterial viability.
- When many mares are examined at one farm over a prolonged period, it is advantageous to 'streak' culture plates immediately.

Interpretation

It is fairly simple to culture and identify the organisms that cause endometritis.

i. Plating on blood agar and one selective Gram-negative medium is adequate, although more sophisticated multiple diagnostic plates are available commercially.
ii. Plates are incubated at 37°C, preferably in a candle jar to provide microaerophilic conditions, and inspected daily.
iii. The practitioner can make therapeutic decisions in most cases simply by inspecting the colonies and making Gram-stained smears from these.

- An indication of the number of colonies must be included in the laboratory report.
- Pure cultures are more significant than mixed ones.

iv. The following organisms, in significant numbers, must be considered pathogenic:[52]
  - β-Hemolytic streptococci.
  - Hemolytic *Escherichia coli*.
  - *Pseudomonas* spp.
  - *Klebsiella* spp. (certain capsular subtypes are more significant than others).
  - *Monilia* (*Candida*) spp.
  - Some *Staphylococcus* spp.

Other organisms, when isolated repeatedly, are occasionally suspect in the presence of inflammation. However, α-hemolytic streptococci, staphylococci and various enteric organisms other than those listed above should generally be viewed as contaminants.

Culture results must always be correlated with cytological findings and it is important that the specimens for each procedure be taken at the same time.

- When cytological findings are persistently positive and cultures are negative, the interpretation is that the cause of the inflammation remains to be determined.
- Other causes of inflammation include reflux of urine into the uterus, pneumovagina, and hypersensitivity to antibiotics or chemicals infused into the uterus, feces, and semen.
- When cultures are positive and cytological findings are repeatedly negative, contamination of the culture is the usual conclusion.

REPRODUCTIVE MANAGEMENT OF MARES

The prime objective in managing an equine breeding program is the delivery of adequate numbers of viable spermatozoa into the genital tract of healthy mares at an appropriate time to ensure the maximum opportunity for fertilization. The major obstacles to attaining this objective are:

- Failure to properly coordinate the physiologic breeding season of horses with the breeding calendar imposed by various breed registries.
- Failure to properly detect estrus and determine the optimum time for breeding.
- Failure to identify and correct reproductive abnormalities of mares.
- Failure to deliver viable semen.

These objectives must be properly addressed to achieve a program yielding maximum fertility. Further management is then required to maximize the foaling rate and minimize neonatal loss.

Teasing (testing) programs for breeding mares

Veterinarians can provide a valuable service to clients by evaluating the teasing program. There are almost as many ways to tease mares as there are breeding establishments. Selecting the proper approach or combination of methods that suits the farm layout and personnel is a challenge. Observation and recording of data are essential to a successful teasing program.

The more familiar the personnel become with the idiosyncrasies of individual mares, the more effective they can be. It is an advantage, therefore, to have the same people tease the mares each day.

- It usually is most productive to handle mares individually, teasing them in stalls, over a teasing board, or loose.
- Variations in restraint and approach should be tried continually. Supplemental procedures, such as group teasing, can be helpful.

- A stallion can be penned where the mares are free to approach on their own. With proper control, some stallions can be led into or near fields of mares.
- It must be remembered that some mares do not show estrus on their own, and these 'loose' teasing methods must be only adjuncts to a careful individual teasing program.

Stud farms with dedicated teaser stallions will recognize the value of a teaser that is suitably aggressive but can be handled safely and easily. The good teaser will not become frustrated but will remain interested in mares presented to him.

Some breeders have success with stallions running loose with mares. Either a pony stallion too small to breed horse mares or a stallion with some mechanical alteration to prevent coitus is employed. A surgical technique to produce retroversion of the penis caudally has produced useful teaser stallions but has very questionable ethics.

- Vasectomized stallions are not acceptable teasers to run with mares. Repeated intromission, even without fertile ejaculates, creates significant irritation and contamination in most mares.

Reproductive management of maiden mares

As a group, maiden mares should have the highest degree of potential fertility. Assuming normal reproductive development, they have the best resistance to bacterial contamination and tolerate marginal breaches of management better than barren mares do.

Specific problems with maiden mares mainly relate to the following:

1. Estrus detection.
   - Psychological factors may prevent normally cycling maiden mares from exhibiting estrus, and great patience is required to determine the proper time for breeding.
   - A firm but gentle approach to handling such mares is the method of choice.
   - Tranquilization sometimes is indicated to adapt maiden mares to a routine, particularly for a first natural service. However, use of tranquilizers should not be a substitute for schooling.
2. Breeding.
   - Young mares are often nervous and unfamiliar with breeding routines, especially teasing and natural service.
   - Forcible restraint of mares for teasing and breeding may establish habits that adversely influence their entire reproductive life.

3. Adjustment to life as a broodmare.
   - Fillies with extensive athletic careers or show-circuit backgrounds may be difficult to convert to broodmares.
4. Management and historical aspects.
   - Anabolic steroids administered during athletic training are detrimental to fertility. Although there is no doubt that prolonged use of glucocorticoids, anabolic steroids, or similar compounds may delay the onset of fertile cycles, there is a tendency for farm personnel to use prior medication as an excuse for reproductive failures of all kinds.
   - After long periods of confinement, rigidly scheduled training, or other established routines, many maiden mares deteriorate in condition on retirement to the breeding farm. Special handling, feeding, and close observation may alleviate this problem. Turning a nervous filly out into a large pasture with mature barren mares almost guarantees the filly will receive physical punishment, be located at the bottom of the pecking order, and receive inadequate nourishment.

A complete reproductive examination of all maiden mares before breeding is advisable.

i. Attention should be directed to the size and function of the ovaries and uterus during rectal palpation.
ii. The pelvic canal should be explored for size and impingement by old traumatic episodes.
iii. The vaginal examination should, in addition to the routine inspection, evaluate remnants of the hymen that might cause problems in breeding.
   - A persistent hymen is simply treated by stretching or incision.
   - A totally imperforate hymen is rare.
   - An imperforate hymen traps mucus and uterine secretions in the cranial vagina.
iv. Uterine cultures of maiden mares may be required before breeding on some farms.
   - The chance of endometritis occurring in a maiden mare is remote.
   - In the absence of clinical signs of inflammation, a positive culture should be viewed skeptically.
   - Occasionally, young mares have pneumovagina and concurrent vaginitis, cervicitis, and even a vulvar discharge. Such cases respond quickly to a Caslick operation (see p. 184).

Breeding maiden mares by natural service presents a challenge even to experienced handlers. The unpredictability of the mare poses a potential for injury to the stallion, mare, and attendants. After suitable restraint is applied, before breeding the mare with a valuable stallion it is wise to allow a teaser stallion to mount the mare a few times. A breeding roll, which limits intromission, is advisable when breeding small mares to large stallions.

Reproductive management of foaling mares

Following prolonged suppression of pituitary and ovarian function by gestation, mares respond with a dramatic, fertile, cycling state after foaling. The first postpartum estrus ('foal heat') occurs quickly and, coupled with rapid uterine involution, the mare can conceive within 9–15 days after parturition. Following foal heat, most mares continue to cycle at normal intervals.

Although foal heat is entirely physiologic, much controversy exists over the value of breeding mares at this time. There is concern over the higher incidences of embryonic death and abortion following conception at this first estrus (see p. 178). Additionally, the belief that mating mares during foal heat influences subsequent cycles adds to the confusion.

The seasonal effect on foaling mares had been largely overlooked. In northern hemisphere mares, 97% ovulate by 20 days post partum, and 43% ovulate by day 9. The mean interval from foaling to first ovulation is around 10.2 days (±2.4 days).[53]

- The effect of season on foaling mares is evident in the interval to first ovulation.
  - ❏ Mares foaling in January and February show a 33% incidence of ovulation by day 10.
  - ❏ 55% of mares foaling in March ovulate by day 10.
  - ❏ Mares foaling in April and May have 65% and 83% ovulation rates, respectively, by the tenth day.
- Use of artificial lighting for pregnant mares during winter may be worth considering in stud management to avoid mares developing lactation anestrus after foaling.
- Conception rate, foaling rate, and pregnancy losses are not significantly different among mares bred at first estrus and those bred at subsequent heats if the uterus is free of intrauterine fluid at the time of breeding on foal heat.
- There are variations between years and among farms, but the cumulative totals are remarkably similar.

The interval from foaling to conception in mares bred during foal heat is shorter by 18 days compared with those bred on subsequent cycles. This indicates that breeding during foal heat, particularly in mares that foal late, is in fact advantageous.

Conception rates tend to be 14% higher in mares bred after postpartum day 10 than in those bred on or before postpartum day 10. Because of this, methods

delaying foal heat to improve fertility rates have been evaluated. Foal heat can be delayed in mares by the administration of progesterone 150 mg in combination with 10 mg of 17β-estradiol given daily for 6–10 days, or altrenogest (0.044 mg/kg for 8 days) in combination with prostaglandin 10 mg on postpartum day 9. Treatment is begun the day after foaling. More mares become pregnant (82%) when ovulation occurs after day 15 postpartum than when ovulation occurs before day 15 (50%).[35]

Delaying foal heat not only delays the first postpartum ovulation but also allows time for the elimination of uterine fluid. When uterine fluid is detected during the first postpartum ovulatory period, fewer mares become pregnant (33%) compared with the mares bred when fluid is not detected (84%). Mares with uterine fluid detected during breeding do not have appreciably larger uterine dimensions compared with those mares that do not have fluid.

- It is therefore advisable to perform a reproductive ultrasound examination prior to breeding to determine if there is fluid accumulation.
- Mares with intrauterine fluid during foal estrus should be treated appropriately before breeding or should not be bred.
- Mares that are not bred can be given prostaglandin 5 days after the first postpartum ovulation.
  - ❏ This allows more time for uterine involution.
  - ❏ Reproductively normal mares should be clear of intrauterine fluid by 15 days post foaling.

Estrus detection in mares that are nursing foals presents potential problems. The protective nature of some mares is such that they do not exhibit estrus behavior when approached by a teaser stallion. This is a particular problem of mares with their first foal. All the resources of the teasing personnel are needed to note behavioral changes in such mares. Restraint in various forms may be of value. The presence or absence of the foal and its location during teasing are variables to consider.

- Failure to detect estrus by the expected time is an indication for routine ultrasonographic examination of the reproductive tract to monitor cyclical changes and the presence or absence of pathological abnormalities.

A complete genital examination is indicated for all foaling mares before the first postpartum breeding.

- The most appropriate time for examination is the first day on which signs of estrus are strong.
- Cervical or vaginal damage sustained during delivery is detected by vaginoscopy and manual palpation of the vaginal area.
- Suspicious uterine exudates can be noted at this time.

- Ultrasonographic examination of the uterus helps to detect intrauterine fluid accumulations.
  - ❑ Uterine size does not appear to be related to uterine involution and fertility; however, the accumulation of uterine fluid is associated with decreased fertility.
  - ❑ Small quantities of uterine fluid are detected more accurately and more simply by ultrasonographic examination than by rectal palpation.
  - ❑ During estrus, uterine fluid may be spermicidal; when present during diestrus, it may cause premature luteolysis or embryonic death.

Valid reasons for not breeding during foal heat include:

- A history of dystocia during the delivery.
- Retained placenta beyond the accepted normal (see p. 313).
- Persistent purulent exudate.
  - ❑ Uterine or vulvar discharges must be evaluated carefully during the early postpartum period.
  - ❑ Blood may be retained in the uterus until the first estrus and is seen as a mucoid, chocolate-brown discharge. This type of discharge seldom warrants uterine treatment.
  - ❑ Uterine cultures may be used to isolate pathogens when purulent exudate is noted in conjunction with inflammation.
  - ❑ However, culture samples obtained during foal heat should be evaluated carefully because some normally residual organisms are invariably evident.
- Physical damage to the reproductive tract.
  - ❑ Any physical trauma to the birth canal, including the cervix, vagina or vulva, is a strong reason not to breed the mare.
  - ❑ Conception rates are low when active traumatic inflammation and likely infection are present.

- Therapeutic or corrective measures for any factor that affects the fertility must be initiated as soon as possible to improve the chances of conception on the next heat.
- Breeding procedures for foaling mares should be aimed at minimizing trauma and contamination, particularly during foal heat.
- Every effort should be made to minimize the number of natural services.
- Artificial insemination, when permitted, definitely increases conception rates.

Reproductive management of barren mares

Management of mares with a history of endometritis should be directed so that as few matings as possible are used.

- Semen induces an inflammatory response and most mares that are infertile because of endometritis are unable to quickly clear the uterus of the by-products of insemination. It is the prolongation of the normal physiological inflammatory response that renders these mares subfertile.
- If the inflammation persists 5 days after ovulation when the embryo enters the uterus, the inflammatory by-products will damage the embryo resulting in pregnancy loss.
- It is extremely important that the stallion to which barren mares are to be bred is fertile.
- If the mare is to be bred with shipped cooled semen, semen quality must be excellent, otherwise the mare will need to be bred on repeated cycles.
- It is not advisable to breed mares with a history of endometritis with frozen semen as pregnancy rates are poor.

Artificial lighting (see p. 164) is an especially useful aid in managing barren mares.

- The more ovulatory cycles that are available during the breeding season, the greater the chance of returning the mare to production.

Before the mare is bred for the first time in the season, serum progesterone should be measured to ensure that the mare has ovulated at least once that year. Repeated breeding of mares with a history of endometritis resulting from repeated mating during the transition phase into the cyclic season induces a prolonged uterine inflammation that will almost inevitably interfere with pregnancy.

The cause of the infertility should be diagnosed prior to the breeding season (see Figs 5.45–5.48 for investigative protocols).

- A complete reproductive examination including an endometrial biopsy should be performed during the summer or early autumn of the previous year.
- As the endometrium undergoes seasonal changes and the mare has been sexually rested, a biopsy taken in January or February (northern hemisphere) or July or August (southern hemisphere) may not be diagnostic.
- Histological findings such as inflammation and lymphatic lacunae will likely resolve with time if semen, feces, urine or air does not challenge the uterus.

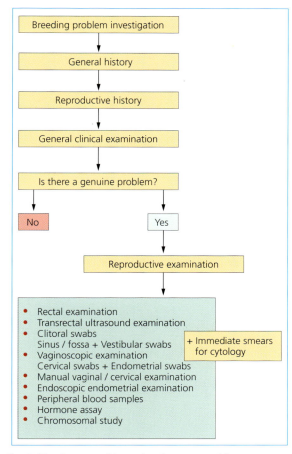

Fig. 5.45 Suggested investigative protocol for a suspected breeding problem.

- As treatments vary depending on the type of endometritis, it is extremely important to discover the cause of the infertility prior to instilling antibiotics or counterirritants/chemicals into the uterus.
- Antibiotic treatment is not benign and can cause secondary infections with yeast or fungi if used indiscriminately.

- Not all infertility is due to the mare. Data on the stallion must be obtained, especially if the mare was bred the previous season with either shipped cooled semen or frozen semen.
- It may be that the infertility was due to poor-quality semen or breeding at the inappropriate time.
- If there are questions about either, it may be advisable to breed the mare to a known fertile stallion.

Contraception

See p. 41.

INFERTILITY IN THE MARE

Fertile: able to conceive and carry the fetus to full term; sometimes used to include the production of a useful offspring.
Infertile: unable to conceive or carry a fetus to full term; sometimes used to include the failure to produce a viable useful offspring.
Sterile: incapable of fertilization or reproduction; sometimes used to imply total and complete infertility (i.e. untreatable).
Barren: not pregnant at the end of the breeding season.

Infertility is the most common reproductive complaint of horse owners. It can be a perplexing problem for the veterinarian as identification of the cause is frequently difficult. Owners may not keep accurate records, the mare may change owners, the stallion may be infertile, or reproductive management may be poor. New technologies, such as the use of fresh cooled semen or frozen semen to breed mares, have complicated and, in some cases, increased the incidence of infertility. Proficiency at rectal and ultrasonographic assessment of the reproductive organs is essential if maximal fertility is to be achieved. New advances in reproductive physiology are being made and the veterinarian needs to keep abreast of these if improvements in fertility rates are to be improved.

The inherent fertility of a mare is a function of:

1. The age of the mare.
   - There is a higher conception rate and higher fertility in younger horses than in older ones, and after 12 years of age there is a significantly lower fertility.
   - In older mares, conception rates are usually good but detection rates for pregnancy are low, indicating that there is an inherently high embryo loss in the first 4 weeks of gestation.[55]
   - Early embryonic loss (up to day 14) is around 9% in mares under the age of 3 years; in aged mares (>14 years old) this rises to over 60%.
2. Free-ranging horses have a high inherent fertility, whereas early season Thoroughbreds may have a significantly lower natural fertility (unless they are subjected to estrus manipulation).
3. The veterinary attention provided.
4. Studs with experienced stud veterinarians will usually have a higher overall fertility than those not having this provision.

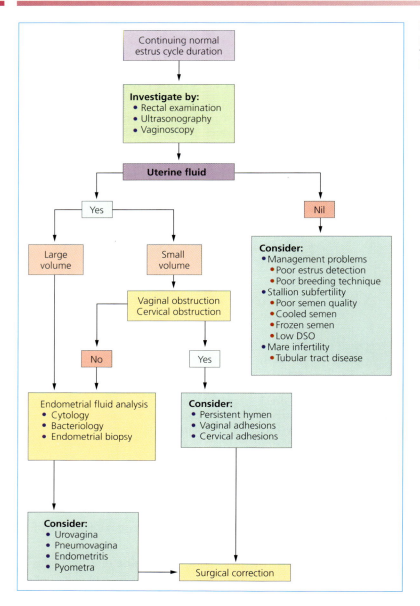

Fig. 5.46 Suggested investigative protocol for mare infertility based on the presence of intrauterine fluid (after Madill and Troedsson[54]).

Fertility is also affected by extrinsic factors, including:

1. Mare management.
   - The ability to detect estrus and to tease the mare effectively.
   - Failure to detect prolonged diestrus may lead to the impression that the mare is pregnant.
   - Mating times not correctly coordinated with ovulation.
2. Stallion management.
   - Over-use of the stallion. A stallion should probably not be used to mate more than two or three mares in any one day; fertility can be lower if it is sustained at this rate.
   - Failure to detect ejaculation (see p. 215).

3. Physiological effects.
   - Individual variations (see below).
   - Inappropriate or incompetent use of artificial insemination.

A systematic approach to identify the nature of infertility is important. The infertility chart presented in Fig. 5.49 provides a summary protocol for the investigation of infertility. The various aspects of infertility are discussed in detail in subsequent sections of this chapter.

A useful approach involves the use of client descriptions of the problem. Three categories can then be recognized:

A. The mare fails to cycle normally.
B. The mare cycles normally, apparently conceives,

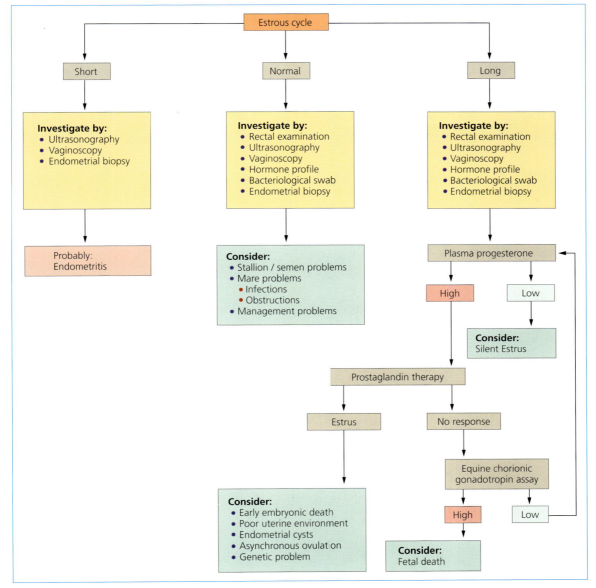

Fig. 5.47 Suggested investigative protocol for mare infertility from a perspective of ovarian size (after Madill and Troedsson[54]).

but loses the pregnancy between 35 and 90 days.

C. The mare cycles normally and, if she conceives, she loses the pregnancy before 35 days (early embryonic loss).

The most common complaint is (A), the failure to cycle normally (or at all). This usually reflects a problem with the hypothalamic–pituitary–gonadal axis which governs follicular development and ovulation. Failures of this system may be caused by:

- Seasonal effects (physiological state).
- Developmental anomalies.
- Abnormal endocrine function.
- Other causes.

Details of the diagnostic characteristics involved are given in Table 5.4.

In both other categories (B, C), the mare appears to cycle properly and then loses the pregnancy, either through failure to conceive or failure to sustain the pregnancy. In these cases the tubular genital system is usually the cause of the problem.

Early embryonic loss is a major factor in the fertility of the horse. Much of this loss is accepted as a natural event, but clearly the causes need to be established before any specific action can be taken to prevent it. Fertilization failure, in the face of normal stallion fertility, actually accounts for a relatively small proportion of the total infertility. Early pregnancy loss, as

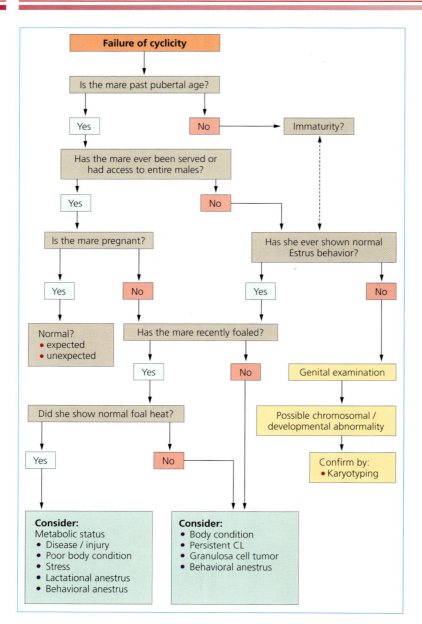

Fig. 5.48 Investigative protocol for mares that fail to cycle or have irregular cyclicity.

in type B, has been associated with an endocrine failure (inadequate plasma progesterone), but there is little supportive evidence for this concept, and current thinking implicates disorders of the tubular tract or systemic release of prostaglandin due to unrelated illness, such as colic.

Diagnostic details concerning type B and C infertility appear in Table 5.5.

Although absence of estrus is sometimes difficult to detect and confirm, some horses are reported to show persistent estrus. Such mares show some or all of the behavioral patterns characteristic of estrus, such as clitoral winking, squatting and frequent urination in the presence of geldings or stallions. While this is

sometimes associated with reproductive abnormalities, others have no such problem (at least it is not detectable by any current means). These cases are presumed to be behavioral problems that have little or nothing to do with the estrous cycle.[56] Some explanations for this are centered around urogenital inflammation or vaginal or vulvar tumors (or other space-occupying lesions).

> - In many cases there is no detectable explanation and these are very difficult to manage.

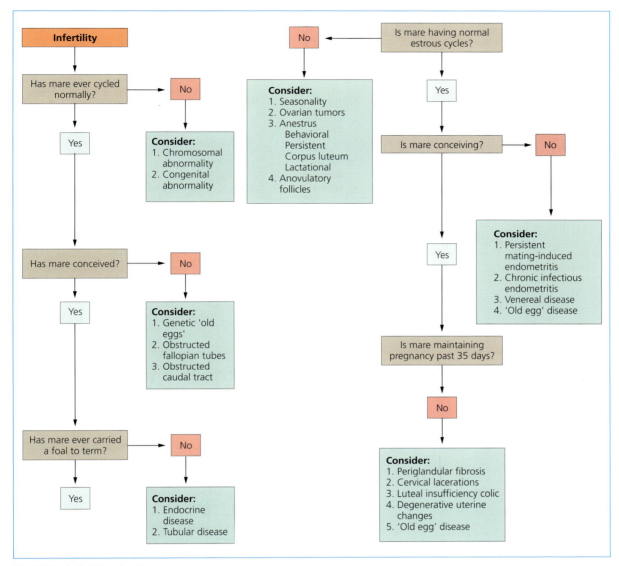

Fig. 5.49   Infertility chart.

MARES THAT FAIL TO CYCLE

By definition, the complete reproductive cycle includes a period of estrus, concluding with ovulation, and a period of diestrus when progesterone levels are elevated.

- A mare that has never cycled can be assumed to have a serious (probably incurable) genetic or developmental abnormality.
- Observing periodic estrous behavior does not prove cyclicity.
- Evidence that ovulation is occurring can be obtained from sequential data from:
  ❑ Ovarian palpation.
  ❑ The presence of a corpus luteum as shown by ultrasonography.
  ❑ Elevation of serum progesterone levels.
- Presumptive evidence of ovulation includes firm uterine and cervical tone and the presence of follicular activity on the ovaries.
- One of the most common causes of interruption of the cycle is pregnancy.
  ❑ Accurate pregnancy examination techniques are critical to successful infertility management.
  ❑ Pregnancy must always be ruled out before other diagnostic procedures commence.

Table 5.4 Findings and differential diagnosis in nonpregnant, noncycling mares (C, cervix; V, variable; R, relaxed; T, tight)

Ovaries	Season	Tubular tract	Behavior	Other findings	Probable cause
Normal-size follicles present	Summer	Excellent tone, CT	Rejects stallion		Prolonged diestrus CL
Normal size, active	Spring	Poor tone, CR	Passive or irregular estrus	Speculum: CV pale, dry; progesterone <1.0 ng/ml	Transition from anestrus to ovulatory stage
Small, inactive	Winter	Flaccid, CR	Passive or irregular estrus	Speculum: CV pale, dry	Winter anestrus
Very small, inactive	Any	Uterus infantile	Passive	Small body size; athletic; good-looking	Gonadal dysgenesis/ testicular feminization
One ovary enlarged, the other one smaller than normal	Any	Variable (flaccid)	Masculine aggression; nymphomania; irregular constant estrus/ anestrus	No ovulation fossa; one large ovary; inhibin increased if granulosa cell tumor	Secreting ovarian tumor

Table 5.5 Early pregnancy loss

Cause	Comment
Persistent mating-induced endometritis (delay in uterine clearance)	• Inconsistent demonstration of inflammation makes diagnosis difficult • Fluid in uterus 24–48 hours after breeding • If mare conceives, she most commonly loses the pregnancy before 35 days
Failure of endometrial glands	• Extensive periglandular fibrosis in biopsy specimens is highly correlated with this
Lymphatic lacunae	• Mares may lose pregnancy between 40 and 90 days if they conceive
Cervical incompetence	• Mares may lose pregnancy early (45–90 days) or later (after 6 months), depending on the severity of the lesion
Luteal/progesterone insufficiency	• Supplemental progesterone is possibly beneficial. • Does appear to be effective in cases of endotoxemia or other causes leading to systemic release of prostaglandin
External factors (nutrition/stress/heat)	• Difficult to document
Chromosomal and genetic factors	• 'Old egg disease' in mares >18 years of age

DEVELOPMENTAL ABNORMALITIES

Chromosomal abnormalities

Profile
• A chromosomal abnormality may be suspected in a mare of breeding age with primary infertility and (profound) permanent gonadal hypoplasia.
• The karyotypes of the normal mare and stallion are 64,XX and 64,XY, respectively.
• Horses of all domestic breeds have the same number, size and shape of chromosomes.
• Chromosomal abnormalities, especially of the sex chromosomes, have been associated with infertility in the horse.

❑ The most commonly reported chromosomal abnormality of the horse is 63,X0 gonadal dysgenesis, in which only a single sex chromosome is present.

❑ The equine condition is analogous to Turner's syndrome in humans.

❑ A number of other chromosomal abnormalities have also been reported in the mare.

- Gonadal dysgenesis is caused by an error in chromosomal segregation, either during the initial development of the zygote (mitosis nondisjunction) or during gamete formation (meiotic nondisjunction).
- Horses with gonadal dysgenesis develop as phenotypic females because of the absence of the Y sex chromosome.
- No breed predilection has been observed.

Clinical signs

- Characteristic clinical findings include:
  ❑ Extremely small ovaries (usually less than 1 cm in diameter), with no germinal tissue.
  ❑ Infantile uterus often no more than a thin band of tissue (Fig. 5.50).
  ❑ A flaccid, pale, dilated cervix.
  ❑ The external genitalia are female, but the vulva may be smaller than normal and there is no clitoral hypertrophy.
  ❑ Persistent anestrus or irregular periods of behavioral estrus. The mare may stand to be mated.
  ❑ Some affected mares appear small in stature.

Diagnosis

- Diagnosis is made by karyotyping.
  ❑ Karyotyping is essential to confirm the diagnosis, because not all mares with hypoplastic ovaries have abnormal chromosomes or are infertile.
  ❑ Chromosome analysis can be performed on any tissue with actively dividing cells.

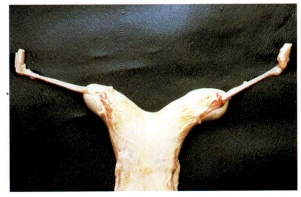

Fig. 5.50 Chromosomal abnormality (63,X0) of genital tract. Note very small ovaries and under-developed uterine horns and body.

❑ A fresh blood sample, collected into acid citrate dextrose or lithium heparin, may be sent by overnight courier to a laboratory specializing in animal karyotyping. The chromosomal structure is identified by the use of electron microscopy.

SEASONALITY

Seasonal effects on the reproductive cycle are a common cause of failure to cycle or of abnormal cycles in the winter and spring. The reproductive cycle of the mare can be divided into four periods:

- Anestrus.
- Transition into the breeding season.
- The physiological breeding season.
- Transition out of the breeding season.

Photoperiod (daylight hours) triggers the natural onset and cessation of reproductive activity in mares. The anestrous period occurs in November, December and January in the northern hemisphere, and during the months of May, June and July in the southern hemisphere. The transition into the breeding season lasts from February until mid-April in the northern hemisphere, and from August to mid-September in the southern hemisphere. This lengthy transition period presents economic difficulties for the horse-breeding industry because 1 January has been designated arbitrarily as the date from which foals are aged (1 August in the southern hemisphere). Breeders are compelled to strive for earlier foaling, even though this is generally incompatible with the natural reproductive physiology of the mares.

In the winter, the content and secretion of gonadotropin-releasing hormone from the hypothalamus are drastically reduced. Shortly after the winter solstice, gonadotropin-releasing hormone secretion begins to increase through mechanisms that are not completely understood. Follicle-stimulating hormone increases, presumably in response to the increase in gonadotropin-releasing hormone, and follicles begin to develop on the ovaries. During this time little if any luteinizing hormone is secreted because the gene for synthesis of this hormone is essentially turned off. The pattern of follicular growth during vernal (spring) transition is relatively predictable, with increased size and numbers of follicles.

- The first several follicles that form in vernal (spring) transition do not normally ovulate, although they may reach normal preovulatory size (>30 mm diameter).

An average of 3.7±0.9 follicles that reach a size of 30 mm or greater but which do not ovulate during the transition phase are produced. These follicles are not capable of producing steroid hormones and do not produce estrogen. This leads to reproductive inefficiency because it is difficult to know whether a given follicle is competent and will ovulate during this time of year.

- Monitoring the development of a follicle over time may be useful in determining the eventual status and outcome of a transitional follicle because the growth rate of follicles destined to regress is considerably slower than that of a follicle that eventually ovulates.

Shedding of the long winter hair coat in spring is another rough indicator of impending ovulation as shedding is closely associated with reproductive renewal. Although it is not known what factors contribute to the eventual development of the first competent follicle, it is clear that this follicle, destined to be the first to ovulate in the year, is reasonably steroidogenically competent. The development of the first ovulatory follicle is accompanied by a surge of estradiol in the peripheral plasma that is followed a few days later by a surge in luteinizing hormone.

Transition period

The ovaries of mares in late transition are usually very active and have several follicles of varying sizes and maturity. The transition period can be accompanied by long periods of erratic ovarian function and estrous behavior.[57] The associated prolonged estrous behavior can last from 1 week to 4 months or more. Owners of mares who are unfamiliar with this seasonality of the reproductive cycle will typically assume that the mares are ovulating and may breed them during this time. There is little or no hope of conception, as almost none of the follicles will in fact ovulate.

Management

Artificial lighting protocols
Artificial light, applied 60 days before the intended breeding season, is the best method of shifting the vernal (spring) transition forward from April to February (northern hemisphere).

- Light added at the end of the day, to provide a total of 14–16 hours of light daily, results in the resumption of cyclicity in 60–75 days.
- Mares exposed to lights from 1 December usually cycle by 15 February (northern hemisphere). (In the southern hemisphere mares are placed under lights on 1 July to commence cycling in late August.) It has become common practice in some areas to place mares under lights from as early as the beginning of November instead of December

to encourage cyclicity within 60 days. Mares placed under lights from early November experience their first ovulation at essentially the same time of year as mares placed under lights in December to in mid-February.[3]
- Older mares (>18 years of age) will take longer to begin cycling. Too much light (>16 hours per day) may actually delay the onset of cyclic activity.

A number of lighting schemes have been advocated.

1. The classical photostimulation technique
   - This is the conventional standard approach used for mares in winter anestrus and consists of a light treatment (14.5 or 16 hours of 100-lux white light), beginning around the winter solstice and ending around mid-April. After such treatment, cyclicity occurs in 70–80 days.
   - If the mare is intended to be bred in mid-February, the lighting regimen is instigated in late November to early December.
   - If the mare is to be bred in March, she can be placed under lights beginning around the winter solstice.[8,9]
   - The minimum intensity of light required to stimulate cycling appears to be 2 foot-candles. Most lighting systems provide 12–15 foot candles of light.
     - ❏ A 100-watt incandescent bulb placed in a 3.66 × 3.66-m box stall is most commonly used.

   - A general rule of thumb is that, if you can easily read a newspaper in all areas where the mares are housed, there is adequate light. This must include all corners and overhangs.

   - Breeders who wish to expose mares to artificial photoperiod in a paddock situation instead of in individual stalls, should consider the shape and size of the paddock and the strength, type, number of lights and their height and angle.
     - ❏ Placing eight 1000-watt metal halide floodlights at a height of 6.1 m (20 feet) in a paddock measuring 25.6 × 20.1 m (84 × 66 feet) successfully achieves the desired illumination.
2. Low-intensity lighting technique
   - The minimum intensity of light required to stimulate cyclicity is only 10 lux; this only represents the light produced with a 20-watt white incandescence bulb in a 3.5 m² box stall.[58]
     - ❏ Mares subjected to this low intensity of light beginning at the winter solstice for 14.5 hours daily have plasma progesterone concentrations higher than 1 ng/ml by

62±6 days (mean±SEM). This is virtually identical to mares subjected to high-intensity light (100 lux for 64±15 days).

❑ Under this regimen mares resume cyclicity in mid- to late February.

• The number of days of increased light required to advance the first ovulation of the year is also less than previously reported.[58]

❑ Mares subjected to 14.5 hours of light daily for 35 days starting at the winter solstice (21 December) resume cyclicity at the same time as mares subjected to artificial light for 60 days (76±4 days).

3. High-intensity regime

• The mare is subjected to a burst of light in the middle of the night during the photosensitive window.

• Mares subjected to a 1-hour burst of high-intensity light (100 lux) 9.5 hours after sunset (generally between 2 and 4 a.m.) for 60 days is sufficient to advance the first ovulation.

• The effectiveness of this protocol suggests that mares have a period in their circadian rhythm in which they are uniquely sensitive to light. It appears to be related to the time of dusk, and occurs 8–10 hours after the onset of darkness.

• Using a low-intensity burst is much less effective: 1 hour of 10 lux of light during 35 days only advances cyclicity in half of the mares.

HORMONAL METHODS FOR INDUCING CYCLICITY

Although photoperiod is the most efficient non-hormonal method for manipulating (advancing) the first ovulation of the year, hormonal treatment schemes (see Table 5.6) added to the end of the lighting regime can advance the first ovulation or can also be used to synchronize the first ovulation in a group of mares. The efficacy of progesterone or progestin treatment in regulating estrus and ovulation depends on the stage of the transition period and follicular status at the onset of treatment.[59]

• Before treatment is instigated several 25–35-mm follicles should be present on the ovaries; these can be induced by the use of photoperiod stimulation. Exposure of mares to artificial lighting for at least 45 days before administration of progesterone increases its effectiveness.

Table 5.6 Hormonal methods used to hasten first breeding season ovulation (IM, intramuscular; IV, intravenous; SC, subcutaneous; PO, by mouth; hCG, human chorionic gonadotropin; GnRH, gonadotropin-releasing hormone; $PGF_{2\alpha}$, prostaglandin $F_{2\alpha}$)

Drug	Dosage	Route	Purpose	Combined treatment	Treatment length (days)
Progestins					
Progesterone	150 mg	IM	Suppress estrus	Give late in transition or after mares have been under 14 hours of light for 45 days	10–14
Altrenogest	0.044 mg/kg	PO			
Estrogens					
17β-Estradiol	10 mg total	IM	Suppress follicular growth	Combined with daily progestin therapy	10
Prostaglandins					
Dinoprost	5–10 mg	IM	Induce luteal regression	Used with progestin treatment or with progestin and estradiol	One injection on last day of progesterone treatment
Cloprostenol	100–250 µg				
Prostianol	7.5–15 mg				
Ovulation inducers					
hCG	1500–4000 IU	IV	Induce ovulation	Give late in transition when follicle >35 mm; edema in uterus	One injection only
Deslorelin	2.2 mg	SC	Hasten follicular growth and ovulation		
Dopamine antagonists					
Sulpiride	200 mg	IM	Induce follicular growth and hasten ovulation during transition	2 weeks of 14.5 hours light in January then start treatment	10–35
Domperidone	440 mg	IM			

- In general, however, the later in the transition period the drugs are administered, the higher the likelihood that the mare will ovulate after treatment.
- Early in the anestrous period, when the ovaries are small and inactive, progesterone or progestins are ineffective in inducing estrus.

Progesterone

- Daily intramuscular administration of 150–200 mg of progesterone in oil or 0.044 mg/kg altrenogest administered by mouth for 10–15 days usually stops prolonged estrous activity within 2 days. Following the last treatment, mares usually exhibit the onset of estrous behavior within 1–5 days.
- Prostaglandin should be administered on the last day of progesterone/progestin therapy to lyse any corpora lutea that might be present on the ovaries.
- Ovulation occurs within 7–10 days.[60]
- Human chorionic gonadotropin administered on day 2 of estrus assists ovulation.[61]
- In about 90% of mares in the late transition period, fertile ovulation, with normal conception rates, can be induced by intravenous injection of 3000–3500 IU (although doses can be as low as 2000 IU) of human chorionic gonadotropin (luteinizing hormone), provided that:
  ❑ There is a follicle >35 mm in diameter.
  ❑ The mare has shown estrous behavior for at least 3 days.
- Under this regimen mares will ovulate 1–6 days after treatment. This is about 7 days sooner than in mares that do not receive human chorionic gonadotropin.
- Pregnancy rates should be normal in such treated mares, confirming that the ovulation is natural and potentially fertile.

Synchronization of ovulation by progesterone and estrogen

- Synchronization of the first ovulation (or any ovulation during the cyclic season) is best accomplished by a 10-day course of once-daily injections of both:
  ❑ Progesterone in oil (150 mg/day intramuscularly).
  ❑ 17β-Estradiol (10 mg/day intramuscularly).
- The addition of estrogen to daily progesterone treatment results in homogeneity of the follicular population and uniformity of follicular growth.
- Treatment is most effective if given late in transition after mares have been under lights for 45–60 days.[62]
- Prostaglandin should be given on the last day of the steroid treatment.

- Mares will ovulate within 8–10 days from the last treatment.[62,63]

- This steroid combination should be used with caution in mares from which uterine bacteria have been isolated as they may develop pyometra or endometritis during the treatment.

Dopamine antagonists

The temporal relationship between changes in daylight hours and prolactin production in the anterior pituitary gland has stimulated interest in the use of dopamine antagonists for hastening the first ovulation.[63]

- Dopamine is a neurotransmitter produced in the brain. It has been suggested that dopaminergic neurons actively inhibit prolactin and the secretion of gonadotropin-releasing hormone. The dopamine concentration in cerebrospinal fluid is lower during the breeding season than during the anovulatory season and levels appear to be inversely correlated with plasma luteinizing hormone and prolactin.
- Mares subjected to artificial light in winter anestrus exhibit an increase in the secretion of prolactin. Administration of ovine prolactin during anestrus results in rapid follicular growth. It is thought that prolactin has a direct or indirect effect at the level of the ovary.
- Administration of the dopamine antagonist drugs sulpiride or domperidone to mares in January was found to effectively advance the first ovulation of the year, but not all mares responded and the first ovulation occurred over a wide timespan.[64,65]
- Extending day length to 16 hours daily for the 2 weeks prior to administration of sulpiride results in a tighter and shorter interval to first ovulation.
- Mares that receive 16 hours of light beginning mid-January for 2 weeks (or until the mares ovulate) prior to twice daily injections of sulpiride (0.5 mg/kg intramuscularly twice daily) ovulate 12–22 days after the start of sulpiride treatment.[65]

Synthetic hormone

- A synthetic gonadotropin-releasing hormone agonist (deslorelin) that is administered as a subcutaneous pellet has been used in Australia to advance the first ovulation of the year.
  ❑ A single implant placed every other day for up to 6–8 dosages, late in transition, may be needed.
  ❑ The cost of this procedure may be prohibitive in many cases.

CYCLIC ABNORMALITIES

Spontaneous prolongation of the corpus luteum (persistent corpus luteum)

Profile

- The lifespan of the corpus luteum may be prolonged by a variety of causes including:
  - Failure of secretion of prostaglandin in amounts adequate to induce lysis.
  - Presence of an immature corpus luteum from a diestrus ovulation that occurred shortly before prostaglandin release.
  - Early embryonic death after maternal recognition of pregnancy.
  - Chronic uterine infection, resulting in destruction of the endometrium and therefore a diminished prostaglandin release.
- If untreated, the corpus luteum may persist for 2–3 months. If ovulation occurs 1–4 days before endogenous prostaglandin release on days 15 or 16 of the estrous cycle (diestrus), the mare will show no signs of estrus.
- The immature corpus luteum (4 days or less from ovulation) is unaffected by prostaglandin and produces more progesterone in the face of destruction of the older corpus luteum.

Clinical signs

- This syndrome may be suspected clinically in mares that do not express normal estrous behavior during the physiologic breeding season.
- Failure to exhibit estrous behavior for up to 60 days after the last estrus.
- The uterus is firm and tubular on palpation and the cervix closed.
- Follicles are palpable, and both follicles and a corpus luteum are usually visible on ultrasonography.
- It must be differentiated from the syndrome of mares with silent heat.

Management

- Administration of prostaglandin or its analogs are specific therapy.
  - Natural prostaglandin (dinoprost tromethamine) may be given intramuscularly at a dose of 5–10 mg.
  - Prostaglandin analog, cloprostenol, may be given intramuscularly at a dose of 125–250 µg (0.5–1 ml).
- The response to prostaglandin depends on:
  - The age of the corpus luteum. There will be no response if the corpus luteum is less than 5 days old.
  - The follicular activity on the ovary at the time of administration.
  - If follicles are <35 mm in diameter, estrus will occur between 2 and 5 days after injection, with ovulation 4–8 days later.
  - If a large follicle (>35 mm in diameter) is present when prostaglandin is given, estrus may occur as early as 24 hours after injection, with the mare ovulating shortly after; in rare instances, the mare may ovulate without showing signs of estrus.
  - If there is a follicle >40 mm on the ovaries at the time prostaglandin is administered, it is advisable not to breed the mare as pregnancy rates may be lower, possibly due to the advanced age of the ovum.

Behavioral anestrus ('silent heat')

Profile

- Behavioral anestrus is a perceived cyclic abnormality that is not related to reproductive endocrine activity.
- Mares may fail to exhibit estrous behavior when they are in physiologic estrus and may be cycling quite normally.[66]
- This most commonly occurs in maiden mares, mares that are retired from long performance careers and protective foaling mares.
- Because highly nervous, primiparous and protective mares are particularly affected, it is sometimes regarded as a psychological disorder.[67]
- Frequently there is no stallion on the farm, making identification of estrus near impossible. The use of artificial insemination using cooled, shipped semen or frozen semen in circumstances when estrus cannot be detected makes timing very difficult. The mare may be inseminated at the wrong times in her cycle, resulting in low to zero conception rates.
- Previous administration of anabolic steroids can have profound long-term effects on reproductive behavior even though there may be normal ovarian activity.[68] This iatrogenic problem should not be mistaken for true behavioral anestrus.

Clinical signs

- Protective or frightened mares will strike, kick or run when presented to a stallion even though they are in physiological estrus.
- Others may be passive and show no detectable behavioral estrus.

Management

- Problem mares should be presented individually to the teaser, preferably restrained in a stock, while applying a lip chain or twitch. Most mares will exhibit subtle changes in behavior while they are in estrus, so keen observation skills are important.

- Estrus may be identified in these mares by performing repeated ultrasonographic examinations of the reproductive tract in conjunction with vaginal speculum examinations to identify relaxation of the cervix (see reproductive examination procedures, p. 133).
- Measuring progesterone concentrations in plasma samples collected every 5–6 days can be used to identify when the mare is in estrus.

- Plasma progesterone is <1 ng/ml during estrus.

Note:
- This method should not be used to identify estrus prior to the first ovulation of the year as plasma progesterone concentrations in all samples will be <1 ng/ml.

Postpartum (lactational) anestrus

Profile

- Postpartum (lactational) anestrus occurs in mares occasionally, most frequently in mares that foal in February and March.[69] It is an uncommon condition.[70]
- Mares may take 60–90 days before they resume cyclicity. Over 95% of mares will show estrus within 3 weeks of foaling. Some then fail to cycle normally thereafter.
- It is more common in older mares and more so in those with poor or mediocre body condition.
- The problem appears to be more related to photoperiod, nutritional status and body condition than to lactation itself.[71] Physical and physiological stress also appear to be important.[72] Causative factors include:
  - ❏ Prolongation of luteal phase (i.e. suspension of luteolysis). This is the most common type that follows an apparently normal foal heat at around 7–21 days.
  - ❏ Development of a persistent corpus luteum after the foal heat with subsequent inactivity of the ovary.
  - ❏ No ovarian activity at all after parturition. The mare effectively passes directly into deep ovarian inactivity.

Clinical signs

- The mare exhibits normal estrous behavior during foal heat and then does not return to estrus at the normal interval. Alternatively, in the less common forms there is no evidence (either hormonally or behaviorally) of estrus following foaling.

- On rectal examination, the ovaries are small, firm and contain only very small follicles.
- The uterus is flaccid and cervix is open.
- Plasma progesterone concentration is <1 ng/ml.
- The condition can last for 1–3 months (or, rarely, even longer).

Management

- The anestrus caused by postpartum or post foal-heat persistence of the corpus luteum will respond to prostaglandin injections, with estrus following normally thereafter.
- Once the true anestrus clinical status of ovarian inactivity is established there is little that can be done apart from improving the nutritional status and reducing stressors.
- Occasional mares have responded to administration of gonadotropin-releasing hormone through a continuous infusion pump by resuming cyclicity in 10–14 days after the start of treatment.
- The condition may be prevented by subjecting the suspect or liable case to a short period of additional light, followed by sulpiride injections which may hasten ovulation (see seasonality above, p. 163).
- It is advisable to place early foaling mares whose projected foaling dates are prior to 15 March under 14.5 hours of light beginning in early December and sustained for 2 months.
- Domperidone (a dopamine antagonist) may induce follicular activity in mares with no corpus luteum present (i.e. progesterone <1 ng/ml). The medication can be administered orally once daily until ovulation occurs.

Anovulatory follicles

Profile

- Failure of ovulation is a normal physiologic event during the spring and autumn transition periods (see above, p. 120).
- A mare may develop a dominant follicle that does not ovulate during the physiologic breeding season. These structures are referred to as either anovulatory, hemorrhagic or persistent follicles and are not to be confused with the large anovulatory follicles that develop during the spring or fall transition.[73]
- Mares that experience this problem may do so over a number of estrous cycles.
- An incidence of 5% has been reported in pony mares, although it does not appear to occur as commonly in mares.
- The cause of ovulation failure has been suggested to be endocrine in nature, either from a lack of sufficient pituitary gonadotropin stimulation to induce ovulation or from insufficient estrogen production from the follicle itself.

- The significance of an anovulatory follicle is that the oocyte is not released.

Clinical signs and diagnosis

- Mares with anovulatory follicles exhibit abnormal estrous behavior and prolonged inter-ovulatory intervals.
- Mares remain in estrus for a prolonged period lasting 7–15 days.
- Most affected mares eventually cease exhibiting signs of estrus once the rim of the follicle develops luteal tissue.
- An affected dominant follicle may reach a size of 10 cm or greater and is identified by repeated ultrasonographic examination of the ovaries during estrus. The dominant preovulatory follicle appears to grow normally but, instead of ovulating, it continues to enlarge.
- Ultrasonographic examination (see Fig. 5.51) reveals scattered free-floating echogenic spots within the follicular antrum that tend to swirl during ballottement of the ovary. Over time, the contents of the follicular antrum begin to organize into fibrous bands or may form a gelatinous, hemorrhagic mass within the follicular lumen. The outer rim (4–7 mm) may contain echogenic luteal tissue.
- On rectal palpation, the structure may feel like a preovulatory follicle or corpus hemorrhagicum and can sometimes be confused with a granulosa cell tumor. Mares with an anovulatory follicle, however, will maintain cyclicity and will have a normal-sized contralateral ovary. The ovulation fossa is palpable and the size of the affected ovary will return to normal within 60 days.
- Aspiration of the follicular contents yields bloody fluid when there are echogenic particles.
- Mares with this condition usually progress into a luteal phase that is either normal or prolonged.
- The majority of anovulatory follicles regress in 4–6 weeks.
- Suspect anovulatory follicles can be identified by measuring plasma progesterone 5–7 days after the mare stops showing signs of estrus.
- Blood progesterone concentration will be low (in the range 1–5 ng/ml).

Management

- Some of these mares will respond to prostaglandin and will return into estrus. Unfortunately, a good number will repeat the process during the subsequent estrus.
- A few anovulatory follicles may ovulate if human chorionic gonadotropin or gonadotropin-releasing hormone is given. Unfortunately, most do not respond.
- Pregnancy does not usually occur if a persistent follicle spontaneously ovulates or is induced to ovulate. This is likely a result of degeneration of the oocyte over time.
- Pregnancy will not occur if the follicle becomes hemorrhagic or luteinized without ovulating.

Persistent estrus (nymphomania)

Profile

- Prolonged or persistent estrus or estrus-like behavior or strong estrus behavior at abnormally short intervals (often as little as 3 days).
- Although many mares are presented for investigation of persistent or abnormally active sexual behavior, some of theses cases are due to nonreproductive disorders.[74]
- Some are due to psychological behavior patterns and have nothing at all to do with reproductive status.
- It is important to separate those that do have a reproductive disorder from those that do not. Most of the former are treatable while most of the latter are difficult or impossible to treat.

Clinical signs

- Prolonged, persistent or short interval repeated, noncyclical display of normal estrus signs, such as elevation of the tail, clitoral 'winking' and frequent urination with stallion receptivity.
- Anestrous mares (winter seasonal ovarian inactivity) are usually passive to the teaser stallion.

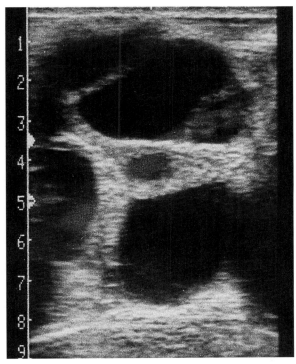

Fig. 5.51 Ultrasonogram of multiple anovulatory follicles in a mare.

- Transitional mares often have irregular and sometimes unusual behavior patterns. Multiple large follicles may be present but these fail to ovulate (see p. 120).
- Social dominance by a mare in a group.

Differential diagnosis

- Behavioral problems/psychosis (disobedience, resistance or aggression).
- Nonreproductive disorders:
  ❑ Urinary tract infection/inflammation (urethritis/vaginitis/cystitis) with repeated urination.
  ❑ Lameness, orthopedic disorders.
  ❑ Poor or inadequate handling/training.
- Prolonged estrus of early season transition period prior to the establishment of normal cyclicity.[17]
- Estrous behavior during pregnancy.
- Granulosa cell tumor.
  ❑ Infertility/noncyclicity/abnormal behavior with one enlarged ovary and one very small inactive one possibly due to inhibin secretion.
  ❑ Progesterone production (diestrous behavior).
  ❑ Testosterone/estrogen-secreting tumor (persistent estrus, virilism and masculine behavior). Most affected mares have elevated testosterone
- Iatrogenic administration of anabolic steroids.

Diagnosis

- Clinical signs are usually well recognized. The mare shows persistent estrus behavior with an apparently over-sexed mentality. Sometimes the mare may become masculine and aggressive.
- A detailed behavioral diary should be kept to establish the cyclical nature of the problem. Closed-circuit television monitoring of the mare can be helpful in eliminating and handling behavior problems.
- Repeated reproductive examinations involving rectal and ultrasonographic examinations (every alternate day) and hormone profiles (plasma progesterone) every fourth day are helpful.
- Repeated teasing of the mare at least every other day by a stallion.
- Test therapy with progestogen (such as altrenogest at 0.044 mg/kg daily by mouth or 150 mg progesterone per day by intramuscular injection) will suppress normal cyclicity for the duration of treatment.
- Definitive diagnosis by histological examination.

Treatment

- Treatment must be directed at the cause.
- Transitional estrus usually settles once normal ovarian activity is established (see p. 120).
- Routine ovariectomy of an obviously abnormal ovary may be curative, but removal of both ovaries may not resolve the behavior if it is caused by other factors.

OVARIAN TUMORS

Granulosa (thecal) cell tumor

Profile

- Granulosa (thecal) cell tumor is by far the most commonly reported neoplasm of the equine ovary.[75]
- Granulosa cell tumors are almost always unilateral, slow-growing and benign. They can be small or large and have characteristic functional properties (producing diagnostically significant hormones) as well as ultrasonographic and palpable features.
- The tumor destroys the remaining normal ovarian tissue in the affected ovary and the functional nature results in a typical (diagnostic) hormone profile that is responsible for the (almost) complete atrophy of the contralateral ovary.[76]

Clinical findings and diagnosis (see Fig. 5.52)

- The signs are dependent on the hormone profile produced.
- Affected mares exhibit a variety of signs:
  ❑ Constant or irregular estrus.
  ❑ Stallion-like behavior, including mounting mares in estrus, aggressiveness, squealing and striking, is a relatively common sign.
  ❑ Changes in muscle distribution to a stallion-like physique may be seen if the condition is prolonged (even in mares that show no stallion-like activity).
  ❑ Anestrous behavior with no detectable cyclicity occurs in about 25% of cases.[70,76]
  ❑ Rarely, a mare may have a granulosa cell tumor and continue to exhibit normal estrous cycles and ovulate from the other ovary.
- Rectal palpation reveals a grossly enlarged ovary with no palpable ovulation fossa. The contralateral ovary is usually small, firm and inactive.

> Note:
> - A mare that has a single grossly enlarged ovary that has a normal cycling contralateral ovary with regular ovulation at the normal interval is more likely to have an ovarian hematoma, teratoma or cystadenoma than a granulosa cell tumor.

- Ultrasonography often reveals a multicystic or honeycomb structure (see Fig. 5.53). A few cases appear as dense, lobulated, smooth masses or appear as a solid ovarian mass with a single, large fluid-filled cyst.[77]
- Mares may develop the tumor during pregnancy and may not have any problem with the

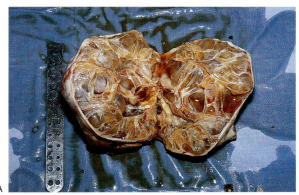

A

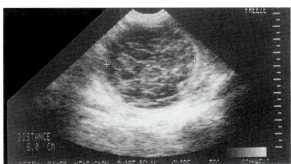

B

Fig. 5.53 (A) The gross specimen of a granulosa cell tumor illustrating the multilocular nature that imparts the characteristic ultrasonographic features. (B) Ultrasonographic of a granulosa cell tumor.

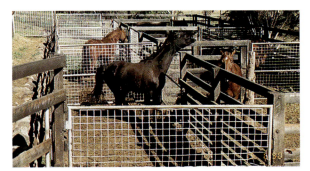

Fig. 5.52 Granulosa cell tumor (mare showing stallion-like behavior).

pregnancy; they will, of course, have considerable abnormalities (including postpartum anestrus) after foaling.

> - It is most unusual for an affected mare to conceive even if she does ovulate from the contralateral normal ovary, although it can occur.

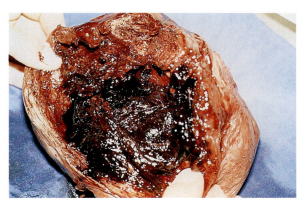

Fig. 5.54 An abnormal granulosa cell tumor that is filled with blood. Histological examination confirmed the tumor; the behavior and hormone profiles were highly suggestive of the condition but the ultrasonographic appearance was not typical.

- Some tumors may contain one or more hematomas within the stroma (Fig. 5.54); the homogeneous ultrasonographic appearance is distinctive.[77]

Granulosa cell tumors must be differentiated from other space-occupying conditions that present with an enlarged ovary such as:

- Cystadenoma.
- Germ cell tumor.
- Lymphoma/lymphosarcoma.
- Ovarian hematoma.

> - Mares with hematomas continue to cycle normally every 18 days; the contralateral ovary is active, the uterus will have tone during diestrus and the ovulation fossa of the affected ovary can be palpated.

Granulosa (thecal) cell tumors are diagnosed by a combination of:[78]

- History.
- Behavior.
- Rectal palpation.
- Ultrasonography.[79]
- Hormone assay.
- Laparoscopy.

Diagnostic tests

Clinical diagnostic assays for the detection of a granulosa cell tumor include the measurement of inhibin, testosterone, and progesterone.

- Inhibin is elevated in approximately 90% of mares with a granulosa cell tumor. It has been suggested that inhibin produced by the tumor is responsible for the inactivity of the contralateral ovary through the suppression of pituitary follicle-stimulating hormone release.[78]

- Serum testosterone levels may be elevated if a significant theca cell component is present in the tumor. Testosterone is elevated in approximately 50–60% of affected mares and is usually associated with stallion-like behavior.[76,78]
- Progesterone concentrations in mares with a granulosa cell tumor are almost always <1 ng/ml, since normal follicular development, ovulation and corpus luteum formation do not occur.

A diagnosis of granulosa cell tumor in a non-pregnant mare can be assured if:

- Inhibin concentration is >0.7 ng/ml.
- Testosterone concentration is >50–100 pg/ml.
- Progesterone concentration is <1 ng/ml.

Pathological features:
- The gross appearance of granulosa cell tumors is reasonably consistent.
- The diameter may vary from 6 to 40 cm (or more), but most are 10–20 cm wide.
- On cut section, multiple cystic structures and a yellowish stroma between cysts are evident.
- Cysts may contain blood, blood-tinged fluid or, most often, straw-colored serum-like fluid.

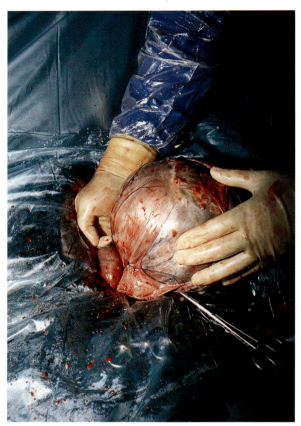

Fig. 5.55 Surgical removal of a granulosa cell tumor. These tumors can be extremely large and their weight may be an advantage for the surgeon in stretching the ovarian pedicle.

Treatment

- Surgical removal of the affected ovary (Fig. 5.55) is the only effective treatment for secreting ovarian tumors.
- Surgical approaches for tumor removal include colpotomy, flank and ventral midline laparotomy and laparoscopy (see below). These are described in detail in standard and advanced surgical texts.

Prognosis

- The prognosis for fertility after successful removal of a granulosa cell tumor is favorable.
- Metastasis is extremely rare.[75]
- Most mares will cycle within the next 9 months, although it may require up to 18 months in the occasional mare.
- If ovariectomy is performed during the winter, resumption of cyclic activity is usually delayed by the natural seasonality of the mare.[76]

Failure to remove the ovary carries risks of:
- Serious behavioral problems (even in those tumors that are not secretory at the time).
- Future discomfort/colic associated with ovarian ligament traction.
- Hemorrhage from ruptured ovarian ligaments caused by the enlarged ovary.
- Rare metastasis.

Cystadenoma, adenomas and adenocarcinoma

Profile

- Nonsecretory tumors are rare and benign and are not considered to be hormonally active.
- Equine ovarian adenomas are of epithelial origin and are usually formed from the surface of the ovulatory fossa or oviductal fimbriae.
- They are usually unilateral, and unilobular or multilobular.
- If cystic, they are referred to as cystadenomas (Fig. 5.56).

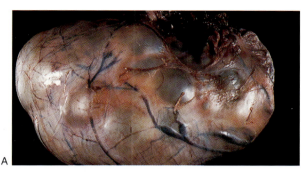

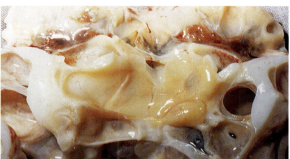

Fig. 5.56 Ovarian cyst adenoma. Note the multiple follicle-like cysts throughout the ovary (A) and yellow tissue in the stroma (B).

- Cystadenomas occur unilaterally and the contralateral ovary is normal.
- On rare occasions, adenomas metastasize and are classified as adenocarcinoma.

Clinical signs
- There are no effects on the estrous cycle.
- The abnormal ovary is identified on rectal palpation and ultrasonography.
- The ultrasonographic appearance of the affected ovary may include one to many cyst-like structures.
- Mares with adenocarcinoma generally have a history of weight loss, ascites and/or recurring abdominal pain from abdominal metastasis.

Management
- Surgical removal is recommended as the mare may exhibit episodes of abdominal pain if the tumor becomes quite large.
- Cystadenoma has not been reported to metastasize.

Teratoma/germ cell tumor

Profile
- Teratoma is the second most common ovarian tumor.
- They are benign, nonsecretory tumors that arise from germ cells.

- Teratomas contain misplaced embryonic structures, such as bone, skin, teeth, cartilage, nerves, blood vessels, and hair.
- They are solid or contain large cystic spaces occasionally lined with squamous epithelium.

Clinical signs/diagnosis
- Mares with ovarian teratoma continue to cycle and ovulate from the contralateral unaffected ovary.[80]
- It is unlikely that teratomas will interfere with fertility unless they are large enough to cause the reproductive tract to become dependent in the abdomen.
- Surgical removal is indicated.
- Ovarian teratoma is discovered most commonly during routine rectal examination.
- The ovary feels firm and enlarged, with rough, irregular surfaces.
- Ultrasonographically the tumor has a mixed appearance, depending on the distribution of fluid and tissue structures.
- Differentiation from other nonsecretory ovarian tumors is difficult without excision.

Dysgerminoma

Profile
- Dysgerminoma is an extremely rare tumor composed of a uniform population of cells that resemble primordial germ cells.
- They are generally considered to be malignant, metastasizing rapidly to both the abdominal and thoracic cavities.

Clinical signs/diagnosis
- The neoplasm is usually smooth and relatively soft, or lobulated with multiple cysts containing gelatinous fluid.
- Neither rectal palpation nor ultrasonography shows any characteristic features.
- Hypertrophic pulmonary osteopathy (Marie's disease) has been found in conjunction with this malignant neoplasm, causing subperiosteal new bone formation (with pain on palpation), weight loss, stiffness, and edema of the extremities.
- It is difficult to differentiate from other nonsecretory causes of ovarian enlargement.

Treatment
- If the tumor can be detected before metastasis, the affected ovary should be removed (see below).

OVARIECTOMY

Ovariectomy is the removal of one or both ovaries, either normal or abnormal. Removal of both ovaries is performed in:

- Performance mares that become unmanageable when in estrus and which are not regarded as suitable for breeding purposes.
- Production of mares used as jump mares in artificial insemination programs.
- Disease states such as granulosa cell tumors which usually only affect one ovary.

SURGICAL METHODS FOR OVARIECTOMY

The method chosen depends on the reasons for ovariectomy, the relative health of the mare and the facilities available. The techniques are described in standard surgical texts.

Normal mare with normal ovaries

Colpotomy
- Via an internal vaginal incision with the use of écraseurs to crush the arterial blood supply to the ovaries to allow their removal.
- The procedure is performed on the standing sedated mare with epidural anesthesia.
- This method is not applicable to enlarged ovaries.

Laparoscopic ovariectomy
- The development of the laparoscope and the technical skill means that ovaries can be removed safely via a laparoscopic technique (Fig. 5.57).[81]
- This method is not practical for large ovarian tumors.

Laparotomy
- Ventral midline approach under general anesthesia.
- Flank laparotomy in the standing sedated mare under local anesthesia.

Abnormal/enlarged ovaries (including tumors of the ovaries and ovarian hematoma)

- Laparotomy is usually the method of choice because the weight of the enlarged ovary makes exteriorization much simpler.
- Laparoscopic methods can be performed but inevitably mean that the excised ovary must in any case be removed via a flank laparotomy incision.

MARES THAT CYCLE, CONCEIVE AND LOSE PREGNANCY AFTER 35 DAYS

Early pregnancy loss is the cause of significant reduction in reproductive performance in horses. The causes of these losses are numerous and varied (see Table 5.5, p. 162). Losses that occur in the late embryonic and early fetal period (35–60 days) are discussed here.

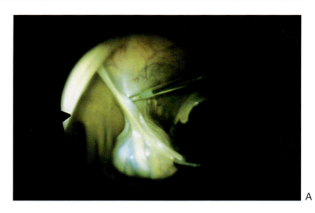

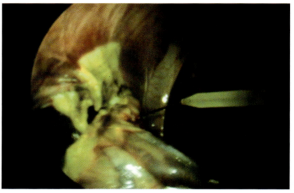

Fig. 5.57 Ovariectomy via laparoscopy is a useful new method that avoids general anesthesia. It is only feasible for smaller ovaries. (A) shows local anesthetic being injected into the pedicle; (B) shows the layers of an endoloop ligature after bipolar cautery. Slides courtesy of J Walmsley.

- Successful conception in these cases indicates that the hypothalamic–pituitary–gonadal axis has functioned properly and that the tubular tract has been normal up to a point.
- Pregnancy failure in these mares can be considered as a defect in the tubular tract.
- Endometritis, a major contributor to this problem, is described on p. 178.
- Mares with persistent mating-induced endometritis will cycle normally and, if they conceive, most commonly lose their pregnancy before 35 days (see p. 178).

Failure of the endometrial glands

Profile
- Advanced periglandular fibrosis is highly correlated with pregnancy loss between 35 and 80 days.[40]
- The specific mechanism for interference of glandular secretion has not been defined. However, the concept that periglandular fibrosis has a significant effect on early pregnancy survival is widely held.

Clinical signs
- Repeated history of early embryonic death between 35 and 80 days.

Diagnosis
- Definitive diagnosis is made histologically.
- Endometrial samples will contain widespread moderate to severe periglandular fibrosis.

Treatment
- There is no known treatment. However, many affected mares are placed on supplemental progesterone therapy and there are anecdotal reports of successful pregnancies.

Cervical incompetence

Profile
- Single or multiple cervical lacerations are usually associated with parturition, commonly resulting from the delivery of a foal before complete cervical dilation has developed or by forcibly extracting a foal without adequate lubrication.[82] Tears may also occur during resolution of dystocia by mutation or fetotomy. Lacerations sometimes occur spontaneously during apparently normal deliveries. Mares may conceive and lose their pregnancy after 45 days or they may develop chronic endometritis.
- Cervical lacerations usually involve the mucosa and fibromuscular layers of the cervix.
- Bruising and tearing of the fibromuscular layer may occur without mucosal defects.
- The lacerations may be either full or partial thickness and may involve only a portion of the length of the cervix or run the entire length of the cervix.
- The damage may involve the vaginal mucosa, muscular layer, and/or the cervical mucosa.
- The earliest indications may be related to infertility.

Clinical signs
- Mares not conceiving after repeated breeding.
- Chronic endometritis.
- Pregnancy loss between 45 days and 4–5 months.

Diagnosis
- Diagnosis of cervical laceration requires careful manual palpation of the entire cervical canal between finger and thumb, preferably when the cervix is tightly closed. The condition is only rarely diagnosed with other methods of examination.
- The severity of the defect is best identified by vaginal palpation of the cervical canal during diestrus when the cervix should be tightly closed.

If the cervical canal is overstretched, one to two fingers will pass through it during diestrus.
- Edematous mucosal folds may cover and mask the laceration.
- Vaginal endoscopy (or direct examination with an illuminated vaginal speculum) is a useful aid to diagnosis, but tears can easily be missed by direct visual examination.

Management

Cervical laceration
- If the external os is damaged it can be repaired surgically.
- Some reports indicate that a defect limited to the external os of the cervix does not need to be repaired unless 50% or more is damaged, whereas others indicate the lesion should be surgically repaired if the lesion incorporates 25% of the external os.
- It is difficult and sometimes impossible to correct an overstretched cervical body. This lesion may occur if a foal is delivered forcibly through a cervix that is not totally dilated at parturition.

Cervical adhesions
Cervical adhesions can occur as a result from damage to the cervical mucosa following:

- Prolonged dystocia.
- Fetotomy.
- Infusions:
  - ❑ Acidic antibiotic solutions such as aminoglycosides that are neither buffered nor diluted with saline.
  - ❑ Iodine.
  - ❑ Povidone iodine solution.

Treatment
The ability of the cervix to close completely to prevent ascending infection is the primary determinant of whether a cervical laceration needs to be surgically repaired.

- Often, newly formed adhesions can be broken down manually.
- Various ointments, including antibiotic/steroid ointments, vitamin A and D ointment, and vitamin E ointment, have been rubbed into the cervical canal after mucosal damage to prevent adhesions.

Partial-thickness tears (or full-thickness tears of a small portion of the cervix)
- These may be allowed to heal by second intention.
- The cervix should be assessed after 30 days post partum, during the luteal phase when progesterone dominance is high and the cervix should be tightly closed.

- If the cervix is tightly closed, no further treatment is needed, and the mare can be bred.
- Cervical tone should be monitored throughout the pregnancy to be sure that with the growing weight of the fetus and uterine fluids that the cervix maintains its tight seal.
- If the mare aborts as a result of cervical incompetence, surgery to repair the laceration should be made prior to attempts at re-breeding.

Full-thickness and full-length tears

- These often affect future fertility in spite of surgical correction.
- Full thickness tears of more than half the length of the cervix or full-length, partial-thickness tears are best managed by surgical repair (Fig. 5.58).[83-85]
- Suturing of lacerations is difficult and should be performed 4–8 weeks after foaling once inflammation subsides.
- The cervix should be assessed for degree of natural healing. A healthy bed of granulation tissue without signs of inflammation should be present, prior to attempting repair.
- There is a high failure rate if inflammation or dead/necrotic tissue is present at the time of surgery.

Technique

The mare should preferably be in early or late diestrus at the time of surgery so that mucosal folds are not excessive and thereby obscuring the limits of the laceration.

- Epidural anesthesia is required and injection of local anesthetic just dorsal to the cervix often increases the amount of caudal retraction possible and therefore makes the procedure easier to perform.
- Special long-handled (40–50 cm) instruments are required to perform these surgeries.
- A three-layer closure is preferred (Fig 5.58):
  - ❏ First layer: this everts the mucosa of the cervical lumen.

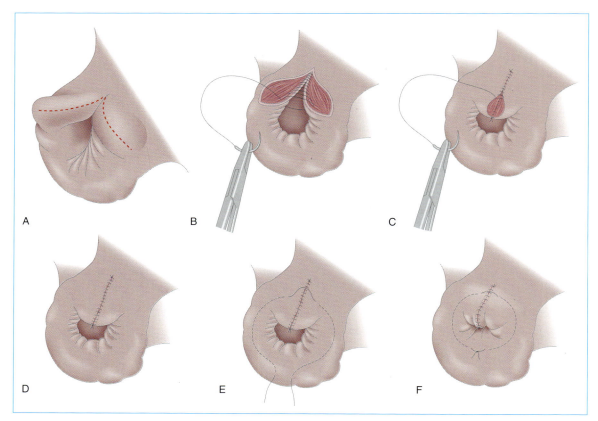

Fig. 5.58 Cervical laceration repair. The operation is performed on the standing mare and the cervix is retracted caudally as far as possible. (A) A full-thickness tear. The first incision is made along the full length of the tear from its most anterior extent to beyond the natural end of the cervix. (B) The deep mucosal layer is closed with simple continuous sutures starting from the most cranial point. (C) The muscular and the outer mucosal layers are closed carefully with simple continuous sutures. (D) Once completed, the cervix should be completely intact and the operation site should be covered in steroid antibiotic cream to try to limit any adhesion formation. (E) Cervical incompetence may be treated by placement of a submucosal circlage 'purse-string' suture. (F) This can be tied in a fashion that permits release and retying without having to replace the suture itself.

❑ Second layer: this apposes the fibromuscular layers.

❑ Third layer: this everts the external mucosa of the cervix in the vagina.

- Application of a combined corticosteroid and antibiotic ointment to the repaired laceration following surgery may diminish the scar tissue that forms in the cervix (scar tissue and cervical adhesions are the most common long-term sequelae of the surgery).
- The repaired laceration should not be manipulated for a minimum of 4 weeks postoperatively. This delay may be problematic in view of the tendency to adhesions, etc.
- Evaluation of the repair is performed preferably under progesterone dominance during the luteal phase (diestrus). At that time, the cervix may be digitally palpated to assess surgical success.
- If the repair is successful, one should allow 30 days from the surgery date if artificial insemination is used.

Note:

- Mares should not be bred within 90 days postoperatively if natural service is used because the stallion's penis may enter or damage the cervix.
- Cervical competence should be monitored throughout the pregnancy to determine if tone is adequate. Some clinicians will treat mares with cervical lacerations with supplemental progesterone during their pregnancies to help increase cervical tone.
- Mares with severely scarred cervices or mares with multiple lacerations that are not amenable to repair may be subjected to cervical cerclage treatment. The cerclage should be placed following early diagnosis of pregnancy; however, success at maintaining pregnancy is only fair. Postbreeding antibiotic treatment and oxytocin administration is recommended, since most mares with cervical incompetence tend to have ascending infections and endometritis is common.

Prognosis

- Mares that undergo fetal death during pregnancy may either tear the cerclage suture and cause severe damage to the external os of the cervix, or are unable to deliver the dead foal, resulting in septicemia and possibly even death.

- The risks should always be explained to the owner prior to attempting this procedure.

- Postsurgical fertility of young mares is relatively high following good repair.
- However, it is not uncommon for mares who have had a torn cervix at one foaling, and have subsequently healed or been surgically repaired, to lacerate the cervix again on the subsequent foaling due to the decreased elasticity of the scar tissue that forms during the healing process.
- Repeat lacerations are usually amenable to another surgical repair procedure.
- If attempts at repair are not economically feasible, or are unsuccessful, the mare can be successfully entered into embryo transfer programs as a donor.

Luteal/progesterone insufficiency

Profile

- Prior to 80 days' gestation, removal of the ovaries or failure of the corpora lutea to produce progesterone, will result in abortion.
- Rapid decline in progesterone concentrations causes loss of uterine and cervical tone, and consequent loss of the conceptus. It has long been considered logical, therefore, that partial failure of the corpus luteum could reduce the absolute amount of progesterone needed to maintain pregnancy. As a result, many protocols for supplementing progestins have been devised in an attempt to prevent early pregnancy loss, especially in mares with a history of such loss. The value of these schemes is unproven. Nevertheless, owners often expect supplementation when there is a convincing reproductive history.
- Progesterone supplementation in mares with histories of endometritis (see p. 178) or lymphatic lacunae (see above) may be contraindicated as progesterone may aggravate the problem.

  ❑ Supplemental progestin does appear to be warranted in pregnant mares that are experiencing endotoxemia.
- Prostaglandins are released from the gastrointestinal tract during colic.

  ❑ In mares that are less than 90 days pregnant, these prostaglandins cause lysis of the corpus luteum and so induce abortion. After 90 days, the placenta becomes the dominant structure, producing progestins that maintain pregnancy for the remainder of gestation and prostaglandins do not then induce abortion.
- Progesterone therapy may inhibit premature uterine contractions and so may be beneficial during the second and third trimesters of pregnancy in mares that have placentitis, colic or severe systemic disease.

Clinical signs

Reasons for placing mares that are less than 30 days pregnant on progestins include:

- History of early pregnancy loss at previous breeding.
- Low plasma progesterone concentrations on days 5, 8 and 12 of gestation.
  - Values less than 4–6 ng/ml are usually considered low.
- Ultrasonographic visualization of uterine edema at the early pregnancy examination (between days 14 and 28).
- Colic.
- Accidental administration of prostaglandin.[86]

Management

- Mares in late gestation, showing signs of colic, anorexia or those with a vaginal discharge may benefit from progestin supplementation.
- Endotoxemic mares in early pregnancy should receive 0.044 mg/kg altrenogest daily (by mouth).[87]
- The progestin can be removed slowly after 90 days of gestation when the fetoplacental unit begins to produce progestins, which serve as an effective source of 'progesterone' and naturally sustain the pregnancy
- Systemically ill mares in later gestation require a double dose of altrenogest (0.088 mg/kg daily by mouth).

MARES THAT CYCLE AND EITHER DO NOT CONCEIVE OR LOSE THEIR PREGNANCY BEFORE 35 DAYS

Endometritis

Profile

- Endometritis is the most common cause of embryonic loss before 35 days in mares that cycle normally.

Endometritis can effectively be classified into three categories:

Category 1: persistent mating-induced endometritis.
Category 2: chronic infectious endometritis.
Category 3: sexually transmitted endometritis.
- Categories 1 and 2 most commonly affect older (pluriparous or nulliparous) mares.
- Young mares may also experience these problems, particularly if they have cervical incompetence (insufficient relaxation during estrus) or have had a previous foaling injury resulting in contamination of the uterus with air, feces, or urine.

- Category 3 (sexually transmitted) endometritis may occur in any mare that is bred with semen contaminated with the incriminating organism.
- The reproductive tract has a mucosal immune system similar to that of the respiratory tract.
- Bacteria, yeast, semen and contaminants, such as feces and urine, are cleared from the uterus by a combination of:
  - Cellular (neutrophil phagocytosis) and immunological processes (IgG, IgA, and opsonization) that kill bacteria.
  - Physical drainage of the by-products.
- If any of these processes malfunctions, the mare may or may not be able to overcome the infection.
- As the mare ages, physical and immunological changes make her more susceptible to uterine infection. Treatments that may have been used successfully in earlier years may, therefore, not be as effective as the mare ages.
- The reproductive history of the mare and a physical examination may provide the most productive information for determining the cause of endometritis. The physical examination should be performed during the physiologic breeding season, preferably within 30 days of the last breeding.
- After prolonged sexual rest, the susceptible mare may have cleared the inflammation on her own.
- Mares that have persistent mating-induced endometritis may develop chronic infectious endometritis if they are bred repeatedly, if conformational defects are not repaired or if intrauterine antibiotics have been used excessively.

Persistent mating-induced endometritis

Profile

- Transient inflammation is a normal physiological response to breeding, foaling, examination of the reproductive tract or contamination.[88]
- Normal, fertile mares clear the inflammation from their uterus within 12 hours of insult.[89]
- Mares susceptible to persistent, postmating endometritis have an intrinsic inability to evacuate uterine contents following contamination during breeding.[90,91]
- Prolonged uterine inflammation following breeding ultimately leads to early embryonic loss.
- A uterus that is located ventral to the pelvis contributes to the problem.[92]

Numerous studies indicate that suppressed uterine contractility is a primary defect in the susceptible mare.[93] It is not known if the defect is a structural defect in the muscle cell itself, or is due to an abnormal response to hormonal or neural signaling.

The persistence of inflammatory debris within the uterine lumen results in accumulation of neutrophils,

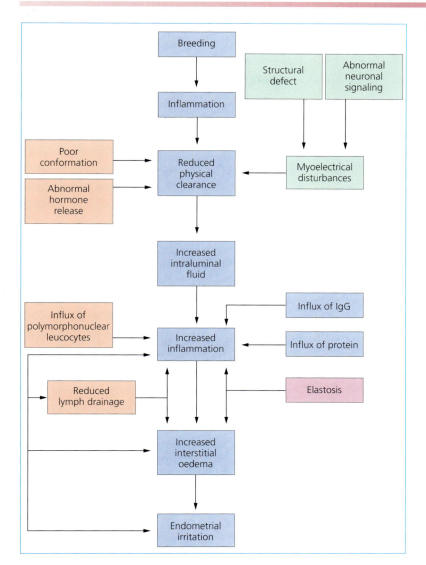

Fig. 5.59 Pathogenesis of persistent mating-induced endometritis.

immunoglobulins and protein in the uterine lumen. This instigates a vicious cycle of fluid accumulation, interstitial edema and endometrial irritation (Fig. 5.59). The longer the process continues the higher the likelihood the endometrium will be damaged, enabling bacteria to attach to the epithelium. Excessive interstitial edema may result from either prolonged inflammation or elastosis of the arteriole walls. The lymphatics may become overwhelmed from the excessive edema and may not be able to drain the tissues of the excessive edema and cellular matter.

Clinical signs
- Pluriparous mares older than 14 years of age with poor perineal conformation are most prone to persistent postmating endometritis.
- Maiden mares (either old or young) may develop endometritis because the cervix does not open sufficiently during estrus. The cause for this cervical malfunction is not known.

- Many susceptible mares will have minimal signs of inflammation *prior* to breeding, only to flare after breeding.
- Fluid accumulation occurs in the uterine lumen 12–36 hours after breeding.
- Perineal anatomy that allows fecal, urinary, or air contamination, is commonly a significant factor.
- Mares may experience early pregnancy loss, may not be found pregnant at the 14-day check after repeated breedings, or may lose the pregnancy as early as 14–16 days.

After repeated breedings, bacteria and neutrophils may be recovered from the uterus.

The typical history of a pluriparous mare with persistent mating-induced endometritis is that she has conceived and foaled successfully for 3–4 years, after which time she has difficulty conceiving.

The typical history for older (12–14 years of age) nulliparous (maiden) mares is that, following a successful performance career, they have difficulty conceiving. The latter group of mares may be bred more often with shipped cooled semen or frozen semen so the quality of the semen also needs to be investigated.

Diagnosis

- Reproductive examination after breeding usually shows characteristic signs of fluid accumulation.
- A presumptive diagnosis is made on past breeding history.

Ultrasonography of the uterus 12–36 hours after breeding reveals fluid within the uterine lumen (Fig. 5.60) and in more severe cases intramural edema after ovulation. The fluid is not palpable via the rectum.

A complete physical and reproductive examination should be performed prior to breeding.

1. Physical examination
   - Body condition score.
   - Perineal conformation from both lateral and caudal aspects.
2. Reproductive examination
   - Rectal examination.
   - Ultrasonography.
   - Vaginal speculum examination.
   - Digital examination of the cervix.
   - Uterine cytology.
   - Uterine bacteriological culture.
   - Uterine biopsy.

> Note:
> - Findings from the reproductive examination may differ, depending on when the examination is performed during the breeding season.

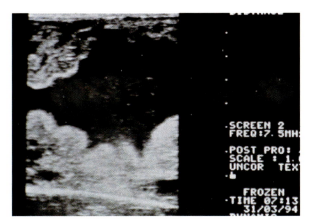

Fig. 5.60 Accumulated fluid in the uterine lumen and the endometrial wall 12 hours after ovulation, arising from persistent mating-induced endometritis.

- After prolonged sexual rest during winter, a susceptible mare usually has:
  - A negative culture.
  - May or may not have neutrophils on cytology.
  - Slight inflammation with or without lymphangectasia on biopsy (commonly a IIa for a biopsy score).
- After repeated breeding during the spring this same susceptible mare may have:
  - Bacteria recovered from the uterus.
  - Fluid accumulation within the uterine lumen during diestrus or after breeding.
  - Possibly a vaginal discharge.

These variations may be perplexing to owners who may assume that the culture was not properly performed at the beginning of the breeding season.

- Owners should have a layman's understanding of the pathogenesis of the disease otherwise mares may be bred repeatedly during the transitional or physiological breeding season.
- Repeated breeding of these mares without postmating treatment may induce severe endometrial irritation resulting in bacterial colonization.

Treatment

- Treatment should be delayed until 4 hours after breeding to ensure that viable sperm are not prematurely washed from the uterus.
- Treatment should be conducted before 8 hours because the uterine inflammatory response in reproductively normal mares is greatest between 8 and 12 hours after breeding.
- The longer the seminal by-products remain in the uterine lumen, the greater the inflammatory response and the greater the endometrial damage.[89] Therefore, treatment is directed at rapid removal of fluids.

Technique

i. Uterine lavage with 1–3 liters of warmed saline or lactated Ringer's solution between 4 and 8 hours after breeding and administration of 10–20 IU of oxytocin (administered intravenously or intramuscularly) 4–8 hours after breeding.[94–96]
ii. If fluid is present in the uterine lumen 24 hours after breeding, the procedure can be repeated.
iii. The number of uterine lavages should be minimized after ovulation to avoid iatrogenic transfer of bacteria from the vestibulum to the uterus after the cervix has closed.

Mares that have lymphatic lacunae in addition to persistent mating-induced endometritis may be treated with a combination of oxytocin treatment between 4 and 8 hours after breeding, and cloprostenol (250 μg) at 12 and 24 hours after breeding. Natural prostaglandins or their analogs should not be given after ovulation as they will adversely affect progesterone concentrations and pregnancy rates.

- The prostaglandin analog induces uterine contractions for 5 hours, thereby assisting lymphatic drainage.
- The oxytocin causes strong uterine contractions for 20–40 minutes and assists in the physical drainage of the uterine lumen via the cervix.

Management

A full reproductive examination should be carried out on any mare that does not conceive after two or three breedings with postbreeding treatment.

- Particular attention should be paid to the perineal conformation.
- Abnormalities, including vestibulovaginal reflux of urine, sunken perineal bodies, cervical tears or rectovaginal fistulas, must be repaired.

Sexual rest for 45–60 days may be warranted in mares that have:

- Chronic, active inflammation of the endometrium.
- Severe lymphatic lacunae.
- Fluid accumulation at their 14-day pregnancy examination.

Prognosis

As the disease is a continuum of degenerative changes and as the mare ages, older mares repeatedly treated with uterotonic drugs may not become pregnant.

Lymphatic lacunae

Profile

- Uterine lymphatics normally reabsorb edema that accumulates within the uterine wall during estrus, as well as clear particulate matter from the uterine lumen that is not cleared through the cervix.[97]
- Lymphatics do not contain muscle within their walls and therefore drain passively.
- Lymph is pumped along the vessels through rhythmic contractions of the uterine smooth muscle.

Clinical signs

- Mares with lymphangectasia retain edema within the uterine wall after ovulation. These mares have a doughy, thick-walled uterus on rectal palpation.
- Poor lymphatic drainage may contribute to uterine fluid accumulation in mares with persistent mating-induced endometritis.

Diagnosis

- Rectal palpation is typical.
- On ultrasonographic examination of the uterus after ovulation, a 'cartwheel' appearance is visualized when the uterus is scanned (see Fig. 6.8); the 'cartwheel' appearance normally disappears before ovulation.
- Histologically, lymphatic lacunae are present.

Management (see also p. 196, uterine therapy)

A suitable treatment regimen is:

   i. 4–8 hours after breeding:
- Uterus is lavaged with saline.
- 20 IU of oxytocin are administered intravenously.

  ii. 12 hours after breeding:
- 1 ml of cloprostenol is injected intramuscularly.

 iii. 24 hours after breeding:
- Ultrasonographic examination of the uterus carried out to detect fluid within the uterine lumen.
- A second uterine lavage is performed if fluid remains.
- A second injection of cloprostenol is given if the mare has not ovulated.
- If there is excessive uterine edema *without* fluid in the uterine lumen and the mare has not ovulated, only cloprostenol is given.
- Prostaglandins cause the uterus to contract for about 5 hours. Prolonged uterine contractions stimulate lymph flow through the vessels.
- Prostaglandins should not be administered anytime after ovulation as they may interfere with progesterone production by the corpus luteum.
  - ❏ If sustained uterine contractility is necessary to facilitate lymphatic drainage and prostaglandins must be administered after ovulation has occurred, then supplementation with progesterone is recommended. Progesterone supplementation should begin 2–3 days post ovulation; if the mare becomes pregnant, supplementation should be continued at least until day 45 of pregnancy, when accessory corpus luteum function is well under way.[98]

Prognosis

Some mares with moderate to severe lymphatic lacunae may become pregnant, but about half of them will abort between 3 and 5 months.

Chronic infectious endometritis

The reproductive history of the mare and a physical examination may provide the most productive information for determining the cause of endometritis.

- Mares exhibiting chronic, severe endometritis have histories of long-standing inflammatory changes.
- Their reproductive histories may include:
  - ❏ Repeated treatments with intrauterine antibiotics (see p. 196).
  - ❏ Repeated breeding the same season.
  - ❏ Poor perineal conformation.
  - ❏ An incompetent cervix during estrus (failure to relax completely).
  - ❏ Persistent mating-induced endometritis.
- The mares are susceptible to endometritis because they have a breakdown in uterine defense mechanisms that allow the normal genital flora to contaminate the uterus and develop into persistent endometritis.
- Bacteria commonly isolated in severe, long-standing cases include:
  - ❏ *Streptococcus zooepidemicus*.
  - ❏ *Escherichia coli*.
  - ❏ *Pseudomonas* spp. or *Klebsiella* spp.
  - ❏ Yeasts and fungi.
- The physical examination should be performed during the physiological breeding season, preferably within 30 days of the last breeding.
  - ❏ After prolonged sexual rest, the susceptible mare may have cleared the inflammation spontaneously.
- Mares that have persistent mating-induced endometritis may develop chronic infectious endometritis if they are bred repeatedly (see above) and particularly if conformational defects are not repaired or if intrauterine antibiotics have been used excessively.

Diagnosis

- The severity of the endometritis is best confirmed histologically.
- Moderate to severe, focal to diffuse lymphocytic or plasmacytic inflammation is usually reported.
- Lymphangectasia may be mild to severe.

Management

- Correction of predisposing causes is an important first step in all cases.
- Correction of damaged external barriers.
- Judicious use of systemic antibiotics, local antibiotic or disinfectant therapy.

Treatment

- Treatment of chronic infectious endometritis is difficult and frequently unsuccessful.
- Mares with chronic endometritis have been treated with intrauterine antibiotics combined with uterine lavage or systemic antibiotics with or without uterine lavage (see section on intrauterine therapy, p. 196).
- Some mares after treatment with intrauterine antibiotics may develop fungal or yeast infections.

- Sexual rest for a minimum of 45 days is often the most effective treatment, especially in severely affected mares.
- Counterirritant therapy in these mares has been used successfully.

Chronic endometritis due to fungi or yeast

When fungi or yeasts are isolated from the uterus, prolonged intrauterine treatment with antimycotic drugs may be needed.[99]

Technique

Conservative therapy may be successful as a first attempt at treatment. A suitable protocol is:
  i. Lavage the uterus daily for 3–5 days during estrus with either:
     - A saline–vinegar mixture (10 ml of vinegar to 1 liter of saline).
     - A mixture of povidone iodine and saline (20 ml of povidone iodine concentrate to 1 liter of saline).

> - The lavage fluids need to be instilled and then removed from the uterus as the cervix and vagina may be sensitive to the vinegar or iodine.

  ii. A uterine biopsy is taken a minimum of two weeks after conclusion of treatment to determine the severity of the inflammation and to identify fungal spores or yeast within the endometrium.
  iii. If yeast or fungi are identified within the endometrium or they are isolated from the uterus during the next estrus:
     - The organism is identified and sensitivity tests performed so that the best antimycotic drug can be used.
  iv. Treatment with the most appropriate drug is instigated on the first day of estrus and continued for a minimum of 10 days through the early postovulatory period.
     - The mare is sexually rested during the next estrus.
  v. If no organisms are isolated from the uterus during the second estrus post treatment, the mare may be bred and it is probably useful to lavage her uterus after breeding.
  vi. Antibiotics should be avoided in these mares following breeding.

> - It is not uncommon to isolate a streptococcal species from the uterus after the mare has been treated for fungal or yeast infections; many of these mares have incompetent immune processes in some respect.

Sexually transmitted endometritis

See sections on contagious equine metritis (p. 193) and equine viral arteritis (p. 259).

Pyometra

Profile

- Pyometra is an occasional sequel to infections of the tubular genital tract.
- Large volumes of inflammatory debris accumulate in the uterus and there is a concurrent retained functional corpus luteum during the normal breeding season.[100]
- Abnormalities of the cervix (adhesions or inflammation) are a logical possible cause but many cases have no such problems. Furthermore, the pyometra itself may be a predisposing cause of cervical inflammation and adhesion development.
- Older mares that are prone to uterine infections (through poor functional bacterial protection or through inadequate natural uterine defense mechanisms, or both) are more susceptible.
- Little is known of the true etiopathogenesis.

Clinical signs (see Fig. 5.61)

- Palpable enlargement of the uterus with a 'doughy' solid feel.
- Noncyclicity due to a prolonged luteal phase. However, some affected mares cycle regularly or irregularly.
- Bacteriological culture of the uterine fluid sometimes reveals mixed growths of bacteria, which may or may not include pathogens, but in other cases the fluid is sterile.
- Systemic signs are rarely present but some mares may be lethargic.
- Cervical and uterine adhesions are common.

Differential diagnosis

- Pyometra must be differentiated from metritis and endometritis because the diseases have a considerably different reproductive prognosis.
- Pregnancy.
- Mummification of a fetus.

Diagnosis

- Rectal examination and ultrasonographic examination are helpful but the reproductive history is probably the most important factor.
- Hematological and biochemical analyses are usually not remarkable. There is little systemic response that reflects in changes in blood parameters.
- Endometrial biopsy is essential to establish a prognosis before any attempt is made at long-term treatment.

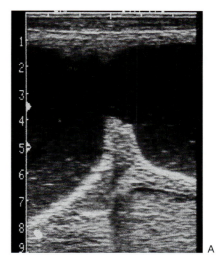

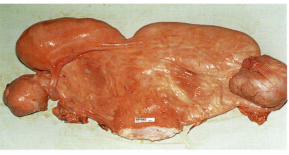

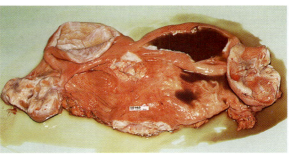

Fig. 5.61 Pyometra. (A) Ultrasonographic appearance of a uterus affected with pyometra. Note the floccular fluid material with a heavy deposit. (B) Necropsy specimen showing entire uterine body with ovaries and grossly enlarged uterine horns. The mare was infertile. (C) Same specimen of the uterus of the same mare as in (B), showing red/brown purulent contents. Histopathological examination showed complete loss of normal uterine structures with severe fibrosis.

Treatment

- Once established the condition is very difficult to treat.
  - ❑ Uterine flushing and evacuation is essential.
  - ❑ Appropriate antibiotics are logical but somewhat disappointing.
- The prognosis for future breeding is virtually nil because the consequent endometrial atrophy is profound and irreversible.

- Recurring fluid accumulation is common.
- In cases where the cervix is badly scarred and fluid accumulation occurs repeatedly, creation of a surgical cervical laceration may allow fluid to drain from the uterine lumen. This, of course, is a salvage procedure, and these mares have no useful reproductive potential unless entered into embryo transfer or in vitro fertilization programs.

- Cycling mares and those with a short history of pyometra, particularly if there is limited endometrial atrophy, have a slightly better chance of reproductive cure.

Other causes of early embryonic death

These include:

- Oviductal obstruction.
- Embryonic defects.
- Stress resulting in prostaglandin release.
- Poor nutrition.
- Advancing age.

Egg viability diminishes as the mare gets older and this contributes significantly to infertility ('old egg disease'). Unfortunately, this aspect of infertility is difficult to investigate or diagnose without using the latest reproductive techniques such as embryo transfer or oviductal flush (see p. 221).

INJURIES/DISORDERS/DISEASES OF THE VAGINA, VESTIBULE AND VULVA

Vulvar laceration and vulvar insufficiency

Vulvar lacerations are a common aftermath of foaling.

- With extensive pressure on the labia during foaling, circulation of the vulva may be disrupted, resulting in vulvar necrosis.
  - ❏ Failure to open the previous year's Caslick operation adequately is a frequent cause.
- Small tears in a previously sutured dorsal vulvar commissure may occur at the time of breeding.
- These are usually of no consequence to the mare's health or fertility at that mating.
- Depending on perineal conformation, repair of the Caslick vulvoplasty may be necessary.
  - ❏ If the laceration is severe, the inflammation must be resolved before repair is attempted.
- Immediate care should include cleansing of the laceration and administration of systemic antimicrobials and tetanus toxoid.
- The damage may reduce the amount of vulvar tissue and require a deeper closure than the simple Caslick procedure.
- In the worst cases, more healing time is allowed and repair should be delayed until after the mare is mated.

Caslick's operation

Caslick's operation (Fig. 5.62) is probably the most important procedure in the treatment of pneumo-

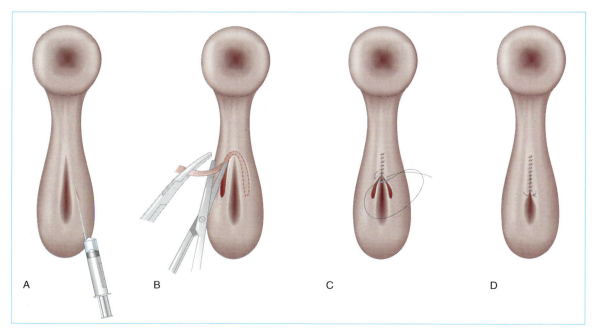

A   B   C   D

Fig. 5.62 Caslick's operation (vulvoplasty).

vagina and infertility caused by infection of the genital tract. With numerous foals, loss of condition and aging, the shape of the perineal area of the mare changes. There is usually an insidious loss of fertility, but continuous contamination of the breeding tract with air and fecal material lowers the mare's uterine tone and resistance to infection and, as the mare ages, so creates a lowered plane of fertility.

- Careful adherence to the measurements and calculation required to define the Caslick index (see below) removes much of the doubt as to whether a mare will or will not benefit from the surgery.

- Mares requiring Caslick's operation should always have the vulvar dorsal commissure carefully closed and kept closed.
- Failure to be meticulous about this reduces fertility.

Caslick index

Calculation and measurements

Caslick score = (length of vulva in cm) × (angle of declination)

Interpretation
- Values of less than 150 are associated with a normal anatomical arrangement. Fertility is best in mares with a score of 100 or less. The Caslick score naturally increases with age.
- Continuous evaluation is essential especially if loss of body condition occurs.

- A Caslick operation must be performed when the dorsal vulvar commissure is located more than 4 cm (1.5 inches) dorsal to the pelvic floor.
- The vulvar lips should be sutured such that the 'new' dorsal vulvar commissure is preferably at the level of the pelvis and not further than 1 cm ventral to the pelvis. Mares sutured below this point may reflux urine.
- Endometritis secondary to pneumovagina may resolve spontaneously after the operation.
- Natural defense mechanisms are effective after eliminating the continued irritation from air and external contaminants.
- Once pneumovagina is corrected, a mare must remain sutured for the remainder of her reproductive life. Therefore, once a mare has been Caslicked once, she requires a Caslick operation every year thereafter. This includes mares that have been Caslicked for performance reasons, since the vulvar seal is disrupted once the Caslick is opened for breeding or foaling reasons. So, in young mares, even if perineal conformation

is normal, a previous Caslick operation requires follow-up procedures every successive breeding season.
- Incision and resuturing for breeding and foaling are necessary; a delay in re-suturing of as little as a few days may allow re-infection.

Technique

i. The mare is restrained in stocks/chute (or behind a doorway) and twitched or tranquilized (an α_2-adrenoceptor agonist, such as romifidine or detomidine, with butorphanol or acepromazine is effective and safe).
ii. The tail is wrapped in a plastic sleeve and held to one side (either by an assistant or by tying it to the post).
iii. The rectum is manually evacuated to reduce the risks of defecation during the procedure.
iv. The vulva and perineum are carefully cleaned with soft soap and water or a dilute surgical scrub.

- Strong, irritating antiseptics and surgical spirits should be avoided.

---

v. The labial margins are infiltrated with local anesthetic (2% lignocaine hydrochloride or mepivicaine) using a 22-gauge (or smaller) needle.
vi. The tissues should be distended sufficiently to stretch the skin along the labial margins.
vii. An 8–10-mm strip of mucosa and skin is then removed along the mucocutaneous junction with sharp scissors.
  - Because the vulva will need to be opened at foaling time (and possibly at breeding time), it is important that no more than an 8–10-mm strip of mucosa and skin is removed from the stretched labial margin during the initial procedure.
  - Removal of a strip narrower than 8 mm may lead to gaps between the adherent labia, especially at the dorsal commissure.
  - Care should be taken to ensure that an uninterrupted raw surface is obtained from 1 cm ventral to the pelvic floor up to and including the dorsal commissure.
viii. The raw edges of the right and left labia are sutured together, starting at the dorsal vulvar commissure.
ix. Nonabsorbable monofilament (nylon or polypropylene) is the preferred suture material.
x. Various suture patterns, including simple-continuous, interrupted, and vertical mattress, have been used successfully. All are effective if sutures are placed carefully no more than 8 mm apart.

- With repetition of the procedure, excessive scarring and loss of plasticity of the tissues occur; it is therefore important to perform the surgery with the utmost care.

Additionally, the 'breeding stitch' is sometimes used:

  i. A single suture of umbilical tape is placed sufficiently dorsal to allow intromission and protect the ventral aspects of the closed labia.
  ii. However, it cannot protect the vulva effectively and still allow intromission by the stallion.
  iii. This suture also carries the danger of trauma to the stallion's penis at the time of mating.
  iv. Its usefulness is therefore very limited.

Management

- At the time of foaling (and possibly at the time of breeding) the vulvar cleft must be re-opened and re-sutured immediately to prevent laceration of the vulva and ingress of infection or contamination.
  ❏ Re-opening of the vulva should be left as close as possible to foaling to prevent contamination of the vagina and cervix thereby preventing ascending infection, which can occasionally lead to infection of the placenta and even premature foaling and/or abortion.
  ❏ The procedure is simply performed following the infiltration of local anesthetic as above. The 'healed scar' is cut directly upwards with sharp scissors.
- Quite frequently the Caslick suture is re-opened 20–30 days before foaling, but it is better to reduce this to 7–10 days if good supervision is available before foaling.
- Mares should have Caslick repairs carried out as soon as possible after foaling.
  ❏ Delay may be necessary if the fetal membranes have not been passed.

Vestibulovaginal sphincter insufficiency

If labial and vestibular sphincter function is not re-established by a Caslick procedure, surgical reconstruction of the perineal body is indicated. The vulvar and vestibular sphincters can become incompetent as a result of repeated stretching during repeated foaling or second-degree laceration. Perineal body reconstruction restores the integrity of the vestibular sphincter by reducing the diameter of the vestibule and surgically enlarging the perineal body dorsoventrally and craniocaudally.

Perineal reconstruction (vestibuloplasty)

Pouret's technique (Fig. 5.63)

  i. The mare is restrained in stocks (or with a suitable protective kickboard or door) and sedated (with an α_2-adrenoceptor agonist such as romifidine or detomidine and butorphanol).
  ii. Epidural anesthesia is preferred (the technique for this is described in standard surgical and anesthesia texts), but local infiltration can be used.
  iii. The tail is wrapped in a plastic sleeve so that all hair is covered and held or fastened to one side or raised over the mare's back.
  iv. The rectum is thoroughly evacuated manually and a tampon of rolled cotton or gauze sponges placed in the rectum to prevent expulsion of feces into the surgical field during the procedure.
  v. The animal's perineum and vulva are scrubbed thoroughly.
  vi. The mare's tail and buttocks and the stocks are then draped.
  vii. Two stay sutures of umbilical tape or long-jaw Balfour retractors are used to provide retraction of the vulvar lips.
  viii. An incision is made along the mucocutaneous junction of the dorsal labia and the dorsal commissure and a triangular section of mucosa is then dissected from the dorsum and dorsolateral aspects of the vestibule.
      - The apex of the mucosal triangle is located at or near the vestibulovaginal junction and the base of the triangle at the mucocutaneous junction of the labia.
      - This triangular section of mucosa is then removed.
      - **Care must be used in the submucosal dissection not to enter the rectum.** If the rectum is entered, the defect should be closed immediately with sutures that invert the rectal mucosa into the rectum, and then dissection is continued.
  ix. The incised edge of the mucosa of the right side of the vestibule is then sutured to the incised edge of the left side of the vestibular mucosa with a simple-continuous pattern of no. 2-0 polypropylene.
  x. The raw surfaces dorsal to this suture line are apposed with simple-interrupted 'quilting' sutures of polypropylene.
  xi. Suturing must proceed from deep layers to superficial layers, alternating first the continuous line in the mucosa, then the 'quilting' sutures above.
  xii. The skin of the perineum and vulva are closed as for the Caslick procedure.
  xiii. Complete healing of deep tissues takes 4–8 weeks; complete sexual rest is mandatory during that time.

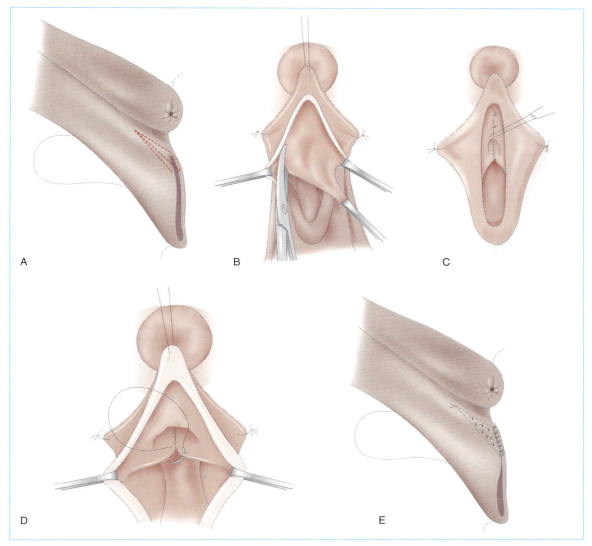

Fig. 5.63 Perineal body reconstruction (extensive vulvoplasty/episioplasty). The procedure is best performed in the standing mare with epidural or/and local infiltration of a local anesthetic. (A) A single incision is made along the skin–mucosa junction from the dorsal commissure to the lower third of the vulva. (B) The roof of the vestibule is exposed by retraction of the labiae and a triangular-shaped piece of the mucosa is removed from this area. The dorsal commissure is retracted caudally while the skin incision is extended anteriorly to the level of the vestibular seal. (C) Horizontal mattress sutures are laid to reinsert the mucosa into the vestibule. (D) The deep tissues are apposed using simple interrupted sutures while the dorsal commissure is drawn gently backwards. (E) Finally, the vulva should be in a more vertical position with the anus in a more forward position. In effect the surgery reconstructs part of the perineal body.

Vaginal laceration/rupture

Injuries to the mare's vaginal vault may be caused by breeding or foaling accidents.

- Vaginal lacerations have frequently been attributed to a discrepancy between the stallion's penis and the mare's vagina.
  - ❏ For this reason, a breeding roll sometimes is used to maintain distance between the mare and stallion.
- ❏ However, this type of injury occurs more commonly with some stallions than others and may relate also to copulatory behavior as well as to penis size.
- ❏ Unless a mare is examined after detection of fresh blood at the vulva or on the stallion's penis, the possibility of vaginal rupture and contamination of the peritoneal cavity may easily be overlooked.
- Vaginal lacerations incurred during breeding

most commonly involve the cranial dorsolateral vaginal wall close to the cervix.

❑ They are generally less than 5 cm long and accompanied only by minor transient hemorrhage.

❑ Most of these injuries would pass unnoticed except for the presence of fresh blood on the stallion's penis after dismounting.

❑ Such lesions have minimal clinical significance, although the associated hemorrhage mixed with semen could have the same effect as hemospermia, which has been associated with reduced fertility.

❑ Spontaneous healing is rapid and complete, and most lesions are virtually undetectable by the next estrous cycle.

❑ Peritonitis is a potential consequence to full-thickness lacerations due to vaginal flora, contamination from the penis and seminal fluid entering the abdominal cavity at the time of injury. The mare should be monitored carefully for the next 72–96 hours for signs such as fever, depression, colic, and anorexia. Appropriate treatment for acute peritonitis should be instituted should these signs occur.

• Severe vaginal lacerations during breeding can occur, involving rupture of the vaginal wall with eventration of bowel or the urinary bladder.

❑ Most commonly this affects the dorsal aspect of the cranial vagina.

❑ Speculum examination usually reveals a ballooned vagina and ragged dorsal bleeding tear in the anterior vagina; air may aspirate into the abdominal cavity with the introduction of the speculum.

❑ Discovery of the injury by manual palpation or speculum examination of the vagina warrants prompt preventive antimicrobial therapy.

❑ The peritoneal cavity is contaminated with bacteria from the stallion's penis and mycolic acid from sperm cells.

• Vaginal rupture may also be caused by the foal's foot or by obstetric manipulation.

❑ The vagina may rupture at any point from the cervix caudally, but the dorsal wall is the most susceptible to perforation by the foal's feet.

• Cranial vaginal ruptures communicate directly with the peritoneal cavity; however, bowel seldom eventrates through a laceration in this location.

❑ The risk of eventration of abdominal viscera can be reduced by preventing the mare from lying down by cross-tying.

❑ Continuous observation for at least 48 hours is advisable.

❑ Medication to prevent straining can be administered, or a tracheotomy tube inserted to reduce the effects of straining.

❑ If vaginal rupture is overlooked, the mare

usually becomes depressed 2–3 days after breeding and shows signs of acute peritonitis (fever, depression, abdominal guarding, and reluctance to move).

• If a portion of bowel eventrates through the defect, it should be washed with normal saline solution containing antimicrobials before replacement in the abdominal cavity.

• Protection of the damaged loop is critical, particularly if the mare is to be transported to a referral hospital.

• The bowel is simply placed in the anterior vagina and a saline- and antiseptic-soaked tampon of cotton introduced before suturing the vulva closed.

• This will permit transport for about an hour without sedation and for about 2 hours with sedation. Measures to stop or limit straining are helpful.

• If the bowel is undamaged and can be safely returned to the abdomen, the vagina should be flushed with 500 ml of saline solution containing a nonirritating antimicrobial.

• If injury to the intestine is significant, the mare must be referred to a specialist center where surgical enterectomy and management of the inevitable peritonitis can be performed.

• If the prolapsed gut has been badly damaged or if a large amount has eventrated, or if the referral center is too far away to allow quick transfer (within 1–2 hours), the only option is to salvage the foal and humanely euthanize the mare.

• When the ventral wall of the vagina is lacerated, herniation of abdominal viscera frequently occurs.

• If eventration occurs before delivery of the foal, it complicates the delivery severely.

• Vigorous attempts to deliver the foal vaginally lead to further serious trauma and contamination of the bowel and peritoneal cavity.

• Immediate cesarean section is indicated.

• If surgery can be performed quickly (i.e. within an hour or two) the edges of the laceration should be apposed with absorbable sutures using epidural anesthesia in the standing mare.

- Unless surgical repair of vaginal damage can be achieved easily and quickly, it is probably counterproductive.
- After repair of a vaginal tear, a Caslick operation reduces the possibility of air aspiration into the peritoneal cavity.

Vestibulovaginal reflux (urine pooling)

Pooling of urine in the cranial vaginal vault (vestibulovaginal reflux) and subsequent bathing of the uterine lumen as urine flows through the cervix is a well-recognized cause of reduced fertility in mares, which, if uncorrected, leads to infertility. Vaginitis, cervicitis, and endometritis are common secondary consequences. This can be a difficult and complicated problem, particularly in older mares, and should always be carefully checked in prepurchase examinations.

- It is always more obvious when the mare is in estrus.

Etiology
Factors that affect the integrity of the vulvar or vestibulovulvar sphincter and predispose to vestibulovaginal reflux include:

- Abnormal conformation.
  - ❏ With the anus positioned cranial to the vulva.
  - ❏ Collapsed sacroiliac girdle. The mare has a flat croup as viewed laterally allowing the weight of the uterus to drag the urethral opening anteriorly so that urine can flow anteriorly into the anterior vagina.
  - ❏ Lack of slope downwards and backwards from the urethral opening to allow natural drainage at urination.
  - ❏ Conformation is usually worse in older pluriparous mares.
- Weight loss (loss of body condition).
- Relaxation of the reproductive tract during estrus.
- Injury to pelvic nerves usually as a result of difficult foaling.
- It is not uncommon for large, pluriparous mares to pool urine after foaling.
  - ❏ The weight of the postpartum uterus pulls the vaginal compartment cranially and ventrally.
- Fragility and 'thin' mucosa surrounding the urethral opening.

When vestibulovaginal urinary reflux first occurs, mares may still conceive if urine is evacuated from the vaginal fornix before breeding.

- Sexual rest and improved physical condition occasionally alleviate the problem.
- Resolution occurs in most postpartum mares after uterine involution.

- When the vestibulovaginal reflux persists, however, moderate-to-severe endometritis results such that, with time, chronic endometrial changes are detectable by uterine biopsy.

Clinical signs (see Fig. 5.64)
Vestibulovaginal reflux should be suspected in mares that:

- Repeatedly fail to conceive.
- Are old, thin and infertile.
- Have poor external/perineal conformation.
- Have ultrasonically detectable uterine fluid accumulations before and after ovulation.

Diagnosis

- Because mares usually do not pool urine in their vagina during diestrus, diagnosis of vestibulovaginal reflux by vaginal speculum examination is best performed during estrus. Visualization of urine pooling may not be evident on every examination, so repeated speculum examinations may be required to confirm the diagnosis. Urination, defecation or exercise prior to examination can result in urine draining from the vaginal fornix due to increased abdominal pressure.
- Fluid in the vaginal fornix may be confirmed as urine by visual inspection of color or by biochemical testing (osmolality and urea content).
- Presence of urine crystals on endometrial cytology slides.

Treatment

- When vestibulovaginal reflux is diagnosed initially, sexual rest, improved nutrition, or external conformation modification (i.e. perineal body transection) may alone resolve the problem.
- If the condition recurs, surgical correction is indicated.

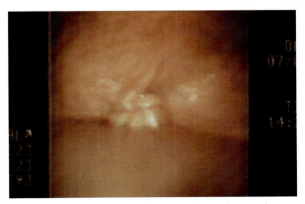

Fig. 5.64 Urine pooling in the anterior vagina can be seen clearly with an endoscope.

• Urethral extension and its variations are the most commonly performed and apparently most successful procedures for this problem. These operations are designed to create a mucosal tube from the urethra to the mucocutaneous junction so that urine is voided to the exterior rather than into the vestibule.

Technique

Method 1[101]

Following restraint, sedation and preparation as described for perineal body reconstruction, the bladder is catheterized with a no. 30 French Foley catheter to prevent urine flow through the surgical site.

i. Balfour retractors or umbilical tape stay sutures in the vulva provide retraction.
ii. The membranous transverse fold over the urethra is grasped with forceps and split into dorsal and ventral layers with a scalpel.
  • The incision is continued caudally along the ventrolateral aspects of the vestibule to within 1 cm of the mucocutaneous junction of the labia.
  • The mucosa is undermined dorsally and ventrally to create two mucosal layers.
  • Sufficient dissection is necessary to allow the edges of these layers to be pulled to the midline with minimal traction.
iii. The mucosal layers are then sutured right side to left side with three separate suture lines to create a mucosal tube that lengthens the urethra.
  • The ventral mucosal layers are apposed using a continuous horizontal or vertical mattress pattern of no. 2-0 polypropylene.
  • The raw dorsal surfaces of the ventral layer are apposed and the cut edge is everted ventrally.
  • This suture line must be placed carefully so that a complete seal is obtained.
  • **Urine leaking through this layer dissects between and through the dorsal suture line and leads to fistula formation.**
iv. The ventral suture line is over-sewn with a simple-continuous pattern of no. 2-0 polypropylene placed in the submucosal tissue between the dorsal and ventral layers.
v. The dorsal shelves are then apposed using a continuous vertical or horizontal mattress pattern of no. 2-0 polypropylene. The mucosa of this layer is everted dorsally.
vi. The Foley catheter is removed after completion of surgery.
  • Alternatively, a one-way valve, such as a Heimlich valve, may be attached to the Foley catheter and the catheter left in place to reduce straining and to ensure emptying of the bladder for the first 48 hours after surgery.

Note:
• Some mares do not empty their bladder properly after surgery.
• Careful and repeated postoperative rectal examinations are necessary to ensure that the bladder does not become overfilled and atonic, possibly rupturing.
• Tetanus prophylaxis and antimicrobial and anti-inflammatory therapy is administered.

Method 2[102]

i. Following restraint, sedation, epidural anesthesia and surgical preparation, the midline caudal border of the transverse fold over the urethra is grasped with Allis tissue forceps and retracted caudally.
ii. A horizontal transverse incision is made in the submucosa 2–4 cm cranially from the caudal border of the transverse fold.
iii. The incision is continued laterally and then slightly dorsally to the vestibular wall and extended to the labia.
iv. Dissection of the vestibular wall flaps is continued ventrally until the cut edges can be reflected without tension past the midline.
v. A continuous modified Connell's suture pattern, using no. 3 polyglactin, is used to appose the submucosal tissue layer.
  • The final configuration is in the shape of a Y, with the apex pointing caudally.
vi. The first suture line begins cranially and laterally at the junction of the transverse fold and vestibular wall incisions and ends at the midpoint of the transverse fold reflection.
  • Cut edges of the transverse fold and vestibular walls are inverted so that denuded tissues are in apposition.
vii. The second suture line begins on the opposite side at the junction of the transverse fold and vestibular wall incisions and is continued to the end-point of the first line and then on the midline to the caudal end of the vestibular wall reflections.
  • The denuded tissues created dorsally by the dissection of the transverse and vestibular folds are allowed to heal by second intention.

Method 3[103]

This method is a simple technique that may be used in mares with ample loose vestibular mucosa.

i. The mare is restrained, sedated and prepared for surgery as above.

ii. A Foley catheter is placed into the bladder via the urethral orifice.

iii. Interrupted horizontal mattress sutures of no. 3.5 or 3 synthetic absorbable material (e.g. polyglycolic acid) are placed in the ventral vaginal mucosa on either side of the catheter so that, as the sutures are placed, the mucosa closes over the catheter dorsally.

iv. Sutures are placed well back from the edge to allow a generous amount of mucosa to 'pucker' over the catheter.

v. The first suture must be placed cranial to the urethral orifice to preclude fistula formation.

vi. Sutures are continued caudally to within 2 cm of the labia.

vii. The tube so created should fit loosely around the catheter and should place minimum tension on the vaginal mucosa.

viii. The tissue dorsal to the horizontal mattress sutures is then trimmed off sharply, leaving four freshly cut edges.

ix. The four edges are then carefully apposed with a suture using similar absorbable material in a simple-continuous pattern.

Outcome and complications

- Success in repairing fistulas is variable.
- The most common complication with all three techniques is continued urine pooling as a result of fistula formation.
- To avoid fistula formation when placing sutures, tension on the tissue by the suture line must be minimal.
    - ❏ This is achieved by radical dissection of transverse fold and vestibular wall flaps.
    - ❏ The suture pattern must also invert the edges of the relocated tissue flaps to appose denuded submucosal tissue, thereby creating a broad seal that reduces the likelihood of fistula formation.
- Mares with scarring of the vestibular walls or atrophic, inelastic vestibular mucosa are unrewarding candidates for these procedures.

Bacterial vaginitis

Inflammation of the vagina of mares almost always occurs in conjunction with endometritis. In the early stages of pneumovagina or vesicovaginal reflux of urine, it is possible to detect vaginal hyperemia and some degree of exudate without concurrent uterine inflammation. It usually is just a matter of time until endometritis follows as an extension of vaginal or cervical involvement (Fig. 5.65).

When pneumovagina alone is responsible for vaginitis, a rapid return to normal should follow correction of the predisposing anatomic defect (see p. 184).

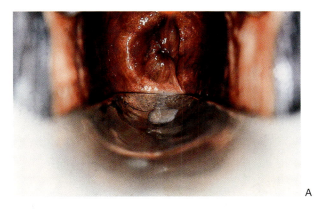

A

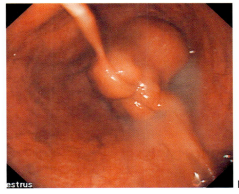

B

Fig. 5.65   (A) An inflamed vagina and cervix from bacterial infection. (B) Cervicitis (endoscopic examination). Note the inflamed external os and purulent exudate over the surface.

If there is no evidence of air aspiration ('vaginal wind-sucking'), consideration should be given to irritating substances or contaminated equipment introduced into the vaginal tract as a cause.

- Chemicals, such as dilute iodine (2% solution) and chlorhexidine (10% stock solution or as a suspension), can cause vaginal mucosal ulceration and necrosis.

Necrotic vaginitis

Profile

- Necrosis of the vagina occurs after dystocias of prolonged duration and is usually associated with excessive manipulation.
- Mares that deliver unattended may also develop the condition if the foal remains in the vagina for a prolonged period.
- Mares will often have concurrent metritis and be septicemic.

Clinical signs

- Mares may have a foul malodorous discharge, may strain severely and squat frequently.
- They will become systemically ill and can develop endotoxemia.

Diagnosis

- Vaginal speculum examination and manual vaginal examination.

Management

- Treatment of mares with this condition consists of broad-spectrum antibiotics given intravenously, application of an antibiotic ointment to the vagina and preventative treatment for laminitis.
- If the vaginal wall necroses and communicates freely with the abdomen, the mare may develop severe peritonitis and/or die acutely.

Prognosis

- Good if identified early and treatment begun immediately.
- Future fertility is good, if the condition is identified early.
- Mares may develop vaginal adhesions or peripelvic abscesses if not treated appropriately. Mares in this latter group may die.

VENEREAL DISEASE

- The control of venereal disease is a very important aspect of stud farm management.[104] All visiting mares must be swabbed (preferably before entering the stud but in any case before mating is allowed).
- Hygiene precautions on studs must be exercised. Each mare and stallion should be handled with separate gloves and boots, aprons, etc. All equipment *must* be sterilized between horses (although this may seem excessive, it is not only sensible but it is responsible).
- Failure to adhere to the protocols in force at the time has the potential to cause serious losses to both mare and stud owner alike.
- A stud that does not insist on the routine precautions of swabbing carries a major risk for the mares that visit. A dirty, unhygienic stud will usually have a low fertility rate and a high disease incidence.

- Because there may be statutory requirements in certain countries, consultation with the governing bodies should be made before deciding on treatment or other control measures.

Coital exanthema

Profile

- Coital exanthema is a disease of the external genitalia caused by equine herpesvirus 3, a virus that is antigenically distinct from equine

herpesvirus 1 or rhinopneumonitis virus.[105]

- Although it is regarded primarily as a venereal disease, grooming, veterinary instruments, and possibly insects may transmit coital exanthema.

Clinical signs (see Fig. 5.66)

- The disease appears 5–7 days after an infected mating (or contact with contaminated breeding equipment) and affects both stallions and mares.
- Clinical signs may develop spontaneously after minor vulvar abrasions, stretching, or episiotomy.
- In such cases, mating should be postponed until healing is complete.
  - ❑ Lesions appear mainly on the vulva and perineal skin of mares and rarely within the vestibule.
  - ❑ Similar lesions occur on the penis and prepuce of stallions, with the most aggressive lesions usually being found on the preputial fold.
  - ❑ Stallions in heavy service may be reluctant to breed, and lesions on the glans penis and urethral process may remain inflamed until breeding is discontinued.
- Vesicles (blisters) 1–3 mm in diameter appear first and rapidly progress to pustules. The pustules become shallow necrotic ulcers.
- Edema, tenderness, and painful urination may be present in the acute (early) stages.
- Healing occurs in 7–10 days in the absence of secondary bacterial infection.
- Permanent loss of pigmentation at the site of healed lesions is common.
- Respiratory disease has been suggested as part of the syndrome after experimental inoculation of horses with the virus. Lesions may rarely occur on the lips and nasal mucosa.

Diagnosis

- Intranuclear inclusion bodies can be demonstrated histologically in affected tissues and in scrapes made from fresh lesions.

Treatment

- Symptomatic treatment with antiseptic creams may prevent secondary bacterial infections.
- Where the disease is secondary to vulvar abrasions or other damage this must be addressed.
- Mares are suitable for mating at the next estrus, and treatment usually is unnecessary.

Prognosis

- The prognosis is excellent although it inevitably means a delay in breeding. The effect on fertility is apparently negligible.
- Healed lesions are not a potential danger.
- Recovered cases are probably immune but it is not known if the virus can be latent.
- In natural outbreaks, the virus has not been associated with abortions.

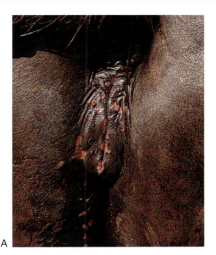

A

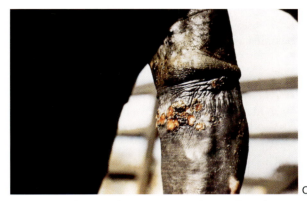

C

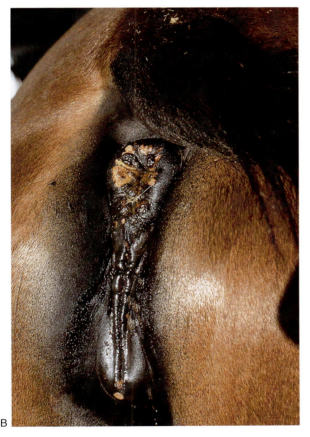

B

Fig. 5.66 (A) Equine herpes virus 3 infection (coital exanthema). The lesions were seen approximately 10–11 days after infected service. (B) Lesions of coital exanthema can affect the anus. These lesions are around 14 days old. (C) Coital exanthema lesions on the preputial reflection of a stallion This is a typical site because it is in the area that is most in contact with the vulvar lips during coitus.

- There is no vaccine for the disease (neither is one necessary).

Contagious equine metritis

Profile

- The disease is caused by infection with *Taylorella equigenitalis*.[106]
- It is a highly contagious venereal disorder that is

transmitted between mares by the teaser or stallion.[107]
- Transmission can also occur through the use of infected semen for artificial insemination.
- Indirect transmission has also been implicated (contaminated water, instruments and via the hands of stud or veterinary staff who handle the infected animals). Nasal transmission between the nose of the teaser and the perineum of the mare is possible also.

- Carrier mares and stallions may show no signs but remain infectious. Transmission between mares does not seem to occur.

For disease control purposes mares are usually classified as:
- High-risk.
  - ❏ Mare has been previously infected.
  - ❏ Mare exposed to risk of infection.
- Low-risk.
  - ❏ Maiden mares that have not been mated previously.
  - ❏ No previous exposure to infection.

This classification dictates the type and site of swabs taken for culture (see below).

> Note:
> - The clinical features, diagnosis, treatment and control outlined below for *Taylorella equigenitalis* are very similar to those used in the management of *Klebsiella pneumoniae* (capsule types 1, 2 and 5) and *Pseudomonas aeruginosa* infections.
> - These are the other major venereal pathogens of the horse in normal stud conditions and can be very difficult to eradicate.

Clinical signs (Figs 5.67, 5.68)

Mares
- Infertility is the most obvious sign. Fertility on an infected stud may fall to 30% or less.
- Severity varies markedly from mild/unapparent to severe/obvious.
- Purulent vaginal discharges (gray-white and profuse) originating in the uterine lumen (acute endometritis) appear 2–4 days after mating.
- Early return to estrus after 7–10 days.
- Chronic cases may show little or no discharge; these are particularly dangerous because they have more deep-seated infection and are more difficult to treat.
- The carrier state may develop after a short course of acute disease or may develop immediately. Carrier state mares show no outward signs but continue to shed the organism for months (or even longer).[108]
- In some carrier mares the infection appears to be restricted to the caudal parts of the genital tract; they may conceive and carry the foal to full term.

Stallions
- Infected stallions and teasers are more often passive carriers with little if any clinical evidence of the infection.
- The bacteria colonize the external genital organs (particularly the urethral fossa and the skin of the penis and inner lining of the prepuce) and possibly the secondary sex glands.

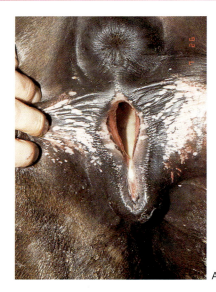

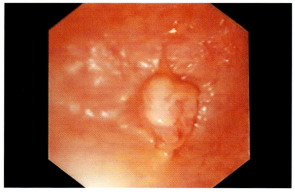

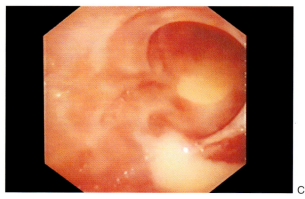

Fig. 5.67 The typical appearance of contagious equine metritis in a mare showing vaginal discharge (A), cervicitis (B) and endometritis (C).

- In rare cases a purulent urethritis may be evident.

Diagnosis
- Endometrial swabs shows many neutrophils with ingested organisms.

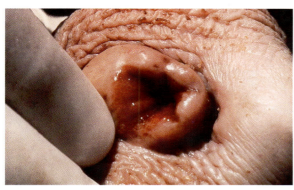

Fig. 5.68 Contagious equine metritis causes little obvious inflammation in stallions, but an acute urethritis and inflammation of the glans penis can be found in recently infected animals.

- Culture of the organism from the clitoral fossa and clitoral sinuses. Culture is difficult because of the microaerophilic nature of the organism and the presence of commensals.

Swabbing

Mares

- Technique[109]
  i. The perineum of the mare is wiped (not washed) with antiseptics.
  ii. A sterile, fine-cotton bacteriological swab with charcoal transport medium is used.
  iii. Full personal hygiene precautions should be taken (hand-washing, gloves and clean apron).
  iv. Swabs can be taken from the clitoral sinuses and fossa, and from the endometrium in early estrus (protected swabs via the cervix) (see p. 151).
  v. Clitoral swabs only are taken from pregnant mares before foaling.
  vi. Swabs with a charcoal transport medium are taken as early in the breeding season as possible and delivered promptly to the laboratory (within 12–24 hours).
  vii. Microaerophilic and aerobic cultures for *Taylorella equigenitalis* and the other two important bacteria, *Klebsiella pneumoniae* and *Pseudomonas aeruginosa*, are routinely performed and reported.
- Interpretation
  i. A negative swab result is satisfactory and this result remains in force until the estrous period in which the mare is mated.
  ii. For low-risk mares the stud can proceed with mating on the basis of an early aerobic culture alone if adequate clitoral swabbing has already been carried out and clinical disease is not suspected. The results of the microaerophilic culture should still be sent to the stud farm so that in the event of a breakdown only limited spread will occur.
  iii. For high-risk mares all results must be known before the mare is mated. Because cultures usually take up to 6 days, the mare is unlikely to be bred at the same estrus as the sampling.
  iv. **If a mare returns to season earlier than expected a full set of swabs must be taken immediately and the mare should not be bred until the results are known.**
  v. Foals born to known infected or high-risk mares should be swabbed before they reach 3 months of age (clitoral/penile and penile sheath swabs are required).

Stallions/teasers

- Technique
  i. Swabs are obtained from the urethra, urethral fossa and penile sheath and if possible from pre-ejaculatory fluid.
  ii. Usually repeat samples are taken because of the risks the stallion faces with mating many mares in one season.
- Interpretation
  i. A positive swab renders the stallion unusable for natural service or semen collection.
  ii. Repeat swabs taken at 7-day intervals after local treatment are required. After three negative tests the stallion may be taken to be free of infection.

Differential diagnosis

Other causes of endometritis have a longer duration and include:

- *Klebsiella pneumoniae* and *Pseudomonas aeruginosa* infections.
- The early return to estrus is characteristic of contagious equine metritis.

Treatment

- Treatment of mares affected by contagious equine metritis does not appear to be effective.
- Usually the acute endometritis is self-limiting and does not warrant antibiotic use. However, there remains the risk of symptomless carriers. About 20% of affected mares become carriers.
- Mares that are persistently positive should be removed from the breeding pool until they are proven clear of infection. This may mean the loss of a whole breeding season (or more).
- Treatment of infected stallions is difficult and involves antibacterial washes and possibly systemic antibiotics.
- Mating cannot be restarted until three sets of swabs have been negative (taken at least 7 days apart).

Dourine

Profile

- A venereally transmitted protozoal disease affecting mares and stallions due to *Trypanosoma equiperdum*. The disease has a characteristically slow, progressive course and a very high mortality rate.[110]
- The disease is restricted to areas of Africa, Central and South America, the Middle East and areas of Asia.
- Strict international disease-control measures are applied to limit its spread. Epidemics occur as a result of introduction of a carrier/early infected horse. The slow course may mask the spread from an infected stallion. True carrier animals exist and show no apparent evidence of infection.

Clinical signs (see Fig. 5.69)

- Onset is insidious with an incubation period of between 1 and 26 weeks.
- Low-grade chronic fever.
- Characteristic urticaria-like 'dollar' plaques of edema develop on the skin of the flanks in particular.
- Muscle wasting and weight loss with later development of neurological signs, collapse and death.
- Mare
  - ❑ A mucoid or purulent vaginal discharge is the earliest sign.
  - ❑ Perineal and vulvar edema slowly extends to the mammary gland and ventral abdomen.
- Stallion
  - ❑ A mucoid or purulent urethral or preputial discharge is the earliest sign.
  - ❑ Scrotal and preputial edema slowly extends to the ventral abdomen and brisket.

Diagnosis

- The clinical signs, epidemiology and history are typical.
- The organism can be identified on smears of discharges, aspirates from plaques, cerebrospinal fluid and blood.[111]
- Serological testing is effective in detecting previous exposure and is used for international control.

Treatment

- Treatment is possible but this conflicts with eradication and control measures.

Prognosis

- Hopeless.
- Cases should be destroyed to avoid further suffering and spread to other horses.

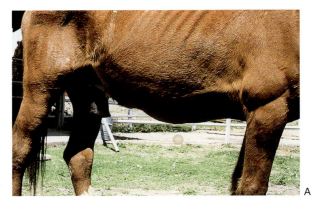
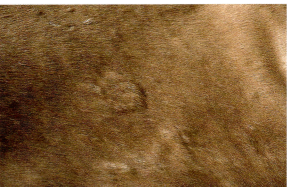
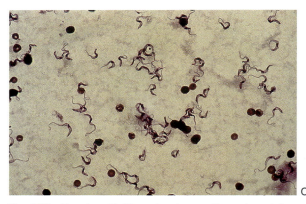

Fig. 5.69 Dourine. Stallions develop penile and scrotal inflammation and edema, often with penile paralysis (A). In the mare, vulvar edema is common and characteristic 'dollar'-sized plaques may be present over the skin of the quarters (B). These contain nests of *Trypanosoma equiperdum* parasites (C). Slides courtesy of K van der Berg.

INTRAUTERINE THERAPY

GENERAL GUIDELINES

In the selection of antimicrobials for intrauterine therapy, various factors must be considered:[112]

1. Susceptibility of the microorganisms.
2. Potential efficacy of the antimicrobial in the intrauterine environment.

3. Concentrations attainable at the site of infection, and the effects of treatment on immediate and future fertility of the mare.

Intrauterine antimicrobial therapy is usually preferred over systemic treatment because the endometrium is a locally infected tissue that is treated most economically by local application of antimicrobials.[113] In general, antimicrobial concentrations are higher in the endometrial layers and last longer after intrauterine treatment than after systemic treatment.[114] If metritis is present, systemic antimicrobials are indicated because they can more easily penetrate the myometrium.[115] Intrauterine antimicrobial treatment may have adverse effects.

- Failure to isolate the causative organism and random selection of antimicrobials lead to therapeutic failure and secondary bacterial or fungal infections.
- Antimicrobial selection should be based on culture and sensitivity results.

> - Unfortunately, in vitro and in vivo efficacy may not always be equivalent. For example, most uterine cultures of *Pseudomonas* show in vitro sensitivity to polymyxin B, yet few mares with endometritis caused by *Pseudomonas* respond well to polymyxin B therapy.

- Sensitivity testing is the only rational guide to antimicrobial selection.
- Endometrial irritation also is a potential problem.

Intrauterine infusions should be administered with sterile equipment and proper aseptic preparation of the mare. Catheters should be passed through the cervix and into the uterine lumen via a speculum or manually to ensure maximal cleanliness. A true aseptic procedure is difficult to achieve.

Uterine size, determined by palpation and ultrasonographic examination, can be used to estimate the volume to be instilled.[116] The objective is to use sufficient volume to achieve uniform distribution in the uterus without excessive backflow through the cervix. This is especially important if expensive drugs are being used.

> - The capacity of a healthy mare's uterus is approximately 100–300 ml.
> - The uterine capacity of an older mare's may be 500–750 ml.

Total infusion volumes of 50–200 ml are usually recommended. Decreasing the volume of antimicrobial solution increases the amount and rate of absorption; therefore, to maintain concentrations in the uterus for longer periods, larger volumes should be infused.[117]

The distribution of the antimicrobials within the uterine lumen and their absorption are also dependent on the specific carrier used to deliver the drugs.[118] Furthermore, certain antimicrobials (aminoglycosides) and antiseptics may be highly irritating to the uterine mucosa. If small volumes of aminoglycosides are to be infused into the uterine lumen, they must be buffered.

> - For example, 1 ml of a 7.5% sodium bicarbonate solution should be used to buffer 50 mg of gentamicin or amikacin.

- Chlorhexidine solution is highly irritating to the endometrium even in dilute (1:10,000) solutions, and may cause endometrial, cervical, and vaginal adhesions.
- Strong irritants, such as Lugol's solution, are contraindicated.
- Povidone iodine preparations may irritate the endometrium unless they are diluted at least 1:10.

The frequency of intrauterine antimicrobial therapy is usually based on convenience.[114,119]

> - For example, therapy could be given as daily infusion for 3–5 days during estrus, 1–3 days after ovulation, or every other day for two to five treatments.[120]

Frequent treatment, sometimes up to four times per day, may be required to maintain therapeutic levels of some antimicrobials.[121]

Exposure to large doses of antimicrobials for brief periods increases the susceptibility of bacteria to killing by leukocytes.[122] This may explain the efficacy of treatment schedules in which antimicrobial levels are allowed to fall below inhibitory concentrations for part of the treatment interval.

Exudate in the uterine lumen may dilute an infused antimicrobial to a subtherapeutic concentration. Release of metabolites and binding of the antimicrobial drug to exudative cells also reduce efficacy. Uterine lavage before the infusion of antimicrobials is therefore a useful method of increasing the efficacy by removing inflammatory by-products and increasing contact of therapeutic agents with the endometrial surface.

When uterine contents are more acidic than plasma, antimicrobials that are weakly acidic reach lower concentrations in the uterine lumen than those that are weakly alkaline. With alkaline uterine contents, the reverse is true. Some antimicrobials (such as aminoglycosides or penicillins) seem to be more active at a high pH and others (e.g. tetracyclines) are more active at a low pH.[123]

Intrauterine antimicrobial therapy for bacterial endometritis may cause complications. The most perplexing problem occurs when treatment for one pathogen allows the proliferation of another that often is more difficult to manage than the original. A common example of this is a streptococcal infection that, after treatment with the appropriate antimicrobial, is followed by the development of a *Pseudomonas* or yeast infection. In these cases, a mixed infection may have existed initially and antimicrobial use merely allowed proliferation of the other organism.

> • This frequently occurs with the use of penicillin. *Pseudomonas* is typically resistant to penicillin, and *Candida* and other yeasts proliferate in its presence.

In other cases, a second organism may be introduced accidentally during the course of treatment for the primary infection. Whatever the cause, the accurate diagnosis of endometritis is important and treatment should be restricted to those mares that definitely require treatment.

- Prophylactic therapy is probably unwise; there may be more problems from the treatment than from the condition.
- Mares with endometritis are especially susceptible to recurrent infection, and uterine infection may recur after it has been initially eliminated by treatment. Inappropriate medication may make subsequent management more difficult as bacterial resistance and other organisms may be significant.

Additional factors that may contribute to failure of therapy include:[124]

1. Drug antagonism/incompatibility
   - Drug compatibility is an important principle of therapy. The polypharmacy approach of multiple antibacterials and antiseptics mixed together may be of no therapeutic value and could be much more harmful.
2. Drug resistance
   - Veterinarians have a responsibility to use antibacterial agents with due care and with appropriate recognition of the wider implications of resistance.
   - Inappropriate courses and doses are often the major instigating factor for antibiotic resistance.

ANTIMICROBIALS AND ANTISEPTICS

Guidelines for the intrauterine use of various drugs are listed in Table 5.7.

Uterine irrigation

- Uterine lavage with large volumes of saline solution is useful in the treatment of endometritis and acute postpartum metritis.

- Uterine lavage may produce therapeutic effects by mechanically removing bacteria and debris, by stimulating the uterus to contract and expel foreign material, and by irritating the endometrium, causing the migration of neutrophils into the lumen.
- Uterine irrigation may be used before or after breeding (see below), and used in combination with oxytocin[125] and/or prostaglandins.[96,126]
- Intrauterine plasma (see below) (and/or antimicrobials) has improved pregnancy rates in mares with endometrial disease.[127]

Technique (see Fig. 5.70)

i. Uterine lavage can be accomplished with a no. 24–30 French Foley catheter with an 80-cm autoclavable flushing catheter.
ii. Sterile physiologic saline solution is infused, 1 liter at a time, by gravity flow and then recovered by siphoning into a container for inspection.
iii. The opacity of the recovered solution indicates the amount of inflammation in the uterine lumen.
iv. Measurement of the recovered fluid or ultrasonographic examination of the uterus ensures that all fluid has been recovered.

> • This is important because the mare may have an impaired ability to clear the uterus spontaneously.

v. If fluid remains, 10–20 IU of oxytocin are administered intravenously or intramuscularly, or an intramuscular injection of prostaglandin (cloprostenol 250–500 µg) can be given to stimulate myometrial contractions and therefore encourage emptying of the uterine lumen.
vi. Uterine lavage with saline solution should be repeated until the recovered fluid is clear.

Plasma infusion

Plasma provides immunoglobulins and complement, which are the major proteins involved in the opsonization of bacteria in the uterus. Intrauterine plasma infusion appears to be beneficial in mares with chronic and chronic-active endometritis.[128] Pregnancy rates of lactating and barren mares may also be improved by intrauterine plasma infusion and antibiotics administered 12–36 hours after breeding.[129]

Technique

- Proper preparation of plasma for uterine infusion requires aseptic withdrawal of blood and addition of heparin at 5–10 U/ml of blood.

Table 5.7 Guidelines for administration of intrauterine drugs

Drug	Dose per infusion	Comments
Antibacterials		
Amikacin	2 g	Used for *Pseudomonas*, *Klebsiella*, and persistent Gram-negative organisms
Ampicillin	3 g	Use only the soluble product
Carbenicillin	6 g	Broad spectrum
Gentamicin sulfate	2 g	Excellent Gram-negative spectrum, buffer with bicarbonate or large volume of saline (200 ml); used for *Klebsiella* spp. infections
Enrofloxacin	3 g	Gram-negative spectrum; used for resistant Gram-negative organisms
Ceftiofur sodium	1 g	Gram-positive and -negative spectrum; used for resistant organisms
Penicillin (sodium or potassium)	5 million units	Used for Gram-positive organisms (e.g. *Streptococcus zooepidemicus*)
Neomycin	4 g	Gram-negative organisms (*Escherichia coli* and some *Klebsiella* spp.)
Ticarcillin (±clavulanic acid)	6 g (±200 mg)	Gram-positive and Gram-negative organisms
Penetrating agents		
EDTA-TRIS (1.2 g of sodium EDTA with 6.05 g of TRIS per liter of water, titrated to pH 8.0 with glacial acetic acid)	250 ml, then 3 hours later infuse antibacterial solution	EDTA binds Ca^{2+} in bacterial cell walls, making cell wall permeable to antibacterials
Dimethylsulfoxide (5% stock solution)	50–100 ml	Does not appear to be effective as a carrying agent; possibly associated with inducing uterine fibrosis
Antiseptics		
Povidone iodine (1–2% stock solution)	250 ml	Good irrigation for nonspecific inflammation and for fungal infections; concentrations >10% cause irritation
Antimycotics		
Nystatin	5×10^6 U	Dissolve in 30 ml of 0.9% saline solution, daily for 7–10 days
Clotrimazole	500 mg	Suspension or cream, daily for 1 week
Vinegar	2%	20 ml wine vinegar to 1 liter of 0.9% saline solution; use as uterine lavage
Amphotericin B	200–250 mg	Daily for 1 week

- Because complement is stable for only a few hours at room temperature, prompt separation and infusion are indicated.
- Cold centrifugation is the ideal method of separating plasma.
- If centrifugation equipment is not available, gravity sedimentation is acceptable, particularly if the blood is refrigerated at 4°C during the sedimentation process.
- Plasma can be stored frozen (–20°C) for 100 days or more without losing its opsonic properties.

- Immediately before use, frozen plasma should be thawed by immersion in lukewarm water. Overheating by using hot water or microwave thawing inactivates many of the proteins.

Minimum contamination technique

In this technique, 100–300 ml of semen extender containing antimicrobials (see p. 65) is infused into the uterus immediately before natural breeding.[130]

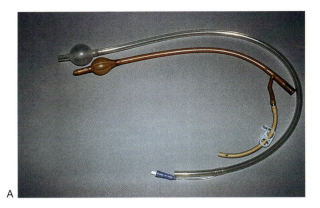

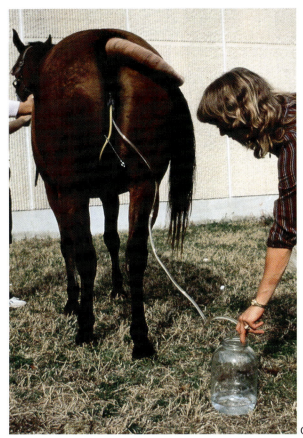

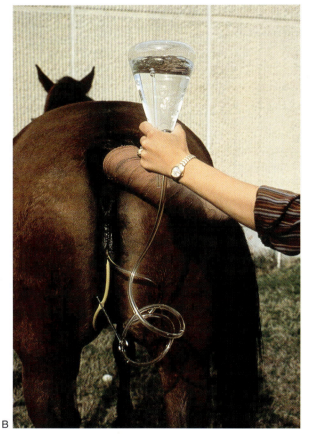

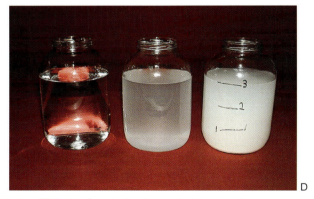

Fig. 5.70 Uterine irrigation. (A) Bivona catheter and Foley catheter. (B) Bottle for uterine lavage held up to allow gravity flow. (C) Collection (siphonage) of irrigation fluids. (D) Efflux from uterine lavage in jars showing sequential reduction in cloudiness.

- The technique has been used in the past, but results have not been consistently convincing.
- The procedure is of questionable benefit when breeding mares with no history of infertility.
- Infusing semen extender into the uterus of mares that have pooled a small amount of urine immediately before breeding may improve pregnancy rates as it dilutes out the urine and improves sperm motility.
- Best results are obtained when stallions infected with *Pseudomonas aeruginosa* or *Klebsiella pneumoniae* are mated with susceptible mares.
- The selection of drugs and their concentrations in the semen extenders is critical because sperm cell viability may be compromised.

APPLICATIONS OF INTRAUTERINE THERAPY

The intrauterine therapies described above can be applied to various types of inflammation, such as chronic endometritis, or persistent mating-induced endometritis (delay in uterine clearance). The following is a short synopsis of the treatment regimens that are used most frequently.

Chronic infectious endometritis

Long-standing infections caused by *Streptococcus zooepidemicus*, *Escherichia coli*, *Pseudomonas aeruginosa*, or *Klebsiella pneumoniae* often result from contamination of the uterus by fecal and genital flora.

- These organisms may also be isolated from the uterus of mares exhibiting persistent mating-induced endometritis after repeated breeding during a season.
- The first therapeutic approach should be to correct any predisposing causes, such as a breakdown of external barriers, by performing Caslick's vulvoplasty, urethral extension, or cervical repair as needed.
- Antimicrobials may be administered by either local or systemic routes.
- Because most antibiotics have reduced efficacy in the presence of inflammatory debris, the uterus should be lavaged before intrauterine treatment if free fluid and inflammatory debris are present.
- Therapeutic guidelines governing the timing and length of treatment are based on clinical observations.
  - ❑ A 3- or 5-day regimen of once-daily uterine lavage followed by intrauterine therapy is most commonly performed.
  - ❑ Systemic drugs are usually administered for 5 days and are given at the prescribed time interval (see Table 5.8).

> Note:
> - The dosages are based on anecdotal reports and may not conform with local regulatory approvals.

- After the infection is cleared, breeding should be limited to a single attempt each estrus.
- A period of 45–60 days of rest from breeding may be helpful to allow recovery from the chronic inflammation.

Yeast or fungal infection

These infections often result from prolonged use of antibiotics in the uterus. They are difficult to treat

Table 5.8 Antimicrobials suitable for the systemic treatment of endometritis

Drug	Dose[a]	Frequency (times daily)
Amikacin sulfate	7 mg/kg	2 (q 12 h)
Ampicillin trihydrate	10–15 mg/kg	2 (q 12 h)
Enrofloxacin	5 mg/kg	1 (q 24 h)
Gentamicin sulfate	2.2 mg/kg	3 (q 8 h)
	3.3 mg/kg	2 (q 12 h)
	6.6 mg/kg	1 (q 24 h)
Procaine penicillin	20,000 IU/kg	1 (q 24 h)
Trimethoprim+ sulfamethoxasole	3 mg/kg + 15 mg/kg (total 18 mg/kg)	2 (q 12 h)

[a]Note that these dosages are based on anecdotal reports and may not conform with local regulatory approvals.

and tend to recur. There are anecdotal accounts of treatment success; however, there are no clinical reports on controlled treatment trials.

- Yeast and fungi may be resistant to various antimycotic drugs. It is prudent to identify the sensitivity pattern of the incriminating yeast or fungi before beginning treatment.
- Antimycotic drugs used include:
  - ❑ Nystatin.
  - ❑ Clotrimazole.
- Uterine irrigation with diluted povidone iodine solution, vinegar, or dilute acetic acid has been used with varying results. Daily intrauterine treatments for a minimum of 10 days have been suggested.

Mating-induced endometritis

(see p. 178)

Mares with persistent mating-induced endometritis (usually ascribed to delay in uterine clearance) are usually free of bacteria before breeding. These mares tend to accumulate fluid within the uterine lumen after breeding in response to the intrauterine deposition of semen.[88]

Free fluid in the uterine lumen

This is detrimental to embryo survival. Several factors appear to contribute to the problem. These include:

- An abnormality in myoelectrical activity.[93]
- Impaired lymphatic drainage.[97]
- A uterus located ventrally in the abdomen resulting in impeded free flow of fluids through the cervix.[92]

Treatment of affected mares is directed at rapid removal of intrauterine fluids after breeding.[94]

- The combination of uterine lavage and administration of oxytocin alone[95] or together with antibiotics after breeding has improved pregnancy rates.[131]

- PGF$_{2\alpha}$ and the analog cloprostenol have also been demonstrated to increase myometrial activity and assist in clearing the uterine lumen of contaminating products.

A suggested treatment regimen is as follows:

i. Lavage of the uterus between 4 and 8 hours after breeding with buffered saline solution or lactated Ringer's solution until the efflux is clear.

ii. Then oxytocin 10–20 IU intravenously or intramuscularly is administered.

iii. Twenty-four hours after breeding, the reproductive tract is examined by ultrasonography to determine if there is any fluid remaining in the uterine lumen or intramurally and to detect ovulation.

iv. If there is intraluminal fluid with hyperechoic particles, the uterus is lavaged a second time and the mare is treated with either oxytocin or cloprostenol. If a small amount of clear fluid is present, the administration of oxytocin or cloprostenol may suffice. Cloprostenol may promote lymphatic clearance of excessive intramural edema because it induces uterine contractions for approximately 5 hours. Myometrial contractions assist in lymph flow by a pumping action on the lymphatic vessel wall. Oxytocin induces strong uterine contractions for only 20–40 minutes and may be most useful for emptying the uterine lumen of free fluid.

v. Treatment should be performed after each mating to be effective. If mares treated 8 and 24 hours after breeding have free fluid in the uterine lumen at 36–48 hours or after ovulation, they should not be treated with cloprostenol as it may adversely affect the corpus luteum.

vi. Mares treated with prostaglandin after ovulation should be supplemented with progesterone (oral or injectable) beginning 2–3 days post ovulation because the function of the corpus luteum may be adversely affected.

- Pregnancy rates in mares with fluid at 36–48 hours appear to be lower than those in mares that respond to treatment.

SYSTEMIC ANTIMICROBIAL THERAPY

Although intrauterine therapy is the preferred treatment for endometritis, there are indications for the use of systemic antibiotics. Higher antimicrobial concentrations throughout the genital tract are achieved with systemic administration rather than with intrauterine therapy.[132]

Systemic treatment is best if antimicrobials are subjected to degradation by conditions in the lumen. Also, systemic therapy eliminates the need to invade the vestibule, vaginal canal, and cervix. The vestibule and clitoral fossa harbor a vast array of bacteria, including potential uterine pathogens, even in reproductively normal mares. These organisms might serve as a source of uterine inoculation when the hand or an instrument is passed through the vulva to cannulate the cervix during intrauterine infusion.[2]

Problems with systemic antimicrobial administration are the quantity of drug needed, the expense of the drug, and, in the case of injectable drugs, reluctance on the part of the animal or owner concerning multiple injections. Antimicrobials that are considered to be effective by the systemic route are presented in Table 5.8.

Note:
- The dosages given in Table 5.8 are based on anecdotal reports and may not conform with local regulatory approvals.

MISCELLANEOUS DISORDERS OF THE TUBULAR GENITAL TRACT

Chromosomal abnormalities

Profile

The diploid chromosome number of the horse is 64. The presence or absence of an XX chromosome arrangement for female and an XY chromosomal arrangement for male governs the genetic determinant of sex. Initiation of gonadal development requires only that either a single X or a single Y is present. Completion of the development of the gonads requires the full complement (XX or XY). Thus, the developing ovary must have precisely two X chromosomes in each cell; similarly, the testis must have an X and a Y chromosome for its normal development and function. A signal from the Y chromosome converts the undifferentiated gonad into a testis; absence of the Y chromosome directs the development to an ovary.

- The female has 31 paired chromosomes and two X (sex) chromosomes that determine the sex as female.
- The male has 31 chromosome pairs and an XY pair of sex chromosomes; the presence of the Y chromosome determines the male character.
- Chromosomal abnormalities occur in either the number of chromosomes present or the presence of an intrachromosomal defect.
  ❏ A missing chromosome is called a monosomy and an extra chromosome is called a trisomy.

Clinical signs

- The most common abnormality is a missing X chromosome (63,X0). This arrangement is characterized by primary infertility and gonadal dysgenesis with a normal female phenotype (outward appearance).
- The mare is usually small in stature, with irregular (or totally absent) estrous cycles and very small ovaries.

Diagnosis

- A presumptive diagnosis can be made on clinical examination and reproductive history.
- All chromosomal abnormalities require specialist diagnosis reliant on karyotyping.

Differential diagnosis

- True hermaphroditism (see p. 81).
- Previous surgical interferences (ovariectomy, etc).

Treatment

- There is none.

Hermaphroditism

See p. 81.

Persistent hymen

Profile

- The hymen usually ruptures during the first year of life. If it does not rupture, fluid produced by the endometrial glands during estrus may accumulate behind the hymen causing it to bulge out through the lips of the vulva.

Clinical signs

- The hymen will appear as a bluish-tinged round tissue that protrudes from the vulva most commonly when the mare is excited or running through the pasture.
- It may not be identified until the mare has her first vaginal examination.

Diagnosis

- Vaginoscopy and manual examination of the vagina.

Differential diagnosis

- Prolapsed bladder.

Treatment

- Pushing one's hand through the hymen can usually rupture it.
- If this is not possible, the mare can be sedated and the hymen cut with scissors.

Prognosis

- Good for fertility once the free intrauterine fluid is resolved.

Endometrial cysts

Profile

- Endometrial cysts are thin-walled, cystic structures filled with fluid (lymph) that arise on the endometrial surface of the uterus[133] and project a variable distance into the uterine lumen (Fig. 5.71).
- Mares over 10 years of age are more commonly affected.
- Two types of cyst have been described but for all practical purposes they are all lymphatic in origin.

Clinical signs

- They are often identified incidentally during rectal or ultrasonographic examination; their main importance lies in their ultrasonographic similarity to an early pregnancy.
- Most cysts are small (<10 mm in diameter) and few in number (1–3).
- Large cysts (they can be up to 10 cm in diameter or larger) can sometimes be palpated per rectum by experienced examiners.
- All have a characteristic and easily identifiable ultrasonographic appearance.
- Occasional small cysts are probably insignificant, but larger ones (>10 mm in diameter) and large numbers may adversely affect fertility. However, most experienced researchers consider that there is no conclusive evidence that they have any adverse effect on fertility or on the viability of the foal.[134] They may reasonably be expected to have some restrictive effects on migration of the embryo before implantation and so may interfere with the signals for maternal recognition of pregnancy.[134]

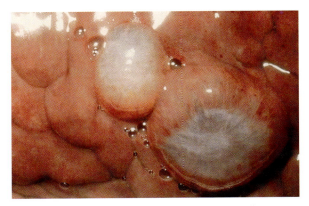

Fig. 5.71 Endoscopic view of a large and a small endometrial cyst in the wall of the uterus, identified during routine ultrasonography.

- Clinical examination of the chorionic surface of the placenta may reveal an avillous area(s) corresponding to the cyst(s) present on the endometrium.

Diagnosis

- Palpation and ultrasonographic recognition of a cystic structure projecting into the lumen of the uterus are characteristic.
- The cysts are typically devoid of any ultrasonographically identifiable structure being totally echolucent.

Differential diagnosis

- The major differential is an early pregnancy.
- Pregnancy will progress while cysts tend to remain static for long periods (or grow very slowly).
- There is no identifiable embryo with a cyst.
- Cysts do not move and so the very early pregnancy can be differentiated from small endometrial cysts by repeated examination over a few hours.

Treatment

- Small cysts are probably insignificant and so can justifiably be left alone.
- Large single cysts can be drained by needle aspiration or ruptured under endoscopic guidance, but there is a high rate of recurrence
- Diathermy ablation is possible[135] and may prevent recurrences. However, this carries the risk of endometrial scarring and adhesions. CO_2:YAG laser ablation causes less damage.[136] Electromicrosurgery using an electric loop has been compared to Nd:YAG laser and an electrosurgical cutting blade. Use of the electric loop was associated with the smallest wound in the endometrial surface, less inflammation at the site of cautery and less granulation tissue.[137]

Prognosis

- There is no evidence that endometrial cysts have any deleterious effect on fertility, but severely affected horses might reasonably be expected to have some difficulty. Of course, the cysts are more common in older mares that might in any case be subfertile.

NEOPLASTIC DISORDERS OF THE TUBULAR GENITAL TRACT OF MARES

Leiomyoma

Profile

- All endometrial tumors are very rare in horses and leiomyoma is the most common of these.
- They usually occur in older mares.

Clinical signs

- Single or multiple nodules within the wall of the uterus (between 2.5 and 15 cm in diameter).
- They are usually identified incidentally at rectal examination because they seldom cause any distinctive clinical signs.
- Occasional slight bleeding if the surface becomes ulcerated.

Diagnosis

- The histological appearance is characteristic although the endoscopic appearance and rectal and ultrasonographic features are much less distinctive.
  - ❏ Ultrasonographically they are solid, highly echogenic structures with a distinct spherical shape.
  - ❏ Rectal palpation identifies a single, or a few, firm spherical masses within the wall of the uterus.

Differential diagnosis

- Hematoma.
- Fibroses/scar.
- Endometrial abscess.

Treatment

- Pedunculated tumors can be removed by diathermy snare via an endoscope or with CO_2:YAG laser excision or cautery.

Prognosis

- Guarded for fertility.
- Removal of the whole tumor may be very difficult, but there is little risk of metastasis.

Benign polyp (uterine/vulvar/vaginal)/papilloma

Profile

- Very benign, slow-growing pedunculated masses, most often developing on the wall of the vestibule or on the vulvar lips.
- Supposedly, they are caused by an undefined papilloma virus. There is no apparent relationship to horses that have had cutaneous viral papillomatosis.
- Usually older mares are affected.

Clinical signs

- A proliferative mass may be seen protruding from the vulvar lips.
- The tumor is usually pedunculated with a relatively narrow neck and little surrounding inflammatory response.
- Sometimes they can reach large sizes and can become secondarily infected.

Diagnosis
- Made on vaginal examination.

Differential diagnosis
- Leiomyoma.

Treatment
- Removal by suturing off the narrow neck.

Prognosis
- Good for fertility after removal.

Squamous cell carcinoma

Profile
Squamous cell carcinoma mainly affects older horses and in particular those with nonpigmented perineal skin. The tumor occurs in two distinct types and at two locations:

- Proliferative (polyp) type. This type most commonly occurs on:
  - ❑ The vulvar lips.
  - ❑ The wall of the vestibule.
  - ❑ The clitoral glans.

> Note:
> - Carcinoma of the clitoris is not dependent on a nonpigmented area of the clitoral region.

- Ulcerative (destructive type). This type most commonly occurs on:
  - ❑ The vulvar lips.
  - ❑ The perineal skin.

Squamous cell carcinoma has the potential to be highly malignant but is seldom so.

- The ulcerative forms have the greatest tendency for local and metastatic spread.
- The local draining lymph nodes are usually the inguinal and iliac nodes. Enlargement of the glands on the affected side is an indication of a poor prognosis.
- There is no merit in early thoracic radiography in mares affected with squamous cell carcinoma.

Clinical signs (see Fig. 5.72)
- Proliferative or ulcerative lesions on or around the perineal skin.
- The tumors may become infected and extensive tissue necrosis is commonly present.
- This gives a fetid odor and persistent dripping of blood and serum/plasma.
- In spite of the large size of some of these tumors they seldom have significant systemic effects and they rarely cause any difficulty with urination.

Rare secondary effects include debility, weight loss and secondary infection of the tumor mass. Metastasis to other organs (notably the vertebral bodies and the lungs) are rare but local extension to the iliac lymph nodes is common. Rectal examination can be useful to determine if this has occurred.

Diagnosis
- Biopsy.

Treatment
- Surgical excision is the treatment of choice for small proliferative lesions on the vulvar labiae or the vestibular wall.

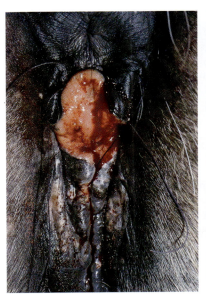 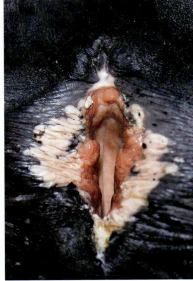 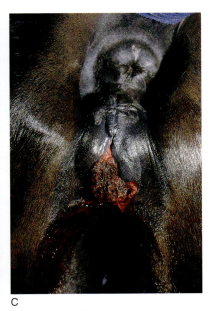

A   B   C

Fig. 5.72   (A) Labial erosive (destructive) squamous cell carcinoma. (B) Ventral commissural and labial squamous cell carcinoma affecting the nonpigmented vulvar lips. (C) Clitoral proliferative squamous cell carcinoma. A similar proliferative form may occur on the vulvar lips or on the vestibular mucosa.

- Cryonecrosis of the surgical wound is sometimes used to widen the area of destruction and minimize the chance of recurrences.
- 5-Fluorouracil applied daily for 3 weeks or until the tumors slough and new skin or mucosa is generated.
- BCG immunomodulation.
- Radiation.

Melanoma

Profile

Melanoma is a common tumor of older gray horses. By far the most common site for their development is the perineum.

The large majority of melanomas are benign and slow-growing. In these cases the main effects are due to their space-occupying nature. However, an occasional tumor is highly malignant and many of these are characterized by diffuse pink or gray tissue dispersed in the normal black material.

Fast-growing lesions and those that are traumatized by the tail or otherwise may ulcerate and produce a thick, black, hemorrhagic discharge. Although this is unsightly it is seldom an indicator of malignancy.

Clinical signs

- Typical black, sometimes ulcerated, lesions in the skin of the perineum are easily recognized.
- Sometimes they can be of sufficient size to cause reproductive difficulty both with mating and with parturition. A few lesions become ulcerated and discharge a tarry black material often mixed with blood.
- The tumors are usually nonpainful.
- The appearance of depigmented areas within the black mass is suggestive of a high malignancy.
- Rectal examination may be required in some cases if there is extensive infiltration of the perineum.

Diagnosis

- The clinical appearance is typical. Lesions are frequently multiple both in the perineum and in other sites, such as the parotid salivary and lymph nodes and the guttural pouches.
- Fine-needle aspiration or surgical biopsy is diagnostic and may establish some important features of growth and mitotic rates.

Differential diagnosis

- Equine sarcoid.
- Localized abscess and foreign-body reactions.

Treatment

- Benign neglect with regular checks and if necessary removal of any troublesome (ulcerative/bleeding) lesions.

- Localized cryosurgical necrosis or even surgical excision can be used on individual lesions.
- Cautery with potassium permanganate may be used to dry the lesions out and so slow their growth and limit the exudation.
- Intralesional cisplatin may be helpful for larger flatter lesions that are not amenable to surgery.
- Autogenous X-irradiated vaccines based on cultured cells have been investigated and may become a significant therapeutic method.
- Oral cimetidine therapy may result in decrease in size of the masses over several months of treatment. Once the maximal reduction in size is reached, therapy is discontinued. If the masses begin to enlarge again, another course of therapy can be re-instituted.

Prognosis

The outlook is generally good but individual lesions can create significant local problems that might even result in euthanasia. There has been little work to define the characteristics of malignancy but a change to paler or even pink tissue is usually regarded unfavorably.

Vascular/muscular hamartoma

Profile

A hamartoma is an abnormal accumulation of a normal cell type in a normal or abnormal anatomical location. The most common hamartomas involve blood vessels (vascular hamartoma) and muscles (muscular hamartoma) but in theory any tissue type can be involved. The main reproductive implication is for vascular lesions in the vagina and for muscular hamartoma of the perineal muscles.

Clinical signs

- A large, progressively enlarging space-occupying mass in the perineal skin or adjacent muscles (depending on the tissue of origin).
- There may be significant distortion of the perineal anatomy (Fig. 5.73).

Diagnosis

- Biopsy reveals a normal tissue type for the tissue involved.

Differential diagnosis

- Melanoma.
- Perineal abscess.
- Perineal hematoma.

Treatment

- No treatment is required.
- Large lesions are invariably very difficult to remove surgically because they are not well defined and are unrecognizable from the adjacent normal tissue.

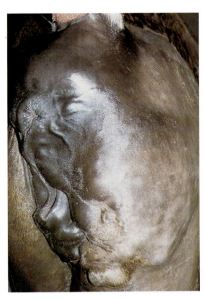

Fig. 5.73 Hamartoma of muscle (semi-membranosus). Note the physical distortion of the perineum.

Prognosis

- Good unless the size interferes with function or perineal conformation.

REFERENCES

1. Pascoe RR. Observations on the length and angle of declination of the vulva and its relationship to fertility of the mare. Journal of Reproduction and Fertility Supplement 1979; 27:299–304.
2. Hinrichs K, Cummings M, Sertich P, et al. Clinical significance of aerobic bacterial flora of the uterus, vagina, vestibule and clitoral fossa of clinically normal mares. Journal of the American Veterinary Medical Association 1988; 193:72–76.
3. Ginther OJ. Reproductive biology of the mare: basic and applied aspects. 2nd edn. Cross Plains, WI: Equiservices; 1992:1–17.
4. Van Niekerk CH, Gerneke WH. Persistence and pathogenetic cleavage of tubal ova in the mare. Onderstepoort Journal of Veterinary Research 1966; 33:195–232.
5. Mitchell D, Allen WR. Observations on reproductive performance in yearling mares. Journal of Reproduction and Fertility Supplement 1975; 23:531–536.
6. Wesson JA, Ginther OJ. Influence of photoperiod on the onset of puberty in the female pony. Journal of Reproduction and Fertility Supplement 1982; 32:269–274.
7. Squires EL. Puberty. In: McKinnon AO, Voss JL, eds. Equine reproduction. Philadelphia, PA: Lea & Febiger; 1992:114–120.
8. Burkhardt J. Transition from anoestrous in the mare and the effect of artificial lighting. Journal of Agricultural Science 1946; 37:64–68.
9. Kooistra LH, Ginther OJ. Effect of photoperiod on reproductive activity in mares. American Journal of Veterinary Research 1975; 36:1413–1419.
10. Hughes JP, Stabenfeldt GH, Kennedy PC, et al. The estrous cycle and selected functional and pathologic ovarian abnormalities in the mare. Veterinary Clinics of North America: Large Animal Practice 1980; 2:225–239.
11. Noden PA, Oxender WD, Hafs HD, et al. The cycle of oestrus, ovulation and plasma levels of hormones in the mare. Journal of Reproduction and Fertility Supplement 1975; 23:189–192.
12. Davis SD, Sharp DC. Intra-follicular and peripheral steroid characteristics during vernal transition in the pony mare. Journal of Reproduction and Fertility Supplement 1991; 44:333–340.
13. Palmer E, Jousset B. Urinary oestrogen and plasma progesterone levels in non-pregnant mares. Journal of Reproduction and Fertility Supplement 1975; 23:213–221.
14. Allen WR. Endogenous hormonal control of the mare's oestrous cycle. In: Proceedings of the 9th Bain-Fallon Memorial Lectures 1987; 2–13.
15. Irvine CHG. The non-pregnant mare: a review of some current research and of the last 25 years of endocrinology. Biology of Reproduction Monograph 1995; 1:343–360.
16. Evans MJ, Irvine CHG. The serum concentrations of FSH, LH and progesterone during the oestrous cycle and early pregnancy in the mare. Journal of Reproduction and Fertility Supplement 1975; 23:429–433.
17. Neely DP. Reproductive endocrinology and fertility in the mare. In: Neely DP, Liu IKM, Hillman RB. Equine reproduction. Princeton Junction, NJ: Veterinary Learning Systems; 1983:12–37.
18. Osborne VE. An analysis of the pattern of ovulation as it occurs in the annual reproductive cycle of the mare in Australia. Australian Veterinary Journal 1966; 61:149–154.
19. Withrow JM, Sargent GF, Scheffrahn NS, et al. Induction of male sex behavior in pony mares with testosterone propionate. Theriogenology 1983; 20:485–490.
20. Squires EL. Estrus detection. In: McKinnon AO, Voss JL, eds. Equine reproduction. Philadelphia, PA: Lea & Febiger; 1993:186–195.
21. Lieux P. The relationship between the appearance of the cervix and the heat cycle in the mare. Veterinary Medicine 1970; 65:879–893.
22. Rossdale PD, Ricketts SW. Events leading to conception. In: Equine stud farm medicine. London: Baillière Tindall; 1980:1–119.
23. Easley J. External perineal conformation. In: McKinnon AO, Voss JL, eds. Equine reproduction. Philadelphia, PA: Lea & Febiger; 1993:20–24.
24. LeBlanc MM. Clinical examination of the reproductive system: the mare. In: Radostits OM, Mayhew IGJ, Houston DM, eds. Veterinary clinical examination and diagnosis. Philadelphia, PA: WB Saunders; 2000:674–691.
25. Asbury AC. Examination of the mare. In: Colohan PT, Moore JN, Merritt AM, et al., eds. Equine medicine and surgery. 5th edn. Mosby; 1999:1088–1094.
26. LeBlanc MM. Vaginal examination. In: McKinnon

AO, Voss JL, eds. Equine reproduction. Philadelphia, PA: Lea & Febiger, 1993:221–224.

27. Neely DP. Evaluation and therapy of genital disease in the mare. In: Neely DP, Liu, IKM, Hillman RB. Equine reproduction. Princeton Junction, NJ: Veterinary Learning Systems; 1983:53–55.

28. McKinnon AO, Voss JL, Squires EL, et al. Diagnostic ultrasonography. In: McKinnon AO, Voss JL, eds. Equine reproduction. Philadelphia, PA: Lea & Febiger; 1993:266–302.

29. McKinnon AO, Carnevale EM. Ultrasonography. In: McKinnon AO, Voss JL, eds. Equine reproduction. Philadelphia, PA: Lea & Febiger; 1993:211–220.

30. Ginther OJ. Ultrasonographic imaging and reproductive events in the mare. Cross Plains, WI: Equiservices; 1986.

31. McKinnon AL, Squire EL, Voss JL. Ultrasonic evaluation of the mare's reproductive tract. Part 1. Compendium of Continuing Education for the Practicing Veterinarian 1987; 9:336–345.

32. McKinnon AL, Squire EL, Voss JL. Ultrasonic evaluation of the mare's reproductive tract. Part 2. Compendium of Continuing Education for the Practicing Veterinarian 1987; 9:472–482.

33. Gastal EL, Gastal MO, Ginther OJ. The suitability of echotexture characteristics of the follicular wall for identifying the optimal breeding day in mares. Theriogenology 1998; 50:1025–1038.

34. Adams GP, Kastelic JP, Bergfelt DR, et al. Effect of uterine inflammation and ultrasonically detected uterine pathology on fertility in the mare. Journal of Reproduction and Fertility Supplement 1987; 35:445–454.

35. McKinnon AO, Squires EL, Harrison LA, et al. Ultrasonographic studies on the reproductive tract of postpartum mares: effect of involution and uterine fluid on pregnancy rates in mares with normal and delayed first postpartum ovulatory cycles. Journal of the American Veterinary Medical Association 1988; 192:350–353.

36. Hinrichs K. Ultrasonographic assessment of ovarian abnormalities. Proceedings of the American Association of Equine Practitioners 1990; 36:31–40.

37. Ricketts SW. Endometrial biopsy as guide to diagnosis of endometrial pathology in the mare. Journal of Reproduction and Fertility Supplement 1975; 23:341–345.

38. Ricketts SW. The technique and clinical applications of endometrial biopsy in the mare equine. Veterinary Journal 1979; 7:102–106.

39. Ricketts SW. Histological and histopathological studies of the endometrium of the mare. Fellowship thesis, Royal College of Veterinary Surgeons, London; 1978.

40. Kenney RM. Cyclic and pathological changes of the mare endometrium as detected by biopsy, with a note on early embryonic death. Journal of the American Veterinary Medical Association 1978; 172:241–262.

41. Doig PA, Waelchli RO. Endometrial biopsy. In: McKinnon AO, Voss JL, eds. Equine reproduction. Philadelphia, PA: Lea & Febiger; 1993:225–233.

42. Ricketts SW. The barren mare. In Practice 1989; 11:156–164.

43. Kenney RM. Endometrial biopsy technique and classification according to interpretation. Proceedings of the Society of Theriogenology 1978;14–25.

44. LeBlanc MM. Endoscopy. In: McKinnon AO, Voss JL, eds. Equine reproduction. Philadelphia, PA: Lea & Febiger; 1993:255–258.

45. Knudsen O. Endometrial cytology as a diagnostic aid in mares. Cornell Veterinarian 1964; 54:415–422.

46. Gadd JD. The relationship of bacterial cultures, microscopic smear examination and medical treatment to surgical correction of barren mares. Proceedings of the American Association of Equine Practitioners 1975; 362–368.

47. Wingfield Digby NJ. The technique and clinical application of endometrial cytology in mares. Equine Veterinary Journal 1978; 10:167–170.

48. Brook D. Uterine cytology. In: McKinnon AO, Voss JL, eds. Equine reproduction. Philadelphia, PA: Lea & Febiger; 1993:246–255.

49. Scott P, Daley P, Baird GG, et al. The aerobic bacterial flora of the reproductive tract of the mare. Veterinary Record 1971; 88:58–61.

50. Solomon WJ, Schultz RH, Fahning ML. A study of chronic infertility in the mare utilizing uterine biopsy, cytology and cultural methods. Proceedings of the American Association of Equine Practitioners 1972; 55–68.

51. Greenhoff GR, Kenney RM. Evaluation of reproductive status of non-pregnant mares. Journal of the American Veterinary Medical Association 1975; 7:449–452.

52. Ricketts SW, Young A, Medici EB. Uterine and clitoral cultures. In: McKinnon AO, Voss JL, eds. Equine reproduction. Philadelphia, PA: Lea & Febiger; 1993:234–245.

53. Loy RG. Characteristics of postpartum reproduction in mares. Veterinary Clinics of North America 1980; 2:345–359.

54. Madill S, Troedsson MHT. Breeding soundness examination of the mare. In: Robinson NE, ed. Current therapy in equine medicine 4. Philadelphia: WB Saunders; 1997:505–512.

55. Vanderwall DK, Woods GL. Age related ovulatory dysfunction. In: Robinson NE, ed. Current therapy in equine medicine, Vol. 3. Philadelphia, PA: WB Saunders; 1992:643–644.

56. Sertich PL. Persistent estrus: fact or fiction. In: Robinson NE, ed. Current therapy in equine medicine, Vol. 3. Philadelphia, PA: WB Saunders; 1992:641–642.

57. Ginther OJ. Occurrence of anoestrus, estrus, diestrus and ovulation over a 12 month period in mares. American Journal of Veterinary Research 1974; 35:1173–1179.

58. Guillaume D, Duchamp G, Nagy P, et al. Determination of minimum light treatment required for photostimulation of winter anoestrous mares. Journal of Reproduction and Fertility Supplement 2000; 56:205–216.

59. Allen WR, Urwin V, Simpson DJ, et al. Preliminary studies on the use of an oral progestogen to induce oestrus and ovulation in seasonally anoestrous thoroughbred mares. Equine Veterinary Journal 1980; 12:141–145.

60. Bour B, Palmer E, Driancourt MA. Stimulation of ovarian activity in the pony mare during winter

anoestrus. In: Ellendorff F, Elsaesser F, eds. Endocrine causes in seasonal and lactational anoestrus in farm animals. Boston: Martinus Nijhoff; 1985:85–87.

61. Carnevali EM, Squires EL, McKinnon AO, et al. Effects of hCG on time to ovulation and luteal function in transitional mares. Journal of Equine Veterinary Science 1989; 9:27–29.

62. Loy RG, Pemstein R, Ocanna D, et al. Control of ovulation in cycling mares with ovarian steroid and prostaglandin. Theriogenology 1981; 15:191–199.

63. Bergfelt D. Oestrus synchronization. In: Samper J, ed. Equine breeding management and artificial insemination. Philadelphia, PA: WB Saunders; 2000:165–177.

64. Brendemuehl PJ, Cross DL. Influence of the dopamine antagonist domperidone on the vernal transition in seasonally anoestrous mares. Journal of Reproduction and Fertility Supplement 2000; 56:185–193.

65. Daels PF, Fatone BS, Hansen BS, et al. Dopamine antagonist-induced reproductive function in anoestrous mares; gonadotropin secretion and the effects of environmental cues. Journal of Reproduction and Fertility Supplement 2000; 56:173–183.

66. Grimmet JB. Behavioral anoestrus. In: Robinson NE, ed. Current therapy in equine medicine, 2nd edn. Philadelphia, PA: WB Saunders; 1983:400–401.

67. Hughes JP, Stabenfeldt GH. Anoestrus in the mare. Proceedings of the American Association of Equine Practitioners 1973:89–96.

68. Skelton KV, Dowsett KF, McMeniman NP. Ovarian activity in pubertal mares treated with anabolic steroids prior to the onset of puberty. Journal of Reproduction and Fertility Supplement 1991; 44:351–356.

69. Loy RG. Characteristics of post partum reproduction in mares. Veterinary Clinics of North America 1980; 2:345–259.

70. Daels PF, Hughes JP. The abnormal oestrus cycle. In: McKinnon AO, Voss JL, eds. Equine reproduction. Philadelphia, PA: Lea & Febiger; 1993:144–160.

71. Heeneke D, Potter GD, Krieder JL. Body condition during pregnancy and lactation and reproductive efficiency in mares. Theriogenology 1984; 21:897–909.

72. Neucshaefer A, Bracher V, Allen WR. Prolactin secretion in lactating mares before and after treatment with bromocriptine. Journal of Reproduction and Fertility Supplement 1991; 44:551–559.

73. Ginther OJ, Pierson RA. Regular and irregular characteristics of ovulation and the interovulatory interval in mares. Journal of Equine Veterinary Science 1989; 9:4–12.

74. Sertich PL. Persistent estrus: fact or fiction. In: Robinson NE, ed. Current therapy in equine medicine 3. Philadelphia, PA: WB Saunders; 1992:641–642.

75. Meagher DM, Wheat JD, Hughes JP, et al. Granulosa cell tumors in mares: a review of 78 cases. Proceedings of the 23rd Annual Convention of the American Association of Equine Practitioners 1977; 133–143.

76. Stabenfeldt GH, Hughes JP, Kennedy PC, et al.

Clinical findings, pathological changes and endocrinological secretory patterns in mares with ovarian tumours. Journal of Reproduction and Fertility Supplement 1979; 27:277–285.

77. Hinrichs K, Hunt PR. Ultrasound as an aid to diagnosis of granulosa cell tumor in the mare. Equine Veterinary Journal 1990; 22:99–102.

78. McCue PM. Review of ovarian abnormalities in the mare. Proceedings of the 44th Annual Convention American Association of Equine Practitioners 1998; 125–133.

79. Frazer GS, Threlfall WR. Differential diagnosis of enlarged ovary in the mare. Proceedings of the 32nd Annual Convention American Association of Equine Practitioners 1986:21–28.

80. Hughes JP, Stabenfeldt GH, Kennedy PC. The estrus cycle and selected functional and pathological ovarian abnormalities in the mare. Veterinary Clinics of North America 1980; 2:225–239.

81. Palmer SE. Ovariectomy: laparoscopic technique. In: White and Moore, eds. Current techniques in equine surgery and lameness. 2nd edn. Philadelphia: WB Saunders; 1998:217–224.

82. Aanes WA. Cervical laceration(s). In: McKinnon AO, Voss JL, eds. Equine reproduction. Philadelphia, PA: Lea & Febiger; 1993:444–449.

83. Brown JS, Varner DD, Hinrichs K, et al. Surgical repair of the lacerated cervix in the mare. Theriogenology 1984; 22:351–359.

84. Evans LH, Tate LP, Cooper WL. Surgical repair of cervical laceration and the incompetent cervix. Proceedings of the American Association of Equine Practitioners 1979; 483–486.

85. Robertson JT. Cervical lacerations. In: White NA, Moore JN, eds. Current practice of equine surgery. Philadelphia, PA: Lippincott; 1990:696–699.

86. Daels PJ, Besognet B, Hansen B, et al. Effect of progesterone on prostaglandin F_2 alpha secretion and outcome of pregnancy during cloprostenol-induced abortion in mares. American Journal of Veterinary Research 1996; 57:1331–1337.

87. Daels PF, Stabenfeldt GH, Hughes JP, et al. Evaluation of progesterone deficiency as a cause of fetal death in mares with experimentally induced endotoxaemia. American Journal of Veterinary Research 1991; 52:282–289.

88. Troedsson MHT. Uterine response to semen deposition in the mare. Proceedings of the Society of Theriogenology 1995; 130–135.

89. Katila T. Onset and duration of uterine inflammatory response of mares after insemination with fresh semen. Biology of reproduction monograph 1: Equine reproduction 1995:515–517.

90. Troedsson MHT, Liu IKM. Uterine clearance of non-antigenic markers (51Cr) in response to a bacterial challenge in mares potentially susceptible and resistant to chronic uterine infections. Journal of Reproduction and Fertility Supplement 1991; 44:282–288.

91. LeBlanc MM, Neuwirth L, Asbury AC, et al. Scintigraphic measurement of uterine clearance in normal mares and mares with recurrent endometritis. Equine Veterinary Journal 1994; 26:109–113.

92. LeBlanc MM, Neuwirth L, Jones L, et al. Differences

in uterine position of reproductively normal mares and those with delayed uterine clearance detected by scintigraphy. Theriogenology 1998; 50:49–54.

93. Troedsson MHT, Liu IKM. Multiple site electromyography recordings of uterine activity following an intrauterine bacterial challenge in mares susceptible and resistant to chronic uterine injection. Journal of Reproduction and Fertility Supplement 1993; 46:307–313.

94. Troedsson MHT, Scott MA, Liu IKM. Comparative treatment of mares susceptible to chronic uterine infection. American Journal of Veterinary Research 1995; 56:468–472.

95. LeBlanc MM. Oxytocin: the new wonder drug for treatment of endometritis? Equine Veterinary Education 1994; 6:39–43.

96. Pycock JF. Assessment of oxytocin and intrauterine antibiotics on intrauterine fluid and pregnancy rates in the mare. Proceedings of the American Association of Equine Practitioners 1994; 19–20.

97. LeBlanc MM, Johnson RD, Calderwood Mays MB, et al. Lymphatic clearance of India ink in reproductively normal mares and mares susceptible to endometritis. Biology of Reproduction Monograph 1995; 1:501–506.

98. Gunthle LM, McCue PM, Farquhar VJ, et al. Effect of prostaglandin administration postovulation on corpus luteum formation in the mare. SFT proceedings, San Antonio 2000:139.

99. Dascanio J. How to diagnose and treat fungal endometritis. Proceedings of the 46th Annual American Association of Equine Practitioners 2000:316–319.

100. Hughes JP, Stabenfeldt GH, Kindahl H, et al. Pyometra in the mare. Journal of Reproduction and Fertility Supplement 1979; 27:321–329.

101. Brown MP, Colahan PT, Hawkins DL. Urethral extension for treatment of urine pooling in mares. Journal of the American Veterinary Medical Association 1978; 173:1005–1007.

102. McKinnon AO, Belden JO. A urethral extension technique to correct urine pooling (vesico vaginal reflux) in mares. Journal of the American Veterinary Medical Association 1988; 192:647–650.

103. Shires GM, Kaneps AJ. A practical and simple surgical technique for repair of urine pooling in the mare. Proceedings 32nd Annual Convention American Association of Equine Practitioners 1986:51–56.

104. Horserace Betting Levy Board (UK). Codes of practice on control of infectious disease. Newmarket: R&W Publications; 2000.

105. Troedsson MHT. Diseases of the external genitalia. In: Robinson NE, ed. Current therapy in equine medicine 4. Philadelphia, PA: WB Saunders; 1997: 512–516.

106. Powell DG. Contagious equine metritis. Advances in Veterinary Science and Comparative Medicine 1981; 25:161–166.

107. Powell DG. Contagious equine metritis. Equine Veterinary Journal 1978; 10:153–159.

108. Hughes JP. Contagious equine metritis: a review. Theriogenology 1979; 11:209–216.

109. Ricketts SW. Vaginal discharge in the mare. In Practice 1987; 12:117–123.

110. Robertson A, ed. Handbook on animal diseases in the tropics. London: British Veterinary Association; 1976:207–209.

111. Parkin BS. The demonstration and transmission of the South African strain of *Trypanosoma equiperdum* of horses. Onderstepoort Journal of Veterinary Research 1948; 23:41–57.

112. Asbury AC. Endometritis in the mare. In: Morrow DA, ed. Current therapy in theriogenology 2. Philadelphia, PA: WB Saunders; 1986:718–722.

113. Davis LE, Abbitt B. Clinical pharmacology of antibacterial drugs in the uterus of the mare. Journal of the American Veterinary Medical Association 1977; 170:204–207.

114. Bennett DG. Therapy of endometritis in mares. Journal of the American Veterinary Medical Association 1986; 188:1390–1392.

115. Gustafsson BK, Ott RS. Current trends in the treatment of genital infections in large animals. Compendium of Continuing Education for the Practicing Veterinarian 1981; 3:147–152.

116. Neely DP, Liu IKM, Hillman RB. Evaluation and therapy of genital disease in the mare. In: Equine reproduction. Princeton Junction, NJ: Veterinary Learning Systems 1983:41–56.

117. Allen WE. Plasma concentrations of sodium benzyl penicillin after intrauterine infusion in pony mares. Equine Veterinary Journal 1978; 10:171–173.

118. Bretzlaff KN. Factors of importance for the disposition of antibiotics in the female genital tract. In: Morrow DA, ed. Current therapy in theriogenology 2. Philadelphia, PA: WB Saunders; 1986:34–39.

119. Threlfall WR, Carleton CL. Treatment of uterine infection in the mare. In: Morrow DA, ed. Current therapy in theriogenology 2. Philadelphia, PA: WB Saunders; 1986:730–737.

120. Bretzlaff KN. Factors of importance for the disposition of antibiotics in the female genital tract. In: Morrow DA, ed. Current therapy in theriogenology 2. Philadelphia, PA: WB Saunders; 1986:34–39.

121. Allen WE, Clark AR. Absorption of sodium benzyl penicillin from the equine uterus after local Lugol's iodine treatment, compared with absorption after intramuscular injection. Equine Veterinary Journal 1978; 10:174–175.

122. McDonald PJ, Wetherall BL, Pruul H, et al. Postantibiotic leukocyte enhancement-increased susceptibility of bacteria pretreated with antibiotics to activity of leukocytes. Review of Infectious Disease 1981; 3:38–44.

123. McGowan JE. Outline guide to antimicrobial therapy. Oradell, NJ: Medical Economics Books; 1982:212–243.

124. Bennett DG. Diagnosis and treatment of equine bacterial endometritis. Journal of Equine Veterinary Science 1987; 7:345–352.

125. LeBlanc MM, Neuwirth L, Mauragis D, et al. Oxytocin enhances clearance of radiocolloid from the uterine lumen of reproductively normal mares and mares susceptible to endometritis. Equine Veterinary Journal 1994; 26:279–282.

126. Combs GB, LeBlanc MM, Neuwirth L, et al. Effects of prostaglandin $F_{2\alpha}$, cloprostenol and fenprostalene on uterine clearance of radiocolloid in the mare. Theriogenology 1996; 45:1449–1455.

127. Asbury AC. Infectious and immunologic considerations in mare infertility. Compendium of Continuing Education for the Practicing Veterinarian 1987; 9:585–592.

128. Asbury AC. Uterine defense mechanisms in the mare: the use of intrauterine plasma in the management of endometritis. Theriogenology 1984; 21:387–393.

129. Pascoe DR. Effect of adding autologous plasma to an intrauterine antibiotic therapy after breeding on pregnancy rates in mares. Biology of Reproduction Monograph 1995; 1:539–543.

130. Kenney RM, Bergman RV, Cooper WL, et al. Minimal contamination technique for breeding mares: technique and preliminary findings. Proceedings of the American Association of Equine Practitioners 1975; 21:327–335.

131. Rasch K, Schoon HA, Sieme H, et al. Histomorphological endometrial status and influence of oxytocin on the uterine drainage and pregnancy rate in mares. Equine Veterinary Journal 1996; 28:455–461.

132. Ott RS. The efficacy of uterine treatment with antimicrobial drugs. In: Morrow DA, ed. Current therapy in theriogenology 2. Philadelphia, PA: WB Saunders; 1986:39–42.

133. Kenney RM, Ganjam VK. Selected pathological changes of the mare's uterus and ovary. Journal of Reproduction and Fertility Supplement 1975; 23:335–339.

134. Ellis BE. Prevalence of endometrial cysts and their effect on fertility. Biology of Reproduction Monograph 1995; 1:527–532.

135. Brook D. Electrocoagulative removal of endometrial cysts in the mare. Journal of Equine Veterinary Science 1987; 7:77–81.

136. Blikslager AT, Tate LP, Weinstock D. Effects of neodymium:ytrium aluminium garnet laser irradiation on endometrium and on endometrial cysts in six mares. Veterinary Surgery 1993; 22:351–356.

137. Leib B, Bartmann CP, Supperle H, et al. Comparison of thermal injury zones and wound healing of the equine endometrium subsequent to minimal invasive Nd:YAG laser- and electromicrosurgery II. Histological and immunohistological investigations of the endometrium. Pferdeheilkunde 2001; 17:688–689.

Chapter 6
MATING
Michelle LeBlanc,
Cheryl Lopate

Pregnancy begins with delivery of the sperm to the ovum. There are several ways in which sperm can be delivered to the egg, including:

- Natural (paddock) service.
- Supervised mating.
- Controlled mating.
- Artificial insemination, using:
  - ❑ Fresh semen.
  - ❑ Chilled fresh semen.
  - ❑ Frozen semen.

NATURAL SERVICE

Management of the teaser depends on the type and number of teasers available on the farm; for further discussion, see p. 77.

Each mare is an individual, and her specific teasing and estrus behavior must be learned in order for teasing to be properly utilized in a reproductive program. Teasing behavior will also change with the season. Mares will often be ambivalent to the teaser or stallion during winter anestrus, with signs of good standing heat increasing during the transitional period, becoming most reliable when normal cyclicity is occurring and then decreasing again during the fall transition.

Breeding by natural service[1]

On small studs and in some breed associations – most notably the Thoroughbreds – natural service is the only acceptable method of breeding. If natural service is utilized, the stallions and mares must be carefully managed.

> - The safety of the mares, stallions, and handlers is of the utmost importance.

The goal of any breeding program is to breed each mare once only, with all mares conceiving from that breeding.

- It is important to manage the mares so that they are bred the fewest number of times per cycle and have the highest conception rate possible.
- Stallions must be carefully managed so that their libido is maintained and they are not over-used such that their fertility declines.

The advantages of natural service are:

- It is less labor-intensive than artificial insemination.
- The mechanics of the process are proven.
- The number of mares bred to each stallion is limited so that one stallion's genes will not be over-used.

The disadvantages of natural service are:

- The danger of disease transmission.
- Injury to mare, stallion or handlers may occur.
- The number of mares to be bred is less than with artificial insemination.
- The number of sperm delivered to the mare is not known.

Natural service requires that the stallion physically mates with the mare.

- A mare must be teased on a regular basis to establish her reproductive receptivity (heat).
- Some mares that are in estrus are not receptive to the stallion. This usually affects:
  - ❑ Maiden mares.
  - ❑ Timid mares.
  - ❑ Mares that have had a bad experience during a previous breeding.

Mares may not be receptive until they become accustomed to new surroundings. A strange environment or unusual circumstances (handler changes, etc.) can have a marked effect on the mare's display of estrus.

The facilities

- The breeding shed should be large enough for movement of the mare, the stallion, and their handlers (see p. 16).
- There should be good, firm, nonslippery footing (Fig. 6.1).
- There should be an exit route for both the mare and the stallion should problems arise.
- The mare should be hobbled or breeding boots put on her rear feet and a twitch applied (Fig. 6.2).
  - ❑ Mares that are not receptive or are badly behaved may require sedation, but particular care should be taken to ensure that such a mare is indeed in estrus.

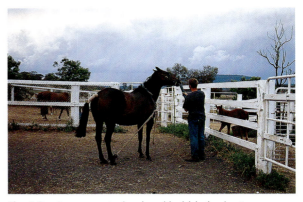

Fig. 6.2 A mare restrained and hobbled prior to breeding. A nose twitch and hind foot boots may be required to avoid possible injury to the stallion.

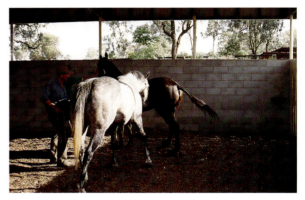

Fig. 6.3 A receptive estrous mare raising her tail to one side prior to service.

- ❑ Care should be taken to not rely completely on the hobbles for protection of the stallion, since mares can still kick effectively even with hobbles on.
- The tail can be tied to one side if quick-release knots are used both on the tail and around the neck of the mare, so that the tail can be released easily if the stallion should become entangled. Otherwise, the tail can be allowed to hang.
  - ❑ Receptive mares will raise their tails out of the stallion's path, and, as long as the tail is wrapped, the mare's tail hairs will not become entangled with the stallion's penis (Fig. 6.3).
  - ❑ Minor lacerations of the glans from tail hairs can result in hemospermia and lowered overall fertility. Paddock mating more often causes injuries of this type.
  - ❑ Should lacerations occur, the breeding process may be painful for the stallion and he may become less enthusiastic.

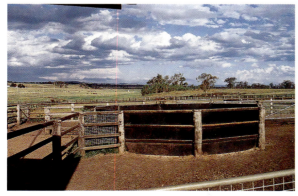

Fig. 6.1 The floor/surface of the breeding area must be 'nonslip'.

Personnel

- One person should handle the mare.
- A second person should handle the stallion and a third person should assist the stallion during intromission (Fig. 6.4).
  - ❑ Mares that have a 'breeding stitch' (not a Caslick's suture, see below) in place at the time of mating should have this stitch moved out of the way by the same person who assists in intromission. A breeding stitch is simply a suture that is inserted to restrain the vulvar lips and limit vulvar flaccidity and the risks of damage to the Caslick site. This will prevent any injury to the stallion's penis by the stitch. In the event that the vulva is damaged during service it is routinely repaired immediately afterwards.
  - ❑ The same person can keep a hand on the base of the penis to palpate for urethral pulsation and confirm that ejaculation has occurred (Fig. 6.5).
  - ❑ Some stallions do not like having their penis handled in any way, making this third person's job unnecessary.

Preparation of the mare for breeding

- i. When the mare is found to be receptive and ready to be bred, her tail should be wrapped and the perineum washed with mild soap and warm water and rinsed thoroughly (Fig. 6.6).
  - ❑ The vulva and hairs surrounding the perineum should be dried thoroughly.
  - ❑ A fresh bucket and wash material are used for each mare to reduce the incidence of disease transmission.
- ii. Mares that have had a previous Caslick's operation (vulvoplasty; see p. 184) should be

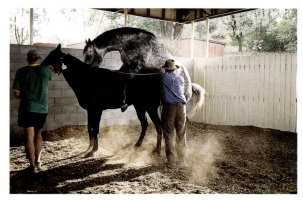

Fig. 6.5 Checking for urethral pulsations will confirm ejaculation.

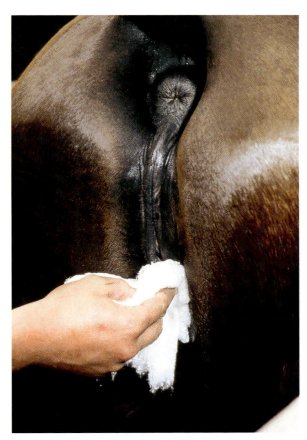

Fig. 6.6 Washing the perineum with warm water and careful drying of the vulvar area (including the inner margins of the vulvar lips) should precede coitus.

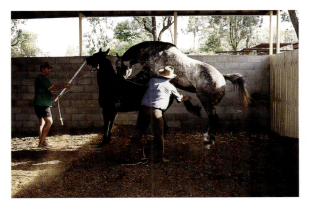

Fig. 6.4 Assistance with intromission will help to minimize potential injury during coitus but some stallions may not accept this.

examined to determine if there is adequate area for penetration without the risk of tearing the vulva or injuring the stallion's penis.
- ❑ If there is insufficient room for safe natural service, the suture should be opened and adequate time allowed for all bleeding to

cease before the mare is bred. Damage occurring during service should be repaired immediately afterwards.

❏ If there is still suture material in place, this must be removed carefully so that fecal material or other contamination is eliminated and there is less risk of injury to the stallion.

❏ Additionally, a breeding roll can be used to prevent the penis from entering too far and thereby tearing the mare.

Preparation of the stallion

i. At the start of the breeding season, the penis, fossa glandis and urethral diverticulum should all be cleaned carefully. Suitable swabs, etc. will be required for disease control.

ii. The stallion's penis should be washed with warm water prior to breeding (Fig. 6.7).[2,3]

❏ Warm water and mild soap should be used and the penis rinsed thoroughly. This procedure tends to be stimulatory in most stallions.

❏ Once the penis is thoroughly cleaned and rinsed it should be dried.

❏ After the initial washing of the season, only water should be used.

❏ If the penis becomes excessively dirty, a mild soap can be used, again whenever considered necessary.

iii. After covering the mare, the penis should be washed again to rinse any contamination derived from the mare.

❏ A dismount semen sample can be obtained for evaluation by gently stripping the penis down towards the glans as the stallion dismounts. Although it is not nearly as accurate as the sperm-rich portion of the ejaculate, this allows some evaluation of the semen.

❏ At a minimum, motility can be evaluated, and it can be confirmed that ejaculation did occur.

The stallion book

See p. 76.

Minimal contamination breeding technique

i. Only one covering per estrous cycle is usually permitted.

ii. The mare must be in estrus with a mature follicle.

iii. Human chorionic gonadotropin (luteinizing hormone; 1500–3000 IU) or a deslorelin implant is administered 24 hours before mating.

iv. Both mare and stallion are thoroughly cleaned with soap and warm water and dried carefully with a sterile paper towel.

v. The mare's uterus is filled with about 100–200 ml of warmed semen extender with antibiotic added. The amount of extender used will depend on the size of the mare's uterus.

vi. Mating is fully supervised to ensure rapid and effective intromission and ejaculation.

> Note:
> - Administration of oxytocin to mares affected by chronic endometritis (see p. 178) 4–8 hours after mating can improve conception rates.
> - This is presumed to be mediated through stimulation of uterine drainage.

ARTIFICIAL INSEMINATION

Artificial insemination has become a normal procedure in stud medicine. However, there are still major problems associated with both the ethical aspects (it is not an accepted procedure in the Thoroughbred) and the relatively poor cryoprotection of sperm in frozen semen compared with other domestic species.

There are significant advantages in the use of artificial insemination, but there are also disadvantages. Artificial insemination includes the use of:

- Fresh semen.
- Chilled semen.
- Frozen semen.

The methods commonly used for semen collection in modern stud practice are outlined on p. 62. Although there are other, cruder, methods (such as the

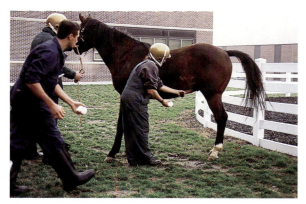

Fig. 6.7 Washing the penis with warm water prior to breeding. Chemicals and strong soap should not be used.

use of vaginal sponges), these are becoming less acceptable as the technology of semen collection and use improves. It is important to realize that the correct collection of semen, precise handling of the ejaculates and the management of the mare are all vital if first conception pregnancy rates are to be kept acceptably high.

Most breeding programs that use artificial insemination incorporate the administration of an ovulatory agent and repeated ultrasonographic examinations of the reproductive tract to time ovulation. Both should be used in breeding programs if mares are to be bred with cooled or frozen semen. If the stallion resides on the farm with the mares, it is not uncommon to breed the mares with fresh semen every other day until they stop exhibiting estrous behavior. This breeding protocol is not recommended if the mare has a history of persistent mating-induced endometritis. The technique of artificial insemination is similar with fresh, fresh-cooled or frozen semen with the exception of the delivery system. Most commonly, mares are bred with an artificial insemination pipette attached to a syringe when fresh or cooled semen is used. An artificial insemination gun or a flexible catheter for deep inseminations into the uterine horn may be used with frozen semen.

Use of an ovulation-inducing agent

- Ovulation can be timed with reasonable accuracy by administering either human chorionic gonadotropin or deslorelin.
- Most mares are given the ovulatory agent when the dominant follicle is 35 mm in diameter (normally on the second or third day of estrus) and endometrial folds are present in the uterus.[4]
- The size of the follicle affects the mare's ability to respond to human chorionic gonadotropin. Most mares will not respond if the dominant follicle is smaller than 35 mm. Some Warmblood mares will not respond with a 35-mm follicle, especially if it is present on the first day of estrus. In these mares, it may be best to administer human chorionic gonadotropin on the second or third day of estrus when the dominant follicle is 38–45 mm and there are prominent endometrial folds.
- The majority of mares ovulate 36–48 hours after intravenous administration of 1500–3000 IU of human chorionic gonadotropin.
- Deslorelin, a synthetic gonadotropin-releasing hormone agonist, designed as an implant, under the same criteria, induces ovulation in mares on average 41–48 hours after it is inserted.[5]
- The response to deslorelin does not appear to be so dependent on follicular size. It may be given when the dominant follicle is as small as 30 mm in diameter.
- Some mares that are implanted with deslorelin have a prolonged inter-estrous interval between 28 and 45 days if they do not conceive. Removal

of the implant between 42 and 48 hours after it was inserted prevents this problem from occurring. Placing the implant in the submucosa of the vulvar lips facilitates implant removal.

Ultrasonographic changes in the reproductive tract

Ultrasonographic examination of the reproductive tract during estrus is extremely useful in timing ovulation because estrogen causes the uterus and follicles to undergo characteristic ultrasonographic changes.

As the mare nears ovulation, the follicle changes from a round to a tear-drop (pear) shape and the rim of the follicle becomes hyperechoic (appearing whiter).[6]

> - The increase in echogenicity of the follicular rim is more common than the change in shape of the follicle.[6]

- Follicular fluid becomes more echogenic immediately prior to ovulation.
- Care must be taken when interpreting the follicular shape as the ultrasound operator can cause the follicle to change shape by placing too much pressure on the ovary during the rectal examination.
- With the rise in estrogen on the first or second day of estrus, the uterus becomes edematous. Endometrial folds are visible and appear as a 'cartwheel', bicycle spokes, or 'tiger stripes' on the ultrasound screen (Fig. 6.8).

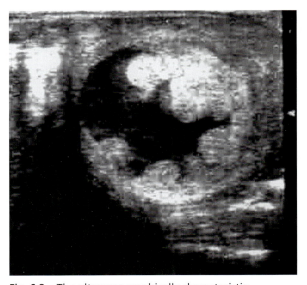

Fig. 6.8 The ultrasonographically characteristic 'cartwheel' or 'bicycle spoke' appearance of the estrous uterus.

- At 24–48 hours before ovulation, estrogen levels begin to decline, causing the image of the 'cartwheel' to break up.
  - ❏ As the edema decreases, the uterus develops a more homogeneous appearance.
- At 6–12 hours before ovulation, the ultrasonographic image of the dominant follicle changes from spherical to 'pear' shape, the follicular wall thickens and the density of the follicular fluid increases (see Fig. 5.30c).

Insemination techniques

The equipment required for insemination varies, depending on the type and volume of the semen to be used (frozen straws, 0.5–5 ml).

- An insemination pipette attached to a syringe (one-piece plastic plunger without a rubber tip), or an artificial insemination gun and disposable sheath may be used.
- All equipment should be kept at 37°C.
- Clean (preferably sterile) scissors are needed for cutting semen packages after thawing.

The mare must be prepared for insemination before the semen is thawed.

The procedure is always carried out using a sterile technique.[7] This is important both for hygiene and for fertility.

i. The mare is restrained suitably to ensure the safety of the operator.
ii. The tail is wrapped in a disposable plastic sleeve and bandaged to ensure that it does not slip during the procedure. It should be held to one side during the procedure.
iii. The perineal area is washed with soap and warm water and then dried with a clean towel. This is repeated two or three times to ensure that the lips of the vulva are clean, while ensuring that there is minimal contamination of the vestibule with soap, etc. Thorough rinsing with warm water is essential because many soaps and surgical scrubs are spermicidal or irritant to vaginal mucosa.
iv. If the mare is to be bred with fresh or cooled semen, the semen is drawn up into a sterile, nontoxic plastic syringe (rubber plungers can be spermicidal[8,9]) and fixed to a sterile insemination pipette.

Note:
- Cooled semen does not need to be warmed before breeding unless it has been extended in a cream gel extender.
- The semen supplier will usually supply documentary advice on the preparation of the semen.

v. The operator applies sterile obstetrical lubricant to the gloved hand/arm.
vi. The tip of the insemination pipette is covered by the hand, which is then inserted into the vagina of the mare.
vii. Once the fingers locate the cervix the index finger is used to guide the pipette tip into the cervix and then the pipette is passed approximately 1 cm into the uterus.
viii. The semen is injected slowly into the uterus ensuring that the whole dose is used. The pipette tip should be introduced well into the uterine body to decrease the risk of the semen spilling back through the cervix into the vagina.
ix. The hand is withdrawn and the tail bandage removed.

Management of mares to be bred with shipped, cooled semen

To breed mares successfully with shipped, cooled semen, and to minimize disappointments and financial losses, all parties involved need to cooperate in order to coordinate the semen shipments with the timing of the mare's ovulation. Before shipping semen, the attending veterinarian or a representative for the veterinarian should clarify several points with the stallion manager:

- The cost of stallion collection.
- The cost of preparing the semen for shipment, the number of collections provided gratis (if any), the cost of shipping semen tanks by air, and when and how the semen tanks must be returned.
- The days of the week the stallion is collected.
- Times during the breeding season when the stallion will not be available.
- The longevity of the semen.
- First-cycle conception rate of the stallion.
- The method of air transport used (same-day air or overnight shipment).

The breed registry requirements, and the number and timing of postinsemination clinical (pregnancy) examinations must be established. The attending veterinarian should clearly explain to the client the problems involved with shipping cooled semen. A pamphlet or notes explaining the process and logistics of the procedure can provide helpful information for clients, especially during a busy time of the year.

First-cycle conception rates tend to be lower with shipped semen than with natural breeding or with artificial insemination with a stallion housed at the same facility as the mare. Also, breeding management is more intensive and veterinary costs are higher. Stabling all mares to be bred with shipped cooled semen at a single facility, such as a veterinary clinic or suitable broodmare farm, saves the veterinarian time and the client money, compared with daily calls to the individual mare owner's farm. Many mare owners do not have a stallion to tease their mares nor are they familiar with the signs of estrus. Keeping the mares at a facility with a teaser stallion avoids this problem.

The highest pregnancy rates are achieved when mares are bred within the 24 hours before ovulation using semen of high fertility.[10] The quality of the semen to be used is clearly of paramount importance: stallions of low fertility usually have much lower conception rates than those with high inherent fertility. Furthermore, the handling of the semen is critical; failure to prepare it correctly as well as poor subsequent handling can make the process very disappointing. Important historical data that can be used to decide when to order a semen shipment include:

- Knowledge of the specific idiosyncrasies of the mare's estrous cycle, especially the number of days she is in estrus.
- The day and with what size follicle the mare typically ovulated in previous cycles. Once the mare owner has decided on the approximate week to breed the mare, the stallion manager should be notified; this notification should be no later than the first day of estrus.

Estrus can be determined by presenting the mare daily to a stallion or by performing ultrasound examinations of the reproductive tract every other day if no stallion is available. Serial serum progesterone can also be measured to determine where the mare is in her cycle. Vaginal examinations to determine the degree of cervical relaxation complement the ultrasound examinations. This is not a regularly repeated feature because the procedure can increase the contamination rate. Beginning on the second day of estrus, the mare's reproductive tract should be examined daily by rectal palpation and ultrasonographically.

- When the dominant follicle reaches 35 mm in diameter, semen should be ordered and a hormone administered to induce ovulation.
- The shipment of semen usually arrives within 24 hours. Particular care must be taken with weekend shipments, which can be significantly delayed.

This management method is not successful with all mares because some ovulate from a 30–35-mm follicle. The combination of the mare's history and the use of a stallion to identify estrus is critical for success in these cases.

If the mare's reproductive cycle is not known and she has a slowly developing dominant follicle, or if a mare historically ovulates from small follicles, semen should be ordered based on the mare's progression through that particular estrus. Either human chorionic gonadotropin or deslorelin is then given when the mare is bred or when semen is ordered.

The mare should be prepared for breeding before the semen tank is opened.

- When the semen tank is opened, the operator must immediately identify that the semen is from the correct stallion.

All but 1–2 ml of semen is used for insemination (see below for procedure and techniques of artificial insemination). Progressive motility is then determined from the remaining sample after it has been warmed to 37°C for 2–5 minutes.

- Progressive motility should be >30%.
- If the semen is not properly warmed, the percentage of progressively motile sperm determined may be erroneously low.

The insemination dose should contain at least 500 million progressively motile, morphologically normal sperm. The data derived from this examination are recorded and sent to the stallion's stud manager.

Twenty-four hours after insemination, the reproductive tract should be examined for intrauterine fluid accumulation and for ovulation. If fluid is present in the lumen, postbreeding treatment is warranted. If the mare does not ovulate within 36 hours of the insemination, she should be rebred.

Note:
- It is not uncommon for two bags of semen, each containing one dose of semen, to be sent in a shipment. Controversy exists as to whether both bags should be used for one insemination or whether the second bag should be refrigerated for 24 hours and introduced into the mare's uterus the next day. If the latter procedure is performed, the second bag must be placed in a covered Styrofoam cup at the back of the refrigerator until it is used.
- Many stallions have <30% progressively motile sperm if their semen is chilled for 48 hours or more, but the sperm have good motility if the semen is chilled for less than 24 hours.
- If semen is to remain chilled for more than 24 hours, longevity data should be obtained prior to its use.

If a mare is bred at the appropriate time over two estrous cycles with chilled semen from a fertile stallion and still does not conceive, a breeding soundness evaluation should be performed (see p. 128). Information on the stallion's first-cycle conception rates for that breeding season should also be obtained. Complete and thorough breeding records must be kept for the mare and of the quality of the semen inseminated, so that, in the event of failure, a cause can be identified.

Management of mares to be bred with frozen semen

Breeding mares with frozen/thawed semen often results in a significantly lower first-cycle pregnancy rate than that attained with either fresh semen or fresh cooled semen. Equine semen appears far less tolerant of the freezing process than bull semen. There is large variability among stallions in the ability of their semen to withstand freezing and thawing. There also appears to be some variation within an individual stallion in its ability to tolerate freezing and thawing at different times of the year and for different ejaculates.

- First-cycle pregnancy rates of 31–73% have been reported.
- The best (highest) conception rates are achieved using frozen semen from stallions of known fertility in young mares of known fertility which are examined every 6 hours, given human chorionic gonadotropin and inseminated before and/or directly after (within 4–6 hours) ovulation.
- To obtain the best pregnancy rate, frozen semen should be inseminated during the period from 12 hours before ovulation until 6 hours after ovulation.

There are various ways in which a mare can be managed during the insemination period, depending on the facilities and organization at the breeding farm.

- The examination of the reproductive tract should consist of manual palpation and ultrasonography.
- The maturing follicle should be evaluated for size and shape, and the uterus evaluated for endometrial folds, edema, and the presence of intraluminal fluid (see p. 217).
- An ovulatory agent (human chorionic gonadotropin or deslorelin) should be given to induce ovulation.

The ultrasonographic changes in combination with an ovulatory agent and rectal examinations performed at a minimum of every 12 hours and preferably every 8 hours will produce the greatest accuracy in the timing of ovulation.

The procedures described below can be adapted to local conditions.

If a mare is inseminated 36 hours after she receives human chorionic gonadotropin or deslorelin, there is a good chance of her being close to ovulation. However, there is a risk of missing the ovulation if the mare ovulates early. The following regime helps overcome this possibility:

- The reproductive tract is evaluated daily during early estrus until the follicle has reached 35 mm in diameter and endometrial folds are visualized ultrasonographically.
- Between 1500 and 3000 IU of human chorionic gonadotropin are then injected intravenously or a deslorelin implant is placed subcutaneously. The reproductive tract is carefully examined.
- Thereafter, the mare is examined 24 and 36 hours after hormone treatment.
- If, at 24 hours, the mare has ovulated, she should be inseminated immediately. If the follicle is still present 36 hours after hormone treatment, the mare should be inseminated.
- The reproductive tract should be re-examined ultrasonographically 8–12 hours after insemination. If the mare has not ovulated, she should be re-inseminated.

This regime reduces the period of intensive monitoring and, with a maximum of two inseminations, it should be effective for most mares. The system may be modified to accommodate an individual mare's estrous cycle and rate of follicle development.

Semen is usually packaged in 0.5–5-ml straws or in plastic or aluminum packets. The date of collection and the stallion's name should be printed on each package. Information on the method for thawing the semen and expected post-thaw motility should accompany the semen. Straws must be handled carefully as pregnancy may be reduced if the semen contacts tap water, detergents, or disinfectants.

- Temperature fluctuations and exposure to air or sunlight should also be avoided.

Thawing procedures vary, depending on the freezing method. Directions for thawing methodology should always accompany the semen shipment.

- Most straws are thawed in one or two water-baths at 37–48°C. The water-bath(s) must be large enough that the straws are completely submersed while they are being thawed.
- Only one insemination dose should be removed from the liquid nitrogen tank at a time. It should be placed quickly into the water-bath and left for the recommended time.
  - i. The label on the straw must be examined to ensure that the semen is from the correct stallion.
  - ii. If there is more than one dose in the canister, the canister should not be lifted above the neck of the tank.
  - iii. The straw must be dried well after it is removed from the water-bath.
  - iv. The label on the straw must again be examined to ensure that the semen is from the correct stallion.

v. Thawed semen that is not used for insemination must be discarded. Any attempt to re-freeze the thawed semen by re-immersing it in the liquid nitrogen will kill the sperm.

Semen can be transferred from a straw into an insemination pipette by many methods:

- It can be drained into a warmed receptacle and then sucked into a syringe.
- It can be left in the straw and directly inseminated into the mare using an artificial insemination gun.
- It can be drained into a syringe that is attached to a pipette.

Once thawed, the mare should be inseminated without delay because the semen will be irreparably damaged by unnecessary temperature fluctuations.

The reproductive tract must be examined 12–24 hours after insemination. If the mare has not ovulated, she should be inseminated again.

Whereas it is well established that 500×10^6 progressively motile sperm are required for optimal pregnancy rates using fresh semen,[11] the minimum breeding dose to optimize pregnancy rates is unknown for frozen semen, and it may be stallion-dependent. Insemination with dosages of 150 to 350×10^6 progressively motile spermatozoa (post thaw), performed close to ovulation, have been reported to result in acceptable pregnancy rates.[12,13]

It is therefore important that a small drop of semen from each dose used for insemination be evaluated at least for motility.

- The recommended dose varies from stallion to stallion, on the method of freezing the semen, on the country of origin and on the individual technicians freezing the semen.
- Doses ranging from 100 to 500 million progressively motile sperm have been suggested.
- Most investigators suggest that there be a minimum of 25% progressively motile sperm after thawing and warming to 37°C for at least 3 minutes.

Insemination of thawed sperm may induce a severe inflammatory reaction in some mares. These mares accumulate fluid within the uterine lumen after insemination. If fluid is visualized by ultrasonography, it is advisable to perform a uterine lavage by introducing Hartmann's solution or 0.9% saline solution until the efflux is clear and then administering oxytocin systemically.

EMBRYO TRANSFER

The practice of embryo transfer is widespread in many other large animals and, of course, man. In the horse, there have been major obstacles in the development of the technique, including:

- Nonacceptance of the offspring by certain breed societies, notably the Thoroughbred.
- Poor response to efforts to induce superovulation with hormone drugs, which means that multiple embryos are less often obtained in mares.

As a result, there has been a disappointing development of the technique over the last 20 years; however, as acceptance increases and technological advances are made, the procedure is likely to become an important stud technique. There are increasing numbers of commercial organizations that will undertake the procedure. Recently, technology that allows the short-term storage and transportation of equine embryos has been developed. This allows embryos to be collected in the field and then shipped to a centralized embryo-transfer facility for transfer into a suitable surrogate recipient mare. The ability to successfully ship embryos provides veterinarians with the opportunity to offer an embryo-transfer service to their clients without the burden of maintaining recipient mares.

The advantages of the procedure include:

- Mares can be bred during their performance careers without problem, and mares as young as 2 years of age can be bred. This improves the number of foals a mare can deliver during her 'breeding' life.
- Mares that are incapable for any reason of sustaining a pregnancy (e.g. older mares and those with physical or hormonal difficulties such as cervical incompetence, gross physical pelvic obstruction, or habitual early embryonic death) can be bred effectively using a surrogate mother.
- Improved numbers of genetically superior foals can be born to a single mare (by contrast, twin pregnancies are usually regarded as catastrophic, with a high rate of abortion or neonatal failure; see p. 242).
- Mares that consistently have twin ovulation can be bred effectively either by using two surrogate mothers or by re-implanting a single embryo.

Superovulation is commonly used in bovine, caprine, and ovine breeding programs with embryo transfer. In the horse, the result of superovulation is very disappointing. Not only are fewer ova shed, but fertilization rates are lower in multiple ovulating mares than in those with a single ovum.[14,15] Recent advances have, however, resulted in improved superovulation techniques.

- Twice-daily injections of 25 mg of crude equine pituitary gonadotropin, starting on day 6–8 after ovulation with an ovulation-inducing dose of human chorionic gonadotropin when the majority of the follicles have reached 35 mm in diameter, have been used to produce an average of 7–10 ovulations with a 50% viability ratio.[16]

In vitro fertilization of equine ova has so far proven largely disappointing, but some progress is likely to be made in this area also.[17] Artificial splitting of early embryos has recently been reported; and the first cloned foals have recently been born.[18]

Embryo-transfer techniques[19]

Management of donor mares

- The donor mare is bred (either naturally or by artificial insemination) in the normal fashion during estrus.
- The date of ovulation is noted and identified as day 0.
- Embryos are recovered between days 6 and 9 post ovulation.
- A collection catheter with an inflatable cuff of 50–75 ml is inserted into the uterus via the cervix; after the cuff is inflated the catheter is drawn firmly backwards so that the cervix is effectively sealed (Fig. 6.9).
- 1–2 liters of a specially formulated solution (usually modified Dulbecco's solution; i.e. phosphate-buffered saline with 1% fetal calf serum or newborn calf serum with penicillin 100 U/ml and streptomycin 100 mg/ml; warmed to approximately 36°C) are slowly introduced, under gravity feed alone, into the uterus via the catheter.
- The solution is drained immediately into a suitable sterile receptacle through a 0.75-mm embryo filter.

- The procedure is repeated three to four times (with simultaneous gentle massage of the uterus per rectum) before the catheter is deflated and removed.
  - ❏ Massage through the rectum aids in the suspension of the embryo in the flush medium and enhances recovery of fluid.
- The majority of the fluid infused into the uterus should be recovered. It should be clear and free of cellular debris or blood.
- At completion of the flush, fluid within the filter cup is poured into a sterile search dish with grid and a small amount of flush medium is used to rinse the filter.

Recovery, quality control and transport of embryos

- The fluid flushed from the uterus is carefully examined under a stereoscopic microscope using ×15 magnification to identify any embryo in the solution. There is usually only a single embryo (or at most two).
- Once an embryo is identified, it is washed by transferring it sequentially through several (3–10) 1-ml drops of holding medium which is an enriched formulation of the flush medium.
- After washing, the embryo is placed into a small Petri dish containing holding medium, and the embryo is examined at high magnification (×40–80) and graded on a scale of 1 (excellent) to 4 (poor). Some individuals have five grades, the fifth grade being for grossly degenerated embryos.

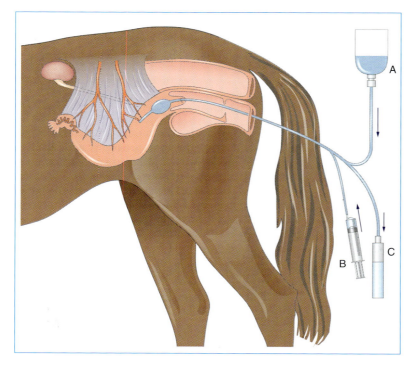

Fig. 6.9 Schematic drawing of nonsurgical recovery of embryos. (A) Fluid culture medium. (B) Air syringe to inflate cuff to ensure a good seal. (C) Aspiration of medium hopefully containing embryos.

- Identified embryo(s) are assessed carefully to ensure that they are normal for their age and to help assess the probability of maintenance of the pregnancy following transfer.[20]

Factors that affect the recovery and quality of the embryos include:

- The date of recovery relative to ovulation.
  - ❑ Recovery at 5 days is very unrewarding (10%).
  - ❑ Recovery rates of 70–80% can be expected at day 7 or 8 after ovulation.
  - ❑ After day 9, embryo viability falls significantly.
  - ❑ Embryos recovered at day 6 appear to be the best for freezing purposes.[21]
  - ❑ Embryo quality is graded on a scale of 1–5 (1=excellent, 5=grossly degenerated).[22]
  - ❑ Embryos of grades 3–5 carry a poor or hopeless prognosis for pregnancy when implanted (even if this is done immediately) and are not generally suitable for cryopreservation (freezing).
  - ❑ At 6–7 days the embryo should be about 0.2–0.4 mm in diameter.
- The quality of the semen and the method of insemination.
  - ❑ Significant differences are found in embryo recovery and quality from the use of different insemination methods and semen extenders.[23] Stallions with inherently low fertility would be expected to have a lower recovery rate.[24]
- The reproductive health and history of the mare.
  - ❑ Again this is fundamental to the recovery of embryos.[25] Mares with an abnormal uterine environment (inflammation, infection, fibrosis) present an inhospitable environment for the embryo even if only for a few days or hours and may decrease the chances of a successful transfer.

Equine embryos can be stored for up to 24 hours and will remain viable in transit if maintained at 5°C. This allows shipment of the embryo to a centralized embryo-transfer facility, which provides a suitable recipient mare.

Equine embryos can be stored in a tissue culture medium called Ham's F-10. Prior to use, the Ham's F-10 must be buffered by diffusing a mixture of 90% nitrogen, 5% oxygen and 5% carbon dioxide gas through the medium for 3–5 minutes. The medium is then supplemented with 10% newborn calf serum, penicillin and streptomycin. A new enriched medium is now available that does not require gas diffusion prior to its use. This facilitates field use and extends shelflife.

The embryo is added to the medium, and the container with the embryo is placed in a larger vessel that also has medium in it. The tops of the containers are sealed with paraffin wax and shipped in an equitainer used for shipment of cooled semen.

Management of the recipient mare

Recipient mares must be healthy and have no reproductive problems. Younger mares are preferred and 3–8-year-olds are probably best suited to the role. A full clinical and breeding soundness examination is compulsory.

Although nonsurgical transfer (i.e. via the cervix with manual catheterization using a guarded pipette or Cassou gun system) is technically the simplest procedure, surgical embryo transfer historically has a better success rate.[26] However, with the development of new insemination rods and clinical practice, nonsurgical transfer rates can equal those of surgical transfer rates.[27,28] In fact, most commercial operations are switching over to nonsurgical techniques. It seems that the highest overall percentage 'hold' is around 70–75%.[29] Subclinical infections and/or endometrial irritation during the procedure (bearing in mind that transfer is performed during diestrus) may significantly affect nonsurgical transfer. The overall pregnancy rates for fresh transfer are close to first-time conception rates for normal mating; thus in this area at least there may be less scope for improvement. Results from frozen embryos are disappointing compared with those in many other species.

Surgical embryo transfer is a specialized technique that involves a flank incision or may be performed more simply with specialized laparoscopic techniques.[30] It is unlikely that nonspecialist centers will undertake this procedure.

- Embryos are usually transferred between 6 and 8 days of age.
- Transfer of 9-day embryos is much more unreliable, possibly because of their apparently increased size, and fragility.[21]

A vital part of the procedure of embryo transfer is the synchronization of the donor and the recipient.

- Failure to correctly synchronize the age of the embryo with the recipient carries a much lower success rate.
- For maximum success, the donor and the recipient should ovulate within 24 hours of each other, but results are somewhat improved if the recipient ovulates 1–3 days after the donor.
- Success is decreased if the recipient ovulates before the donor.
- Synchronization of estrus and careful ovarian assessment is vital for success.
- If frozen embryos are to be used, synchronization may be easier as the ovulation of each mare can be accurately identified. However, there may be losses from the freezing process itself.

Methods for freezing and thawing of equine embryos are well established. Usually the embryos are assessed for quality (see above) and most are stored in culture medium for 12–24 hours before freezing.[31] Inevitably there is a lower pregnancy rate when embryos are stored in this fashion.

- Cryopreservation of equine embryos is a highly specialized technique involving storage in liquid nitrogen at −196°C.
- The loss of embryo viability is still higher than for many of the other species in which these techniques are commonly practiced; further research is therefore needed.

- The techniques of in vitro fertilization involving surgical or laparoscopic aspiration of ova from preovulatory follicles are not yet well established in horses, but there are reports of successful pregnancies.[15]

REFERENCES

1. Rossdale PD, Ricketts SW. Equine stud farm medicine. 2nd edn. London: Baillière Tindall; 1980:126–130.
2. Bowen JM, Tobin N, Simpson RB, et al. Effects of washing on the bacterial flora of the stallion's penis. Journal of Reproduction and Fertility Supplement 1982; 32:41–45.
3. Jones RL, Squires EL, Slade NP, et al. The effect of washing on the aerobic bacterial flora of the stallion's penis. Proceedings of the American Association of Equine Practitioners 1984:9–16.
4. Samper JC. Ultrasonographic appearance and the pattern of uterine edema in mares. Proceedings of the 43rd Annual American Association of Equine Practitioners 1997:189–191.
5. Meyers P, Wolfgang J, Trigg T. Acceleration of ovulation in the mare with the use of the GnRH analog, desorelin acetate. Proceedings of the 40th Annual American Association of Equine Practitioners 1994;13–14.
6. Gastal EL, Gastal MO, Ginther OJ. Ultrasound follicular characteristics for predicting ovulation on the following day in mares. Theriogenology 1998; 49:257–262.
7. Kenney RM, Bergman RV, Cooper WL, et al. Minimal contamination techniques for breeding mares: technique and preliminary findings. Proceedings of the American Association of Equine Practitioners 1975:327–336.
8. Jones WE. Toxic agents in equine AI procedures. Equine Veterinary Data 1984; 5:219–221.
9. Broussard JR, Roussel JD, Hibbard M, et al. The effects of Monoject and AirTite syringes on equine spermatozoa. Theriogenology 1990; 33:200–204.
10. Palmer E. Factors affecting stallion semen survival and fertility. Proceedings of the Tenth International Congress on Animal Reproduction and Artificial Insemination 1984:377.
11. Householder DD, Pickett BW, Voss JL, Olar TT. Effect of extender, number of spermatozoa and hCG on equine fertility. Equine Veterinary Science 1981; 1:9–13.
12. Vidament M, Dupere AM, Julienne P, et al. Equine frozen semen: freezability and fertility field results. Theriogenology 1997; 48:905–917.
13. Leipold SD, Graham JK, Squires EL, et al. Effect of spermatozoal concentration and number on fertility of frozen equine semen. Theriogenology 1998; 49:1537–1543.
14. Douglas RH. Review of induction of superovulation and embryo transfer in the equine. Theriogenology 1979; 11:33–46.
15. Palmer E, Bezard J, Magistrini M, et al. In vitro fertilization of the horse. A retrospective study. Journal of Reproduction and Fertility Supplement 1991; 44:375–384.
16. Alvarenga MA, McCue PM, Squires EL, et al. Improvement of ovarian superovulatory response and embryo production in mares treated with equine pituitary extract twice daily. In: Katila T, Wade J, eds. Equine embryo transfer. Havermeyer foundation monograph 5. Newmarket: R&W Publications; 2000:38.
17. Morris L. Artificial reproductive technology in the horse. Proceedings of the British Equine Veterinary Association Congress, Birmingham, 2000:121.
18. Hinrichs K, Shin T, Love CC, et al. Comparison of bovine and equine oocytes as host cytoplasts for equine nuclear transfer. In: Katila T, Wade J, eds. Equine embryo transfer. Havermeyer foundation monograph 5. Newmarket: R&W Publications; 2000.
19. Squires EL. Embryo transfer. In: McKinnon AO, Voss JL, eds. Equine reproduction. Philadelphia: Lea & Febiger; 1992:357–367.
20. McKinnon AO, Squires EL. Morphological assessment of equine embryos. Journal of the American Veterinary Medical Association 1988; 192:401–406.
21. Squires EL, Cook VM, Voss JL. Collection and transfer of equine embryos. Animal reproduction laboratory bulletin no. 1. Fort Collins: Colorado State University; 1985.
22. Slade NP, Takeda T, Squires EL, et al. A new procedure for the cryopreservation of equine embryos. Theriogenology 1985; 24:45–58.
23. Squires EL, Amman RP, McKinnon AO, et al. Fertility of equine spermatozoa cooled to 5 or 20°C. Proceedings of the International Congress of Animal Reproduction and Artificial Insemination, Dublin, 1988:297–300.
24. Douglas RH. Review of induction of superovulation and embryo transfer in the equine. Theriogenology 1979; 11:33–46.
25. Cook VC, Squires EL. Results from a commercial embryo transfer programme. Equine Veterinary Journal Supplement 1985; 32:405–408.
26. Iuliano MF, Squires EL, Shideler RK. Effect of age of embryo and method of transfer on pregnancy rate. Theriogenology 1985; 31:631–642.
27. Foss R, Wirth N, Schiltz P, et al. Nonsurgical embryo transfer in a private practice. Proceedings of the Annual Convention of the American Association of Equine Practitioners 1999; 45:210–212.
28. Vanderwall DK. Current equine embryo transfer techniques. Proceedings West Coast Equine Reproduction Symposium 2001:115–122.

29. Squires EL, Juliano MF, Shideler RK. Factors affecting success of surgical and non-surgical equine embryo transfer. Theriogenology 1982; 17:35–41.

30. Neal H, Morris L, Wilsher S, et al. Laparoscopic embryo transfer. Proceedings of the British Equine Veterinary Association Congress, Birmingham 2000:117.

31. Carnevale EM, Squires EL, McKinnon AO. Comparison of Ham's F10 with CO_2 or Hepes buffer for storage of equine embryos at 5°C for 24 hours. Journal of Animal Science 1987; 65:1775–1781.

Chapter 7
PREGNANCY

Michelle LeBlanc,
Cheryl Lopate,
Derek Knottenbelt

The objective of a successful reproductive program is to produce the maximum possible number of live, healthy and athletic foals each year from the pool of mares at stud.[1] After an uneventful delivery, the foal should grow into a productive adult. The economic consequences of a good or bad fertility for a stud are incalculable. Failure to realize the potential of a valuable stallion results in a poorer value and an economic downturn; the converse is also true. The benefits of successful progeny are easy to appreciate. In stud medicine, assessment of fertility is taken to include the realization of athletic performance of the progeny. Without a successful progeny record even the best performing stallion will inevitably end up with a lower commercial value/reputation than a stallion whose progeny consistently achieve success in the chosen performance arena.

- A survey carried out of the wastage in the Thoroughbred industry in the UK revealed that over 45% of mares sent to stud failed to produce a useful foal. This included about 22% that failed to conceive, 10% that delivered dead or nonviable foals, and a further 14% that had foals that were never named (thus implying that they were not of suitable quality or that they had died).[2]
- This represents a significant infertility rate in the Thoroughbred breeding population that must have a significant bearing on the industry itself.
- There is little evidence of similar surveys for other breeds, but it is quite likely that certain of the categories reported in this study are typical of other breeds also.

In order to maximize the potential of breeding programs, the breeder and the veterinarian must have a good understanding of:

- The estrous cycle.
- The characteristics of a normal pregnancy.
- The factors involved in a normal or successful delivery and the management of:
  - ❑ The stallion.
  - ❑ The mare.
  - ❑ The neonatal foal.

EARLY EVENTS

Pregnancy occurs as a result of fertilization of an oocyte with a spermatozoon, and subsequent maturation of the ensuing embryo with its passage into the uterus (Fig. 7.1).[3–5] The ovum has undergone one meiotic division close to ovulation and the first polar body is typically extruded before it enters the oviduct. Fertilization of the oocyte with a single spermatozoon occurs in the ampulla of the oviduct; this stimulates

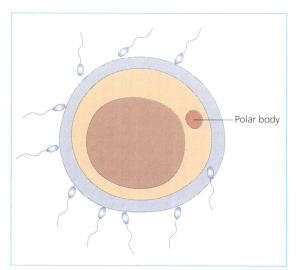

Fig. 7.1 Fertilization of the oocyte. A single spermatazoon will penetrate the oocyte, blocking the penetration of further spermatozoa.

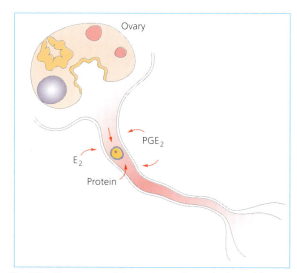

Fig. 7.2 Transport of the embryo through the oviduct. This is facilitated by the production of prostaglandin (PGE$_2$), oxytocin, local hormones (E) and proteins by the ovary, endometrium, oviduct, and embryo.

the completion of meiosis and the early development of the embryo. The embryo enters the uterus as a compact morula 5–6 days after ovulation. The uterine proteins and secretions provide a suitable environment for the developing embryo.

Typically, only fertilized eggs will pass from the oviduct into the uterus. The mechanism that allows a fertilized egg to enter the uterus, but precludes an unfertilized one, is unknown.[6,7] Prostaglandin E$_2$ (PGE$_2$), oxytocin and local hormones, or even proteins produced by the embryo and/or uterine tube themselves, may stimulate embryo transport (Fig. 7.2).

Once the embryo enters the uterus, it sheds its original outer coating (the zona pellucida) and develops a new smooth capsule as a result of the action of uterine proteins or secretions.[8] This capsule protects the embryo during its stage of active migration through the uterus. The capsule is not shed until the amnion is complete, at around day 20 of pregnancy, thereby providing protection to the embryo proper until its placental protection is produced. The capsule may also provide protection from maternal white blood cells and antibodies.

Although a chemical factor associated with early pregnancy (early pregnancy factor) can be recognized as early as 48 hours after conception,[9] the pregnancy is very unstable at this stage and so its use for pregnancy diagnosis is probably not helpful. The embryo migrates through the entire uterus from day 6 until day 15–16 post ovulation.[10] Movement is maximal between days 11 and 14. The migration appears to be necessary for maternal recognition of pregnancy. The embryo contacts the entire endometrial surface repeatedly as a result of uterine contractility and continues until the size of the embryo precludes its movement, along with an increase in uterine tone due to persistently high levels of progesterone. The cessation of movement of the embryo is called fixation (Fig. 7.3) and typically occurs at the base of one of the uterine horns.[11,12] The embryo is thought to produce factors that prevent release of PGF$_{2\alpha}$ from the endometrium, thereby allowing maintenance of the corpus luteum within the ovary. The developing embryo will begin to produce estrogens at about day 12 of pregnancy. Estrogens may increase the mobility of the embryo. The production of estrogen from the embryo and progesterone from the primary corpus luteum results in a marked increase in tone in the uterus.[13] This is one of the cardinal diagnostic signs of early pregnancy.

Maternal recognition

Maternal recognition of pregnancy occurs between days 14 and 16.[14–16] This is the point at which PGF$_{2\alpha}$ would normally be produced to result in regression of the corpus luteum and the instigation of the next estrous cycle. In the pregnant mare this does not occur and so the next cycle is suspended. PGF$_{2\alpha}$ is normally produced by the endometrium and is carried by the local circulation to the ovary with the corpus luteum, resulting in the latter's demise (Fig. 7.4).[17–20] The embryo must be present in the uterus for maternal recognition of pregnancy. It has yet to be proven if the embryo produces a factor that blocks or inhibits PGF$_{2\alpha}$ production by the endometrium. Movement of the embryo along the endometrial surface until days 15–16, when it becomes fixed within one of the horns, blocks the release of PGF$_{2\alpha}$ from the endometrium. Blockage of PGF$_{2\alpha}$ release maintains the corpus luteum. The embryo must have access to at least 50%

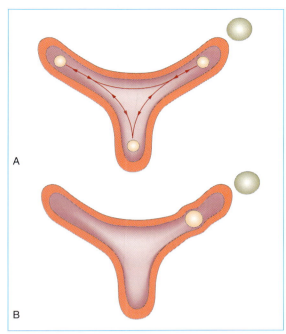

A

B

Fig. 7.3 Embryo motility and fixation. (A) Mobility phase: in early pregnancy when uterine tone is good and the embryo is small, uterine motility moves the embryo along the entire lumen of the uterus. Embryonic factors produced by the embryo and/or endometrium are released, resulting in maternal recognition of pregnancy. The embryo will migrate throughout the entire uterus many times. (B) Fixation phase: as uterine tone increases and embryonic size increases, the embryo becomes trapped in the uterine lumen. Fixation usually occurs near the body/bifurcation junction (more rarely in the body or tip of a horn).

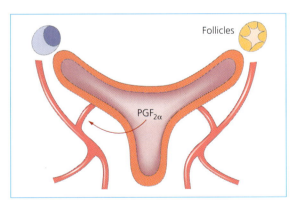

Fig. 7.4 Luteolysis. $PGF_{2\alpha}$ is produced by the endometrium, released into the local circulation and carried to the ovary, resulting in the demise of the corpus luteum.

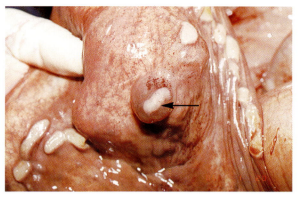

Fig. 7.5 Endometrial cups (day 70). Note the normal interrupted ring of cups on the uterine wall. The arrow indicates an endometrial cup implanted on a uterine cyst.

mare's uterus between days 10 and 20 of pregnancy. It has been suggested that the continuation of the corpus luteum (through blocking of $PGF_{2\alpha}$ secretion) results in maintenance of the pregnancy.

- The equine conceptus is called an embryo until day 40 of pregnancy and is called a fetus thereafter.[21] At or immediately before delivery it is commonly referred to as the foal.
- Attachment of the placenta to the endometrium occurs gradually, beginning around days 36–40 of pregnancy, and continues until day 150 when placentation is complete.
- Around day 25 of pregnancy, endometrial cup formation begins.[22] The endometrial cup cells are specialized trophoblasts produced by the developing conceptus that form the chorionic girdle, an annular band of tissue which invades the epithelium of the uterus starting at about 35–38 days of pregnancy. There is a generous supply of lymphatic vessels in the area of the endometrial cups; this is probably important for the transport of lymphatic fluid involved in the immune recognition of the embryo by the maternal immune system. The endometrial cups can be seen on the endometrial surface as pale shallow cups of tissue in the pregnant horn. The endometrial cups produce equine chorionic gonadotropin (eCG; formerly known as pregnant mare serum gonadotropin). The cups continue to increase in size until day 70 of pregnancy at which time they begin to degenerate (Fig. 7.5). They will continue to produce eCG until days 120–150 when degeneration is complete; they then cease functioning completely. eCG is also thought to assist in immune regulation during early pregnancy.
- During the first 3 weeks of pregnancy the yolk sac is the predominant structure of the newly forming placental unit. At around day 30 of pregnancy, the formation of the allantois begins

of the uterine lumen for maternal recognition of pregnancy to occur.

Estradiol, estrone and uteroferrin concentrations increase significantly in the lumen of the pregnant

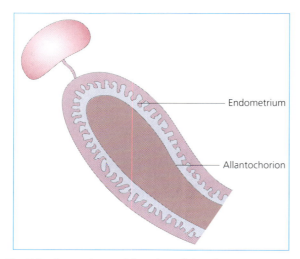

Fig. 7.6 Formation and function of the placenta. Microvilli are formed by the allantochorion and invade the endometrium to form a link between the maternal and fetal circulations in the placenta. Microcotyledons transport nutrients to the fetus and waste products from the fetus.

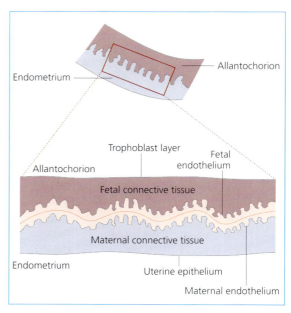

Fig. 7.7 The six layers of the placenta.

to dominate the placental unit. The yolk sac is visible through the second month of pregnancy. The allantois and the chorion will fuse and attach to the endometrium to form the placenta, which will be present for the remainder of the pregnancy. The formation of the placenta occurs slowly. The entire endometrial surface is encompassed with placental attachment by day 80 of pregnancy. The allantochorion will invade the endometrium by the attachment of tiny finger-like structures known as microvilli or microcotyledons (Fig. 7.6).[23] These tiny invasions of the endometrium allow fetal nutrition and facilitate waste management and transference of substances (proteins, hormones, etc.) across the placental membranes. Microvilli are initially noted by day 40 of pregnancy and continue to develop beyond day 100. They provide for the exchange of nutrients, blood, oxygen, and other molecules between the mare and the fetus (Fig. 7.6).

Placentation in the mare is described as epitheliochorial.[24,25] This term is used to describe the fact that the maternal endometrial epithelium and the fetal chorion are intact and this has implications for the function of the placenta.

There are six layers involved in the placenta of the mare (Fig. 7.7):

- The maternal vascular endothelium (lining of the blood vessels on the maternal side).
- The maternal connective tissue.
- The uterine epithelium.
- The trophoblast layer.
- The fetal connective tissue.

- The fetal vascular endothelium (lining of the blood vessels on the fetal side).

- The thickness of the placental attachment decreases as pregnancy length increases, allowing for more efficient transport of the necessary nutrients and molecules in both directions as the fetus increases in size and its nutrient demands and waste products increase.

Between the microvilli are the uterine glands. These glands produce proteins and secretions, sometimes called uterine milk, which facilitate maintenance of early pregnancy and the exchange of molecules to and from the maternal and fetal circulation.

ENDOCRINOLOGY OF PREGNANCY[26]

The hormonal profile during the first 2 weeks of pregnancy is similar to that of the non-pregnant mare (Fig. 7.8). The differences in hormone concentrations start at day 14, when prostaglandin would normally increase with a subsequent decrease in progesterone. It is the maternal recognition of pregnancy that accounts for the continued production of progesterone because prostaglandin is not released. Maternal recognition of pregnancy has been described on p. 228. The primary corpus luteum (corpus luteum of ovulation) is the sole source of progesterone until day 35.

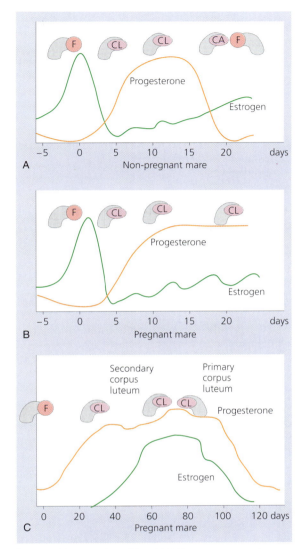

Fig. 7.8 Hormonal profile of (A) the nonpregnant mare and (B) the pregnant mare during the first 20 days of pregnancy, and of (C) the pregnant mare during the first 120 days of pregnancy. F, follicle; CL, corpus luteum; CA, corpus albicans.

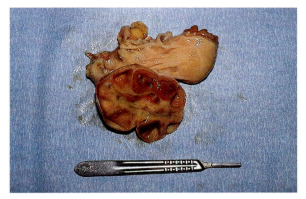

Fig. 7.9 Multiple corpora lutea may assist the maintenance of the early pregnancy prior to the development of a fully functional placenta.

Equine chorionic gonadotropin (eCG)

At day 25 endometrial cup formation begins, followed by the production of eCG from the cup cells at around day 36.[27,28] eCG has biologic activities similar to those of follicle-stimulating hormone and luteinizing hormone. The function of eCG is unclear. It was previously thought that it stimulated development of secondary follicles and the formation of secondary or accessory corpora lutea. However, experiments have established that continued rhythmic secretion of follicle-stimulating hormone during pregnancy stimulates growth of secondary follicles.[29,30] The luteinizing hormone-like component of eCG causes luteinization and/or ovulation of already mature follicles. This

luteinization is considered to be responsible for the rise in serum progesterone concentrations observed between days 40 and 70. eCG stimulates primary and secondary corpora lutea to continue producing progesterone until days 100–120 of pregnancy. By 150–200 days of gestation all corpora lutea will have regressed. The supplemental progesterone produced by the secondary corpora lutea assists in the maintenance of pregnancy until the placenta is fully functional (Fig. 7.9). eCG may be also involved in the formation of an immunoprotective barrier that slows rejection of the 'foreign' fetal cells during the first half of gestation[31].

The estrous cycle is blocked by eCG for the duration of the life of the endometrial cups. Once pregnant beyond 38–40 days, mares do not return to estrus until 110–130 days from the original ovulation date. Abortion, whether from natural causes or induced, does not alter this course.

- Assessing eCG concentrations can be used to diagnose pregnancy.[32]

Progesterone and progestins during pregnancy

For the first half of gestation, progesterone from luteal tissue supports pregnancy. Luteal progesterone levels peak at about day 100 and subside to baseline by about day 180–200. After day 200, levels of progesterone in the dam's serum are negligible. Small amounts of progesterone can be identified in the dam's serum after 305–310 days of gestation. This late rise in progesterone peaks at about 5 days prior to parturition.

The combination of fetus and placenta makes significant contributions to the endocrine patterns of pregnant mares. The unit is responsible for the production of progesterone, progestins, estrogens, and relaxin. Before day 60, a small amount of circulating progesterone and 5α-pregnanes (progestins) are produced by the fetoplacental unit. At around day

90, serum concentrations of 5α-pregnanes increase, only to level off at about 180 days of gestation. Concentrations remain relatively constant in maternal serum until days 305–310 of gestation when they begin a dramatic rise, peaking about 5 days before parturition.[33]

The rise in progestins in the last 3 weeks of gestation is thought to be associated with maturation of the fetal adrenals. Uteroplacental progestin production rises in late gestation, concurrent with an increase in fetal pregnenolone output probably from the fetal adrenals which increase in weight during the last month of gestation. The decline in plasma progestins over the last 1–2 days prepartum occurs in parallel with a substantial surge in fetal plasma cortisol and maturation of the equine fetus.[34]

Estrogens

Estrogen remains relatively low in pregnant mares until day 35, when it suddenly increases. It is produced by ovarian luteal tissue and reaches levels exceeding those during estrus. Presumably its rise is associated with secretion of eCG. Ovarian sources of estrogens gradually subside by about day 120.

The fetoplacental unit also produces significant levels of estrogens, some of which are derived from the fetal gonads and some from the placenta.[35]

There are eight types of estrogenic compounds produced by the fetoplacental unit. A second surge in estrogens occurs around day 60 of pregnancy when estrogens synthesized by the fetoplacental unit appear in the circulation. A massive rise continuing from day 70 to day 100 is only likely to occur in mares with normal fetal development. Estrogen production appears to follow gonadal size closely, peaking at about day 210–240, and gradually decreasing, though still detectable, as gestation continues to term. The elevated levels of conjugated estrogens can be used as a pregnancy test in the horse by immunoassay of blood, urine or milk from day 45 to term (Fig. 7.10).

- Measuring levels of total estrogens in the blood or urine of the pregnant mare can assess fetal viability.
- Depending on the stage of pregnancy, either total estrogens or eCG can be measured to determine the normality of fetal development (Table 7.1).
- eCG is also believed to be involved in stimulating estrogen production from the ovaries in early pregnancy (beginning at day 35 of pregnancy). eCG is thought to stimulate estrogen production through its ability to invoke luteal steroidogenesis.

Summary of hormonal events of pregnancy

Equine chorionic gonadotropin (eCG)

- eCG is secreted by the endometrial cups. It is detectable as early as day 35, peaks around day 60 and then gradually falls, to disappear by day 125.
- eCG has follicle-stimulating hormone and luteinizing hormone properties.
- eCG drives the formation of secondary corpora lutea (through its luteinizing effects)[36] from the

Table 7.1 Equine chorionic gonadotropin and total estrogen concentrations during pregnancy

	Days of gestation			
	35–120	90–200	200–240	240–300
Equine chorionic gonadotropin (pg/liter)	5–30	5–30	<1	<1
Total estrogen (pg/ml)	<50	50–175	175–250	250–400

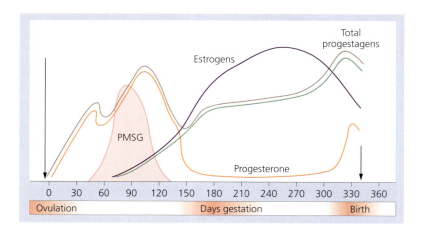

Fig. 7.10 Estrogen elevation in blood, urine or milk can be used as a test of a viable pregnancy after day 45. eCG, equine chorionic gonadotropin.

large number of follicles that form from the action of pituitary follicle-stimulating hormone.

- The luteinizing effects result in the rise in serum progesterone concentrations between day 40 and day 70 and may also be responsible for some of the antirejection effects that enable the embryo to survive rejection by the uterine environment.
- Measurement of eCG is a useful indicator of pregnancy between day 40 and day 120.
- The estrous cycle is blocked by eCG production from the endometrial cups. This explains why, once a mare is pregnant beyond 40 days, she will not return to estrus until the cups regress at around day 120 from the ovulation date. Once formed, the endometrial cups persist up to day 120 whether pregnancy is maintained or not. Therefore, false-positive pregnancy tests (for eCG) are possible if the mare has lost the pregnancy after day 40.
- During the period when the endometrial cups are dominant, neither prostaglandin nor saline infusions will be effective in inducing a fertile estrous cycle.

- Because therapeutic abortion cannot be induced between day 40 and day 120, decisions for manipulation of estrus and pregnancy must be made before day 35–40. This is particularly important for a twin pregnancy (see p. 242); if a twin pregnancy is detected after day 40 there is little chance that the mare can be bred for several months and will probably mean that the season is lost.

Progestins (progestogens)

- The fetoplacental unit (comprising the fetus itself and the placenta) produces progestins.
- In the early stages of pregnancy (before day 60) the fetoplacental unit produces a small amount of progesterone.
- Small amounts of progesterone can be detected in the mare's blood before 5 months and after 10 months.[37] However, total progestins remain high for the duration of the pregnancy; this is due to the secretion of other progestins (such as 5α-pregnane) by the fetoplacental unit.
- Serum progesterone assay (in which total progestins are assayed) may therefore be used to indicate pregnancy after day 60.
- The rise in total progestins in the last month of pregnancy corresponds with maturation of the fetal adrenal glands. Increases in fetal adrenocorticotropin in late gestation stimulate the fetal adrenal glands to produce pregnenolone. The fetal adrenal glands cannot convert progesterone to cortisol as it is lacking the enzyme 17α-hydroxylase needed for conversion.

Therefore, pregnenolone is converted to progesterone which is likely reduced to progestins within the fetoplacental unit.[38]

- A premature rise in progestins (before 305 days) indicates fetal stress or precocious maturation, whereas a drop is usually observed in fetal demise.[34,39]

Estrogens

- From day 35, the concentration of estrone sulfate in the mare's blood increases. This is also reflected in a urinary increase.
- Estrone sulfate is predominately secreted by the developing fetus and the fetal membranes.[40]
- Estrone sulfate is an index of fetal viability as well as of pregnancy. Because this hormone is produced only by a viable fetus, any drop in urinary estrone sulfate concentration (and less sensitively in the mare's blood) between day 60 and term should be viewed as indicating fetal death/compromise. Almost no foal is viable when this occurs.

Fetal cortisol

The equine fetus only matures in the last week of gestation. Inducing parturition before this time will result in a premature foal that likely dies in the first few days of life.[41]

DIAGNOSIS OF PREGNANCY

Safe, early and reliable diagnosis of pregnancy is an essential part of stud farm management, without which overall fertility rates would probably be much lower. There are obvious advantages to establishing that a mare is pregnant and that the pregnancy is (at least at the stage of the examination) normal. Early embryonic death is a relatively common event in mares (see p. 240) and the development of a pseudo-pregnancy may seriously affect the future fertility of the mare. A standard protocol of diagnosis therefore needs to be used to define the best stages at which to confirm a pregnancy. Early loss of a pregnancy or a nonpregnancy-related cessation of cyclicity might result in serious financial loss for the owner. However, at least if the problems can be defined early, suitable measures may be taken to re-establish a pregnancy. Furthermore, one of the most important aspects of diagnosis is the detection of twin pregnancy at a stage at which manipulations are possible (or at least so that reproductive cyclicity can be restarted completely).

Pregnancy can be diagnosed by a variety of methods.

Absence of estrus

A diagnosis of pregnancy may be suspected by nonreturn to estrus at 17–21 days post ovulation. In a breeding mare, the absence of estrus must be regarded as strongly suggestive of pregnancy. However, not all mares that fail to demonstrate estrus will be pregnant because of a variety of factors, including, but not limited to, early embryonic death or retained corpus luteum.

False-positives and false-negatives are common when estrous behavior alone is monitored.

- Estrous behavior may be 'silent' or at least not overtly visible in mares that are out of contact with stallions.
- The length of the estrous cycle is sufficiently variable to make this an unreliable method.
- Nonpregnant mares (particularly lactating mares with foals at foot early in the season) may not return to estrus after mating, thereby giving the impression of pregnancy.
- Some mares will show prolonged diestrus due to persistence of the corpus luteum.
- Pregnant mares may show estrous behavior.
  - ❏ The implications for this are obvious.
  - ❏ A mare in this state might be restrained to allow mating to take place or she might be subjected to hormonal treatments. Either of these procedures could result in the loss of a normal pregnancy.

Rectal examination (see Table 7.2)

Rectal examination after 30 days is probably the most economical method of diagnosis, but the experience and skill of the operator are important factors. There are important (unavoidable) risks involved in the rectal examination of any horse.

- Palpation of a 16–19-day pregnancy will indicate the existence of good to excellent uterine tone (the uterus feels singularly firm and turgid), and the cervix will be tightly closed (Fig. 7.11).
- By day 20 the embryonic vesicle can be palpated by an experienced practitioner using rectal examination only. However, it is difficult to determine if twins are present at this stage of the pregnancy by palpation alone, especially if they are unilaterally fixed (see p. 242).
- At day 20–21 there is a palpable ventral bulge at the uterine bifurcation, uterine tone is very good to excellent and the cervix is becoming narrow and elongated.
- By day 30 the ventral enlargement of the pregnant horn is quite prominent. Uterine tone directly surrounding the bulge is decreased, but tone in the tip of the gravid horn and of the entire nongravid horn is very good to excellent. The size of the bulge continues to increase, while the tone surrounding it decreases with time.
- By day 50 the uterine fluid involves the mid-uterine horn and the uterine body at the bifurcation. The uterine horn tips still have good to excellent tone. The cervix remains tightly closed throughout the pregnancy.
- As the pregnancy progresses, the uterus increases in size and gravitates into the abdominal cavity. The ovaries may be noticeably closer together (more towards the midline). Because the fetus is small and there is significant fluid surrounding it, actual palpation, or ballottement, of the fetus is not usually possible until much later in the pregnancy. The uterus of a mare with a pyometra (see p. 183) may be mistaken for a pregnancy of

Table 7.2 Palpation and ultrasound findings in diagnosis of early pregnancy

| | Days of gestation | | | | | |
	12–16	16–18	18–24	24–30	30–60	60+
Uterine tone (0 = flaccid, 5 = excellent)	3	4	5	5	5 (nonpregnant horn) 4 (pregnant horn)	5 (nonpregnant horn) 4 (pregnant horn)
Vesicular bulge	Absent	Slight difference in uterine diameter	Present	Present	Fluid-filled pregnant horn	Fluid-filled pregnant horn; partial distention of nonpregnant horn
Cervix	Closed	Tightly closed	Narrow and elongated		Tightly closed	
Ultrasound	Round vesicle	Round, oblong or triangular vesicle	Triangular vesicle; trophoblast/ embryo visible	Ovoid vesicle; heartbeat visible	Irregularly round vesicle; embryo/ fetus evident	

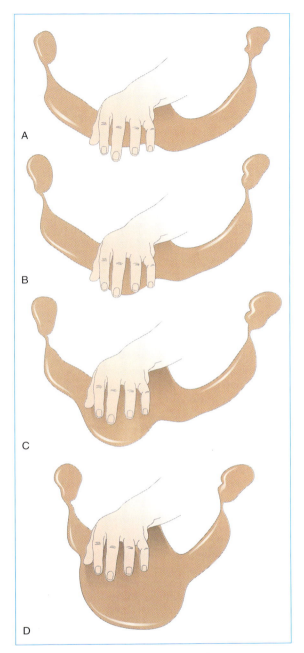

Fig. 7.11   Rectal examination of an early pregnancy at: (A) 33 days; (B) 42 days; (C) 60 days; (D) 90 days. The obvious palpable characteristics are: characteristically excellent uterine tone; a ventral bulge in the pregnant horn; a narrow elongated cervix.

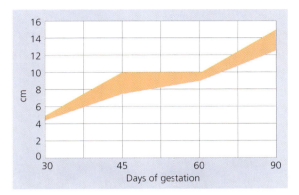

Fig. 7.12   Diameter of the pregnant horn containing the conceptus between gestation days 30 and 90 in a Thoroughbred mare.

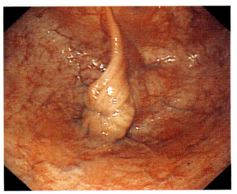

Fig. 7.13   The vaginoscopic appearance of a pregnant (closed) cervix.

of a fetus by comparison with standard measurements for head or limb size (see Fig. 7.12).

Vaginal examination

Direct visualization of the cervix using a vaginoscope (or an endoscope), or direct palpation, can be used to aid the diagnosis of pregnancy.[42]

Vaginoscopic examination has largely been replaced by rectal palpation. Nevertheless, detectable changes are obvious at an early stage. In early pregnancy the cervix has a pale appearance and is tightly closed.[43] It is frequently pulled to one side in the vagina (Fig. 7.13).

Ultrasonographic examination (see Table 7.2; Fig. 7.14)

The value of ultrasonographic examination for the diagnosis and assessment of pregnancy is undisputed; it is probably the most important advance in our ability to monitor pregnancy.[44] Its ability to detect very early pregnancy with a high degree of accuracy (with an experienced operator) means that fertility rates can be

70 days or more, but the uterus will have a doughy 'dull' feel, which is quite atypical of a pregnancy.

- Rectal palpation of the fetus is easily performed beyond 120 days of pregnancy, as the fetal size increases in relationship to the volume of uterine fluid. It becomes increasingly easy to identify the fetus and so it may be possible to estimate the age

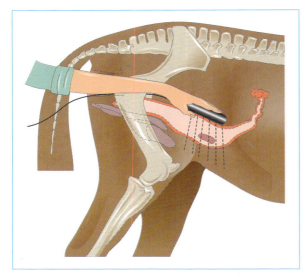

Fig. 7.14 Diagrammatic representation of transrectal ultrasonographic diagnosis of pregnancy.

significantly improved.[45] Modern ultrasound machines are small, portable and robust. The definition obtained by these is often remarkable and very subtle changes can easily be detected. Apart from its obvious benefits in pregnancy diagnosis, ultrasonography is routinely used to investigate uterine and ovarian health and status. The procedure itself has no known dangers, although the risks of rectal examination should never be ignored.

Although ultrasonography can aid in pregnancy diagnosis, it is not a replacement for rectal palpation, because ultrasonography cannot measure uterine and cervical tone, or the presence of some abnormalities of the broad ligaments, ovaries, uterus and cervix, which are important factors in the determination of the normality of a pregnancy. Additionally, a solitary uterine cyst may be confused with a vesicle, resulting in the misdiagnosis of pregnancy. Early embryonic death may be difficult to distinguish using either palpation or ultrasonography until sufficient changes occur to differentiate it from a normal pregnancy.

- Before day 14. Examination for pregnancy before day 14 requires careful examination of the uterus with a high quality 5- or 7.5-MHz ultrasound transducer. Ultrasonography can be utilized to evaluate pregnancy between days 9 and 16 before any detectable palpable changes will be present. The ultrasonographic characteristics of the early embryonic vesicle are shown in Fig. 7.15. The embryonic vesicle is about 2 mm in diameter on days 8–9 of pregnancy.
- Days 16–19. From a practical standpoint, ultrasound examination can often be delayed until days 18–20. The embryonic vesicle is typically 15 mm at 15 days of gestation.
- Day 18. The ultrasound evaluation will reveal a slightly elongated or triangular shape to the vesicle and the outline is less regular.
- Days 19–20. The trophoblast will be noted first on the ventral surface of the vesicle. It will subsequently slowly migrate dorsally as the yolk sac regresses and the allantois develops beneath the embryo.
- Days 20–21. The trophoblast will slowly migrate dorsally.
- Days 24–50. A heartbeat is evident in the embryo proper on average around day 24. This is the first time at which fetal viability can be assessed.
- Days 28–50. The trophoblast is seen near the middle of the vesicle and by day 40 it is near the dorsal edge of the vesicle. At this time the umbilicus begins to elongate and the fetus will gravitate ventrally again, reaching the bottom of the vesicle by day 50.
- Days 50–180. The increasing size of the fetus makes it more difficult to image the whole structure; however, the fetal fluids and individual anatomical parts can almost always be identified.
  - ❏ The sex of the foal can be confirmed at around days 55–75, and sometimes much later.
  - ❏ The age of the fetus can be established by reference to standard measurements for orbital diameter, etc. If the date of service is known, the maturation and growth status of the fetus can be established. Retarded growth can be established early and the pregnancy can be classified as high risk.
  - ❏ The volume and nature of fluid surrounding the conceptus can also be calculated by ultrasonographic measurements, which is more useful in late-term pregnancy (see Fig. 7.18).
- By day 180 of pregnancy, the fetus can be examined by transabdominal ultrasound as well as transrectally (Fig. 7.16). Visualization of the heartbeat is often easier with transabdominal ultrasonography. The mare's abdomen may need to be clipped to facilitate this examination.

- One of the most significant benefits of ultrasonographic examination is the early diagnosis of twin pregnancy, which enables measures to be taken to address the problem before much time is lost.
- Manual examination carries a much lower rate of detection; nor can it monitor the results of fetal destruction in twin reduction (see p. 235).

Hormone tests

Pregnancy diagnosis can also be made by hormonal means. These tests are indirect indicators of pregnancy

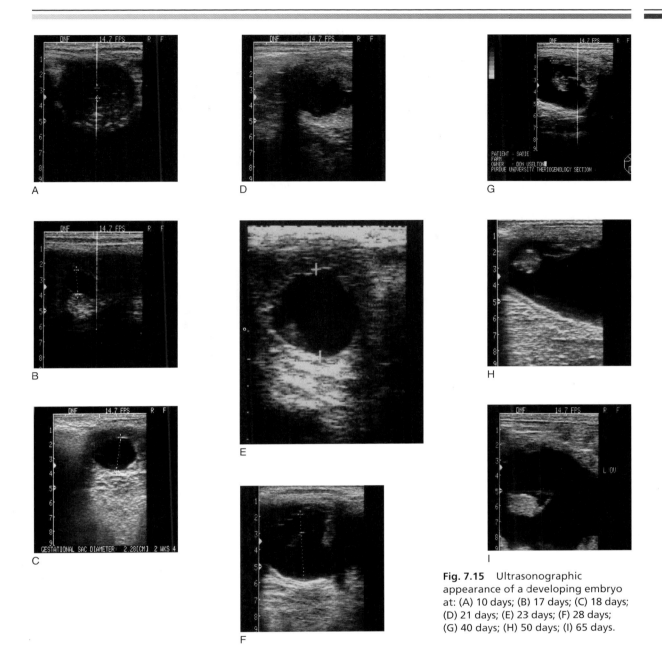

Fig. 7.15 Ultrasonographic appearance of a developing embryo at: (A) 10 days; (B) 17 days; (C) 18 days; (D) 21 days; (E) 23 days; (F) 28 days; (G) 40 days; (H) 50 days; (I) 65 days.

and can be misleading when used on their own; they are therefore regarded as unreliable and should not be used as the sole source of pregnancy determination.

Progesterone concentrations

Progesterone concentrations can be determined easily and quickly in blood or milk samples and the results are probably better than reliance on absence of estrus alone.[46] The test kits are accurate and suitable for use in practice. Progesterone can be measured in a practice laboratory using an ELISA kit.

- At 18–20 days post ovulation, pregnant mares should have a peak progesterone concentration above 2 ng/ml, while a nonpregnant mare should be returning to estrus and have a progesterone concentration below 2 ng/ml. Progesterone concentrations range from 4 to 10 ng/ml in most mares in early pregnancy. However, not all mares with these concentrations will be found to be pregnant, and some pregnant mares have lower progesterone concentrations for short periods.
- Progesterone concentrations may increase considerably after day 20. A persistently elevated progesterone after days 17–21 post ovulation is suggestive of pregnancy; however, progesterone may remain elevated in:

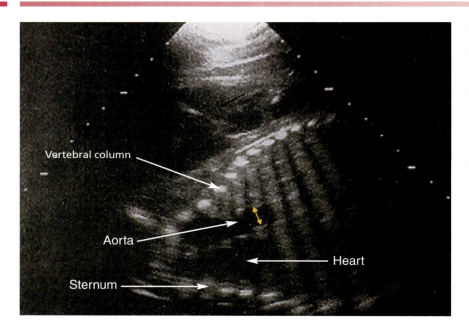

Fig. 7.16 Transabdominal ultrasonogram of a 6-month fetus obtained by placing the probe on the ventral abdominal wall on one side of the midline. The mare's skin surface is at the top of the picture and the foal's thoracic vertebrae and rib pattern are obvious (arrows). The foal is of course lying on its back at this time. Note also the fetal heart open and aorta (label), which can be clearly seen during the examination.

❑ Cases of delayed double ovulation.
❑ Retained corpus luteum.
❑ Following early embryonic death.[37,46]

- Progesterone concentrations remain elevated until days 150–200 of pregnancy and then decline. After day 200 they may be as low as <2 ng/ml and should not be used as the sole means of pregnancy determination.
- During the last month of pregnancy, progesterone levels increase slightly until 5 days prior to parturition.

eCG concentrations

As described previously (see p. 228), the fetal trophoblasts that invade the maternal endometrium produce detectable levels of eCG at around days 35–38. These cells form the endometrial cups, which maintain their function of stimulating secondary ovulations until around day 60 when maternal rejection causes their remission. The cup cells begin to degenerate after about day 75 and finally cease to function at around day 120.

Estimation of the blood concentrations of eCG by ELISA, latex agglutination or hemagglutination inhibition is therefore most applicable between day 45 and day 90, but can still be of value up to day 120.

- Because the levels of eCG reflect the function of the endometrial cups, concentrations of this hormone can provide reliable estimations between day 45 and day 120 of pregnancy.[47]

False-positives may result from early embryonic death. False-negatives may result from samples being taken before or after eCG concentrations are detectable or, interestingly, from mares with mule fetuses.

- Early embryonic death that occurs prior to endometrial cup formation (before days 32–35) will result in a return to estrus within 21–28 days. However, if endometrial cup formation has started, and eCG production has begun, follicular development and secondary corpus luteum development will occur whether the mare remains pregnant or if the pregnancy is lost. Because the supplemental corpus luteum will have formed, the mare will not return to estrus until endometrial cup degeneration is complete, which is usually around 120–150 days from ovulation. Therefore, if eCG test kits are utilized to determine pregnancy status without rectal confirmation of pregnancy, a false-positive pregnancy test is possible.

Estrogen concentrations

- Historically, urinary estrogens were measured by the Cuboni test. This qualitative chemical assay for estrogens was technically demanding and has been replaced by much more accurate tests.
- Biological tests using mice or guinea pigs are no longer ethically acceptable (or necessary) as a means of pregnancy testing of mares.

The concentration of estrogen in urine, blood or feces can be used to diagnose pregnancy after day 60 up to full term[48–50] using standard ELISAs for conjugated estrogen determination.

- Although a minor and insignificant maternal increase in estrogens is common between 35 and 60 days (as a result of pulsatile secretion of follicle-stimulating hormone), conjugated estrone sulfate concentrations can be used to diagnose pregnancy after day 60.[51]
- Estrogen concentrations increase until days 180–240 days of pregnancy reaching their peak in blood (and urine) around 150 days and then slowly decline until birth.

In contrast to other indirect indicators of pregnancy, estrogen levels are good indicators of fetal viability. Death of the fetus results in an immediate decrease in circulating estrogen concentrations.[2]

- If a mare in late gestation begins to lactate, fetal viability may be established by measuring estrone sulfate, although ultrasonographic examination can provide much more information. As long as the approximate stage of pregnancy is known, the serum estrogen concentration of the dam can be compared to the normal range of values for that stage of pregnancy.

Summary of pregnancy diagnosis

- Although ultrasonography has revolutionized pregnancy diagnosis, it is not a replacement for rectal palpation. Ultrasonography cannot measure uterine and cervical tone, nor can it detect the presence of some abnormalities of the broad ligaments, ovaries, uterus and cervix, which are important factors in the assessment of a pregnancy.
- Additionally, a solitary uterine cyst may be confused with a vesicle, resulting in the misdiagnosis of pregnancy.
- Early embryonic death may be difficult to distinguish using either palpation or ultrasonography until sufficient changes occur to differentiate it from a normal pregnancy.
- Estrogen concentrations in blood and urine are useful adjuncts to assess fetal viability when other means are not practicable.
- Pregnancy is most accurately diagnosed using a combination of rectal palpation and ultrasonography (see Table 7.3).[52–54] The benefits include the ability to:
  - ❑ Diagnose pregnancy accurately by days 14–16 post ovulation.
  - ❑ Diagnose a twin pregnancy in a very early stage.
  - ❑ Accurately determine the age of the

Table 7.3 Methods and accuracy of pregnancy diagnosis

	Days of gestation	Accuracy
Ultrasonography	14 to term	Very high
Rectal palpation	18–20 to term	High
Nonreturn to estrus	17–21 post ovulation	Low to moderate
Increased progesterone	17–21 post ovulation	Moderate
Increased equine chorionic gonadotropin	45–120	Moderate to high
Total estrogens	90–100 to term	Moderate to high

pregnancy if accurate breeding dates are not available.
  - ❑ Determine fetal viability.
  - ❑ Monitor fetal and placental development, with early determination of abnormalities occurring in the pregnancy.
  - ❑ Determine fetal sex between 55 and 75 days of pregnancy.

ASSESSMENT OF THE FETUS

DETERMINATION OF FETAL SEX

Determination of fetal sex is becoming more significant and can be performed with a reasonable degree of accuracy between days 55 and 75.[55] In order to perform this procedure it is important that:

- The operator is experienced. Experience can be gained during normal ultrasonographic examinations carried out between 59 and 65 days.
- The pregnancy is between 55 and 75 days. Proper timing is essential!
- High-quality ultrasound equipment is used.
- Adequate restraint and rectal techniques are used (to avoid risks of injury to mare and operator and allow a relaxed examination).
- There is subdued external light so that the image can be clearly seen.

When undertaking the examination it should be noted that:

- The genital tubercle appears as a bi-lobed structure approximately 2 mm in diameter (Fig. 7.17).
- The genital tubercle is located close to the umbilicus in the male fetus and under the tail in the female fetus. The difference is quite distinctive to an experienced operator.
- Prior to day 53 the sex of the fetus cannot be determined because the genital tubercle is situated between the hind legs of both males and females.

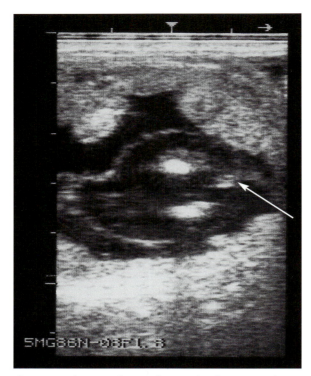

Fig. 7.17   Ultrasound scan of an equine fetus at 60 days showing the genital tubercle of a female foal (arrow) (slide courtesy of J. Pycock).

- After days 68–70 it may not be possible to image the whole fetus, making it harder to determine the location of the genital tubercle.

The fetus can be sexed using transabdominal ultrasonography later in gestation by the experienced operator after 9 months of pregnancy. The landmarks at this stage are the mammary glands, prepuce and penis in the male and the mammary glands, vulva and clitoris in the female.

EARLY EMBRYONIC LOSS

Early embryonic loss is defined as the loss of the conceptus before 40 days from fertilization.[56] Embryo loss can occur at any stage in the first 40 days of gestation (both before and after the earliest ultrasonographic detection).

- The rates of actual fertilization in mares are estimated to be between 90% and 95% in young fertile mares bred to fertile stallions and around 80–90% in older (subfertile) mares.[57]
- The earliest diagnosis of pregnancy is made through ultrasonographic examination. This technology has resulted in an increase in the diagnosis of early embryonic loss.

In most cases the mare has been diagnosed as 'in foal' at ultrasonographic and rectal examination at

12–17 days. Between 7% and 16% of equine pregnancies diagnosed by rectal examination are believed to terminate in early embryonic loss,[58] but the upper limit of the range rises to 24% if diagnosis of pregnancy is made by ultrasonographic means.[59]

- The highest losses occur in the first 10–14 days post ovulation.[60]
- Losses after day 12–13 are progressively less with advancing time.

In the case of twin ovulations it is difficult to confirm that the apparent extra loss in twin ovulating mares is due to failure of fertilization or to failure of the embryo at a later stage (days 7–10).

- There is evidence to suggest that, in mares with twin ovulations, less than half ultimately have twin pregnancies.

There is little information on the extent of early embryonic loss in the various breeds.

Etiology

Many causes for early embryonic loss have been implicated or proposed, including:

1. Genetic factors, which are probably the most common overall cause of loss.
   - Chromosomal abnormalities (with a fatal genetic combination) have been a regular and understandable cause of embryonic loss.[61]
   - Mares bred to stallions with karyotypic abnormalities (e.g. 63/X0, 65/XXY, 64/XY) show a higher rate of embryonic loss.
   - Late fertilization with aging sperm or an aging oocyte may also be involved.
   - A significant proportion of embryos will have accidental or inherited genetic abnormalities that are not consistent with life and the embryo can die at an early developmental stage.
2. Maternal management, age and health status (including nutritional status and extent of stress).
   - The rate of loss within the first 14 days for young healthy mares is around 25%, but in older mares this rises to 60%.
   - Subfertility appears to be a major factor in early embryonic loss.[62] Older mares have a higher rate of embryo abnormalities and so would be expected to suffer significantly from early embryonic loss.[63]
   - Mares bred on foal heat have higher rates of loss than those bred at the subsequent estrus.
   - Low body weight and a low nutritional plane prior to mating, and acute food deprivation involving significant weight loss result in increased embryonic death. Lactation may have a direct effect on the survival of the embryo or there might be an indirect effect involving nutritional stresses.

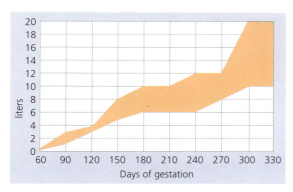

Fig. 7.18 Graph showing the volume of fluid surrounding the conceptus between 60 days gestation and full term as calculated from ultrasonographic measurements.

- Any type of illness, injury or other stressor (e.g. chronic laminitis) is believed to be a significant cause of early embryonic loss.
3. Uterine environmental problems.
  - Uterine disease has long been regarded as a cause of early embryonic loss and it is reasonable to suppose that a hostile uterine environment would cause problems such as:
    - ❑ Delayed uterine involution.
    - ❑ Infection or other inflammation.
    - ❑ Atrophy (see p. 148).
    - ❑ Accumulated intrauterine fluid (including lochia and inflammatory fluid or exudate) (Fig. 7.18).
  - The effect of endometrial (lymphatic) cysts is controversial but in some cases they may cause loss. Endometrial cysts are more commonly found in older mares and are far less common in ponies. Mares with one or two cysts (even large ones) may breed normally; multiple cysts can result in embryo loss, although this may not reflect the presence of cysts.[64] Large or multiple cysts may inhibit embryo mobility and thereby block maternal recognition. Alternatively, the fibrosis/nesting commonly seen in mares with multiple endometrial cysts may result in improper emptying of the lymphatics and glands resulting in improper uterine protein and a hostile environment for the embryo.
  - Embryo loss may be due to an abnormal uterine environment, such as that associated with chronic inflammation, uterine fibrosis and lymphatic stasis[65] (Fig. 7.19).
4. Endocrinological factors.
  - Alterations in the hormones that are responsible for the maintenance of pregnancy (see p. 230) may be involved, but the cause of these alterations may be difficult to establish.

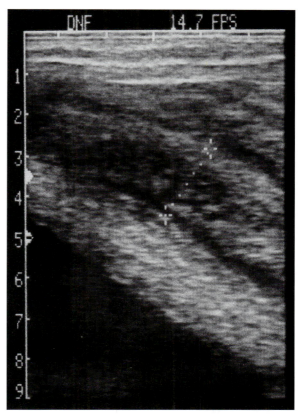

Fig. 7.19 Accumulation of fluid between the placenta and the endometrium typical of placentitis (dotted line).

5. Abnormalities of embryo location.
  - Embryos that develop 'upside down' (the normal embryo develops centrally on the floor of the vesicle and gradually moves upwards were thought to be abnormal, but there is no abnormally high failure rate.
  - Fixation of the embryo within the body of the uterus rather than at the base of one of the horns (regardless of the location of the subsequent fetus) means that the conceptus is not palpable per rectum and may even be missed during ultrasonographic examination. The majority of these pregnancies fail.
  - Fixation of the embryo in the distal regions of the uterine horns is likely to fail.

Diagnosis

Following a diagnosis of pregnancy either from ultrasonographic examination (between day 14 and day 25) or manual examination, the mare is found not to be pregnant at around day 40. The ultrasonographic features of the abnormal embryo can sometimes be identified and the value of ultrasonography cannot be overstated.

- An abnormally large vesicle at day 17 (often over 30 mm in diameter, and often with an abnormal or irregular shape) may be associated with embryonic loss, but some embryos certainly survive.

- Small vesicles (<4 mm at day 13) that fail to reach 20 mm in diameter by day 20 commonly fail to survive.[66] This may be due to failure to induce production of the pregnancy-sustaining antiluteolytic signals. In general, vesicles that on days 13–15 are 1 day or more smaller than the normal size-for-age have a high incidence of failure. Accurate measurement is therefore essential and suspicious vesicles should be re-examined at 2-day intervals.
- Anembryonic vesicles are invariably small for their gestational age. Vesicles that fail to develop an embryo by day 20 or are not readily visible at day 24 (usually of a size consistent with a 21-day gestation) will inevitably fail. Thus, if an embryo is not visible by days 24–27 the pregnancy should be terminated to avoid time loss.
- Abnormal accumulations of fluid can be seen around the developing embryo.
- Loss of heartbeat.
- Decrease in embryo size or failure to continue to develop normally.

Management

In the event that an abnormal embryo is identified (see above), a decision must be taken either to continue monitoring its progress (or otherwise) or to abort it immediately to avoid wasting time. The pregnancy can be terminated easily at this stage with a prostaglandin, and the remains of the conceptus should be flushed out of the uterus to avoid it acting as a nidus of infection if it is not promptly expelled following prostaglandin administration.

Reduction of twin pregnancies can be a problem with respect to the remaining embryo. Following reduction of a twin embryo, the surviving embryo often continues to normal term, but there is a high rate of early loss and so continued monitoring must be undertaken. The reduction procedure is most successful if carried out during the first 14–17 days when the embryos are still mobile (see p. 245).

Mares that habitually suffer from early embryonic loss should be carefully examined to establish if there is any identifiable reason for this. The use of exogenous progesterone (150 mg daily) or progestogen (0.044 mg/kg daily) is controversial but some specialists believe it to be useful when the survival of the pregnancy is in jeopardy. Under these conditions, hormone treatment should be maintained until the next ovarian follicle has ruptured and its corpus luteum can then take over maintenance of the pregnancy.

In general, in mares that are found to have a threatened pregnancy, the problems associated with embryo loss mean that it is probably better to start again and ensure uterine health and a healthy viable conceptus at a subsequent mating.

TWINNING

> - All mares should be evaluated for twin pregnancy regardless of whether multiple ovulation was noted at the time of breeding. This has become standard practice in almost every stud.

In the vast majority of cases, twin pregnancies in the mare result from dizygotic (separate) ovulations.[67]

- Identical twins resulting from a single fertilized ovum are particularly rare in horses.[68]
- The incidence of twins is higher in certain breeds. In the Thoroughbred and Draft breeds, 16% of total ovulations will result in twin conceptions. The proportion is lower in other breeds.[69] Pony mares have a relatively low incidence of double ovulation.
- Multiple ovulations are more common in older mares than in younger mares and are also more common within 80 days of foaling.
- Mares that tend to double-ovulate will usually do so over multiple subsequent cycles and from one year to the next, and they therefore remain prone to twin pregnancy.

The ovulations may occur within 24 hours of each other (synchronous ovulation), or more than 24 hours apart (asynchronous ovulation).[70]

- The twins may fix in the same horn (unilateral or unicornual twins; Fig. 7.20) or in both horns (bilateral or bicornual twins; Fig. 7.21).
- If the ovulations are synchronous, the vesicles appear to be of similar size on ultrasound examination, whereas for asynchronous ovulations the vesicles may be significantly different in size.
- In mares that are examined very early in pregnancy (days 12–14 post ovulation), the second vesicle may be too small to be noted on examination if the ovulations are asynchronous.
- It is essential that follow-up examinations be performed on these mares 2–4 days later, so that a twin pregnancy can be identified before the embryos become implanted.

The mare has the ability to reduce twin pregnancy spontaneously in approximately 75% of cases of unilateral twins and in 15% of cases of bilateral twins.[71]

- Twins that fix unilaterally (Fig. 7.20) have a membrane that is shared between the two vesicles. This membrane does not function as a nutrient supply; thus, as the vesicles grow, their demand for nutrients quickly outgrows the supply (often before day 40). In this case, one,

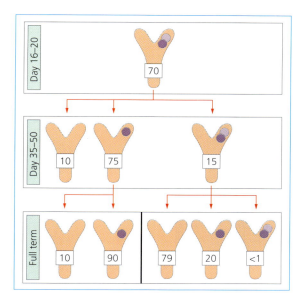

Fig. 7.20 The outcome of unicornual twin pregnancy (the twin embryos are implanted in the same uterine horn) in the mare. In spite of up to 70% of twin pregnancies being unicornual, only 1% will result in natural full-term births.

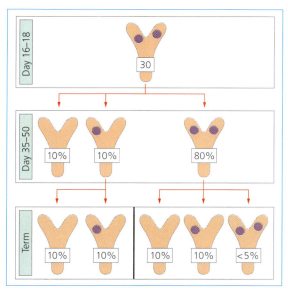

Fig. 7.21 Outline of the incidence and distribution of bicornual twin pregnancy (the embryos are fixed in different uterine horns) in the mare. Only 30% of twin pregnancies are bicornual; of these, the large majority will produce only one full-term foal or will be barren.

or sometimes both, vesicles will succumb. If one vesicle survives, the fact that it was adjacent to a twin for the first 40 days does not cause it any harm.

- In the case of bilateral twins (Fig. 7.21), abortion usually occurs significantly later in gestation,

when overcrowding compromises the uterine space and both of the fetuses cannot be adequately nourished.

- In some cases of bilateral twins, one fetus may mummify and the second twin may continue on to full term.

Natural twin reduction can be expected to occur in around 60% of all cases[72] and is dependent on:

- The relative location of the embryos at the time of fixation in the uterine wall.
- The extent of synchrony of the two ovulations (one may survive at the expense of the other because it is fertilized at an ideal stage; the other may be an older oocyte or an older sperm).
- An obvious disparity between the sizes of the two embryos; the larger one is probably the more viable.

Natural reduction is more common when there is a greater than 4 mm^3 size difference, ovulations are asynchronous by more than 24 hours and one of the embryos had a poor endometrial contact.

Few twin fetuses will survive to term. Those that do survive to term are often born weak or stillborn and may require considerable intensive care and may succumb even with this type of care. These foals are small and are often dysmature due to the space and nutritional constraints of twin pregnancy.

Complications associated with twin pregnancy include:

- Dystocia.
- Retained placenta.
- Delayed uterine involution.
- Reduced fertility following abortion or birth of twin fetuses.

- For these reasons, twins are considered undesirable and attempts to reduce one or both twins should be attempted when the diagnosis is made.
- Ignoring the presence of twins is poor stud farm management.

The best stage at which to identify the presence of twin pregnancies is at 14–15 days when the embryo is still mobile. This requires the use of a meticulous ultrasonographic examination of the whole uterus.

- The mare should be adequately restrained such that a complete and thorough examination can be performed. A hasty examination under unfavorable conditions may be misleading and is poor practice.
- A high-quality 5-MHz ultrasound machine should be used and hard-copy pictures or video recordings should be taken for subsequent study and record.

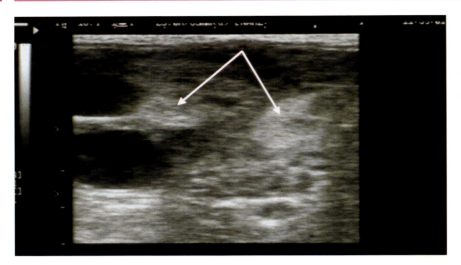

Fig. 7.22 Two corpora lutea suggestive of twin ovulation. In these circumstances, the uterus should be scanned extremely thoroughly to establish whether or not a twin pregnancy exists.

- Measurement of all suspected vesicles should be made to rule out endometrial cysts at subsequent examinations. Vesicles increase in size daily, whereas cysts do not.

The ultrasonographic detection of twin (or even triple) maturing follicles will often alert the clinician to the possibility of a subsequent twin pregnancy. However, in some cases, two follicles may be adjacent to each other and recorded as a single ovulation. In other cases, an asynchronous ovulation may have occurred which was not noted during the prebreeding assessment. The presence of uterine cysts can confuse the diagnosis.

- Careful manual and ultrasonographic examination of both ovaries at the time of pregnancy diagnosis will allow the number of corpora lutea to be counted. This may also support the possibility of a twin pregnancy (Fig. 7.22).

Adjacent twin embryos may be difficult to distinguish on some examinations.

- Usually, there is a dividing membrane that is visible between the vesicles; however, depending on the orientation of the transducer over the embryos, this membrane may not always be evident.
- The size of twin embryos is usually larger than a singleton of the same age. However, with asynchronous ovulations this may not be so evident.
- If it is unclear whether adjacent embryos exist, repeat examination should be performed in 24–48 hours.
- Additionally, in all mares diagnosed with singleton fetuses, re-evaluation should be performed before day 30, so that, if a mistake has been made and twins have been missed,

the pregnancy can be terminated or the twins reduced before endometrial cup formation occurs.
- Bilateral twins are easier to diagnose because of the space between them.
- A solitary uterine cyst may resemble an embryo if it is of similar size and shape (Fig. 7.23). In this case, the embryo (true) may be reduced, leaving the cyst in the uterus. On re-evaluation, the cyst will be found in the same location and will be the same size.

Methods for differentiating cysts from pregnancies are:

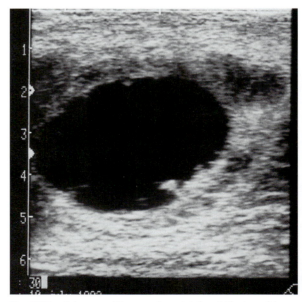

Fig. 7.23 A large solitary endometrial cyst that could on cursory examination be mistaken for a pregnancy.

- Repeated ultrasonographic evaluation over several hours if the embryo(s) are still in the mobile phase. Embryos will move, whereas cysts will remain in the same place at every examination.
- Re-evaluate the mare ultrasonographically in 24–48 hours. Embryos grow in size and change shape (as they age) whereas cysts grow very slowly, such that a change in this short time-span would not occur.

In mares with multiple cysts, re-evaluation is usually required to determine which are cysts and which are embryos prior to embryo reduction. In mares that have been evaluated by ultrasound prior to breeding, any cysts, their sizes and locations should be recorded and mapped, so that subsequent pregnancy examinations will be more accurate.

Management of a twin pregnancy

If a twin pregnancy is diagnosed during ultrasonographic examination, some method of termination of one or both pregnancies should be seriously considered.[73,74]

- Examination at days 14–16 of pregnancy with mobile embryos will allow one vesicle to be manipulated to the tip of a horn or to the cervix where it can be manually crushed[75] (Fig. 7.24).
- Alternatively, the embryo can be crushed against the pelvis or the ultrasound probe (Fig. 7.25). The mare should have a relaxed rectum if crushing is to be performed; this will often require sedation.
- In cases of bilateral fixation, manual reduction can be performed up to 30 days of pregnancy. In cases of unilateral pregnancy, resorption of both vesicles is common and return to fertile estrus within 2 weeks is likely, especially if reduction is performed following fixation.
- Manual reduction under ultrasound guidance is entirely feasible with care and meticulous rectal examination technique. Experienced stud veterinarians commonly use the technique.

Technique for the manual reduction of twins (bilateral fixation)

i. The mare is restrained effectively.
ii. A lubricated gloved hand is inserted into the rectum and the uterine bifurcation is located.
iii. The hand locates the selected embryo (usually the smallest one as identified by ultrasonographic examination). The palm of the hand is placed over the horn and the fingers passed over the horn to cup the area with the embryo.
iv. The fingers are then tightened, starting with the finger closest to the bifurcation (this prevents

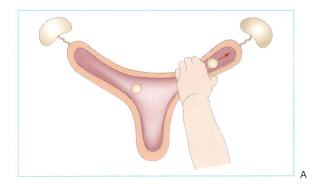
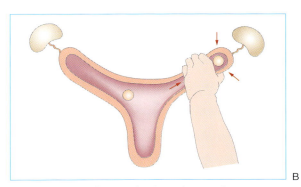

Fig. 7.24 Manipulation of twin embryos prior to crushing/ablation. The smaller embryo is manipulated to the tip of the uterine horn (or towards the internal os of the cervix). This is done by gently milking the uterine horn from the bifurcation side (A). Once the embryo is located at the tip of the uterine horn (confirmed by ultrasound examination), pressure is applied to the lumen using fingers and thumb until the vesicle is felt to pop (B). This can easily be felt through the rectal and uterine walls and satisfactory ablation can be confirmed by ultrasound examination. In cases where the twins are surviving jointly (and are in contact), gentle manipulation between the embryos is used to separate them. This must be performed prior to manipulation of one embryo to the tip of the uterine horn. It is imperative that the mare's rectum is relaxed during this procedure to prevent rectal perforation.

the embryo from being squeezed into the bifurcation).
v. Gentle pressure is applied until the embryo is felt to 'pop'.
vi. Ultrasonographic examination is used to confirm that the embryo is at least 50% of the original size.

Technique for the manual reduction of twins (unilateral fixation)

i. The mare is restrained effectively.
ii. A smooth muscle relaxant (such as hyoscine n-butyl bromide, xylazine, detomidine, or

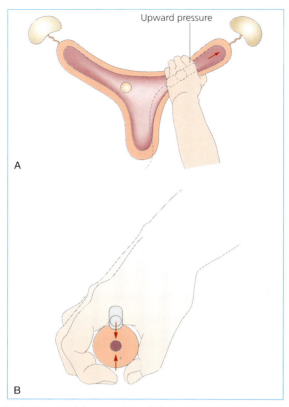

Fig. 7.25 Crushing a twin vesicle against the ultrasound probe. The rectal probe is held parallel to the length of the uterine horn so that the dorsal surface of the uterus is under the palm of the hand, with the probe between the palm of the hand and the uterine wall (A). The fingers curve around the ventral surface of the uterus and upward pressure is applied until the vesicle is seen to pop (B).

propantheline) is administered to allow more detailed palpation. The effects of propantheline commence within 3–4 minutes and are quite profound; the uterus loses tone in 10–15 minutes making examination and twin manipulation less easy. In occasional mares there is a possibility of bowel stasis and colic with this drug.

iii. A lubricated gloved hand is inserted into the rectum and the uterine bifurcation is located.

iv. The wall of the uterus is gently pressed between thumb and forefinger until one embryo is located.

v. The adjacent embryo is located and digital pressure is applied between the two until they are felt to separate.

vi. At this point one embryo might be felt to collapse; if it does not, follow-up ultrasonography can help to locate the smaller of the two.

vii. Quite commonly this procedure results in significant damage to both embryos.

- Reduction of a single vesicle is possible in more than 90% of twins that have not fixed at the time of diagnosis.
- Those mares that resorb both vesicles will return to a fertile estrus within 2 weeks.
- If twin pregnancy is not reduced prior to endometrial cup formation, return to estrus may not occur until the regression of the cups occurs after 120 days.
- In cases where reduction is not possible (fixed, adjacent twins), re-evaluation before day 30 is essential.

If manual reduction is not desired or not possible, the mare can be aborted using a single dose of $PGF_{2\alpha}$ before day 35 of pregnancy, or multiple doses of $PGF_{2\alpha}$ after day 35 of pregnancy. However, if the mare is more than 35 days pregnant when $PGF_{2\alpha}$ is given it is unlikely that she will have a fertile estrus before the endometrial cups have disappeared.

Alternative methods for reducing twin pregnancies

1. Uterine lavage.
   - The embryos or fetuses can be flushed from the uterus. In cases where the pregnancy would be visible to the naked eye, confirmation of pregnancy termination is made by monitoring the effluxed fluid.
2. Embryo harvest (see p. 221).
   - In mares that habitually have a twin pregnancy, and particularly if ovulation cannot be restricted to a single follicle, it may be possible to harvest the embryos using normal embryo-collection methods 7 or 8 days after ovulation.
   - The mare can be re-implanted with a single embryo (following suitable freezing) and managed to maximize the chance of a successful single pregnancy.
   - Alternatively, each harvested embryo may be implanted in surrogate mares.
3. Transvaginal aspiration of the allantoic fluid.
   - In this circumstance, loss of the remaining pregnancy is common as a result of collapse of the fetoplacental unit after the fluid is aspirated from the other pregnancy.
4. Injection of one fetus with potassium chloride, or other noxious substance.
   - This results in fetal death and resorption after day 75 of pregnancy.[76]
   - Alternatively, an injection of an irritating substance (e.g. dilute iodine solution) into

the allantoic fluid will result in fetal death in most cases.

General considerations

In all cases of twin reduction, follow-up examinations should be performed 3–4 days later to ensure that reduction has taken place and that the remaining embryo is viable.

- Re-checking at 2 days can be too early in some cases.
- There is a disappointingly high rate of embryo loss despite normal growth to day 30.
- To minimize this loss it is important to destroy the smaller of the two embryos.[77]

When the abortion of both fetuses is desired, follow-up examination should be performed to ensure that both pregnancies have been terminated.

In cases where no natural or iatrogenic reduction occurs prior to mid-gestation, or a diagnosis of a twin pregnancy is made for the first time at mid-gestation, the mare should be aborted using multiple doses of prostaglandin ($PGF_{2\alpha}$).

- Owners must be made aware that there are increased risks of retained placenta(s) and the possibility of metritis as a result.
- Alternatively, one fetus can be injected with potassium chloride under ultrasound guidance.

- Because of the known risks associated with twin pregnancies, as outlined above, mares with known twin fetuses should not be allowed to continue with the pregnancy beyond mid-gestation.

On rare occasions, triplet or even quadruplet ovulations may occur. Reduction of the unwanted pregnancies may be performed as described above for double ovulation. There is no information on whether the resulting embryos from this circumstance have normal (or altered) viability when harvested by embryo-collection methods (see p. 221).

Some practitioners premedicate mares with flunixin meglumine to minimize local prostaglandin release following twin reduction. Others administer progestogens (progestins) to these mares following reduction, to facilitate maintenance of the remaining conceptus by promoting uterine quiescence and maintaining cervical closure until follow-up examination can be performed. There is no evidence that either of these measures increases the chances of survival of the remaining twin.[78]

A useful protocol for the diagnosis and management of suspected or confirmed twin pregnancy is presented in Fig. 7.26.

MANAGEMENT OF THE HIGH-RISK PREGNANCY

The classification of a pregnancy as high-risk (see p. 360) requires that extra attention be paid to the mare during pregnancy and parturition. A history of a problematic pregnancy during a previous breeding season or problems occurring during the current one are indicators of an impending problem and 'forewarned is forearmed'. With care it is possible to pre-empt significant difficulties and allow the pregnancy to develop to term with the satisfactory delivery of a live, viable, healthy foal.

One of the biggest mistakes is to assume that problems only occur at or near term. Many disasters are due to problems at a much earlier stage. Not only is the foal usually nonviable but there are serious implications for the future fertility of the mare. Therefore, all high-risk mares require regular detailed clinical and hematologic examinations. Regular fetal assessment is essential (see also p. 249).

Continued careful assessment of fetal well-being is an important stud measure.

- Mares that have sustained injuries or been subjected to surgery, or those known to have had infectious disease, are classified as 'high-risk' and are potential candidates for careful assessment of the fetus' state of health throughout the remainder of the pregnancy.[79]
- If the fetus is suspected to be abnormal or induced delivery may be required, knowledge about its health is vitally important. All the available methods for fetal assessment have problems because technology and knowledge have been slow to develop.
- Mares that exhibit precocious mammary development (or even lactation) and those that show vaginal discharge are candidates for regular monitoring of the fetus.

Equine fetal viability is very dependent upon adrenocortical maturation, which occurs only near full term, during the last 5–7 days of in utero development.[80]

- Viable foals may be born as early as day 290 of gestation if the dam experiences a slowly spreading placental insult such as ascending placentitis. However, some foals will have defects in skeletal and other systems that are serious enough to necessitate euthanasia.
- Experimental induction of precocious maturation has been investigated but has largely been unsuccessful. Repeated injection of adrenocorticotropin into the fetus at 300 days of gestation resulted in the birth of precociously mature foals, but the technique is associated with a high risk of abortion.[81]

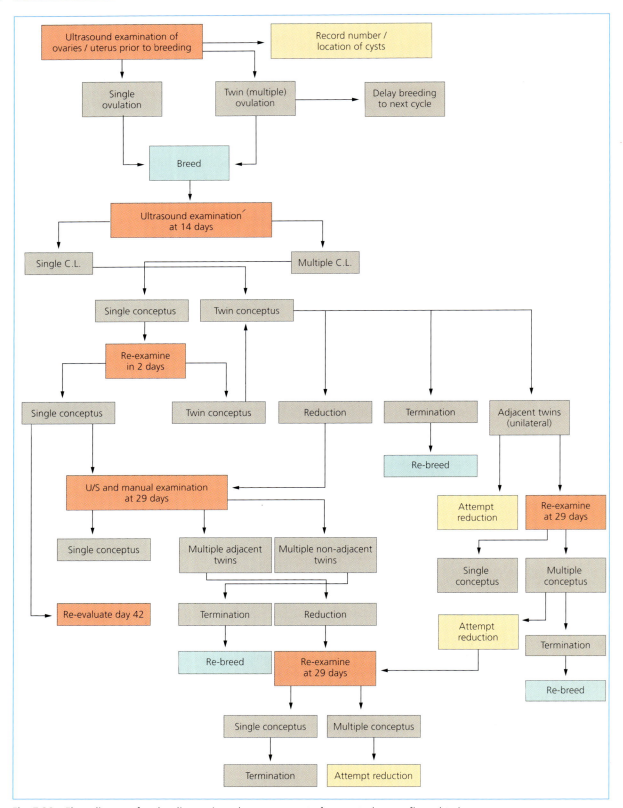

Fig. 7.26 Flow diagram for the diagnosis and management of suspected or confirmed twin pregnancy.

Most clinicians accept that the high-risk equine fetus has a better chance of survival if it remains in the uterus, no matter how severely compromised, because early intervention results in the birth of a premature or dysmature foal that will probably die. In the majority of cases this is the correct decision, but there are circumstances in which it may be better to remove the fetus. Identifying which cases should be induced, and when to intervene, is at best a guess since clinical perinatal medicine is a relatively new discipline in the horse.

FETAL ASSESSMENT

Because the maintenance of a pregnancy is heavily dependent on the status of the fetus, assessment of fetal well-being is critical in the management of high-risk pregnancies.

High-risk pregnancies that are candidates for antepartum evaluation of the equine fetus include those mares that:

- Have had problems in previous pregnancies.
- Develop a vaginal discharge during the pregnancy.
- Carry an increased risk of congenital malformations (e.g. Overo-Paint breedings and Fell ponies).
- Show premature mammary gland development and lactation.
- Develop a serious medical or surgical problem during the later stages of gestation.

A variety of techniques are used for the clinical evaluation of late pregnancy.

Palpation per rectum

This is an insensitive method for assessing fetal well-being because episodes of fetal activity are intermittent and the normally developing fetus may be unresponsive during the examination.

- This is the simplest method for fetal monitoring. In general, however, rectal palpation alone should not be relied upon if there are doubts about the pregnancy.
- In the last 2–3 months, the fetus' head or extremities can usually be appreciated easily per rectum.
- The position of the fetus may be determined.
- If movement is felt, it can safely be assumed that the fetus is alive.
- Reduction of muscular activity (fetal movement) may be reduced naturally in late-term foals.
- Movement can usually be induced by gentle tapping or by a gentle squeeze on a fetal extremity. Movement alone is a poor index, however, as foals may become very still for some

periods and fetal movement in the last weeks of gestation may be naturally reduced.
- An experienced examiner can detect abnormal amounts of fetal fluid and this can be helpful.

Vaginal examination

This is used to assess the degree of cervical softening, the appearance of the vaginal walls and to obtain samples of abnormal vaginal discharges for culture. It is performed in mares suspected of having ascending placentitis, premature placental separation or impending abortion due to twins or an unknown cause.

- Mares identified as having problems because they have precocious udder formation, milk let-down, and in many cases a vaginal discharge in mid- to late gestation, should have a vaginal examination.
- Information gained from a vaginal speculum examination is limited to conditions that involve the cervix, vagina and vestibule. The severity of the disease process or the degree of placental separation cannot be assessed.
- The risks of this procedure are low and the high-risk status of the mare should not necessarily inhibit the full examination.

Collection of blood for hormonal analysis

Analysis of the hormone profile of the mare can be used as an aid to pregnancy diagnosis (see p. 236) and to predict the approximate date of foaling. Hormonal concentrations in maternal plasma are not routinely assayed because a single plasma sample is not diagnostic.[82] Serial blood samples will detect abnormal trends in progestin concentrations in maternal plasma that may be associated with fetal compromise.

- A rapid drop, or a progestin concentration that remains below 2 ng/ml for more than 3–4 days in a mare that is over 300 days of gestation, indicates impending abortion and has been associated with herpesvirus infection,[83] maternal or fetal hypoxia, endotoxemia, and starvation. In contrast, a premature rise in progestin may result in the birth of a relatively mature foal at a gestation of 290–310 days.[81] This has been observed in mares with placentitis and premature placental separation.[34,39,84]
- Circulating estrogen is an important index of fetal viability; this is the only indirect method of establishing that the foal is alive (see p. 237).
- Concentrations of equilin (estrogen) fall dramatically within hours of fetal death.
- Three to four serial samples of plasma taken every other day to measure plasma progestins in

late gestation (>260 days) can be used to identify fetal viability, stress or fetal death.[39]

Fetal and placental ultrasonography

There are two ultrasonographic approaches that can be made:

1. Per rectum. This is used at any stage of pregnancy but it is an invasive procedure and not without risk. However, it is a standard procedure in all forms of equine practice and experienced veterinarians encounter few problems (see p. 236).
2. Transabdominal.[85,86]

Ultrasonographic examination is particularly useful for:

- The detection of twin pregnancy.
- Assessing placental thickness.[86,87] This can be measured accurately in the later stages of gestation via transabdominal or transrectal ultrasonography. Although gross abnormalities are clear indicators of problems, the significance of subtle changes has yet to be established.
  - ❏ Fetoplacental infections cause nearly a third of all abortions or fetal mortality, and 90% of these infections are due to an ascending placentitis.[88] Transrectal ultrasonographic evaluation of the equine placenta is useful in detecting early signs of placentitis.[87] In normal pregnant mares, the uteroplacental thickness cranial to the cervix increases from approximately 0.5 cm to 1.0 cm between 8 and 12 months of gestation. These changes are not evident when mares are scanned transabdominally. In mares with ascending placentitis, the placenta commonly thickens in the area of the cervical star and separates from the endometrium. This results in the uteroplacental thickness being greater than 1.5 cm in diameter and detachment of the placenta in the area of the cervix (Fig. 7.27).[89]
- Assessing the ultrasonographic appearance (echogenicity) and the volume of the allantoic and amniotic fluids (see p. 241). However, there is little information at present as to its clinical significance. Echogenic particles are thought to increase with advancing gestational age.[90]
- Documenting fetal position.
- Measurement of fetal size/age (see p. 235).
  - ❏ The size of the eye (Fig. 7.28), and of the aorta (Fig. 7.16) in particular, have been used to correlate with gestational age.
  - ❏ If the gestational age is not known and the pregnancy is normal, size measurements can provide some guidance on the age of the fetus. Some indication of the expected date of delivery may be obtained.

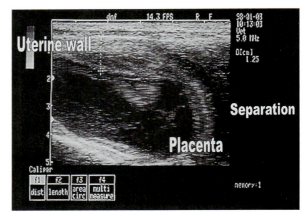

Fig. 7.27 Transrectal ultrasonography of the placenta separated from the uterus, with fluid accumulation between the two.

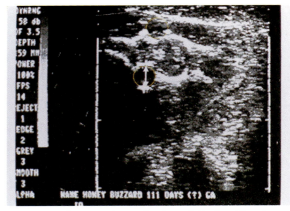

Fig. 7.28 Ultrasound examination of the fetal head provides an accurate measure of the orbital diameter. This can be correlated with fetal age for each breed of horse.

  - ❏ Measurements can be used to predict the birth weight with a good degree of accuracy (subject to the caveat that the body size condition score can be affected if the foal loses weight in utero as a result of placental inadequacy).
- Color flow Doppler studies have been used, but again there is little information on how this technique can be used clinically.
  - ❏ Changes in fetal heart rate have been found to precede fetal death.[90]
  - ❏ Severe abnormalities of cardiovascular function can be detected and measures taken to prepare for an abnormal delivery.

A biophysical profiling system has been developed that provides a useful 'score' for the status of the fetus from 300 days to term using ultrasonographic parameters.[91] It is patterned from the Manning biophysical profile, which measures the likelihood of acute or chronic hypoxemia and asphyxia in human fetuses.[92] The equivalent equine profile evaluates:

- Fetal heart rate.
- Fetal aortic diameter.
- Maximal fetal fluid depth.
- Uteroplacental contact (including contact area and thickness).
- Fetal activity.

A low score indicates an impending negative outcome; however, a high score does not ensure a positive outcome. The biophysical profile is of limited value to the veterinary clinician as only poor outcomes can be predicted. Intervention and prevention are not possible.

Fetal electrocardiography[93–95]

Fetal electrocardiography is a well-recognized technique in horses and provides useful information on the status of the foal's heart and circulation. It can also be used to identify twin pregnancy.[94]

- The technique does have considerable technical limitations but with care can be useful. It should not be used on its own to assess the fetal health (or indeed as a means of pregnancy diagnosis).
- Many specialists do not consider this method to have any advantages over others that are available.

Technique

i. A standard electrocardiograph with EMG filters and a variable sensitivity is required.
ii. A normal base–apex trace is obtained from the mare before attempting any fetal trace. This establishes the rate and rhythm of the mare whose trace will inevitably be superimposed on that of the foal (Fig. 7.29).

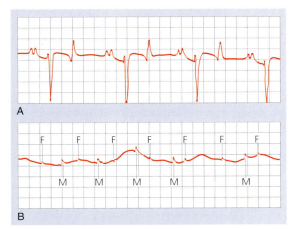

Fig. 7.29 Fetal electrocardiography. (A) Electro-cardiographic trace taken from a mare in the last trimester of pregnancy. (B) Fetal electrocardiographic trace showing the faint recordings of fetal activity (F) with the more obvious maternal activity (M).

iii. The leads are then attached as follows:[96]
- RIGHT ARM on the dorsal midline.
- LEFT ARM on the ventral midline some 10 cm forward of the udder. If this is resented by the mare or if a suitably clear trace is not achieved, the lead can be moved to the left flank or the left stifle.
- The EARTH (ground) lead is usefully placed in the perineal region or in the area just behind the point of the elbow.
- The exact position of the leads may need to be altered to obtain a good trace.[97]

Interpretation

- The fetal heart rate and regularity (or otherwise) of the rhythm can be measured, but usually little else can be established because of the small size of the complexes.
- Increasing the sensitivity of the machine seldom helps as it merely introduces artifacts and magnifies the maternal trace.
- Nevertheless, abnormally high heart rates with dramatic falls thereafter and irregularities have been found to precede fetal death.[98]
- Normal fetal heart rates are quoted as being 60–120 beats per minute. The rate falls significantly as term approaches, whereas that of the mare increases correspondingly.[99]

Amniocentesis

Amniocentesis allows analysis of allantoic or amniotic fluid to be performed but the technique has no material advantages over other methods.[100,101]

- Samples of fluid can safely be obtained using ultrasound guidance to ensure that no vital structures are damaged during the procedure.
- Analysis of the phospholipid content (surfactant) may be helpful in establishing the maturity of the fetus but very little is known at present.
- Abortion is a potential complication.

Changes in mammary secretion electrolytes (see Table 8.1 and Fig. 8.2)

Characteristic changes in mammary secretion electrolytes, the presence of colostrum in the udder and a gestation length of at least 320 days are criteria used by clinicians to time induction of parturition.[102] The first criterion appears to be correlated with fetal maturation.

- During the last week of gestation, potassium and calcium concentrations in mammary secretions rise, whereas sodium concentrations fall.[103] Final maturational processes occur in the fetus concurrent with these maternal changes.

- Mares carrying normal pregnancies that are induced after the calcium concentration in the mammary secretions has risen above 12 mmol/l rarely deliver a dysmature foal if all induction criteria are followed.

Note:
- Electrolyte values must be viewed with caution, especially in ill, pregnant mares, because fetal maturation is not always synchronous with maternal preparation for birth.
- In field cases, electrolyte values may rise prematurely in sick pregnant mares, presumably as a result of hormonal changes induced by disease. In such cases, the udder may decrease in size and electrolyte values revert to levels that are normally associated with that specific time of gestation as the mare recovers.
- If the mare recovers from her illness, the mare many times carries her foal for the normal gestation length.

Fetal blood measurements

Fetal blood measurements provide a theoretical means of assessment of the readiness for delivery. These measures would, of course, require a means of obtaining a fetal blood sample and are therefore not of any practical value.

- Fetal cortisol and tri-iodothyronine concentrations rise and the neutrophil: lymphocyte ratio switches from 1:1 to 3:1.[41,104]

MANAGEMENT OF THE HIGH-RISK MARE

Prerequisites for a successful pregnancy are:

1. Maintenance of a relatively quiescent myometrium.
   - The factors regulating myometrial activity in the mare are still uncertain, but progestin may inhibit myometrial activity.[105]
   - Aborting mares have high concentrations of circulating $PGF_{2\alpha}$, whereas mares that remain pregnant release only small pulses of $PGF_{2\alpha}$ in association with prostaglandin injection.
   - Progesterone in oil, or altrenogest, can be used successfully to prevent abortion in mares in which the pregnancy is at risk due to diseases associated with excess $PGF_{2\alpha}$ secretion. Moreover, flunixin meglumine is ineffective in modulating cloprostenol-induced uterine $PGF_{2\alpha}$ secretion and therefore does not prevent abortion in mares at risk of abortion due to

systemic illness. However, flunixin meglumine may be useful in helping to mediate inflammatory mediators released in response to endotoxemic insult and may therefore be useful in preventing abortion in mares with systemic, endotoxemic disease processes.

2. Adequate nutrition and gas exchange to the fetus.
   - Inadequate or intermittent feeding or fasting mares may result in premature delivery; however, the cause for premature delivery is not clear.
   - Fasting in late gestation causes an increase in PGF metabolite levels in uterine arterial blood and uterine venous blood and a 70% decrease in the arteriovenous plasma glucose difference across the placenta. This results in premature delivery of the foal. Periodic increases in $PGF_{2\alpha}$ production and metabolism by the uterus may sensitize the myometrium to other factors, such as increasing numbers of oxytocin and prostaglandin receptors. It is also possible that the fetus rather than the mare is more adversely affected by food withdrawal.
   - Re-establishment of normal feeding patterns or infusions of glucose cause an immediate fall in uterine PGF metabolite levels and a rise in glucose.

Treatment of ill, pregnant mares during the second or third trimester is limited to supportive medical therapy. The administration schedule, length of treatment and drug dosages have been chosen arbitrarily as there are few studies on treatment efficacy.

An oral progestin or progesterone in oil is commonly given in combination with nonsteroidal anti-inflammatory drugs to inhibit the adverse effects of circulating prostaglandins on myometrial activity and uterine blood flow.

Nonsteroidal anti-inflammatory drugs are administered in mares with endotoxemia, placentitis or with restricted feed intake. The efficacy of these drugs may be limited since they block the increase in plasma PGF metabolites that occurs in pregnant mares near term that are fasted prior to surgery, but not the increase in plasma PGF metabolite levels that occurs after cloprostenol-induced abortion.

Antibiotics appropriate for the isolated organism are frequently administered in cases of placentitis or endotoxemia, and as a preventative measure after surgical procedures; however, little is known about the transfer of antibiotics across the placenta and their effects on the fetus.

- Of the three most commonly used antibiotics in equine practice (gentamicin, penicillin G and trimethoprim sulfadiazine) only trimethoprim sulfadiazine was detected in fetal fluid samples and foal serum collected at parturition when dams of the foals were administered antibiotics during the last 2 weeks of gestation.[106] These were normal pregnancies, however, and the placental barrier was intact. It is not known what drugs will cross the placenta when the barrier is disrupted.

- It is possible that normal maternal–fetal exchange may be altered during placentitis, resulting in antibiotic concentrations in the conceptus that are different from those achieved when the placenta is normal. If maternal–fetal exchange is not different during placentitis, it is unlikely that administration of penicillin or gentamicin will control infection in the fetus.

Tocolytic agents are routinely used in human medicine, but only clenbuterol (a β_2-agonist) has been evaluated in mares.

- Clenbuterol causes a dramatic, but transient, increase in maternal and fetal heart rate at all stages of pregnancy.
- When administered in early pregnancy, clenbuterol causes decreased uterine tone.
- In late pregnancy, changes in uterine tone are either subtle or absent.[107]
- There have been no clinical trials evaluating the ability of clenbuterol to delay or prevent premature parturition in the mare.

> - Clenbuterol may not be effective in inducing uterine relaxation.

SUMMARY OF THE MANAGEMENT OF HIGH-RISK PREGNANCY

- It is possible to identify the compromised equine fetus. However, options for treatment and management are severely limited.
- Because of these problems some veterinary clinicians view antepartum assessment as futile. However, preparation for a high-risk delivery can be made and the mare moved to a suitable facility for delivery or induction of parturition if it is known that the fetus is in distress or that the pregnancy is not normal.
- It is unlikely that there will be major advances in clinical perinatal medicine until the endocrine mechanisms that are involved in the control of fetal maturation are elucidated.

ABORTION

Definition

Abortion is the term applied to the loss of a pregnancy over the gestational age of 150 days; i.e.

after organogenesis is complete and before the limit of viability (300 days).[108] Embryonic loss up to 4 months of gestation has different implications (see p. 240).

Few medical conditions create more acrimony and upset between owners and veterinarians than equine abortion, yet the incidence of abortion in mares is still somewhat higher than in other species.[109]

- The loss of the pregnancy may occur at any stage, but between 8% and 15% of mares diagnosed as pregnant at 50 days are found not to be in foal in late gestation.
- Abortion from 150 days of gestation may result in an obvious loss of the pregnancy, but some fetal deaths are not reflected in any obvious signs.
- If the fetus is retained in the uterus at any stage after 50 days there will be some degree of mummification or autolysis.
- From about day 80 the placenta maintains the pregnancy; therefore fetal death after this stage results in immediate abortion.
- The cause of an abortion can be diagnosed in about 50% of cases if the fetal membranes and the fetus are examined shortly after the event.
- The large majority of abortions are sporadic, but there are very important causes of infectious or epidemic abortion that can be catastrophic in a stud farm situation (e.g. equine herpesvirus 1).

The primary objectives following any abortion in mares are:

- To establish the etiology and thereby the risk to other mares in contact (directly or indirectly).
- To return the mare to health as soon as possible.
- To safeguard the health of the in-contact horses (including the stallion) during subsequent attempts to establish the pregnancy.
- To re-establish a safe pregnancy that will be carried to term and result in a healthy foal.

Etiology

- The incidence of abortion in mares ranges from 5% to 15%.[109]
- Abortion is more common in older mares than in younger ones, possibly because of their lower uterine resistance, greater endometrial fibrosis and a higher incidence of 'small' embryos.
- Most abortions occur sporadically. The exceptions are those caused by equine herpesvirus 1.
- Twinning has been by far the most common cause of abortion in mares,[69] but since the widespread use of ultrasonography this is far less common and is a particularly unnecessary and disappointing cause of abortion.
  - ❑ More than 90% of mares carrying twins abort the pregnancy at some stage (see p. 243).
  - ❑ Ultrasonography of the reproductive tract during early pregnancy has led to a decrease in

twin abortions because it is now possible to identify twins by as early as 12–14 days.
- ❏ One of the two vesicles can be crushed, resulting in a singleton pregnancy.
- Equine herpesvirus infection has been the single most important infectious cause of abortion,[110] although bacterial abortion (from all causes) is relatively more common than that due to herpesvirus 1.
  - ❏ Vaccination of mares against herpesvirus 1 has decreased the incidence of abortion storms from this virus.
  - ❏ Because of the advances in the management of twins and effective vaccination for equine herpesvirus 1, bacterial placentitis is the most common cause of abortion in many breeding centers.
- Other possible causes are mentioned in Fig. 7.30.

Clinical signs

- Often no abortion is noticed at all and the mare is simply found to be nonpregnant at the end of the expected gestation period.
- Usually few premonitory signs are seen.
  - ❏ Probably the most common premonitory sign in protracted abortion (particularly that associated with placental separation or inflammation) is early lactation.
  - ❏ Preterm lactation is always significant in mares and it may continue at a high or low rate for some days or weeks before the abortion occurs.
- Sometimes a mummified fetus is found (consistent with fetal death some months previously), or fetal membranes are seen hanging from the vulva.
- Often the mare may show signs of labor.
  - ❏ Straining and behavioral isolation or distress may be seen but dystocia is seldom a problem.
- Most mares have few postabortion complications.
  - ❏ Most abortions are 'clean' (i.e. the whole fetoplacental unit is delivered without any complications). However, occasionally retained placenta or retained portions of placenta or metritis can develop in which case laminitis and other signs associated with endotoxemia can be serious and often life-threatening.

- Given a full reproductive history and the opportunity to investigate the mare and the fetus (with membranes) fully, a diagnosis can usually be reached in about 50% of cases.[111]
- The value of an examination of the fetal membranes cannot be overstated (see p. 325).

Investigation technique (see Fig. 7.31)

i. The possibility of an infectious cause must be paramount in every case and precautions must be taken to pre-empt the spread of infection.
  - It is wise to examine other in-contact mares before attending to the aborted mare.
  - Careful clinical examinations may help to establish the presence of infectious disease.

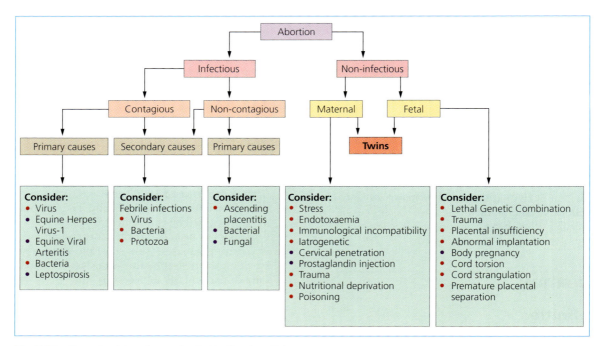

Fig. 7.30 Flow chart for diagnosis of abortion by etiology.

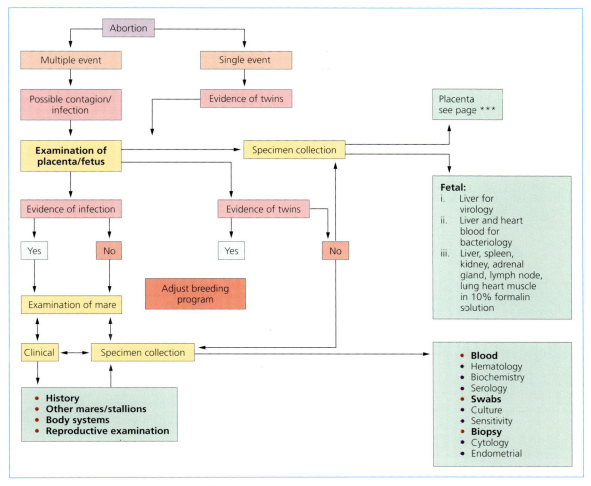

Fig. 7.31   Flow chart for investigation of abortion by etiology.

- The aborted mare should immediately be isolated and the aborted tissues removed to a clean, isolated place away from possible contact with other mares.
ii. A full breeding, management and vaccination history should be taken.
   - Previous disease, accident, injury or stresses are important factors.
iii. The gestational age of the fetus is an important aspect.
   - This can be compared with the fetal size (this obtaining some indication of when the fetus died).
   - The crown–rump length is obtained (Fig. 7.32).
iv. The collection of suitable specimens for laboratory analysis is important.
   - These should be obtained as soon as possible.
   - Poor postmortem technique, delays or poor collection/preservation technique inevitably reduce the chance of a successful diagnosis.[112,113]

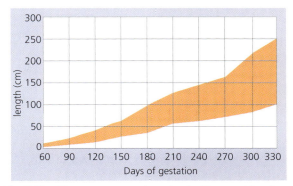

Fig. 7.32   The crown–rump length of a Thoroughbred fetus between 60 days and full term. There is some variation in the length, and different breeds will of course have a different set of parameters.

- The best specimen to send is the undamaged fetus and placental tissues (on ice, but not frozen), but in practice this is seldom feasible.

- All microbiological specimens should be taken with aseptic precautions (both to avoid contamination and to minimize the risk of contagion).
  v. Fetal tissues
  - Small pieces of fetal liver, lung, heart blood, and stomach content are collected for viral culture (virus transport medium) and for bacterial culture (bacterial transport medium).
  - Small representative pieces of fetal liver, lymph node, spleen, lung, heart, gastrointestinal tract, kidney and adrenal gland are placed in 10% formalin solution for histological examination.
  vi. Placental tissue
  - The placenta is carefully weighed and examined for obvious areas of abnormality/discoloration.
  - A portion of the placenta and any obvious areas of abnormality are taken fresh (on ice or in transport medium) for bacterial and viral culture; further specimens of chorioallantois and amnion are placed in 10% formalin solution.

- All formalin-fixed tissues may be sent in one container.
- It is preferable to allow the tissues to fix overnight in 10% formal saline and then to transfer them to a smaller container with two to three volumes of fresh, buffered neutral formalin before shipping.

Interpretation of findings

i. A combination of history, fetal size and fetal status can establish the age of death; this is not always the same as the stage of abortion.
ii. Before the development of fetal immune defenses at about 8 months of gestation, inflammatory changes in the aborted fetus are minimal.
iii. Fetuses aborted before 6 months are usually severely autolysed on delivery.
  - Histological and microbiological examination may be difficult or impossible.
iv. Fetuses aborted between 6 and 8 months of gestation are usually much less autolysed.
  - Fetal and placental lesions are more discernible and the chances of determining the cause improve.[114]
  - Hyperemia, hemorrhage, ischemic focal necrosis, and intravascular and extravascular

bacterial colonies can sometimes be observed microscopically.
v. After 8 months of gestation, discrete inflammatory lesions develop because fetal immune defense mechanisms are present.
  - The lesions are usually nonspecific.
  - Most fetuses aborted as a result of bacterial infections are reasonably fresh and have more discernible lesions then those less developed.
  - Placental lesions are the most diagnostic (see p. 341).
  - Microbiologic culture, impression smears, and histological examination of the placenta help distinguish bacterial and mycotic placentitis.
  - With equine herpesvirus infection, the fetus is aborted quickly and is in a fresh condition. Fetal lesions in these cases are unlike those of any other equine abortion.

Stillbirth/perinatal death

A full-term fetus may die in the immediate peripartum period. This is referred to as neonatal asphyxia. Causes of neonatal asphyxia include:

- Dystocia.
- Premature placental separation.
- Congenital abnormalities (especially of the fetal heart).
- Placental infections.
- Equine herpesvirus 1 or 4 infection.

- Immunoglobulin concentrations in umbilical cord blood may be useful in diagnosing fetal infection.
- In mares, high or rising titers may indicate viral arteritis and leptospirosis, although cautious interpretation is advised in view of the widespread prevalence of these infections.

Effect of maternal illness

- Severe or prolonged maternal illness may significantly compromise the developing foal, even resulting in fetal death.[115,116]
- Embryonic death in early gestation (<55 days) is caused by inadequate progesterone production by the ovaries that occurs secondary to systemic release of $PGF_{2\alpha}$.
- Mares in the second or third trimester of pregnancy that exhibit endotoxemia, placentitis, or restricted feed intake may release prostaglandins into the systemic circulation. This

prostaglandin surge is associated with a dramatic drop in fetal blood glucose concentration and rise in free fatty acid concentrations in the dam.[117] Death of the fetus and abortion ensue if the situation is not rectified quickly. Treatment of these mares is directed at ensuring myometrial quiescence and providing adequate nutrition and gas exchange to the fetus.

Prevention and treatment

In all cases of infectious (not necessarily contagious) abortion, the mare should be treated for endometritis (see p. 181).

Prevention is difficult without the full range of stud management procedures that might be expected to detect significant causes of abortion and so avoid their development.

1. Twinning
   - Twinning is a disappointing cause of abortion because it should be preventable by routine stud management in the first 25 days of gestation (see p. 245).
   - The presence of twins should never be ignored.
   - Twin ovulating mares tend to do so repeatedly; in theory, therefore, it should be possible to breed away from families that are inclined to twinning. It is doubtful if such a practice will ever occur.
2. Endometrial disease
   - Results of uterine biopsy can be used to select against mares that are likely to abort.
   - If endometrial periglandular fibrosis is extensive and severe, the chances that the mare will carry a foal until term decrease appreciably.
   - It is common for mares with widespread fibrosis to become detectably pregnant but to then lose the fetus before 90 days of pregnancy.
3. Infections
   - Equine herpesvirus 1
     - ❑ This remains the most important single infectious agent causing abortion in mares. It also is the most difficult to combat.
     - ❑ Prevention includes routine vaccination, avoidance of stress, and maintenance of closed herds of pregnant mares.
     - ❑ Vaccination programs are usually used with moderate success (see p. 258).
   - Viral arteritis (see p. 259)
     - ❑ Routine vaccination of stallions has been advocated in endemic and high-risk areas.
     - ❑ Breeding of stallions shedding the viral arteritis virus should be restricted to vaccinated or seropositive horses (see p. 259).
   - Bacterial endometritis (see p. 181)
     - ❑ Since the widespread use of vaccinations against herpesvirus and ultrasound detection of twins, bacterial infection remains the most prevalent overall cause of abortion.
     - ❑ Preventing endometritis in barren mares controls bacterial abortion.
     - ❑ Attention must be given to the anatomic changes of the external genitalia that predispose to loss of integrity, contamination, and persistent endometritis.
     - ❑ The short breeding season often necessitates breeding mares that have not completely recovered from bacterial infections. These mares represent the group at highest risk for subsequent bacterial abortion.

DISEASES RESPONSIBLE FOR ABORTION

INFECTIOUS CAUSES OF ABORTION

Equine herpesvirus 1 (Figs 7.33 and 7.34)

Profile
- Equine herpesvirus 1 is the most common infectious cause of abortion in mares.
- The virus also produces respiratory disease and a well-recognized neurological disorder characterized by hind-limb ataxia and paraplegia.
- The virus has a characteristic latency (i.e. it can be harbored without any clinical evidence in an apparently normal horse).
- Equine herpesvirus 4 may also cause abortion but is more often associated with respiratory tract infections only.
- The prevalence varies in different seasons but extensive abortion storms may occur.

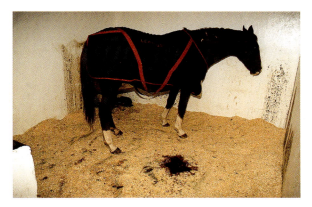

Fig. 7.33 Abortion as a result of equine herpesvirus 1 infection. The whole fetoplacental unit was expelled without difficulty and without significant secondary consequences.

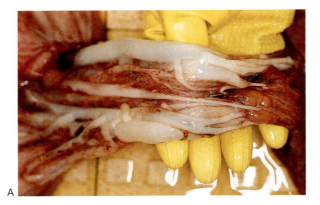

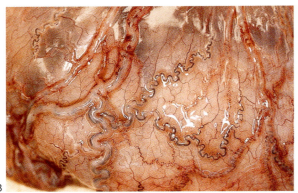

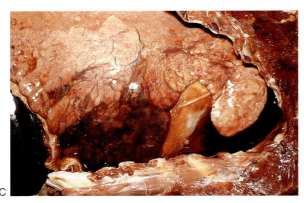

Fig. 7.34 Equine herpesvirus abortion. The placenta is edematous (A, B) and the foal was dead on delivery. If the foal is born alive it commonly dies within a day at most. (C) Pleuritis and pneumonitis typical of herpesvirus infection in neonatal foals.

- The epidemiology of herpes abortion relates to the congregation of mares at studs in late gestation.
- Disease control measures are directed at visiting mares and preventing the introduction of infected animals.
- The virus is transmitted via the respiratory route (through aerosol or fomite contact) and has a characteristically slow spread between horses in contact. Infected fetal membranes, fluids and vaginal discharges are a potent source of infection on stud farms.

Clinical signs

- Late-term abortion[118] (after 5 months but usually around 9 months) occurring 4–14 weeks after infection.
- Abortion occurs without premonitory signs and is characteristically clean (i.e. the foal is delivered wrapped in the intact membranes).
- Occasionally the foal is born alive but is characteristically weak and seldom survives beyond a few hours.

Diagnosis

- History of maternal respiratory infection or contact with infected horses during pregnancy. Possibly history of previous herpesvirus abortions.
- Fetal and placental examination for virus and characteristic changes.
- Focal hepatic necrosis, pleuritis and consolidated pneumonia with severe pulmonary edema.
- Virus isolation from fetal tissues or placenta and blood (in lithium heparin anticoagulant) if the foal is alive. The live foal may have significant antibody at birth (before colostral ingestion).[119]
- Virus identification in tissues with fluorescent antibody test.
- Histological features such as lymphoid necrosis and pneumonitis with focal hepatic necrosis are typically seen. Viral inclusion bodies are seen in many tissues.[120]

Differential diagnosis

Other causes of abortion (see Fig. 7.31).

Treatment

There is no treatment in mares or foals. The disease must be allowed to run its course and the risks of abortion are therefore unavoidable. Prevention and control of spread are therefore vital.

Control

- Immunity to the virus only lasts for 4–6 months and so repeated abortions can occur in successive seasons.
- Vaccination is available and has become standard practice for stud farms. Stud farms usually insist upon vaccination prior to the mare's arrival. On arrival mares should be quarantined for a suitable duration to minimize the risk of breakdowns and dissemination of infection to noninfected mares and stallions.
- Vaccination is not totally protective; latency is still a serious problem, but it does reduce the overall risk.
- Mares should be vaccinated at 3, 5, 7 and 9 months of gestation with a killed herpes vaccine.

Equine viral arteritis

Profile

Equine viral arteritis is caused by a togavirus (RNA). The virus occurs worldwide and there are controls that are in force in some countries to limit its importation and spread. Modern transportation provides ample opportunity for sport horses and breeding stock to become infected. In contrast to the stallion, there is no carrier state in the mare and so the spread of the disease is largely dependent on carrier stallions.

Mares can become infected through:

- Venereal infection from mating with an infected stallion.
- Artificial insemination with semen from an infected 'shedding' stallion.
- Contact with an aborted fetus, fetal membranes or fetal fluids from an infected mare.
- Direct aerosol contact transmission from a horse that has the respiratory form of the disease.

The incubation period is 3–8 days. Although morbidity is quite high in a group of animals, mortality is rare.

Clinical signs

Overt clinical signs range from mild to severe and include some or all of the following:

- Fever, lethargy, depression and anorexia.
- Edema of the limbs and mammary region, with urticaria-like plaques on the skin.
- Conjunctivitis and swelling of the conjunctiva (chemosis).
- Nasal discharge and other signs of respiratory disease.
- Abortion.

Diagnosis

Signs of equine viral arteritis can be difficult to differentiate from rhinopneumonitis and/or influenza and some affected mares show no outward clinical sign until abortion occurs. Usually there is an appropriate history, and the breeding record of the stallion will be supportive of a major problem.

- Laboratory diagnosis is essential and is based on viral isolation and serology.
- Virus may be isolated from nasal secretions, urine, semen and aborted fetuses.
- Animals with subclinical infections are best diagnosed using paired serologic titers taken 14 days apart. Tests available include virus isolation, complement fixation, and ELISA. Complement fixation test is the preferred method of diagnosis using serology.

Note:
- Care must be taken in interpreting results if the animals being tested have been vaccinated, as false-positives may occur.
- If virus isolation from semen is attempted, it is imperative that the laboratory is capable of handling the samples.
- Seroconversion of a mare following mating may be used to diagnose carrier stallions.

Treatment

- Most mares recover spontaneously.
- In mild cases no treatment is necessary; in more severe cases, supportive care may be required.

Control

- Avoid all possible mating with a potentially infected stallion. Imported mares should be placed in strict quarantine until their status is known.
- Blood sample every mare prior to breeding and breed only to a known disease-free stallion.
- All mares in contact with an infected stallion or mare must be isolated and tested for both seroconversion and virus.
- Infected individuals should be isolated for a minimum of 3 weeks beyond recovery.
- Aborted placentas and the associated fluids should be removed immediately and the area disinfected. The placenta may be used to identify virus particles.
- An antiseptic detergent capable of dissolving the lipid envelope of the virus should be used to routinely disinfect all equipment and facilities.
- In most countries with significant breeding programs involving expensive horses, there are statutory measures to prevent its importation or control its spread. There are guidelines for the use of positive stallions and for the vaccination of naïve individuals. Stallions used for breeding that are known carriers must be notified to the mare owner in writing.

If a mare is to be bred to a positive stallion, she must either be vaccinated (at least 21 days before breeding) or be seropositive from a previous exposure. These mares are classified as:
- Category 1 (being bred to a shedding stallion for the first time).
- Category 2 (being bred to a shedding stallion for the second or more time).

Note:
- Equine viral arteritis can be transmitted through infected semen being used for artificial insemination (fresh, chilled and frozen) and through infected embryos.

A modified live virus vaccine is available but may be controlled by state/federal officials.

- Prior to vaccination the mare MUST be blood sampled to establish that she was seronegative before vaccination.
- Vaccination should not be viewed as an alternative to good hygiene and husbandry in the broodmare and the stallion.

Bacterial placentitis (see also p. 338)

Profile

Streptococcus spp. is the bacterium most frequently isolated from aborted fetuses and from placentas with gross lesions. Other commonly encountered organisms are:

- *Escherichia coli.*
- *Pseudomonas* spp.
- *Klebsiella* spp.
- *Staphylococcus* spp.

The fetus may become infected in the following ways:[121]

1. Ascending infection via the cervix.
   - Cervical infections are most common, with lesions observed on the placenta at the cervical star.
   - The infection spreads to the fetus, and organisms can be recovered from many fetal organs. Gross fetal lesions are commonly nonspecific.
   - Abortion is caused by fetal death from septicemia or by expansion of the area of chorionitis (placentitis), resulting in placental insufficiency.
2. Hematogenous spread of organisms, including:
   - *Corynebacterium pseudotuberculosis.*
   - *Salmonella abortus equi.*
   - *Streptococcus zooepidermicus.*
   - *Leptospira pomona.*
3. Introduction of small numbers of bacteria at breeding, including:
   - *Klebsiella pneumoniae.*
   - *Pseudomonas aeruginosa.*
   - *Staphylococcus* spp.
   - *Streptococcus* spp.

- Bacterial and fungal causes cannot be accurately differentiated simply by inspection of the placenta.

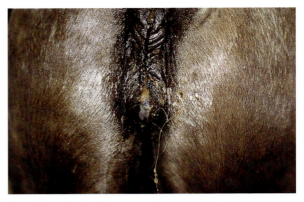

Fig. 7.35 Vaginal discharge in a mare that aborted 4 days later as a result of bacterial (streptococcal) endometritis (placentitis).

- Vaginal discharge and premature lactation are often the first signs of bacterial or fungal abortion (Fig. 7.35).
- When a vaginal discharge is observed, a vaginal speculum examination should be performed to determine the source of the discharge and the extent of cervical relaxation or dilation.
- Transabdominal and transrectal ultrasonography can provide evidence of fetal viability and the degree of placental separation.
- Fetal loss can be established by measuring circulating estrogen in the mare (see p. 238).
- There may be no gross lesions in acute cases of placentitis.
- The placenta may be edematous and heavy, with local areas showing even greater thickening resulting from inflammatory proliferation. The infected chorionic surface is frequently brown, with varying amounts of fibrinonecrotic exudate. Culture and examination of stained smears are necessary for diagnosis.
- Organisms can be recovered from many fetal organs, most consistently from the stomach.[122]

Salmonella abortus equi

Profile

This disease occurs in Europe, South Africa and South America. It was formerly a serious cause of abortion in the USA but has become much less significant.[123] Latent infections are common (as with all pathogenic species of *Salmonella*) and can be activated by stress (transport, disease, surgery, or other less apparent stress).

The organism is spread mainly via contamination of pastures with uterine secretions from aborted mares.

Clinical signs
- Fever, depression and anorexia.
- Occasional diarrhea.
- Abortion occurs some 4–7 days after the sickness develops.
- The fetal membranes are edematous and show petechial hemorrhages and areas of placental necrosis.

Diagnosis
- Culture of organisms from mare, placenta, and fetal heart blood.
- Serodiagnosis of infection is theoretically possible but is not universally available.
- Almost all clinical infections with *Salmonella* spp. cause a moderate to profound leukopenia.

Differential diagnosis
Other causes of abortion accompanied by signs of generalized illness in the mare.

Treatment
There is little that can be done; usually by the time the fever and depression are detected the abortion is inevitable.

Control
- Strict hygiene precautions to avoid spread to other mares.
- Vaccines are available.

Leptospirosis

Profile
- Leptospirosis, once considered an infrequent cause of equine abortion, has been increasingly identified as a causative infection.[124,125] Abortion may be caused by infections with *Leptospira pomona*, *L. bratislava*, *L. grippotyphosa* and *L. icterohaemorrhagica*.
- The incidence of abortion may increase in wet environmental conditions.
- Transmission is thought to occur by contact with wildlife, low-lying or swampy areas, and stagnant water.

Clinical signs
- Abortion in mid- to late gestation
  - ❏ The aborted fetus may be icteric (jaundiced).
  - ❏ Fetal autolysis may suggest that the foal has been dead for some time (often some weeks) before abortion occurs.
  - ❏ Neonatal deaths and stillbirths may occur in cases of abortion in late gestation.
- Systemic signs lasting 3–7 days may be recognized some 2–4 weeks before the abortion, including:
  - ❏ Pyrexia.
  - ❏ Depression and anorexia.
  - ❏ Icterus.
  - ❏ Renal failure (later sign).

Diagnosis
- Leptospiral abortion is difficult to diagnose because mares rarely exhibit clinical signs of disease. A preliminary diagnosis is based on the postmortem findings in aborted fetuses and placentas.
  - ❏ An aborted fetus may have no gross lesions, or it may exhibit icterus and a swollen yellow liver.
  - ❏ Placental lesions are common and varied and may include a thickened allantochorion or an exudate.
  - ❏ Histologically, nephritis and placentitis are commonly observed.
  - ❏ It is unlikely that spirochetes will be identifiable in the fetal tissues.
- Isolation of the organism and serotyping to establish the serovar responsible.
  - ❏ Bacteriological isolation is often very difficult.
  - ❏ Suspected cases may be confirmed by demonstrating the organisms by the immunofluorescence technique or by War thin Starry stain[126] (Silver stain) in fetal kidney and liver and in placental tissues.[124]
- Rising antibody titers are strongly supportive of the diagnosis.
  - ❏ Affected mares often have a high serological titer at the time of abortion because of the delay between infection and abortion.
  - ❏ Serology is based on ELISA and agglutination tests.

Differential diagnosis
- Other causes of fetal icterus and anemia.
- Other causes of abortion (see Fig. 7.31).

Treatment and control
- Prolonged treatment with either intramuscular procaine penicillin G (20,000 IU/kg) twice daily or intravenous oxytetracycline (5 mg/kg) may decrease the shedding period.
- There are currently no approved vaccines for use in horses. In some clinical situations, cattle vaccinations for leptospires have been utilized with success, although there is increased risk of anaphylaxis. The risk/benefits must be weighed in each individual case before employing these vaccinations off-label.
- Management practices of sanitation and hygiene, including elimination of exposure to contaminated feed and water and infective urine, and aborted fetuses, are essential.

Fungal placentitis

- Fungal abortion is very rare.
- *Aspergillus* is the most common fungal cause of placentitis.[127]
- Fungal infection is usually introduced via the vagina and a patent cervix.
- The exudate in fungal placentitis tends to be mucoid, but otherwise this type of placentitis is indistinguishable from bacterial placentitis.
- The chorioallantois is the best specimen of choice for diagnosing mycotic abortion. It is diffusely involved, yellowish, thickened, and leathery and the affected area is clearly demarcated from the normal, reddish-brown chorioallantois. The chorionic surface is necrotic and usually covered with thick, adherent, mucoid exudate.
- The amnion may have irregular necrotic plaques in about 10% of *Mucor* spp. infections.
- The fungal organism may be isolated from a fungal culture of the mare's uterus after delivery of the fetus and placenta.
- Impression smears of the placenta may reveal fungal hyphae.
- Systemic fungal infections have occurred in fetuses delivered from mares with fungal placentitis but skin lesions are not present.

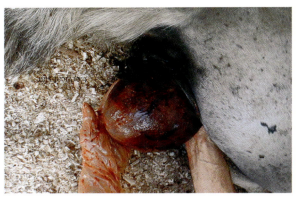

Fig. 7.36   Premature placental separation ('red bag') delivery. This is an absolute emergency requiring immediate attention (see p. 299).

NONINFECTIOUS CAUSES OF ABORTION

By far the most common causes of noninfectious abortion are:

1. Twin pregnancy (see p. 242).
2. Placental abnormalities/insufficiency (see p. 333).
   - When the placenta separates prematurely, a full-term fetus can die from hypoxia or anoxia.
   - Either the allantochorion appears at the vulva with the cervical star intact, or the allantochorion detaches from the endometrium some time before the start of labor.
   - As soon as the condition is recognized, the foal must be delivered immediately (Fig. 7.36).
3. Fetal death from physical trauma (strangulating umbilical cord conditions) (see p. 336).[128]
4. Maternal injury.
5. Maternal endotoxemia.
6. Genetic abnormalities inconsistent with life.
   - Many developmental and structural anomalies have been reported in aborted fetuses.[129]
   - Most abortions occur after 6 months of gestation.
   - Fetuses aborted because of developmental retardation often appear physiologically unable to survive.
7. Iatrogenic interference.
   - Ill-advised or rough handling of the uterus or cervix during rectal or vaginal examinations.
   - Inadvertent administration of abortifacient drugs (see p. 263).
8. Toxic and nutritional disorders.
   - Various plants, anthelmintics, purgatives, and nutritional deficiencies have been incriminated as causes for abortion in mares.
   - Fescue grasses, Sudan grasses, sorghum, and other weeds have been reported to be toxic to the fetus.
   - Phenothiazine derivatives and organophosphates are the anthelmintics most commonly associated with abortion.
   - The most notable nutritional deficiencies involved are lack of selenium and iodine.
   - Little is known about other drugs and plants that may cause abortion.

Fetal mummification

A fresh fetus is most commonly aborted. Mummified fetuses are aborted when one of two fetuses dies in utero and the pregnancy continues, or in cases of bacterial or mycotic placentitis in which the mare is treated with systemic antimicrobials and progesterone. In these cases, if the fetus dies and the cervix remains closed, the fetus is retained. For this reason, practitioners must be cautious about administering antimicrobial and progesterone to pregnant mares with a vulvar discharge.

INDUCTION OF ABORTION

Successful elective induction of abortion requires a basic understanding of the endocrinology of pregnancy and the mechanisms by which pregnancy is sustained.

- From about 5 days after ovulation until around day 37–38, the embryo is solely dependent upon a functional corpus luteum for its survival.

- From day 36 up to around 110 days the endometrial cups secrete eCG, and secondary corpora lutea develop and provide supplementary progesterone.
- By about 80–100 days up to full term, maintenance of the pregnancy becomes dependent upon progestogens derived from placental sources.

The circumstances for elective abortion include:

- The mare has conceived twins (see p. 242).
- The mare has become pregnant from inadvertent/accidental breeding.
  - ❏ Accidental access to stallions.
  - ❏ The wrong stallion or the wrong semen has been used.
- The mare has been purchased recently as an athlete but is found to be pregnant.
- The mare has complications that might threaten her life if the pregnancy were to continue.

Termination during early pregnancy (before 100 days)

- Pregnancy can be terminated within the first 38 days of gestation by a single injection of $PGF_{2\alpha}$.
  - ❏ Abortion occurs about 5–8 days after injection.
- After day 38 (the time of endometrial cup formation), daily prostaglandin injections for 3–4 days are needed to induce abortion.
  - ❏ Estrus and ovulation occur sporadically following this procedure.
  - ❏ It is difficult to breed these mares successfully during the same breeding season.

Termination during late pregnancy (after 100 days)

Mares that are to be aborted after 100 days of gestation must be chosen carefully because the procedure carries a higher risk of uterine damage, dystocia, retained placenta, and other complications.
- The procedure is best limited to pregnancies under 6 months of age for welfare reasons.
- Furthermore, an abortion over 6 months is a harrowing affair for all concerned; the foal is often born alive and should be euthanized promptly.
- Retained placenta is much more common in later pregnancies and this itself can be serious. It is better to leave mares over 6–7 months to carry the foal to full term.

Method 1

Manual dilation of the cervix and irrigation of the uterus with large volumes of warm (38°C), sterile saline solution.

Technique

i. Strict asepsis is required to minimize uterine contamination.
ii. The cervix is dilated by gentle manual manipulation until the fingers enter the space between the allantochorion and the uterus.
iii. Sterile saline is slowly infused into this space causing separation of the placental membranes from the endometrium. The infusion must be slow to allow slow stretching of the myometrium without undue discomfort.
iv. Up to 3 liters may be tolerated.
v. The mare is carefully observed for expulsion of the fetus.
vi. Occasionally the conceptus can be grasped and manually removed from the anterior vagina/cervix.
vii. Antibiotics and intensive care should be supplied for the procedure.

Complications

- Retention of the placenta (particularly in more advanced pregnancies).

Method 2

Endoscopy-guided fetal ablation.

Method 3

Cloprostenol, a prostaglandin analog (250 μg intramuscularly), may be used twice daily to induce abortion in mares between 80 days and 6 months of pregnancy. When it was administered experimentally to mares between 82 and 150 days of gestation, fetal expulsion occurred in all mares following 2–5 daily injections.[105]

- Treated mares usually abort without complications.
- The placenta is usually passed within 4–5 hours.
- If the mare has been treated with progestin to maintain pregnancy, a delay of 48 hours after the last treatment with progestin should be allowed before the cloprostenol regimen is begun. Failure to delay the prostaglandin may result in retained placenta.[105]

- Corticosteroids are not effective in inducing abortion in horses. Large repeated doses are required and this has serious secondary effects on the mare.[130] This procedure should not be attempted in horses.

PREDICTION OF FOALING DATE

Prediction of a mare's foaling date is an important factor in stud farm management. Failure to recognize that a mare is due can significantly reduce the prognosis for the foal. This is especially important in mares that are classified as high-risk. In spite of the availability of published gestation tables and a defined gestational length for horses, foaling is an unpredictable affair and a lot of information needs to be combined if a high rate of fertility is to be achieved:

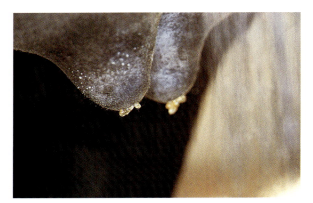

Fig. 7.37 The typical 'wax candles' on the ends of the teats of a mare due to foal within 24 hours.

- Known last service date. In most controlled breeding programs this is known and a fixed expected date can be established using tables.
- Historical duration of gestation. Individual mares often vary in their gestational length. Thus, a mare may 'usually' foal early or late, and if this is combined with the last service date a reasonable prediction can be made.
- Clinical examination:
  - ❏ Udder development, changes in mammary secretions (see p. 270), waxing up of the teats (Fig. 7.37), and pelvic relaxation are late indicators of approaching parturition.
  - ❏ Changes in mammary secretion electrolyte concentrations in the last week of gestation are currently the best predictor for determining foaling date.[102,103] Sodium concentrations in mammary secretions drop and potassium rises approximately 3–5 days before parturition. Calcium concentrations in mammary secretions rise to >12 mol/l (40 mg/dl) approximately 24 hours before foaling (see p. 270)
  - ❏ Changes in body temperature can be used but are less useful than in other species.[131]
- Fetal size and function as determined by ultrasonographic measurements (see p. 235) can be used but are unreliable indicators of readiness for birth or impending delivery.

- Other aids can be used to detect the onset of delivery (see p. 272).

REFERENCES

1. Hearn FP. Factors influencing pregnancy and pregnancy loss from one breeding farm in Ontario. MSc thesis. University of Guelph; 1993:17–19.
2. Jeffcott LB, Hyland JH, MacLean AA, et al. Changes in maternal hormone concentrations associated with induction of fetal death at day 45 of gestation in mares. Journal of Reproduction and Fertility Supplement 1987; 35:461–467.
3. Bezard J, Magistrini M, DuChamp G, et al. Chronology of equine fertilization and embryonic development in vivo and in vitro. Equine Veterinary Journal Supplement 1989; 8:105–110.
4. Betteridge KJ, Eagelsome MD, Mitchell D, et al. Development of horse embryos up to twenty-two days after ovulation: observations on fresh specimens. Journal of Anatomy 1982; 135:191–209.
5. VanNiekerk CH, Allen WR. Early embryonic development in the horse. Journal of Reproduction and Fertility Supplement 1975; 23:495–498.
6. Steffenhagen WP, Pineda MH, Ginther OJ. Retention of unfertilized ova in the uterine tubes of mares. American Journal of Veterinary Research 1972; 33:2391–2398.
7. Betteridge KJ, Mitchell D. Direct evidence of retention of unfertilized ova in the oviduct of the mare. Journal of Reproduction and Fertility Supplement 1974; 39:145–148.
8. Oriol JG, Beresford B, Sharom FJ, et al. Biochemical composition of the equine capsule: a preliminary report. Journal of Reproduction and Fertility Supplement 1991; 44:639–641.
9. Gidley-Baird AA, O'Niel C. Early pregnancy detection in the mare. Equine Veterinary Data 1982; 3:42.
10. Ginther OJ. Mobility of the early equine conceptus. Theriogenology 1983; 19:608–611.
11. Ginther OJ. Fixation and orientation of the early equine conceptus. Theriogenology 1983; 19:613–623.
12. Enders AC, Liu IKM. Lodgement of the equine blastocyst in the uterus from fixation through endometrial cup formation. Journal of Reproduction and Fertility Supplement 1991; 44:427–438.
13. Heap RB, Hamon M, Allen WR. Studies on oestrogen synthesis by preimplantation equine conceptuses. Journal of Reproduction and Fertility Supplement 1982; 132:343–352.
14. Sharp DC. Factors associated with the maternal recognition of pregnancy in mares. Veterinary Clinics of North America: Large Animal Practice 1980; 2:277–289.
15. Sharp DC, McDowell KJ, Weithenauer J, et al. The continuum of events leading to maternal recognition of pregnancy in mares. Journal of Reproduction and Fertility Supplement 1989; 37:101–107.
16. Sharp DC. Maternal recognition of pregnancy. In: McKinnon AO, Voss JL. Equine reproduction. Philadelphia: Lea & Febiger; 1993:486–494.

17. Ginther OJ, First NL. Maintenance of the corpus luteum in hysterectomized mares. American Journal of Veterinary Research 1971; 32:1687–1691.

18. Zavy MT, Mayer R, Vernon MW, et al. An investigation of the uterine luminal environment of non-pregnant and pregnant pony mares. Journal of Reproduction and Fertility Supplement 1979; 27:403–411.

19. Vernon MW, Zavy MT, Asquith RL, et al. Prostaglandin $F_{2\alpha}$ in the equine endometrium: steroid modulation and production capacities during the estrous cycle and early pregnancy. Biology of Reproduction 1981; 25:581–589.

20. Neely DP, Kindahl H, Stabenfeldt GH, et al. Prostaglandin release patterns in the mare: physiological, pathophysiological, and therapeutic responses. Journal of Reproduction and Fertility Supplement 1979; 27:421–429.

21. Douglas RH, Ginther OJ. Development of the equine fetus and placenta. Journal of Reproduction and Fertility Supplement 1975; 23:503–505.

22. Spincemaille J, Bouters R, Vanderplassche M, et al. Some aspects of endometrial cup formation and PMSG production. Journal of Reproduction and Fertility Supplement 1975; 23:415–418.

23. Collins MH. Placentas and foetal health. Equine Veterinary Journal Supplement 1993; 4:8–11.

24. Steven DH. Placentation in the mare. Journal of Reproduction and Fertility Supplement 1982; 31:41–55.

25. Steven DH, Samuel CA. Anatomy of the placental barrier in the mare. Journal of Reproduction and Fertility Supplement 1975; 23:579–582.

26. Ginther OJ. Reproductive biology of the mare: basic and applied aspects. Cross Plaines, WI: Equiservices; 1979.

27. Allen WR, Moor RM. The origin of the equine endometrial cups. I. Production of PMSG by fetal trophoblast cells. Journal of Reproduction and Fertility Supplement 1972; 29:313–316.

28. Squires IL, Stevens WB, Pickett BW, et al. Role of pregnant mare serum gonadotropin in luteal function of pregnant mares. American Journal of Veterinary Research 1979; 40:889–891.

29. Evans MJ, Irvine CHG. The serum concentrations of FSH, LH and progesterone during the oestrous cycle and early pregnancy in the mare. Journal of Reproduction and Fertility Supplement 1975; 23:193–200.

30. Urwin VE, Allen WR. Pituitary and chorionic gonadotrophin control of ovarian function during early pregnancy in equids. Journal of Reproduction and Fertility Supplement 1982; 32: 371–382.

31. Allen WR. The influence of fetal genotype upon endometrial cup development and PMSG and progesterone production in equids. Journal of Reproduction and Fertility 1975; 23: 405–413.

32. Bosu WTK, Turner L, Franks T. Estrone sulphate and progesterone concentrations in the peripheral blood of pregnant mares: clinical implications. Proceedings of the International Congress on Animal Reproduction and Artificial Insemination 1984:78.

33. Moss GE, Estergreen VL, Becker SR, et al. The source of the 5α-pregnanes that occur during gestation in mares. Journal of Reproduction and Fertility Supplement 1979; 27:511–519.

34. Ousey JC, Fowden AL, Rossdale PD, et al. Plasma progestagens as markers of feto-placental health. Pferdeheilkunde 2001; 17:574–578.

35. Raeside JI, Liptrap RM, Milne FJ. Relationship of fetal gonads to urinary estrogen excretion by the pregnant mare. American Journal of Veterinary Research 1973; 34:843–845.

36. Amoroso EC. Ovarian activity in the pregnant mare. Nature 1948; 161:335–356.

37. Holtan DW, Nett TM, Estergreen VL. Plasma progestins in pregnant, postpartum and cycling mares. Journal of Animal Science 1975; 40:251–260.

38. Chavatte P. Biosynthesis and function of corticoids and progestagens in equine pregnancy. PhD thesis, Cambridge University; 1996.

39. LeBlanc MM. What we have learned from an experimental model of ascending placentitis: useful diagnostics. Proceedings West Coast Equine Reproduction Symposium 2002:137–142.

40. Hyland JH, Wright PJ, Manning SJ. An investigation of the use of plasma estrone sulfate concentrations for the diagnosis of pregnancy in mares. Australian Veterinary Journal 1984; 61:123–125

41. Silver M, Fowden AL. Prepartum adrenocortical maturation in the fetal foal: responses to ACTH. Journal of Endocrinology 1994; 142:417–425.

42. Roberts SJ. Gestation and pregnancy diagnosis in the mare. In: Morrow DA, ed. Current therapy in theriogenology. Philadelphia: WB Saunders; 1980:736–746.

43. Rossdale PD, Ricketts SW. Equine stud farm medicine. London: Baillière Tindall; 1980:52.

44. Allen WE, Goddard PJ. Serial investigations of early pregnancy in pony mares using real time ultrasound scanning. Equine Veterinary Journal 1984; 16:509–514.

45. McKinnon AO, Squires EL, Voss JL. Ultrasound evaluation of the mare's reproductive tract: part II. Compendium for Continuing Education 1987; 9:472–482.

46. Hunt B, Lein DH, Foote RH. Monitoring of milk and plasma progesterone for evaluation of post partum oestrus cycles and early pregnancy in mares. Journal of the American Veterinary Medical Association 1978; 172:1298–1302.

47. Chak RM, Bruss M. The MIP test for diagnosis of pregnancy in mares. Proceedings of the American Association of Equine Practitioners 1968:53–55.

48. Terqui M, Palmer E. Oestrogen patterns during early pregnancy in the mare. Journal of Reproduction and Fertility Supplement 1979; 27:441–446.

49. Cox JE, Galina CS. A comparison of the chemical tests for oestrogens used in equine pregnancy diagnoses. Veterinary Record 1970; 86:97–100.

50. Bamberg E, Choi HS, Mostl E, et al. Enzymatic determination of unconjugated oestrogens in faeces for pregnancy diagnosis in mares. Equine Veterinary Journal 1984; 16:537–539.

51. Terqui M, Palmer E. Oestrogen pattern during early pregnancy in the mare. Journal of Reproduction and Fertility Supplement 1979; 27:441–446.

52. Ginther OJ. Ultrasonic imaging and reproductive events in the mare. Cross Plains, WI: Equiservices; 1986.

53. McKinnon AO, Squires EL, Voss JL. Ultrasound evaluation of the mare's reproductive tract: Part II. Compendium for Continuing Education for the Practicing Veterinarian 1987; 9:472–482.

54. Pipers RS, Adams-Brendemuehl CS. Techniques and applications of transabdominal ultrasonography in the pregnant mare. Journal of the American Veterinary Medical Association 1984; 185:766–771.

55. Curran S, Ginther OJ. Ultrasonic diagnosis of equine fetal sex by location of the genital tubercle. Equine Veterinary Science 1989; 9:77–83.

56. LeBlanc MM. Diseases of the embryo. In: Colohan PT, Mayhew IG, Merritt AM, et al, eds. Equine medicine and surgery. 5th edn. Philadelphia: Mosby; 1999:1199–1202.

57. Ball BA, Little TV, Weber JA, et al. Survival of day 4 embryos from young normal mares and aged subfertile mares after transfer to normal recipient mares. Journal of Reproduction and Fertility Supplement 1989; 85:187–194.

58. Bain AM. Foetal losses during pregnancy in Thoroughbred mares: a record of 2562 pregnancies. Irish Veterinary Journal 1969; 17:155–158.

59. Woods GL, Baker CB, Baldwin JL, et al. Early pregnancy loss in broodmares. Journal of Reproduction and Fertility Supplement 1987; 35:455–459.

60. Newcombe JR. Embryonic loss and abnormalities of early pregnancy. Equine Veterinary Education 2000; 12:88–101.

61. Long SE. Genetic wastage in farm animal production. Journal of Animal Breeding 1995; 1:54–60.

62. Ball BA, Little TV, Hillman RB, et al. Pregnancy rates at 2 and 14 days and estimated embryonic loss prior to day 14 in normal and subfertile mares. Theriogenology 1989; 26:611–619.

63. Carnevale EM, Uson M, Bozzola JJ, et al. Comparison of oocytes from young and old mares with light and electron microscopy. Theriogenology 1999; 51:229–230.

64. Eilts BE, Scholl DT, Paccamonte DL, et al. Prevalence of endometrial cysts and their effect on fertility. Biology of Reproduction 1995; 1:527–532.

65. Adams GP, Kastelic JP, Bergfelt DR, et al. Effect of uterine inflammation and ultrasonically detected uterine pathology on fertility in the mare. Journal of Reproduction and Fertility Supplement 1987; 35:445–454.

66. Chevalier F, Palmer E. Ultrasonic echography in the mare. Journal of Reproduction and Fertility Supplement 1982; 32:423–430.

67. Ginther OJ. Relationships among number of days between multiple ovulations, number of embryos and type of fixation in mares. Journal of Equine Veterinary Science 1987; 7:82–88.

68. Ginther OJ. Ultrasonographic imaging and reproductive events in the mare. Cross Plains, WI: Equiservices; 1986.

69. Jeffcott LB, Whitwell KE. Twinning as a cause of fetal and neonatal loss in the Thoroughbred mare. Journal of Comparative Pathology 1973; 83:91–106.

70. Ginther OJ. Relationships among number of days between multiple ovulations, number of embryos and type of fixation in mares. Journal of Equine Veterinary Science 1987; 7:82–88.

71. Ginther OJ. The nature of embryo reduction in mares with twin conceptuses: deprivation hypothesis. American Journal of Veterinary Research 1989; 50:45–53.

72. Pascoe DR. Pregnancy diagnosis and management of twins. Proceedings of the 19th Bain-Fallon Memorial Lectures. Australian Equine Veterinary Association 1997:103–115.

73. Pascoe DR, Pascoe RR, Hughes JP, et al. Management of twin pregnancy by manual embryonic reduction and comparison of two techniques and three hormonal therapies. American Journal of Veterinary Research 1987; 48:1594–1599.

74. Roberts CJ. Termination of twin gestation by blastocyst crush in the mare. Equine Veterinary Journal 1983; 15:40–42.

75. Woods GL, Hallowell AL. Management of twin embryos and twin fetuses in the mare. In: McKinnon AO, Voss JL, eds. Equine reproduction. Philadelphia: Lea & Febiger; 1993:532–535.

76. Rantanen NW, Kencaid B. Ultrasound guided fetal cardiac puncture: a method of twin reduction in the mare. Proceedings of the American Association of Equine Practitioners 1989:173–179.

77. Newcombe JR. Embryonic loss and abnormalities of early pregnancy. Equine Veterinary Education 2000; 12:88–101.

78. Pascoe DR. Management of twin pregnancies by manual embryonic reduction and comparison of two techniques and three hormonal therapies. Journal of Reproduction and Fertility Supplement 1987; 35:701–702.

79. Immegart HM, Threlfall WR. Monitoring gestation. In: Reed SM, Bayly WM, eds. Equine internal medicine. Philadelphia: WB Saunders; 1999:788–790.

80. Rossdale PD, Silver M. The concept of readiness for birth. Journal of Reproduction and Fertility Supplement 1982; 32:507–510.

81. Rossdale PD, McGladdery AJ, Ousey JC, et al. Increase in plasma progestagen concentrations in the mare after foetal injection with CRH, ACTH or betamethasone in late gestation. Equine Veterinary Journal 1992; 24:347–350.

82. Santschi EM, LeBlanc MM, Weston PG. Progestogen, oestrone sulphate and cortisol concentrations in pregnant mares during medical and surgical disease. Journal of Reproduction and Fertility Supplement 1991; 44:627–634.

83. Ousey JC, Rossdale PD, Cash RSG, et al. Plasma concentrations of progesterone, oestrone sulphate and prolactin in pregnant mares subjected to natural challenge with equid herpesvirus-1. Journal of Reproduction and Fertility Supplement 1987; 35:519–528.

84. Rossdale PD, Ousey JC, Cottrill CM, et al. Effects of placental pathology on maternal plasma progestagen and mammary secretion calcium concentrations and on neonatal adrenocortical function in the horse. Journal of Reproduction and Fertility Supplement 1991; 44:579–590.

85. Adams-Brendemuehl C, Pipers FS. Antepartum evaluations in the equine fetus. Journal of Reproduction and Fertility Supplement 1987; 35:565–568.

86. Reef VB, Vaala WE, Worth LT, et al. Transcutaneous ultrasonographic assessment of fetal well being during late gestation: a preliminary report on development of an equine biophysical profile. Proceedings of the American Association of Equine Practitioners 1996; 42:152–153.

87. Renaudin CD, Troedsson MHT, Gillis CL, et al. Ultrasonographic evaluation of the equine placenta by transrectal and transabdominal approach in the normal pregnant mare. Theriogenology 1997; 47:559–573.

88. Giles RC, Donahue JM, Hong CG, et al. Causes of abortion, stillbirth, and perinatal death in horses: 3527 cases (1986–1991). Journal of the American Veterinary Medical Association 1993; 203:1170–1175.

89. Kelleman AA, Lester GD, LeBlanc MM. Ultrasonographic evaluation of a model of induced ascending placentitis in late gestation in the pony mare. Proceedings of the Annual Conference Society for Theriogenology 2000:279–284.

90. Adams-Brendemuehl C. Fetal assessment. In: Koterba AM, Drummond WM, Kosch PC, eds. Equine clinical neonatology. Philadelphia: Lea & Febiger; 1990:16–20.

91. Reef VB, Vaala WE, Worth LT, et al. Ultrasonographic assessment of fetal well being during late gestation: development of an equine biophysical profile. Equine Veterinary Journal 1996; 28:200–208.

92. Manning FA, Morrison I, Lange IR, et al. Fetal assessment based on fetal biophysical profile scoring: experience in 12,620 referred high-risk pregnancies. I. Perinatal mortality by frequency and etiology. American Journal of Obstetrics and Gynecology 1985; 151:343–350.

93. Colles CM, Parks RD. Fetal electrocardiography in the mare. Equine Veterinary Journal 1978; 10:32–37.

94. Parks RD, Colles CM. Fetal electrocardiography in the mare as practical aid to diagnosing singleton and twin pregnancy. Veterinary Record 1977; 100:25–26.

95. Buss DD, Asbury AC, Chevalier L. Limitations in equine fetal electrocardiography. Journal of the American Veterinary Medical Association 1980; 177:174–176.

96. Larks SD, Holm LW, Parker HR. A new technique for demonstration of the fetal electrocardiogram in the large domestic animals (cattle, sheep, horse). Cornell Veterinarian 1960; 50:459–462.

97. Buss DD, Asbury AC, Chevalier L. Limitations in equine fetal electrocardiography. Journal of the American Veterinary Medical Association 1980; 177:174–178.

98. Adams Brendemuehl C, Pipers FS. Antepartum evaluation of the equine fetus. Journal of Reproduction and Fertility Supplement 1987; 35:565–568.

99. Holmes JR, Darke PGG. Foetal electrocardiography in the mare. Veterinary Record 1968; 82: 651–653.

100. Holdstock NB, McGladdery AJ, Ousey JC, et al. Assessing methods of collection and changes of selected biochemical constituents in amniotic and allantoic fluid throughout equine pregnancy. Biology of reproduction monograph series 1: Equine reproduction 1995; VI:21–38.

101. Paccamonti D, Swiderski C, Marx B, et al. Electrolytes and biochemical enzymes in amniotic and allantoic fluid of the equine fetus during late gestation. Biology of reproduction monograph series 1: Equine reproduction 1995; VI:39–49.

102. Leadon DP, Jeffcott LB, Rossdale PD. Mammary secretions in normal, spontaneous and induced premature parturition in the mare. Equine Veterinary Journal 1984; 16:256–259.

103. Ousey JC, Dudan F, Rossdale PD. Preliminary studies of mammary secretions in the mare to assess foetal readiness for birth. Equine Veterinary Journal 1984; 16:259–263.

104. Silver M, Fowden AL, Knox J, et al. Relationship between circulating tri-iodothyronine and cortisol in the perinatal period in the foal. Journal of Reproduction and Fertility Supplement 1991; 44:619–626.

105. Daels P, Besognet B, Hansen B, et al. Effect of progesterone on prostaglandin $F_{2\alpha}$ secretion and outcome of pregnancy during cloprostenol-induced abortion in mares. American Journal of Veterinary Research 1996; 57:1331–1337.

106. Sertich PL, Vaala WE. Concentrations of antibiotics in mares, foals, and fetal fluids after antibiotic administration during late pregnancy. Proceedings of the American Association of Equine Practitioners 1992; 38:727–733.

107. Card CE, Wood MR. Effects of acute administration of clenbuterol on uterine tone and equine fetal and maternal heart rates. Biology of reproduction monograph series 1: Equine reproduction 1995; VI:7–13.

108. LeBlanc MM. Abortion. In: Colohan PT, Mayhew IG, Merritt AM, et al, eds. Equine medicine and surgery. 5th edn. Philadelphia: Mosby; 1999:1202–1207.

109. Mahaffey LW. Abortion in mares. Veterinary Record 1968; 82:681–689.

110. Bain AM. Foetal losses during pregnancy in Thoroughbred mares: a record of 2562 pregnancies. Irish Veterinary Journal 1969; 17:155–158.

111. Dennis SM. Perinatal mortality. Compendium for Continuing Education for the Practicing Veterinarian 1981; S206–S217.

112. Rooney JR. Autopsy of the horse: techniques and interpretation. Baltimore: Williams and Wilkins; 1970:120–134.

113. Acland HM. Abortion in mares: diagnosis and prevention. Compendium of Continuing Education for the Practicing Veterinarian 1987; 9:318–324.

114. Franco OJ. Gross lesions as an aid in the diagnosis of equine abortion. Proceedings of the American Association of Equine Practitioners 1976; 22:257–261.

115. Daels PF, Starr M, Kindahl H, et al. Effect of Salmonella typhimurium endotoxin on PGF-2 alpha release and fetal death in the mare. Journal of Reproduction and Fertility Supplement 1987; 35:485–492.

116. Santschi EM, Sloane DE, Gronwell R, et al. Types of colic and frequency of post colic abortion in pregnant mares: 105 mares (1984–1988). Journal of the American Veterinary Medical Association 1991; 199:374–377.

117. Silver M, Fowden AL. Uterine prostaglandin F metabolite production in relation to glucose availability in late pregnancy and a possible influence of diet on time of delivery in the mare. Journal of Reproduction and Fertility Supplement 1982; 32:511–519.

118. Hyland J, Jeffcott LB. Abortion. In: Robinson NE, ed. Current therapy in equine medicine. Philadelphia: WB Saunders; 1987:520–525.

119. Crandell RA, Angulo AB. Equine herpesvirus-1 antibodies in stillborn foals and weak neonates. Veterinary Medicine 1985; 80:73–77.

120. Acland HM. Abortion in mares: diagnosis and prevention. Compendium of Continuing Education for the Practicing Veterinarian 1987; 9:318–324.

121. Whitwell KE. Fetal membrane abnormalities. In: Robinson NE, ed. Current therapy in equine medicine 2. Philadelphia: WB Saunders; 1987:528–531.

122. Platt H. Infection of the horse fetus. Journal of Reproduction and Fertility Supplement 1975; 23:605–610.

123. Timoney JF, Gillespie JH, Scott FW, et al, eds. The pathogenic bacteria. In: Hagan and Brunner's microbiology and infectious diseases of domestic animals. 8th edn. Ithaca: Comstock Publishing Associates; 1988:80–83.

124. Ellis WA, O'Brien JJ, Cassells JA, et al. Leptospiral infections in horses in Northern Ireland: serological and microbiological findings. Equine Veterinary Journal 1983; 15:317–320.

125. Poonacha KB, Smith BJ, Donahue JM, et al. Leptospiral abortion in horses in central Kentucky. Proceedings of the American Association of Equine Practitioners 1990; 37:397–402.

126. Poonacha KB, Giles RC, Donahue JM, et al. Leptospirosis in equine fetuses, stillborn foals, and placentas. Veterinary Pathology 1993; 30:362–369.

127. Mahaffey LW, Adam NM. Abortions associated with mycotic lesions of the placenta in the mare. Journal of the American Veterinary Medical Association 1964; 144:24–32.

128. Whitwell KE. Morphology and pathology of the equine umbilical cord. Journal of Reproduction and Fertility Supplement 1975; 23:599–603.

129. Whitwell KE. Investigations into fetal and neonatal losses in the horse. Veterinary Clinics of North America 1980; 2:313–331.

130. Alm CC, Sullivan JJ, First NL. The effect of a corticosteroid (dexamethasone), progesterone, oestrogen and prostaglandin $F_{2\alpha}$ on gestation length in normal and ovariectomised mares. Journal of Reproduction and Fertility Supplement 1975; 23:637–640.

131. Cross DT, Threlfall WR, Kline RC. Body temperature fluctuations in the periparturient mare. Theriogenology 1992; 37:1041–1043.

Chapter 8
PARTURITION

Cheryl Lopate,
Michelle LeBlanc,
Reg Pascoe,
Derek Knottenbelt

The duration of pregnancy in the mare is normally said to be between 335 and 342 days.[1] However, there is a naturally wide range of normal gestational length (320–400 days).[2,3] Mares that foal in the early spring (February and March in the northern hemisphere breeding season) tend to have longer gestation lengths than those foaling in late spring and summer. It is believed that there is a period of embryonic diapause (a period of time during which the developing embryo stops growing and simply remains the same size), which may vary in length from a few days to weeks, depending on the individual mare. This may in part account for the natural, well-recognized variability in gestation length in mares.

As a rule, the best place for the fetus is in the mare's uterus until both the mare and the fetus are ready for delivery. Decreased placental function resulting in slower development of the fetus may, however, account for some cases of prolonged gestation, such as foals that are delivered after 365 days of gestation yet are of normal size and similar maturity to their peers who foaled over 30 days earlier.

PHYSIOLOGICAL CHANGES THAT OCCUR BEFORE FOALING[4]

Prior to the delivery of the normal fetus, it must be fully mature and capable of surviving outside the confines of the uterus. All body systems must finalize their maturation in preparation for birth. Increased fetal cortisol secretion in late pregnancy results in maturation of the respiratory and digestive systems. Fetal activity increases significantly in the last few days of the pregnancy. The density of the fetal fluids increases in the last week or two of pregnancy as well.

Signs of impending parturition include:

- Relaxation of the pelvic ligaments and perineum.
- Mammary gland development (Fig. 8.1).
- Waxing of the teats (see Fig. 7.37).
- Changes in mammary gland secretions.

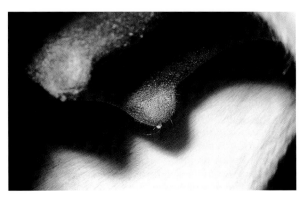

Fig. 8.1 Mammary gland development in a pregnant mare.

Relaxation of the pelvic ligaments and perineum

The ligaments along the tail-head relax and become very soft. Relaxation of pelvic ligaments becomes noticeable from about 2 weeks prepartum and the muscles of the croup and tail-head become progressively more slack, pliable and soft as parturition approaches; this is usually obvious during the day or two before foaling.

Manipulations of this area will result in a wave-like motion of these muscles. The vulva and anus will soften and relax. Lengthening and edema of the vulva may first be noted up to several weeks before foaling and will increase as foaling approaches.

Mammary development and secretions

Udder development begins approximately 1 month prior to parturition, with the most noticeable changes occurring during the last 2 weeks. It occurs earlier in younger mares and later in old, multiparous mares. Final mammary enlargement occurs within 24–48 hours of foaling.

The nature and content of the mammary secretions change slowly over the last month of pregnancy. Initially, the secretions are yellow and watery (serous). As foaling approaches, the secretions thicken and become tenacious, rather like weak honey. This thickening, along with increased mammary engorgement, is indicative of colostrum production. The secretions then change to a thick milky-yellow secretion typical of good-quality colostrum. Milk production may be low with this type of secretion, but as the colostrum is consumed and the secretions become more milk-like the volume will increase significantly.

> • Premature lactation is often a sign of impending abortion; thus mares that produce and possibly leak milk at an early stage in the pregnancy must be carefully assessed.
> • A mare that shows any premature lactation should be classified as 'high-risk' (see p. 252) and full fetal viability testing should be undertaken.

A wax-like secretion may be seen on the teats (see Fig. 7.37). Wax is part of the initial tenacious colostrum fluid produced by the mammary gland. Waxing typically occurs up to 72 hours prior to foaling, although in some mares it may occur up to 2 weeks prior to parturition. There may be only a drop or two of wax or up to several inches of secretions. Some mares may leak colostrum prior to foaling. If the mare is streaming milk for an extended period of time (hours at a time, or several times a day), she should be milked out and the colostrum frozen and saved for the foal, rather than taking the chance that all the colostrum might be lost prior to foaling.

Concentrations of electrolytes in the milk will change in the days before foaling (Fig. 8.2).[5,6] These are useful indicators of fetal maturity and are therefore helpful to some extent in determining foaling dates and in assessing the appropriateness of induced parturition (see p. 279). Milk electrolyte levels have been shown to be potential predictors of foaling (Table 8.1), or at least the times when the mare is unlikely to foal. However, they should not necessarily be relied upon to provide a definite indication of impending parturition.

• Milk electrolytes, and calcium in particular, can be measured colorimetrically or by flame photometer in an aqueous aliquot of the centrifuged specimen of mammary secretion.
• Commercial kits are available to measure calcium levels using a rapid strip dry chemistry test (i.e. water hardness testing kits).[7] These tests are convenient and helpful but were designed to detect calcium concentrations in water (Sofchek, Environmental Test Systems, Elkhart, IN, USA; Titrets Calcium Hardness Test Kit, CHEMetrics Inc., Calverton, VA, USA). The tests need to be calibrated as they are usually working at the limits of their range.

Table 8.1 Alterations in the electrolyte content of mammary secretions in the immediate prepartum period

	Hours prepartum			
	>72	72–48	48–24	<24
Sodium (Na⁺) (mmol/l)	>80	80–65	65–50	<30
Potassium (K⁺) mmol/l	<20	>20–25	25–35	>35
Calcium (mmol/l)	<10	10–20	20–30	>40

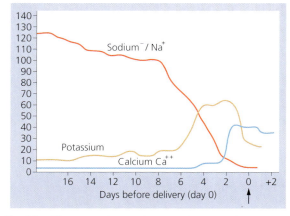

Fig. 8.2 The approximate changes that occur in electrolyte concentrations in mammary secretions in the normal pregnant mare in the days leading up to delivery (day 0, arrow).

- Kits designed specifically for horses are available commercially (Predict-a-Foal Mare Foaling Predictor Kit, Animal Healthcare Products, Vernon, CA, USA).
- The specific equine test strip has been shown to be easier to interpret but had wider variations than the tests using water hardness values.[8]
- An increase in calcium to greater than 10 mmol/l, a decrease in sodium to less than 35 mmol/ml and an increase in potassium to greater than 80 mmol/ml are all indicators of fetal maturity and impending parturition.

ENDOCRINOLOGY OF PARTURITION

Late-term pregnancy in the mare has a unique hormonal environment (Fig. 8.3).[9–11]

- There are high levels of fetally derived estrogen. The levels of estrogens produced by the fetoplacental unit and fetus remain relatively stable until parturition.
- Progesterone rises during the last few weeks of pregnancy with a peak about 5 days before foaling, whereas pregnane levels are decreasing (although they are still found at high levels).[12]
- Both progesterone and the 5α-pregnanes decrease precipitously following parturition and are at baseline levels within 24 hours of foaling.

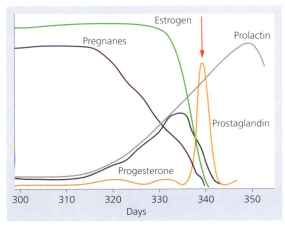

Fig. 8.3 The endocrinology of late pregnancy. Estrogen production begins to fall just before parturition (arrow). Pregnanes slowly reduce over the last 4 weeks of pregnancy and decrease precipitously immediately at parturition. Progesterone gradually increases during the last month of gestation and then falls rapidly after foaling. Prostaglandin is significantly increased during stage 1 of labor with peak concentrations achieved during stage 2. Oxytocin peaks during stage 2 of labor immediately following the prostaglandin surge. Prolactin gradually increases over the last month of pregnancy, peaks at around 30–60 days after parturition and then tapers off over the next 2–4 months.

- The ratio of the declining progesterone concentration to the stable estrogen provides the stimulus for the formation of oxytocin receptors and instigates changes in the muscular ability of the uterus to enable it to contract forcibly.

Relaxin is a hormone produced by the placenta[13] that stimulates relaxation of the pelvic ligaments in the birth canal and cervix. Concentrations of relaxin reach their peak during stage 2 of labor (fetal expulsion).

Prostaglandin F metabolites slowly begin to increase during the last third of pregnancy[14] and increase more significantly during the last 2 weeks. Prostaglandin, which is derived from the fetoplacental unit, reaches peak concentrations at the end of stage 1 of labor; this is partly responsible for cervical relaxation. Concentrations increase again at the onset of stage 2 of labor; this is partly responsible for the onset of coordinated uterine contractions.

Oxytocin is produced in a large surge once the fetus is positioned in the birth canal; this is probably the stimulus for the onset of stage 2 labor. Oxytocin production drops precipitously immediately after delivery. Thereafter it is produced in smaller surges during stage 3 to facilitate placental expulsion.

The ability of the uterine muscle to contract intensely is instigated by a combination of the drop in progesterone during the 24 hours prior to parturition followed by the repeated surges in prostaglandin and oxytocin production.

The onset of lactation is driven by the increasing production of prolactin from the anterior pituitary gland. Significant production is detectable during the last week of pregnancy.

PREPARATION FOR FOALING

Approximately 2 weeks before the anticipated due date, the mare should be moved to her foaling location. A daily and nightly routine should be established and followed without alteration so that she becomes accustomed to the routine and will not be disturbed by these normal occurrences when she is ready to foal.

The mare is remarkably capable of postponing active labor when she does not feel safe or secure. Most mares foal between 11 p.m. and 4 a.m., when there is the least amount of activity surrounding the mare.

- Disturbances in the mare's environment may result in her delaying delivery until she feels comfortable with her surroundings.
- In this situation, the milk calcium level may be greater than 10 mmol/l and foaling may not occur within 48 hours as predicted by the kits (see p. 270).

The mare should be checked twice daily for signs of impending labor and possibly even more frequently as the signs of impending parturition develop. When the mare is very close to foaling she should be monitored frequently for signs of labor. Hourly or bi-hourly visits to the foaling stall/area should be made. For the most part interference should be minimized unless the mare is clearly in trouble. In order to minimize the extent of interference, supervision should be provided through some type of monitoring system (visual, video, alarm).

There are several different types of monitoring systems that can be utilized to minimize the number of physical visits and activity around the mare:

- Video monitoring systems can be set up in the mare stall, with remote TV monitors to evaluate foaling activity. These systems are unobtrusive, but are expensive and they require personnel to monitor the TV system.
- Belt/girth alarm systems, which are activated when abdominal contractions begin, can be strapped to the mare's abdomen. They can be attached to a pager or phone system. False alarms may occur with these systems when the mare grunts or groans when in lateral recumbency.
- Transducers (or magnets) sutured to the vulvar lips are activated when the amniotic sac parts the vulvar lips. However, some mares are irritated by the transducers and will rub against a wall and tear the transducer out. These systems can be attached to a pager or phone system.
- A system utilizing a spirit level attached to the mare's head collar which is activated when the mare lies in lateral recumbency is also available. This system relies upon the movement of the bubble to either end of the spirit level. There is plenty of scope for false alarms with this system when the mare simply lies down to rest.

In the late pregnant mare, some abdominal discomfort may be noted as a result of fetal position, fetal movement and pressure on other abdominal organs. Some term mares may show signs of abdominal discomfort during late gestation as a result of fetal positioning and increased fetal activity just prior to the onset of stage 1 labor.

- This discomfort may be recognized as colic by the owner. It is typically responsive to hand-walking, time, or administration of nonsteroidal anti-inflammatory agents.

As parturition approaches the mare will usually show a decrease in appetite.[15] She may also try to separate herself from the rest of the herd if she is in a group.

Once the process of birth begins, the mare's tail should be wrapped and the perineum washed with clean water, possibly with a mild soap, and then dried off.

If the mare has been previously subjected to a Caslick's operation (Fig. 8.4) she should be examined in stocks, if possible twitched rather than tranquilized.

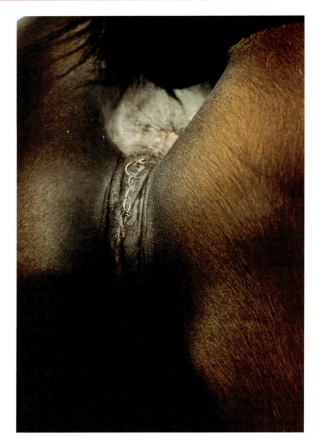

Fig. 8.4 Mares that have been subjected to a Caslick's vulvoplasty operation should be restrained and the sutures removed if still present. A surgical episiotomy usually prevents uncontrolled and unpredictable perineal laceration and delays in delivery.

- After local anesthetic has been infiltrated along the previous incision line, the previously closed vulvar lips are sectioned to return the vulvar opening to its natural dimensions.

As far as possible foaling should not take place into a dirty, wet or muddy environment; stable facilities should be clean and free of any possible infectious agents, and foaling should occur apart from other foaling mares in particular. The management and hygiene involved in the preparation of the foaling box is described in Chapter 1.

- If the mare is to foal inside, a 6 × 6–7-meter loosebox is an adequate area. The mare should be carefully monitored to ensure that she does not foal into a corner.
- If the mare is to foal outside, there should be some shelter for the foal after birth. A clean, dry, grass pasture is ideal.

The flow chart presented in Fig. 8.5 provides a useful protocol for the decisions that need to be made at parturition.

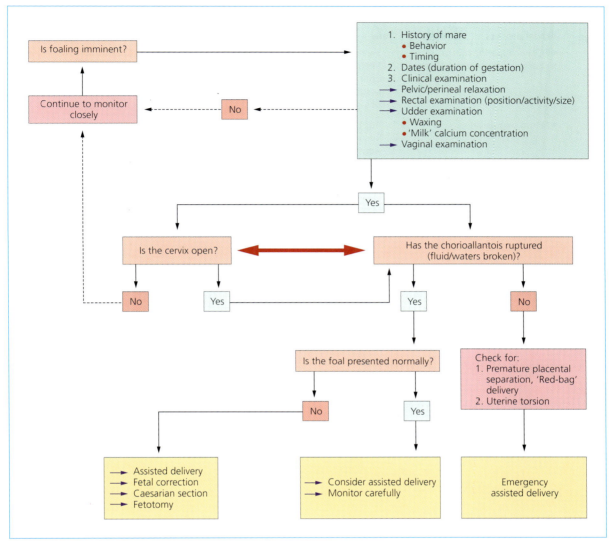

Fig. 8.5   Decision flow chart for parturition.

STAGES AND SIGNS OF LABOR

Labor is classically divided into three stages (see Table 8.2).

Stage 1

This stage involves contraction of the uterus and cervical relaxation. The average duration is about 1 hour, although the range may be from 30 minutes to 6 hours, or longer in some cases. The mare has some ability to control the duration of stage 1 labor; if she is unduly upset or disturbed, she can postpone stage 2 for hours or even days. The fetus takes an active role in its own positioning during stage 1, often becoming noticeably active. Fetal movements can sometimes be seen in the flank as the foal actively rotates from a dorsopubic (upside-down) position (Fig. 8.6) to a dorsosacral (right-side up) position. Rolling by the mare assists in this process of fetal positioning which is required for a normal delivery. Preventing the mare from rolling is not recommended but it is important to distinguish this normal rolling behavior from that associated with severe abdominal pain.

Signs of stage 1

- Rolling, pawing, kicking at the abdomen, looking back at the abdomen (signs commonly attributed to abdominal pain/colic).
- Anorexia. The appetite of many late-term mares is normally reduced. This may have serious implications for overweight ponies liable to the hyperlipemia syndromes.

Table 8.2 Signs and duration of the stages of labor

Stage	Actual process	Signs	Normal duration (average, range)
1	• Cervical/pelvic relaxation • Early uterine contractions	1. Sweating 2. Restlessness 3. Colic/rolling 4. Frequent urination/defecation 5. Dripping of milk	50 minutes (30 minutes to 6 hours)
2	• Fetal expulsion	1. Rupture of fetal membranes 2. Recumbency 3. Active abdominal contractions 4. Delivery of foal	20 minutes (10–60 minutes)
3	Placental expulsion	1. Mild abdominal discomfort/colic 2. Straining 3. Milk let-down	60 minutes (15 minutes to 3 hours)

- Sweating may be noted on neck and flanks.
- Frequent urination and defecation (possibly in an attempt to clear the pelvic canal for the impending delivery).
- Frequent laying down and rising (this can also be mistaken for colic).
- Flehmen response (lifting of the upper lip).

- There are no active or obvious abdominal contractions during this stage.

Stage 1 ends with the rupture of the chorioallantois and the sudden release of a quantity of tan-red colored fluid. This is the 'breaking of the water' or 'water breaking' (Fig. 8.7).

Stage 2

Stage 2 is defined as delivery of the foal. Parturition is an explosive process in the mare, requiring the active participation of the foal. Moribund, weak or dead foals are often problematic as a result of their failure to take an active part in the delivery process.

The average duration of stage 2 is 20 minutes, but it may be as short as 10 minutes or as long as 60 minutes.

Signs of stage 2 (Figs 8.8, 8.9)

- During this stage the mare will usually lie down and have active abdominal contractions.
- While some mares will foal standing up, most adopt lateral recumbency for the delivery.
- When the fetus enters the birth canal it stretches the surrounding tissues, stimulating surges in both prostaglandin and oxytocin. These in turn cause uterine and abdominal contractions to occur (known as Ferguson's reflex).
- The abdominal contractions are very powerful, each lasting for between 15 seconds and 1 minute.

- There will usually be several contractions in succession and then a period of rest (lasting 2–3 minutes) before the next set of contractions.
- The mare may reposition several times during rest periods and may rise to her feet before lying down again.
- Shortly after the waters break, the amnion, which directly surrounds the fetus, is usually presented.
  - ❏ The amnion is a bluish-white sac that commonly looks like a balloon at the vulvar lips.
  - ❏ It is usually wise to ensure that the amnion is removed from the foal's muzzle as soon as the foal's chest clears the pelvic canal so that it can breathe.
  - ❏ Under natural conditions, opposing movements of the foal's head and legs rupture the amnion, resulting in a smaller rush of yellowish allantoic fluid.

Note:
- A strong yellowish brown discoloration of the amnion or amniotic fluid is indicative of meconium staining and should be taken seriously, especially if the foal is also stained. There is a risk that such a foal has been stressed and it may have inhaled meconium-contaminated fluid.
- If a fleshy red-brown structure (the chorioallantois) is presented at the vulva first, this will suggest strongly that there is early placental separation. THIS IS CONSIDERED AN ABSOLUTE EMERGENCY (see p. 299).
- In this event the membrane should be broken manually and the fetus delivered as quickly as possible to prevent oxygen deprivation.
- Details for this procedure are described on p. 299.

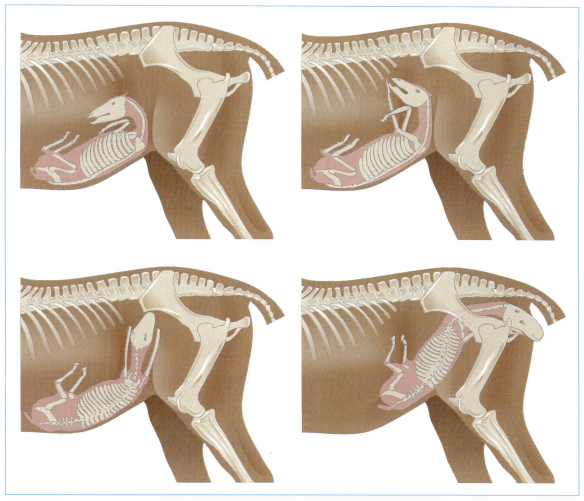

Fig. 8.6 Rotation of the foal in stage 1 of labor. The foal remains in a dorsopubic or dorso-ilial position until stage 1. Rotation of the fetus is an active process involving the mare (through lying down, rolling and rising) and the foal (through rolling and turning).

- As contractions continue, the fetal legs will be seen at the vulvar lips.
  - ❑ Normally, the two front feet are presented first, with one hoof slightly ahead of the other and the head resting on the foal's knees (Fig. 8.10).
- Once the fetus enters the birth canal, contractions tend to occur more frequently until the foal's hips are delivered through the birth canal. Commonly, the mare may rest for several minutes at this time before finally expelling the foal.
- Stage 2 ends with the expulsion of the foal and usually lasts 15–60 minutes.

The decision for interference

Interference in the foaling process is considered appropriate if:

- There is no evidence of strong contractions and/or no progression in the delivery process 15 minutes

after the rupture of the chorioallantois) (water breaking).
- One foot and the head, or two feet and no head, or if only the head are presented at the vulva.
- If the red, velvety surface of the chorionic membrane appears at the vulva instead of the tough, semitransparent, gray amnion before the foal is delivered. This is the so-called 'red bag' delivery. THIS IS A TRUE EMERGENCY SITUATION (see p. 299).
- If rectovaginal perforation occurs. This can be recognized by the foal's leg appearing through the anus of the mare. THIS IS A TRUE EMERGENCY SITUATION (see p. 286).

Immediately post foaling

The umbilical cord will separate on its own either as the foal moves about in trying to rise or when the mare stands up. There is some difference of opinion

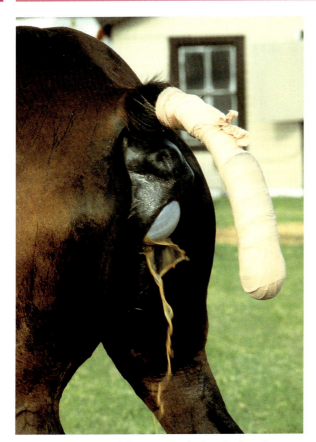

Fig. 8.7 Breaking of the 'waters' during the late first stage to early second stage of delivery.

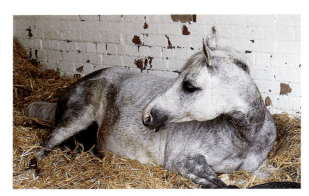

Fig. 8.8 Stage 2 of parturition begins with the mare showing increasing discomfort and 'colic' signs.

about what to do with regard to the umbilical cord.[16] Transfer of up to 1 liter of blood from the placenta back to the foal will occur until the cord breaks. This blood will pass both from the mare to the foal and from the foal to the mare. It is believed by some that this transfer of blood to the foal is important for its immediate well-being during the first few days of life. However, no significant differences in blood volume

have been demonstrated between foals whose umbilical cords were allowed to remain patent for a quarter to half an hour after birth and those whose cords were severed and ligated immediately after delivery. Nevertheless, it is probably best if the umbilical cord is allowed to break naturally. If this occurs immediately after birth, it is not a reason for serious concern. If the mare and foal are both resting quietly, the cord should be allowed to remain intact until the actions of either the mare or the foal result in its spontaneous rupture.

After foaling, the mare should be allowed to rest. The process of labor is extremely strenuous for the mare, and she may lie quietly after foaling for up to 30–45 minutes in some cases. This time is often called the 'period of tranquility' and the mare should not be disturbed during this stage without good reason.

Stage 3

Stage 3 of labor is defined as the passage of the placental membranes and the onset of uterine involution (decrease in size and expulsion of fluid and debris). The duration of stage 3 is usually about 1–3 hours.

- Strong myometrial contractions may induce abdominal pain/discomfort (colic). The mare may lie down and get up repeatedly.

- If there is significant colic-like pain the mare may be hand-walked to prevent self-trauma. However, there are very important causes of colic in newly foaled mares (including cecal rupture, torsion of the large colon, and peritonitis) which should be eliminated before any decisions are made on treatment.

The placenta should be allowed to hang from the vulvar lips (see Fig. 8.11); however, if it is dragging on the ground or hitting the hocks it should be tied up, so the mare does not tear it off or kick at it and so injure the foal.

Once the placenta has been delivered it should be placed in a bag and kept cool or refrigerated until it can be examined by a veterinarian (see p. 328). The veterinarian should examine every placenta in order to:

- Determine if it has been passed in its entirety.
- Evaluate it for abnormalities.

Uterine involution occurs quite rapidly in the mare.

- Within 12 hours after foaling, the uterus is usually only 1.5 times the size of its nonpregnant state.
- In the normal postpartum mare uterine involution is complete by day 15 (see p. 294).

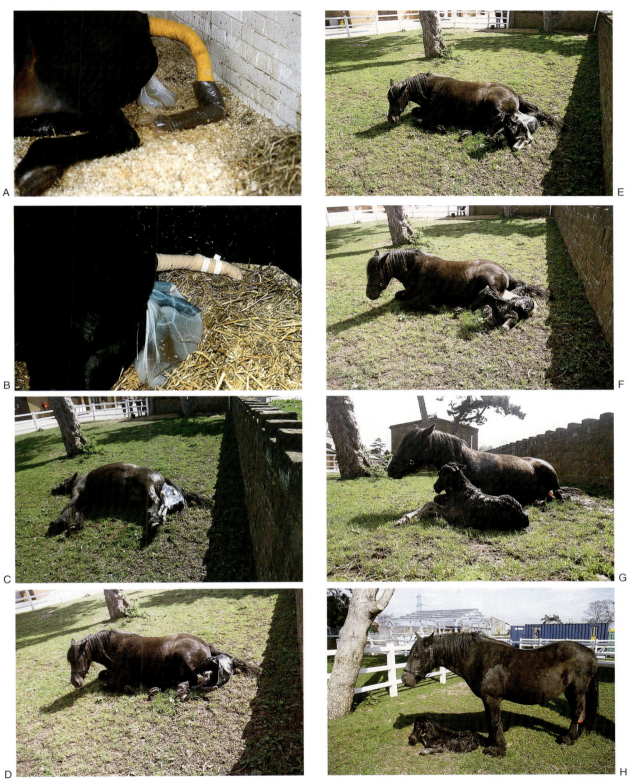

Fig. 8.9 Signs of stage 2 labor. Rupture of the chorioallantois is followed by the appearance of the gray amnion (A). The foal's legs (B) will appear next (one slightly behind the other). Increasing straining delivers the head (C) and the foal's delivery is rapidly completed (D). The mare remains calm and recumbent during the final delivery of the hind legs (E). The foal makes energetic attempts to move towards the head of the mare (F); during this the cord will usually break (G). Once the cord has broken the mare will usually rise and lick/sniff the foal (H).

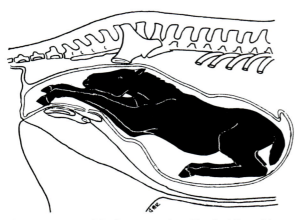

Fig. 8.10 Normal foal presentation. The foal lies with an anterior longitudinal presentation in a dorsosacral position. The front legs are extended and one forelimb is slightly forward of the other. The foal's head rests on its knees.

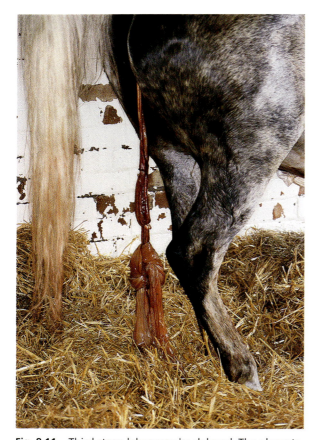

Fig. 8.11 Third-stage labor may be delayed. The placenta should not be forcibly removed, but it can be tied up to minimize the inconvenience. The placenta can be a source of serious infection for the foal.

PLACENTAL RETENTION

Failure to deliver the placenta within 2–4 hours after foaling is usually regarded as a 'retained placenta', but the specific circumstances may be more significant than the time.

In some cases the mare and the placenta will remain healthy for longer without problems, whereas in others there may be serious consequences from retention for less than 1 hour. For example, in Australia many mares that foal in paddocks rather than foaling boxes retain the placenta for 6–8 hours in the colder months without serious consequences.

- It is probably unwise, therefore, to dictate a specific time for placental delivery but rather to carefully assess the mare's state of health and the character of the placental tissues.

In any case, a veterinarian should probably examine all mares that fail to expel the fetal membranes within 3 hours.

- In the event that a veterinarian cannot examine the mare immediately, advice on the possible use of 2-hourly intramuscular injections of 40 IU of oxytocin can be considered.
- There are important unwanted effects from this treatment so consultation with the veterinarian must be made before any treatment is given. In most countries the drug is only available on prescription.

When the mare is considered as being 'not normal', a veterinarian should be called to make further assessments regardless of the time period involved.

Attention should be paid to the health of the mare. In particular, she should be monitored for signs of anorexia (off-feed), depression, fever, or signs of laminitis (shifting weight, rocking horse stance, heat in the hooves and/or increased digital pulses). If any of these signs is present a veterinarian should attend immediately.

Management of retained placenta will be discussed later in this chapter.

POSTNATAL CARE

Care of the foal immediately after birth is critical for its well-being. The protocol for this is described on p. 365. A careful diary of events should be recorded.

The mare should be allowed some quiet time to bond with the foal immediately after delivery. During this time discreet observation can be maintained to ensure that no problems develop as a result of a nervous, apprehensive or aggressive mare, but the mare should not be disturbed until it is clear that there is a strong mutual bonding between the mare and foal. This is especially important for maiden mares or nervous mothers to ensure that abandonment will not occur. In the event that there are behavioral problems, the foal can be separated from the mare by a divider or the mare can be held by a familiar and experienced handler to allow the foal to approach and nurse. In some cases, the mare may need to be sedated before it will allow nursing until the pressure on the full udder decreases and the mare becomes accustomed to the feel of the nursing foal. On rare occasions, rejection of the foal may occur. A nurse mare may be required or the foal may need to be to raised as an orphan. The latter is to be avoided at almost any cost.

After bonding has taken place the mare should be examined for injuries such as perineal lacerations, perforations of the vaginal/digestive tract, or hemorrhage. The mare should be monitored closely for the first 12 hours after foaling, because some internal injuries may not be apparent for several hours. Where necessary vulvoplasty (Caslick's suture) should be carried out as soon as possible.

The mare's udder and perineum (including the thigh regions) should be cleaned and an assessment of both colostral quality and quantity should be made before the foal nurses.

INDUCTION OF PARTURITION

There is no question that the best place for a fetus to be is in the mare's uterus. It has been said that the fetus picks the day it will be born and the mare picks the hour it will be born. Induction of a delivery where the fetus is not yet mature may result in a weak, premature foal that requires intensive care or the birth of a stillborn or a dead fetus.

> • Failure to ensure that the foal is indeed ready for birth and that the mare is in a suitable physiological and psychological state can result in considerable problems.

An induced delivery (and particularly where this is premature) can result in critical problems for both the mare and the foal including:

• Premature placental separation; this is common with induced parturition.

> • The presence of a red, velvety structure at the vulvar lips (see p. 298) or palpation of the chorioallantois lying in the uterine lumen are both indications for emergency manual rupture of the placenta and IMMEDIATE delivery of the fetus.

• Failure of passive transfer (p. 375).
• Dystocia (p. 379).
• Fetal or maternal compromise and death.
• Retained placenta (p. 313).
• Neonatal maladjustment syndrome. This is quite common in foals born by induction even when at full term, and immediate (and often long-term) care is often required for their survival.

There are considerable advantages in an induced parturition but also significant dangers. The procedure should not be undertaken lightly.[17–20] Induction performed by the attending veterinarian provides continuous professional care and monitoring for the mare and the foal. Problems such as premature placental separation and fetal malposition/dystocia can quickly be recognized and dealt with without delay. Furthermore, careful and full preparations can be made in advance and the tendency for mares to foal in the early hours of the morning can be negated.

There are basic rules that can be used to ensure that an induced delivery has the best chance of producing a normal foal with minimal complications to both foal and mare. Careful and thorough assessment of the mare and the fetus are essential if problems are to be avoided rather than created. Mistakes can easily result in the delivery of a nonviable foal.

> Note:
> • It is extremely important that the owner is made aware of the potential dangers, particularly to the possibility that foal pathology may already be present in utero and may result in a nonviable foal which may be incorrectly attributed to the induction process.

It is therefore important to select the cases for induced delivery very carefully based on the whole circumstances and to ensure that the procedure is followed through completely. The decision to induce should be based on specific needs rather than purely on convenience.

Emergency medications and oxygen should be made available in the event that there is a problem. The owner and veterinarian should be fully prepared for the delivery prior to the onset of induction. All the necessary intensive care, resuscitation equipment and obstetric facilities should always be directly available.

Indications for induced delivery

The indications for induced delivery include:

• A classification as a high-risk foaling as a result of mare or foal classification.

- History of difficult deliveries or previous abnormal or problematical foals; thus foaling or situations in which the life of the mare or foal is likely to be in jeopardy can be supervised.
- Habitual or anticipated premature placental separation ('red bag' delivery).
- History of primary uterine inertia resulting in delayed delivery.
- Inability to strain effectively (abdominal muscle, diaphragmatic or tracheal defects).
- Physical deformity of the maternal pelvis, or with a history of previous pelvic injury including old fractures, such that attended labor is critical, impending rupture of the prepubic tendon, or uncontrolled and recurring prefoaling colic. The decision must include the possibility of cesarean section rather than induction of parturition.
- Detectable fetal distress or other life-threatening injury or disease in the foal or the mare.

Note:
- Mares may also be induced for use as nurse mares.
- Inductions should not be performed solely for the convenience of owner or veterinarian.

Criteria for decision

There are five 'rules of thumb' to be followed to provide the best chance for a successful induction:

- There should be colostrum in the udder.
- Gestational age must be between 330 and 350 days. Although the actual gestational age is important, the previous history of the individual mare might suggest that a delay or an earlier induction might be indicated. Thus it is probably not wise to assume normality in a primiparous mare and an assumption based upon the 'normal' gestational duration of the horse is most unwise. Optimal survival is achieved by induction within 10 days of normal delivery date for that pregnancy.
- Pelvic relaxation should be present. The cervix should be relaxing/dilating (as detected by manual examination or vaginoscopy).
- The fetus should be in a normal presentation, position, and posture.
- Mammary secretion analysis is consistent with readiness for birth. The milk calcium level should be >10 mmol/l (>200 ppm).[5,21] A system that provides a score derived from calcium, sodium, and potassium can be used if each of these can be measured accurately (see Table 8.3).[22] This usually requires a laboratory that is equipped to perform specialized testing procedures. It is often worth measuring the IgG concentration if the milk calcium has risen sufficiently to permit induction to determine if passive transfer will be

Table 8.3 Scoring system for mammary secretions[22]

Calcium (mmol/l)	Sodium (mmol/l)	Potassium (mmol/l)	Score (for each electrolyte)[a]
>10	<30	>35	15
5–10	30–50	20–35	10
<5	>50	<20	5

[a] A total score of over 35 suggests a probable safe induction.

normal following delivery. This measurement should be performed again after the foal has been delivered. Assessment of fetal maturity by evaluating mammary secretion concentrations of calcium, sodium, and potassium is described on p. 270.

If any of these criteria are lacking, the chances of having an abnormal delivery or a problem with the foal following delivery are significantly higher.

Methods of induction

There are several methods that have variously been described and are reported to have successful, or at least predictable, outcomes.

Oxytocin injection

Oxytocin can be used in any mare that is over 300 days of gestation. There are several options available:

- Oxytocin may be given either as a 40–60 IU intravenous bolus or added to 1 liter of physiologic saline and administered over 15 minutes (the latter is the preferred method).
- A small single dose (5–10 IU) of oxytocin given intravenously may induce delivery in mares that are close to term. This method can be used repeatedly. It has been used each evening in some cases without any apparent deleterious effects in mares that are 'not quite ready'. In these cases the dose seems to be insufficient to cause certain delivery but is enough to induce delivery when the conditions are right.
- Alternatively, 10–15 IU of oxytocin can be administered intramuscularly or intravenously every 30 minutes until rupture of the chorioallantois (subject to a maximum total dose of 75 IU).

The following should also be noted when oxytocin is being used for induction:

- Intravenous dosing is preferred to intramuscular dosing when low doses of oxytocin are used.
- Abdominal contractions are quite strong with oxytocin inductions.
- Parturition usually begins within 20 minutes of oxytocin administration when 40 IU have been delivered intravenously.

Table 8.4   Prostaglandin drugs available for induction of parturition in horses

Compound	Dose (intramuscular)	Number of injections/intervals
Cloprostenol	250–500 µg	Single dose
Dinoprost	10 mg	Single dose
Prostalene	4 mg	Single dose
Fenprostalene	2–0.5 mg	Two doses, 2 hours apart

- If labor is not progressing normally 20–30 minutes after induction has begun, the mare should be assessed by manual palpation to determine the cause of the problem.
- A mare being induced with oxytocin should not be left unattended until delivery is complete.

Prostaglandin injection

Prostaglandin will also induce parturition.[23] Prostaglandin analogs are preferred but are not generally licensed for use in the mare. Table 8.4 shows the standard doses of prostaglandin drugs available for horses.

- Prostaglandin-induced parturition can also occur quite rapidly and the contractions can be very strong.

Corticosteroid injection

Although dexamethasone at a dose of 100 mg by intramuscular injection every 24 hours for at least 4 days – the mare will foal within 4–7 days – has been used,[24] this method has little to commend it.

- There are significant risks to both mare and foal, one of which is a slow, protracted and often difficult delivery. Furthermore, there is no convincing evidence that preparturient corticosteroids administered to the mare improve the pulmonary function of foals.
- There is no apparent benefit of giving steroid prior to induction to facilitate maturation of the fetus.

- If the cervix is not relaxed, estrogens (5 mg of estradiol cypionate or 10 mg estradiol benzoate) can be administered intramuscularly 24 hours prior to the induction protocol.

CARE OF THE FOAL FOLLOWING INDUCED DELIVERY

If the mare is to be induced, preparation should be made for care of the foal following delivery.

- The presence of a veterinarian for the delivery is mandatory.

- Most inductions are very rapid and quite violent and fetal malposition/posture is relatively common; therefore veterinary assistance is frequently required.

- There is a strong temptation to assume that the foal delivered by induced delivery will be at least as strong, and possibly even stronger, than normal, but this is not often the case.
- Foals delivered by induced parturition should immediately be classified as high-risk (see p. 254) and subjected to the full range of nursing care in order to maximize survival.

DYSTOCIA (ABNORMAL FOALING)

The incidence of dystocia in the mare is relatively small, averaging 1.5–4% in the light horse breeds. Miniature horse mares and draft breeds tend to have a higher incidence of foaling difficulties. Dystocia is more common in the young, primiparous mare than in older, multiparous mares due to increased pelvic diameter. Fetopelvic disparity is uncommon as fetal size is a measure of uterine capacity and this usually relates closely to pelvic size, especially in multiparous mares.

- The primary causes of dystocia are fetal malpresentation, and abnormal position or posture.
- The long extremities of the fetus predispose to malposture and subsequent dystocia.

Dystocia in the mare is always a true emergency[25] because the potential for life-threatening complications for both mare and foal is very high. A general rule that supports interference is lack of obvious progress within 10–15 minutes of the onset of the second stage of labor. Once a clinical assessment has been made a decision needs to be taken on whether to deliver the foal by forced extraction or to delay the interference for another 10–15 minutes. When the cause of the problem can be diagnosed, it is obviously possible to make a logical plan. Other cases that cannot be diagnosed are more of a problem. Most veterinarians will continue with forced extraction as long as there are no obvious reasons to avoid this (e.g. nondilated cervix, gross oversize that will certainly preclude vaginal delivery, etc.).

Placental separation occurs quickly as a result of both the type of placenta and the strong uterine and abdominal contractions characteristic of parturition in the mare. Within an hour of the onset of stage 2 labor, placental separation will begin and consequent progressive fetal asphyxia will develop.

The mare in dystocia is predisposed to laminitis, septicemia, and shock.

> • Veterinary assistance should be called early in the birthing process to minimize complications for both mare and foal.

The mare should be restrained and prepared adequately prior to any obstetric manipulations. All facilities should be available at the outset because time is inevitably precious if a live foal is to be delivered.

- This may require a stock/chute, a large stall or clean, dry, open space.
- There should be adequate and good footing.
- Sedation and sometimes anesthesia will be required to facilitate manipulations.
- Care should be taken not to introduce bacteria or debris into the uterus during the manipulation. The mare should be managed as hygienically as possible. The tail should be wrapped and tied to one side, and the perineum should be carefully washed with mild soap and warm water.

Other medications that are commonly used during or after a dystocia include:

- Spasmolytics such as hyoscine n-butyl bromide and clenbuterol. Clenbuterol is particularly useful in slowing the progression of parturition (e.g. if the mare has to be moved to a hospital for delivery or cesarean section).
- Analgesics such as nonsteroidal anti-inflammatory compounds and opioids such as butorphanol.
- Oxytocin, to stimulate uterine contractions during delivery and postparturient uterine involution.
- Emergency medications for the mare and foal, including steroidal agents, doxapram, epinephrine, and atropine.
- Adequate obstetric lubrication is always required.
  ❏ Carboxymethylcellulose is the standard obstetric lubricant.
  ❏ Mineral oil and soft soap are far less satisfactory.
  ❏ Detergents, etc. must not be used.

Fetal positioning

Three terms are used to describe the location and position of the fetus in relationship to the mare's pelvis and reproductive tract:

1. Presentation. This describes the relationship of the long axis of the foal to the long axis of mare.
   - The normal presentation is anterior longitudinal (see Fig. 8.10).

- Abnormal presentations include:
  ❏ Posterior longitudinal (Fig. 8.12a).
  ❏ Dorsal transverse (Fig. 8.12b).
  ❏ Ventral transverse (Fig. 8.12c).
  ❏ Dorsal vertical.
  ❏ Ventral vertical.
2. Position. This describes the relationship between the dorsum of the fetus and the maternal pelvis.
   - The normal position is dorsosacral (Fig. 8.10).
   - Abnormal possibilities include:
     ❏ Dorsopubic (Fig. 8.13a).
     ❏ Right or left deviation of the head and neck (Fig. 8.13b).
     ❏ Ventral retroflexion of the head (Fig. 8.13c).
3. Posture. This describes the relationship of the fetal extremities to the foal itself.
   - The normal posture is an extended head resting on the carpi of both extended front legs. One leg is usually advanced 5–15 cm ahead of the other to facilitate passage of the shoulders through the birth canal (see Fig. 8.10).
   - Examples of abnormalities include (Fig. 8.14):
     ❏ Flexed joints (Fig. 8.14a–d).
     ❏ Head back or flexed (see Fig. 8.13).
     ❏ 'Dog-sitter' (where the hind limbs are extended forward and hook on to the brim of the mare's pelvis) (Fig. 8.14e).
     ❏ Foot nape (Fig. 8.14f).

Congenital defects/abnormalities

Congenital defects can also result in dystocia.[26,27] There are many possibilities, including:

- Hydrocephalus (see Fig. 8.20A).
- Schistosomus reflexus (Fig. 8.15).
- Fetal anasarca.
- Fetal monsters.
- Arthrogryposis (fused joints) (see Fig. 8.20B).

Management of dystocia

In order to prepare for the management of a dystocia the following information should be obtained:

- Any previous history of problems.
- The length of the mare's gestation.
- How long the mare has been in stage 2 labor.
- Current and past medical problems.
- Intervention that has already been performed on the mare prior to the arrival of the veterinarian.

This information can be written down on the foaling record or any other information record held by the owner or farm manager and so is very quickly assessed by the veterinarian on arrival at the stud.

Before any attempt is made to manipulate or deliver the foal, a careful obstetric examination must be performed to establish the presentation, position,

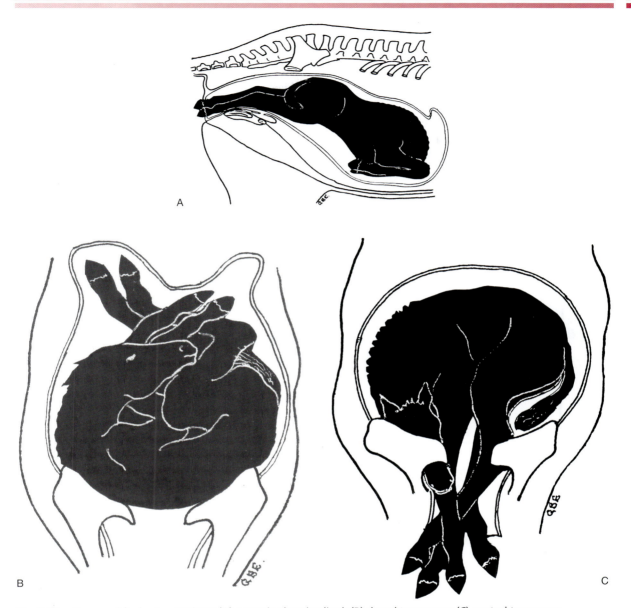

Fig. 8.12 Abnormal foal presentations: (A) posterior longitudinal; (B) dorsal transverse; (C) ventral transverse.

and posture of the foal and whether there are any injuries to mare or foal. The degree of vaginal and cervical relaxation and the viability of the foal can also be established and a sensible plan made for delivery.

> • Delivery should only be attempted when as much information as possible is gained, but there should be minimal delay.

• Epidural anesthesia (Fig. 8.16) is an excellent aid to fetal repositioning.
  ❑ 4–5 ml of 2% lignocaine hydrochloride or 2% mepivicaine hydrochloride introduced in sterile fashion into the epidural space at the level of the first intercoccygeal space is usually sufficient. As a general rule a mare weighing 450–500 kg will require no more than 7 ml of 2% lignocaine hydrochloride.
  ❑ The technique is described in standard texts on anesthesia and surgery.

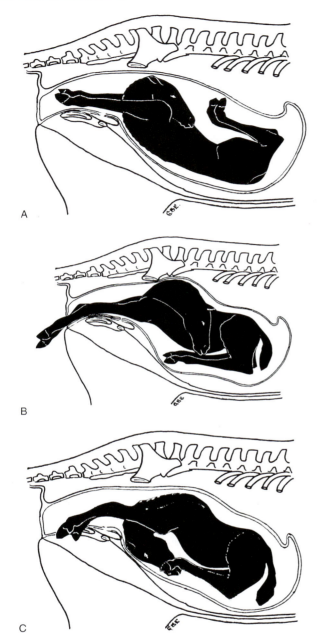

Fig. 8.13 Abnormal foal positions: (A) dorsopubic; (B) left deviation of the head and neck; (C) ventral retroflexion.

- Higher volumes and solutions containing adrenaline should not be used.

- General anesthesia followed by raising the hind end of the mare will facilitate repositioning of the fetus in some cases. Where this facility is possible it is often very worthwhile and minimizes the trauma to both mare and foal.

Usually the foal must be manipulated and repositioned before attempts at extraction can be made (Fig. 8.17). Specific terminology is used to describe repositioning of the fetus:

- Mutation: the return of the foal to a normal position by repulsion, rotation, version, or postural correction.
- Repulsion: the pushing of the foal out of maternal pelvis and back into the uterus prior to repositioning.
- Rotation: the turning of the foal on its longitudinal axis to bring it into a normal dorsosacral position.
- Version: the turning of the foal on its transverse axis to bring it into a normal anterior longitudinal presentation.
- Postural correction: the manipulation of the fetal extremities to prevent them catching on the maternal pelvis.

- Almost all normal deliveries (98%) are anterior presentations, with only 2% posterior or transverse presentations.
- Of dystocia cases, 70% involve anterior presentations, 15% are posterior presentations, 15% are transverse presentations.[28,29]

The correction of abnormal fetal posture involves several steps, including:

- Repulsion of the proximal limb.
- The mid-limb (knee/hock) is then pushed laterally.
- The distal limb (hoof/fetlock) is moved medially.
- Then traction is placed on the distal limb, allowing the limb to be extended into a normal posture so that delivery can be performed.
  - ❏ When the limb is extended, a cupped hand should cover the hoof so that damage to the uterus, pelvis and vagina is prevented.

There are three possible methods of resolving a dystocia:

1. Mutation (manipulation of the fetus to a normal presentation) followed by forced extraction (manipulation and delivery).
2. Fetotomy:[30] division of a dead fetus into smaller deliverable pieces within the uterus with the aid of special instruments that minimize trauma to the mare. This is only applicable when the foal is dead and cesarean section cannot be performed for financial or technical reasons (e.g. on a farm).
3. Cesarean section:[31,32] delivery of the foal (either alive or dead) via laparotomy and uterine incisions.

If possible, mutation using repulsion and repositioning is the ideal method of managing a case

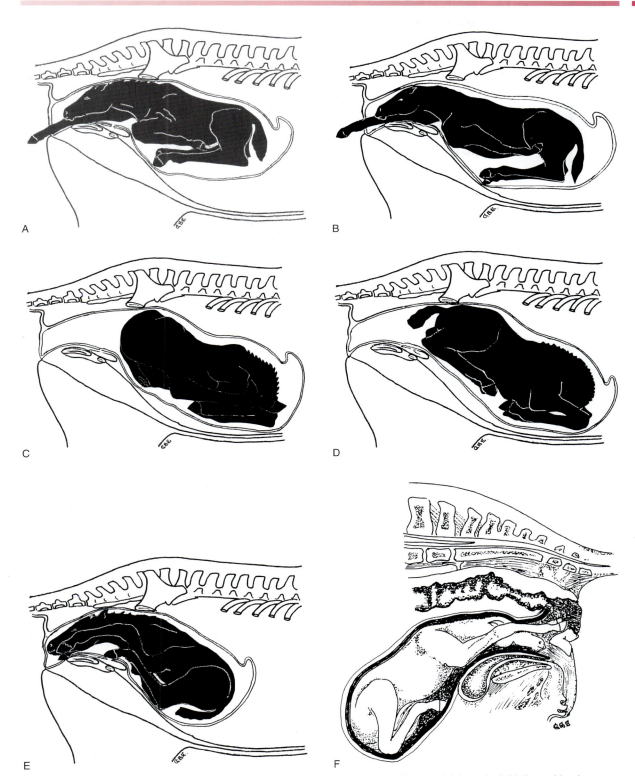

Fig. 8.14 Abnormal foal postures: (A) unilateral carpal flexion; (B) shoulder flexion; (C) breech; (D) bilateral hock flexion; (E) 'dog-sitter' (the hind limbs are under the pelvic rim); (F) foot nape (the feet are over the top of the head/neck and in this case protruding into the rectum, creating a rectovaginal fistula).

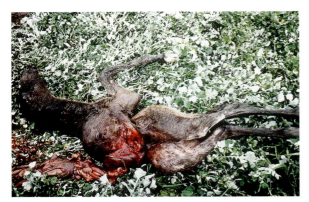

Fig. 8.15 Schistosomus reflexus. This is a fatal complex congenital abnormality that makes normal delivery impossible.

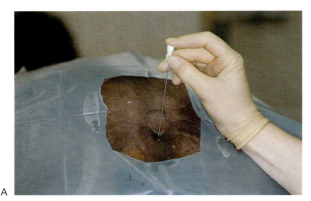

A

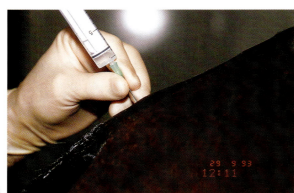

B

Fig. 8.16 Epidural anesthesia is effective and useful for many procedures, including obstetric manipulations.

of dystocia (Fig. 8.18). As fetal malposition is by far the most common reason for dystocia, most cases can be handled in this manner. In some cases, epidural or general anesthesia may be required for this approach to be successful.

Basic rules for managing dystocia

i. All manipulations and investigations must be performed gently to avoid unnecessary trauma to the tissues and to the foal. If the problem cannot be corrected within 15 minutes a different approach must be considered.

ii. Adequate lubrication is extremely important if mutation is to be achieved. Several commercial liquid lubricants are available, as well as a powdered lubricant which can be added to warm water and then pumped into the uterus.

iii. Care should be taken when repelling the fetus so as not to perforate the reproductive tract by the examiner's hand, instruments or a fetal extremity. When applying traction to a foal limb, the hand should be kept over the hoof to prevent any maternal injury.

iv. There should never be more than three people applying traction to the fetus.
- All traction effort should be applied in conjunction with the mare's contractions.
- Traction should not be applied while the mare is resting, except when the foal is becoming increasingly distressed (e.g. when caught in a hip-lock position).

- No motorized/hydraulic equipment or bovine fetal extractors should ever be applied to the foal in an attempt to relieve an equine dystocia.

COMMON MALPRESENTATIONS, POSTURES AND POSITIONS

Most of these can be corrected by repositioning, but others may require cesarean section or fetotomy. Prolonged attempts to correct a malpresentation involving a dead foal may be more traumatic than a simple fetotomy.

Carpal flexion (see Fig. 8.14a)

The knee of the fetus is bent with the hoof pointing towards the rear end of the fetus. This may occur either unilaterally or bilaterally and can usually be resolved by repelling the fetus, elevating the carpus (knee) and then extending the leg.

- Once the carpus is straightened, the leg should be fully extended. The fetus may need to be retropulsed prior to full extension.
- A partial fetotomy involving amputation of the limb can be performed if the fetus is dead and if the carpus cannot be repositioned due to diminished uterine space or ankylosis of the joints.

Shoulder flexion (see Fig. 8.14b)

This occurs when the entire front leg points back towards the back legs of the foal. The condition usually

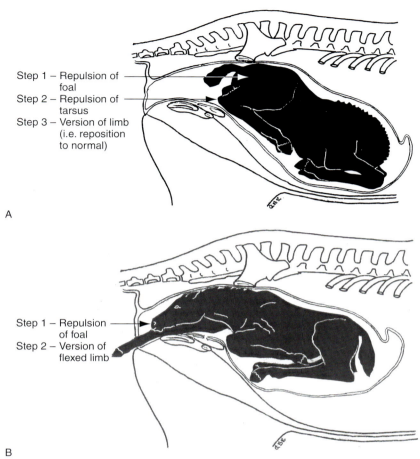

Step 1 – Repulsion of foal
Step 2 – Repulsion of tarsus
Step 3 – Version of limb (i.e. reposition to normal)

A

Step 1 – Repulsion of foal
Step 2 – Version of flexed limb

B

Fig. 8.17   Manipulation of a malpositioned fetus using repulsion, rotation and version.

occurs bilaterally, but it can also occur unilaterally. It can be corrected by converting the posture to a carpal flexion first and then correcting the carpal flexion.

- A good epidural facilitates this type of manipulation.
- There must be adequate uterine capacity to perform this type of manipulation. Easy repulsion of the foal is not always possible due to the contraction of the uterus if the dystocia has been prolonged.
- A partial fetotomy may be required.
- If the foal is alive and there is limited space in the uterus to allow effective mutation, immediate cesarean section provides the best prognosis.

Foot nape (see Fig. 8.14f)

This is the upward displacement of one or both legs above the head. This type of positioning will often prevent fetal delivery and may in turn cause rupture of the dorsal vaginal vault with extension into the rectum. Fortunately, any consequent rupture of the

vagina and rectum is usually retroperitoneal, so there is minimal risk of peritonitis.

- Good epidural anesthesia and adequate lubrication are essential.
- Manipulations are best performed in the standing mare.
- The fetal limb(s) and fetus should be repelled, the limbs repositioned under the head and then the fetus extracted.

Dog-sitter posture (see Fig. 8.14e)

The hind limbs are flexed at the hip and extended under the maternal pelvis. This can be very difficult to correct, especially with a live fetus, as the limbs tend to return to the dog-sitting posture after attempts at repositioning.

- Cesarean section must be considered very early in the correction process. This procedure may justifiably be performed immediately after diagnosis if the fetus is still alive.

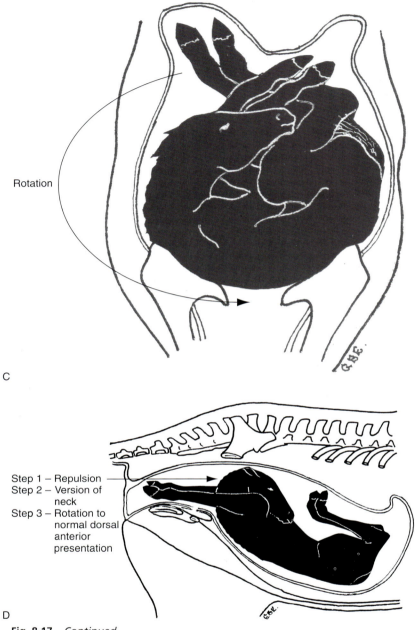

Rotation

C

Step 1 – Repulsion
Step 2 – Version of
neck
Step 3 – Rotation to
normal dorsal
anterior
presentation

D

Fig. 8.17 *Continued.*

- General anesthesia (with hindquarter elevation) and adequate lubrication will facilitate repositioning.
- Once complete fetal repulsion has been achieved, the fetal hind limbs must be pushed away from the pelvic brim. There must be adequate space in the uterus to allow this type of repulsion.
- Once the limb is repelled satisfactorily, it is pushed cranially (towards the head of the mare) so that extension of the hock will occur.
- The same procedure is performed for the opposite limb and the fetus is extracted.
- Care must be taken to be sure the limbs do not return to the dog-sitting posture during extraction. Problems may be encountered during attempts to maintain hock extension, so the posture may not be correctable.
- A fetotomy may be necessary if the foal is dead and repositioning is not possible. Removal of the front half of the fetus will allow either splitting of the pelvis or turning the fetus into a posterior presentation and then extracting it.

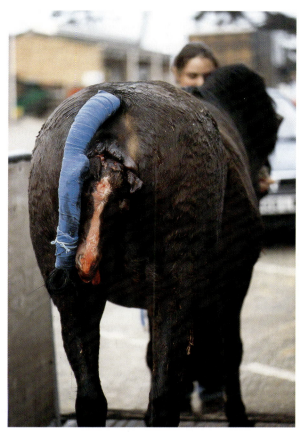

Fig. 8.18 Dystocia with a head presented without either forelimb. This is difficult to correct, but if the foal is alive it is repelled back into the abdomen and the front legs are located and repositioned. If the foal is dead, the head can be removed and then the fetus is repelled to allow limb correction.

Lateral, ventral or dorsal retroflexion of head (see Fig. 8.13c)

The head rests either between the front legs, or to the side of the body, or over the back of the fetus. The length of the fetal neck, the degree of retroflexion and the length of the clinician's arms will all determine the ability to correct this type of malposture.

- First the foal must be repelled; then a snare can be placed around the poll and through the mouth and gentle traction applied to relocate the head in the normal position.
- Alternatively, eyehooks can be utilized without injuring the foal.
- Undue extractive force should not be applied to the head of a live foal.
- Partial fetotomy may be required. Once the head and neck are removed, extraction of the fetus is usually simply achieved.

True breech or bilateral hip flexion
(see Fig. 8.14c)

In this situation, only the tail is presented at the vulva. Hip and hock flexion are usually bilateral. Depending on fetal size and mare size, mutation and fetotomy may be used to resolve these malpresentations.

- Hip flexion is reduced to hock flexion and then the hock flexion is reduced prior to extraction.
- In order to correct these conditions there must be adequate space to manipulate the fetus and sufficient lubrication must be used.
- Cesarean section may be required or may be the most expeditious method to remove the fetus (whether dead or alive).
- In certain cases, multiple fetotomy cuts may be required to remove the fetus.
- An immediate cesarian section is totally justified.

Transverse presentation
(see Fig. 8.12b, c)

Such presentations are fortunately very rare (ventro-transverse presentations are uncommon, and dorso-transverse presentations are extremely rare). They usually occur when the fetus develops the body of the uterus (body pregnancy). Often the fetus is oversized and fetal malformations are common due to the abnormal positioning.

- Diagnosis is based on palpation of the fetus.
- Often the fetus is almost completely out of reach; in other cases, one or two of the foal limbs may be palpable, while the head and neck cannot be located.
- If the foal is alive, immediate cesarean section is recommended because there is rarely adequate room to reposition the fetus.

- If the foal is dead, partial fetotomy may be successful in removing one-half of the foal, then the other half can be repositioned into a longitudinal presentation and extracted. If the fetus cannot be successfully removed within three or four cuts, cesarean section is the preferred method of extraction, even for a dead foal.

FETOTOMY

In some cases, fetotomy (sectioning of the foal into smaller portions for removal) may be the best method to resolve a dystocia. Although sectioning of the foal may seem to be an easy option, it rarely is unless the foal can be delivered quickly with no more than two or three 'cuts'.

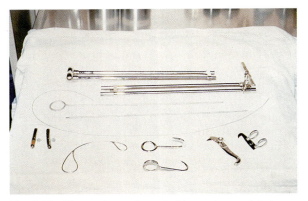

Fig. 8.19 The equipment needed to perform a fetotomy.

CESAREAN SECTION

Cesarean section is often the best method to deliver a live fetus that cannot be easily repositioned (e.g. transverse presentation, 'dog-sitter') or one that is grossly oversize relative to the mare's birth canal. Cesarean section is sometimes necessary in cases of congenital deformity (e.g. schistosomus reflexus, arthrogryposis), due to the difficulty in performing fetotomy.

- Modern surgical facilities will allow a rapid, safe and successful cesarean section, so this should be considered at an early stage.
- The risks associated with the procedure increase significantly with delay.

In order for cesarean section to result in a live foal, the procedure must be carried out promptly, preferably within an hour of the onset of stage 2, because placental separation will be occurring at a significant rate. It is a demanding procedure that requires speed and efficiency for a successful outcome. Having a referral or hospital facility within 15 minutes of the farm will allow for a successful cesarean section (live foal delivered) to be performed in some situations, but by the time problems are recognized the survival of the foal is usually in serious jeopardy. The procedure is, however, highly satisfying when both mare and foal are alive and leave the surgical facility without complications.

- Cesarean section requires general anesthesia and an adequate and sterile surgical facility and surgical team with 24-hour care available. There are major considerations for the staff required for a successful cesarean section.
- Retained placenta is common following cesarean section and fetotomy, due to uterine atony following extended uterine manipulation.

Prolonged fetotomy is potentially disastrous. It is an exhausting procedure for both veterinarian and mare. Nevertheless, it is often the best method to extract a dead foal, because it may require less time to remove the malpositioned extremity than attempting to reposition the foal. If the foal is already dead, it should be delivered by the most direct route possible with every effort made to reduce the stress on the mare.

Performing a safe and efficient fetotomy requires experience and specialized equipment if injuries to the mare are to be prevented. Exposed bones following fetotomy must be adequately covered to protect against accidental injury to the mare.

The minimum equipment necessary to perform a fetotomy safely and adequately includes (Fig. 8.19):

- A fetotome and wire threader.
- A wire introducer.
- A Krey hook.
- A thumb knife.
- Obstetric chains and handles.
- A head snare.
- Obstetric (or Gigly) wire.

- A good 'rule of thumb' is: if the foal can be extracted simply by effecting three cuts or less, a fetotomy may be the best method of delivering a dead fetus.

If the mare is not amenable to fetotomy or there are inadequate facilities, staff or equipment to perform the procedure safely, a cesarean section will probably be required. If the foal cannot be delivered by fetotomy and there is no possibility of safe cesarean section, the mare should be humanely destroyed.

Indications

Cesarean section is indicated when:

- Natural vaginal delivery is either impossible or dangerous.
- The procedure is performed for sound clinical reasons (listed below).
- Gnotobiotic foals[33] are required electively in experimental situations.

The operation should be considered as an alternative to a protracted vaginal delivery or to a prolonged or difficult fetotomy. Given good surgical facilities the procedure may take less time and be far less traumatic and dangerous for the mare than either of the other options for delivery. However, if the facilities are not conducive to safe surgery, cesarean section with recovery of the mare should not be undertaken. The chances of survival are very low under inadequate surgical conditions and the mare may suffer unnecessarily before succumbing to postoperative complications.

Foal problems (see Fig. 8.20)

- Grossly oversized foal. If the foal is alive, a rapid decision is usually possible. If the foal is dead, a decision needs to be taken for cesarean section or fetotomy.
- Fetal malposition that precludes vaginal delivery or might result in a protracted and difficult vaginal delivery with significant danger to mare and foal. For example, a 'dog-sitting' presentation is almost impossible to correct safely. A live foal strongly biases the decision towards cesarean section rather than fetotomy.
- A foal with anatomical abnormalities that preclude vaginal delivery and which cannot be resolved by fetotomy (e.g. fused joints or gross hydrocephalus).

Mare problems

- Previous injury to the pelvis making the pelvic canal too small to allow safe delivery of the foal. This might not be obvious at the time of delivery but should be detectable in a mare with a good clinical history and good stud management from conception to delivery.
- Tumors or other masses. Any gross physical obstructions (such as those caused by muscular hamartoma, perineal melanoma or vaginal leiomyoma) in the vaginal canal and vulva can preclude any possibility of vaginal delivery. These are usually obvious on examination and may present with problems of defecation during the later stages of the pregnancy.
- Previous severe (third-degree) perineal laceration. Injuries that might be rendered incurable if damaged by normal vaginal delivery or where scarring and distortion from surgery prevent any chance of normal delivery.
- Ruptured prepubic tendon (Fig. 8.21). Cesarean section is usually an emergency salvage procedure for these cases. Although cesarean section should not be undertaken lightly, it offers the best chances for a live foal in a mare with full rupture of the prepubic tendon. The mare may have to be destroyed (either immediately before nonsterile removal of the foal) or immediately after delivery of the foal while the mare is still anesthetized.

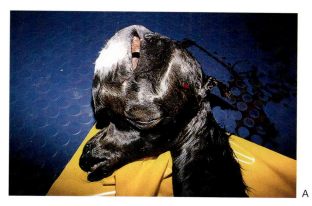
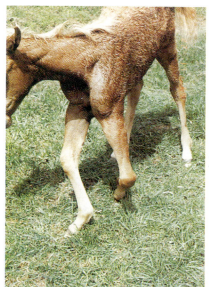

Fig. 8.20   (A) Hydrocephalus. (B) Contracted foal.

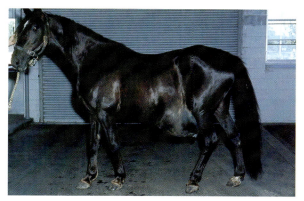

Fig. 8.21   Ruptured prepubic tendon.

- Large ventral hernia (Fig. 8.22). Extensive muscular disruption may render natural delivery difficult and prolonged as the mare might not be able to strain effectively and straining might in any case exacerbate the problem.

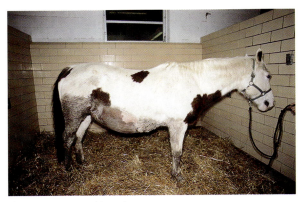

Fig. 8.22 Ventral hernia.

- Expulsive deficiency. Old mares with collapsed ventral abdominal support or with very poor body condition may have little or no abdominal expulsive force. The same circumstances might arise in a mare with a permanent tracheostomy.
- Uterine torsion (see p. 296). Torsion occurring in the last 2 weeks of gestation may well be suitable for cesarean section.

Note:
Elective cesarean section with euthanasia of the mare on delivery of the foal.
- This should be considered when there is no or little prospect of the mare's survival and the foal is still alive.
- Usually the situation involves a distressed and/or critically ill/injured mare which would inevitably carry an unacceptably high risk for conventional surgical delivery.
- This procedure can also be carried out electively when financial or technical constraints such as the nonavailability of suitable surgical facilities conflict with the welfare of the mare.
- After due consideration, simultaneous euthanasia of the mare and delivery of the foal by emergency nonaseptic cesarean section may be undertaken.

Other considerations
- Mares may develop significant adhesions following cesarean section and have lowered fertility.[34]
- The procedure is inevitably expensive (in both financial and labor terms) and the value of the mare and foal may not equate with the total cost of the procedure and the required after care.
- The availability of a suitable surgical facility within a reasonable distance (usually 1–2 hours'

travel is the maximum that is consistent with foal survival). Clearly this time will vary according to the delay prior to the decision to opt for surgery. A significant time advantage may be gained by administration of clenbuterol intravenously to the mare prior to departure. This may inhibit uterine contractions and so delay placental separation.

Note:
- Although this surgery can be performed successfully in the field, there are unacceptable risks associated with postoperative infection in particular. If the foal is already dead, attention should be paid to the mare alone. Her survival may depend heavily on the care she receives before, during and after the procedure.

- If the mare is beyond her economic breeding age, surgery might not be warranted; but, if she has a high sentimental value, surgery remains a viable option. However, successful outcome percentages do fall as mares reach 20–25 years of age.
- All foals delivered by cesarean section are immediately classified as high-risk (see p. 355).

Surgical site considerations

The sites commonly used for cesarean section include:

- Ventral midline.[35] The incision is made through the linea alba, extending from the umbilicus forward a distance of 40–80 cm, and if necessary caudally.
- Paramedian. There is little to commend this site in most cases, but it can be useful when the midline has complications such as previous laparotomy incisions or repair of incisional and umbilical hernias.
- High flank. This incision is made in the sublumbar fossa midway between the last rib and the wing of the ilium. The incision is extended caudally to provide better access. This site is complicated by the underlying abdominal organs (on both sides) and provides little access. This is the preferred site for surgical correction of uterine torsion in the standing mare (see p. 296).
- Low oblique flank (Marcenac).[36] The incision is made in the left flank rather than the right because the cecum adds complication on the right.

Anesthesia and surgical procedure

The specialized anesthesia and surgical procedures are described in standard surgical textbooks. Anesthesia for cesarean section requires special considerations and a skilled anesthetist is important for the mare and the survival of the foal. The circulatory efficiency of the mare is critical to the survival of both mare and foal. Dorsal recumbency in a mare with a heavily gravid uterus adds significantly to the compromise of venous return from the abdomen. The anesthesia should not unduly depress the foal and should allow it to breathe normally from the outset.

The surgical procedure itself carries significant risks and an experienced surgical team is a significant factor in the successful outcome of the procedure.

Postoperative care of the mare

If a live foal is delivered with minimal complications and correct surgical procedures are followed, recovery is good, with many mares being discharged from the surgical facility within 7–14 days.

- Postoperative swelling commonly occurs around the surgical site around the third to fifth day. It may extend along the ventral midline bilaterally either side of a midline incision or laterally ventral to a paramedian or flank incision. The wound is commonly tender to the touch but should be free of significant pain, heat or discharge.
- The mare (and foal) should be confined to a large stable (stall) or stable and yard for exercise.
- Once the foal is strong and has bonded with the mare, twice-daily hand-walking for 10–15 minutes is recommended.
- Regular attention should be paid to the status of uterine involution and if necessary to the placenta (if this was not delivered at the time of surgery). Oxytocin is administered to encourage involution in the early stages but requires to be used with care; complications such as uterine prolapse and inversion of a uterine horn can have serious implications both immediately and for the future fertility of the mare. Uterine flushing is continued until the fluid is consistently clear and free of blood or abnormal exudate.
- Depending on the reason for the operation itself, fluid therapy may be indicated.
- Antibiotics are routinely administered postoperatively for 5–6 days. Usually penicillin is all that is required. Meticulous surgical procedure and careful attention to closure of the uterine incision can usually avoid septic peritonitis. Before being replaced into the abdomen, the uterus should be carefully lavaged to minimize residual infection.
- Particular care must be paid to the possible development of laminitis. Large draught breeds (such as the Shire) seem particularly prone to laminitis after surgery (even in the absence of any detectable metritis).
- It is common practice to administer nonsteroidal anti-inflammatory drugs to control discomfort associated with uterine involution and pain from the surgical site. Due precaution must be taken with respect to gastric ulceration in the foal when these drugs are administered to the mare.
- Postsurgical colic can be avoided through careful attention to feeding. A mildly laxative diet is thought to be helpful.
- Blood samples should be taken repeatedly during the postoperative period to monitor possible developing anemia and sepsis.
- Breeding should be delayed until involution is complete, infection is fully controlled and the mare is otherwise healthy and the incision completely healed.
- Free exercise for the mare should not be permitted for 12–14 weeks after surgery. However, in many cases this is difficult and some compromises between the risks of herniation and wound breakdown and the benefits of exercise and pasture access need to be made.

Immediate postoperative care of the foal

Whenever possible a dedicated team should be available to take care of the foal from the point of delivery. The foal is automatically classified as 'high-risk' and so requires immediate intensive care. If the fetus is dead on delivery it should be removed as quickly as possible from the operation room and stored for postmortem examination.

If the foal is normal and healthy it should be introduced to the mare as soon as she has fully and safely recovered from the anesthesia. Mares may be somewhat reluctant to accept the foal and so extra vigilance must be given to ensure safe bonding and to establish that nursing is taking place.

Immediate procedures that improve survival rates:

i. Once the foal is delivered a sterile clamp (a plastic bag sealer is a useful clamp for this purpose) is applied to the umbilicus and the cord is ligated 5–7 cm from the body wall with sterile umbilical tape.

ii. THE CORD SHOULD NOT BE BROKEN BY TENSION. This may cause blood vessel or urachal damage and may also predispose to umbilical hernia.[37]

iii. Ensure that the airway is clear. There are no special means for airway suction in foals but a downward slope is helpful to drain fluids in the airway towards the pharynx. Administer oxygen by mask or if necessary by positive pressure ventilation.

iv. The exposed umbilical remnants should immediately be soaked in 0.5% chlorhexidine solution. This should be repeated every 6 hours for the first 24–36 hours.[38]

Note:
- It may be useful to leave the vessels intact for a few minutes while the uterus begins to involute (until arterial pulsation is deceased) and breathing begins. During this time there should be no risk to the survival of the foal and attention can be directed at establishing a clear airway and encouraging normal respiration.
- A sterile blood sample can be obtained immediately from the umbilical vessels and subjected to biphasic culture and routine hematological analysis. This may be very useful as an indicator of the health of the foal and cultures with sensitivity will be available within 2 days. In the event that the foal is normal and healthy the wasted samples can be viewed as an insurance policy.
- In the event that the foal is suspected as being a potential neonatal isoerythrolysis candidate, suitable confirmatory tests and cross-matching can be started immediately.
- Navel dipping/soaking with solutions of povidone iodine has been shown to be less effective[38] than with chlorhexidine.
- In any case, strong (7.5%) povidone iodine solutions should not be used as they may cause necrosis of the umbilical tissues.

v. Move the foal to a facility where it can be dried and kept in a warm environment to limit heat loss. Heat loss is a major cause of foal mortality. Foals delivered by nonelective cesarean section will inevitably be weaker and may have few reserves of energy.
vi. Administer colostrum (possibly milked from the mare or from storage) or plasma by stomach tube within 1–2 hours. Alternatively, an immediate plasma transfusion with hyperimmune plasma can be given with full aseptic precautions.
vii. Administer appropriate antibiotics immediately and continue for 4–5 days. Note that antibiotic therapy is easily misused and full courses should always be given.
viii. Tetanus antiserum can be administered if considered necessary. In many studs this is a routine procedure regardless of the vaccination status of the mare and effective passive transfer.

UTERINE INVOLUTION

In order for a mare to foal yearly, the uterus must involute rapidly after delivery of the foal. Additionally, the mare must cycle soon after foaling to produce a foal annually.

Progestogens and relaxin, produced by the placenta, minimize uterine contractility. With placental expulsion, these hormones no longer provide a negative influence on the uterus, thus increasing myometrial contractility.

Additionally, estrogens, which decrease toward the end of pregnancy, begin to increase in conjunction with the first follicular wave within the first few days post partum. Estrogen provides a positive stimulus on uterine contractility, in part by mobilizing oxytocin and prostaglandin receptors.[39] Uterine contractions occur from the tips of the horns towards the cervix, resulting in expulsion of fluid, debris, and bacterial contamination. Increasing estrogen concentrations provide for improved immune function so that the postpartum contamination is controlled and resolved.

- By 15 days post partum, there should be no abnormal fluid or inflammation in the normal mare's uterus.
- The uterine horns are half their pregnant size within 24 hours post partum, and are normal in size by 30 days post partum.
- The endometrium has recovered to its nonpregnant state by day 14 post partum.

In some mares, especially those that have had any manipulations during foaling, may have excessive inflammation to be cleared within the first week after foaling. These mares may require up to 2–3 weeks to clear the inflammation or they may require uterine therapy before resolution of infection or inflammation can occur (see p. 196).

FOAL HEAT

Within a few days of foaling, the mare begins to develop a follicular wave on her ovaries and will develop a preovulatory follicle, such that ovulation will occur between 5 and 20 days from foaling. Signs of estrus will usually be seen between days 5 and 12 post partum. The later in the breeding season the mare foals the shorter the duration of foal heat estrus and the shorter the interval from foaling to ovulation. Most mares will only ovulate one follicle, although some mares will double ovulate at their foal heat, especially if they foal later in the breeding season.

Some mares will not display obvious signs of heat if they are teased in the presence of their foal, as they may be nervous or protective mothers and are more concerned about their foal than showing signs of heat to the stallion. These mares will often break down and show to the stallion if either separated from the foal by a wall, a separate room outside of earshot or are twitched. In other cases, removal of the foal from the mare may result in significant separation anxiety and then the mare will not show signs of estrus until she knows the foal is safe. In these cases, holding the foal within viewing distance, but far enough from the mare to prevent injury should the mare be nonreceptive to the stallion, resolves the problem.

The decision as to whether to breed on foal heat must be based on certain factors:

1. Uterine health

   The mare must be assessed for resolution of the inflammation that normally follows foaling. This is usually best assessed by rectal palpation and ultrasonography of the uterus. The presence of fluid with debris or of a 'doughy' feel to the uterus should preclude breeding at foal heat. Vaginoscopic examination of the vagina and cervix for evidence of inflammation, bruising, fluid accumulation, or urine pooling is recommended for all postpartum mares. Bacteriological culture of swabs from mares on their foal heat is usually not indicated since almost all are contaminated during foaling. Positive cultures are common and may not indicate the need to treat with antibiotics. Most mares will clear their inflammation given adequate time for involution and particularly if a normal estrous cycle can be allowed to pass. Any mare that had a dystocia, retained placenta, or excessive manipulation post foaling should not be bred on foal heat under any circumstances.

2. The time of year

   This is often a factor in the decision to breed a mare at the foal heat. Mares that are foaling very late in the breeding season (June–August in the northern hemisphere; November–January in the southern hemisphere) are often bred on foal heat to try to bring the foaling date earlier the next year, thereby achieving foaling closer to the ideal 1 January (northern hemisphere) or 1 August (southern hemisphere) birth date. If the mare does not become pregnant on the foal heat cycle and, assuming she conceives on the second cycle, she will foal in the same month the next year. Some stud management systems allow the mare to have her foal heat ovulation and then administer prostaglandin around days 18–21. This effectively shortens the period to the second ovulation by approximately 7–10 days (under natural conditions the second heat will occur between days 28 and 32). The alternative is to leave the mare open (unbred) for the season and rebreed early in the season the following year.

3. The type of semen being used

   Mares bred on the foal heat are preferably bred with fresh semen. Use of chilled semen is acceptable, but the breeder should be aware that the fertility of foal heat ovulation is normally only about 50%. Therefore, it is sometimes preferable to delay the first ovulation or shorten the interval to the second ovulation before investing money for transported semen on a reduced fertility cycle. If the mare is to be bred with frozen semen, she should be allowed to pass the foal heat ovulation and then have her second heat naturally. This 30-day heat is the earliest period from foaling before frozen semen is used. Frozen semen is quite irritating to the endometrium and therefore there should be no residual inflammation from foaling prior to breeding with frozen semen.

4. The age of the mare

   Multiparous mares over 12 years of age have a higher conception rate if they are bred following short-cycling (see below) or on their natural second heat. These mares tend to have a more pendulous uterus and are therefore probably slower to clear inflammation and fluid from the uterine lumen.

5. Days post partum

   Some clinicians use day 10 as the minimum time period from foaling that breeding will be allowed. If the mare has normal involution, no obvious abnormal uterine fluid, and no evidence of cervical or vaginal inflammation on speculum examination, then she will be bred as long as ovulation occurs after day 10. If everything else is normal, and ovulation occurs before day 10, the mare will not be bred and, instead, is short-cycled 6 days later (see below). This day 10 cut-off has been set, since it is known that endometrial recovery from foaling is complete in the normal mare by day 15 post partum. If the mare is bred on day 10, the embryo will not enter the uterus before days 15–16. If she is bred before day 10, the embryo may enter a hostile environment because insufficient time has elapsed since foaling. That is not to say that some mares will not conceive if bred before day 10, it is simply difficult to predict fertility before day 15.

Delaying foal heat ovulation

1. Short-cycling

   In order to shorten the interval to the second ovulation, the mare can be 'short-cycled' with a prostaglandin injection administered 6–7 days following the foal heat ovulation. This will effectively shorten the period between successive estrous cycles by about 7–10 days.

2. Hormone manipulation

   In order to delay foal heat ovulation, the mare can be given either oral progesterone alone for 8 days (day 1 of treatment = day after foaling) or progesterone and estradiol for 3–5 days (day 1 of treatment = day after foaling).

Either of these methods is associated with increased fertility when compared with normal foal heat breeding.

Conception rates for foal heat breeding

Pregnancy rates for foal heat breeding are 10–20% lower than for breeding at any subsequent estrus. Also, there is a higher rate of early embryonic death in mares bred at foal heat. These differences may be due to one or a combination of factors including:

- Failure of involution of the uterus or endometrium.
- Delayed uterine clearance.

- It is important that every mare is carefully evaluated as an individual when considering whether foal heat breeding is likely to be favorable or not.

COMPLICATIONS OF PREGNANCY AND PARTURITION

Uterine torsion

Although uterine torsion can occur at any time during late gestation, it usually occurs in the last 3 months of pregnancy,[25,40] but it has been diagnosed as early as 5 months of gestation. Unlike the cow the condition is seldom associated with parturition itself.[41] The cervix is not usually involved. Usually the presenting sign is that of low-grade intermittent colic or slow progression of labor. In a few cases colic (abdominal discomfort) may be more severe. The etiology has not been established but sudden fetal movements, rolling or sudden falls seem logical explanations.

Diagnosis

Diagnosis is based on distinctive rectal palpation of the broad ligaments with one ligament coursing over the top of the uterus and the opposite ligament coursing under the uterus. During rectal examination it should be possible to identify the direction of the torsion (Fig. 8.23).

- If the twist is anticlockwise (viewed from behind the mare), the right broad ligament can be identified stretching to the left over the dorsal surface of the uterus.
- Clockwise torsion reveals the opposite, with the left broad ligament passing across the top of the uterus to the right.
- The amount of rotation may be mild (90°) to severe (>720°).[42] Rotation of over 360° will usually affect the circulation to the uterus, possibly resulting in death of the fetus or damage to the uterus or placenta, which in turn may result in fetal hypoxia.

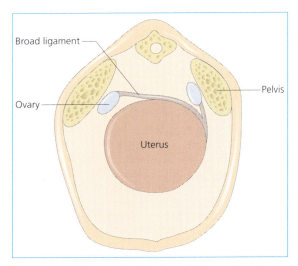

Fig. 8.23 Uterine torsion. The broad ligament on the side to which the uterus is twisted will course ventrally and under the uterus, while the broad ligament of the opposite side courses over the top of the uterus. This diagram illustrates the appearance of a right torsion viewed from behind.

- Vaginoscopic examination is not usually helpful because the cervix or vagina is seldom involved in the torsion.

Treatment

- If the mare is at full term, the cervix is relaxed and the degree of rotation is not too severe so that the fetus can be reached through the cervix, correction of uterine torsion may be made using manual reduction by rocking the fetus.
  - ❏ This method requires considerable upper body strength of the operator, but if the fetal elbow or torso can be reached, it is possible to rock the fetus in a semicircular motion until enough momentum is gained to roll the uterus back into position.
  - ❏ The use of 'detorsion rods' is generally not recommended due to difficulties with the long fetal extremities of foals, but if used properly may be beneficial in some cases.
- Alternatively, the mare can be 'rolled' under general anesthesia using the Schaffer 'plank in the flank' method.[43,44]
  - ❏ This method uses the plank to hold the uterus in one place while the mare is rolled slowly around the uterus (Fig. 8.24).
  - ❏ Several rolls may be required depending on the degree of torsion. If no plank is available the mare can be rolled quickly over and over, the goal being to roll the mare faster than her uterus can roll. This method of rolling often requires a greater number of revolutions for

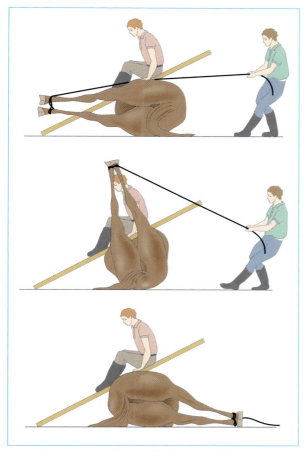

Fig. 8.24   The 'plank in the flank' method for reduction of uterine torsion. The mare is placed in lateral recumbency on the side to which the torsion is directed. In this case the uterus is twisted to the right. Keeping pressure on the plank, the mare is slowly rolled over to the other side.

the same degree of torsion, but does require one less person to help.
- ❑ A complication of either rolling procedure may be uterine rupture or disruption of a blood vessel leading to the uterus.
- ❑ The location of the broad ligaments is assessed per rectum following each roll, to determine if the torsion has resolved.
- Surgical correction, using either a standing flank laparotomy (incision is made on the side of the direction of the torsion) or a ventral midline laparotomy approach with the mare under general anesthesia, is probably the treatment of choice in most circumstances. The benefit of these procedures is that they allow direct visualization of the uterus, broad ligaments and blood supply so that it can be assessed whether any damage to these structures has occurred as a result of the torsion.
- ❑ The procedure requires a surgical facility.

- ❑ A ventral midline approach is the better surgical approach if severe damage is suspected, or if any other abdominal problems are suspected, because it allows for correction of these problems or cesarean section to remove the fetus if this is considered necessary. It also allows direct visualization of the remaining abdominal viscera and subsequent correction of any concurrent conditions or abnormalities.
- ❑ Once the abdomen is entered the uterus is rocked back into a normal position; the position of the broad ligaments is checked before closure to determine that the uterus is in a normal position and no damage has occurred.
- Once the torsion is reduced, the fetus should be assessed for viability.
- If the pregnancy is full term and the fetus is alive, vaginal extraction should be performed slowly to allow the vagina and cervix to relax completely.
- Congestion of the blood vessels and soft tissues following torsion is common.

- Preterm uterine torsions results in immediate classification as a high-risk pregnancy.
- Fetal viability should be monitored carefully over the next 2 weeks, as damage to the uterus, broad ligaments or placenta may result in fetal compromise or asphyxia and subsequent fetal death.

- In the full-term mare, resolution of the torsion is usually evident by a bulging of the allantochorion into the vagina, followed by rupture and development of weaker than usual uterine and abdominal contractions.
- Assistance with delivery should be given when the mare has contractions but excessive pressure should not be exerted. No extractive force should be applied when the mare is resting between contractions.
- Uterine rupture is a significant recognized complication of the condition and of the correction methods.[45]
- The prognosis for the mare and the foal depends on the degree of torsion and the speed and efficiency with which it is corrected. Studies have shown that about 50% of foals and 70% of mares survive surgical management.[40,46]

- When torsion occurs immediately preterm, fetal viability should still be assessed following correction (see p. 249). Additionally, any abnormalities of the uterus or broad ligaments should be assessed.

- In cases where torsion occurs in earlier stages (preterm) of gestation, many clinicians administer progesterone following reduction of the torsion to maintain cervical closure and promote uterine quiescence.

Uterine atony/inertia

Primary uterine atony/inertia is fortunately rare in mares. Secondary uterine atony or inertia due to fatigue of the myometrium may occur following prolonged labor, oversize fetuses or calcium deficiency. Although hydropic conditions are rare, the gross distention of the uterus that arises results in inertia. Most cases are seen in debilitated/weak or old mares or those with systemic illness or metabolic derangement.[47]

Diagnosis

- Usually parturition begins normally but expulsive efforts and uterine contractions fade quickly.
- The condition should be differentiated from an inability to make abdominal effort (e.g. where there is a tracheostomy or an abdominal rupture or ventral hernia).
- Uterine rupture may also present with similar signs.

Treatment

- Assistance should be given before the foal is compromised.
- Oxytocin and fluids containing calcium gluconate should be administered intravenously.

Note:
- Oxytocin should never be administered to mares diagnosed with or suspected to have uterine rupture as the cause of the uterine inertia.

- Excessive force should never be applied. Traction should be applied when the mare is having an abdominal contraction and should stop while she is resting. The exception to this occurs when there is complete absence of contractions. In these cases, the force applied to the fetus should not be excessive, adequate lubrication should be utilized and the position of the fetus and the amount of room in the pelvis should be assessed frequently to be certain that delivery is progressing normally.

Hydrops amnion and hydrops allantois

Hydropic conditions (dropsy) of the fetal membranes, which include hydrops amnion (hydramnios or hydramnion) and hydrops allantois (hydrallantois), are occasionally encountered in mares.[25,48,49] Both can occur simultaneously.

- Hydrops allantois is more common in the mare. It is an accumulation of excessive fluid in the allantoic space and is typically due to abnormalities of the placenta.
- Hydrops amnion is an accumulation of an increased amount of fluid in the amniotic space due to the inability of the fetus to swallow normally. It may be due to abnormalities of the placenta or fetus, such that more fluid is being produced than is being resorbed.[50]

Both conditions are often accompanied by one or more congenital defects in the fetus but it is difficult to be certain whether this is the cause or the effect of the condition. Some reported abnormalities include 'wry neck', ankylosis, hydrocephalus, growth retardation, and ventral herniation. Abnormalities of the placenta, such as placentitis, or abnormalities of the placental vessels may also result in hydropic conditions.

Diagnosis

- Normally, there are 3–7 liters of amniotic fluid and 8–18 liters of allantoic fluid. The normal placenta weighs 2.2–6.4 kg.
- Hydropic conditions usually occur after the seventh month of gestation. In most cases of dropsy, regardless of the type, the accumulation of fluid occurs quite quickly, usually noted as significant abdominal enlargement over a period of days to weeks.[51]
- The abdomen is often markedly distended before veterinary attention is sought.
- In some cases, these mares will be unable to rise due to the pressure on the ventral abdomen and back muscles. Respiration may be labored due to the pressure of the abdominal contents on the diaphragm. There may be signs of colic, herniation or rupture of the abdominal wall.
- Uterine rupture may occur.[52] Rupture of the prepubic or abdominal musculature and ventral edema can be present.
- Rectal palpation reveals a grossly enlarged uterus, often occupying the entire palpable abdominal cavity. It may be difficult to locate and palpate the fetus due to the increased amount of fluid surrounding it and the increased thickness of the placental membranes.
- The foal may be grossly abnormal, often appearing anasarcous (water belly with extensive subcutaneous edema). The prognosis for the foal is poor and most effort should be directed to saving the mare.

Treatment

- Treatment of both conditions involves either abortion or induction of parturition. Manual dilation of the cervix will usually result in abortion. This can be performed over a period of 15–30 minutes. If the mare is at, or close to, term (within 30 days), induction of parturition with oxytocin can be attempted.

- Assisted delivery is invariably still required because there is uterine inertia from overstretching of the uterus.
- Drainage of fluid from the abdomen should be conducted in a controlled manner if possible, such that:
  - ❑ The fluid balance is not grossly disrupted too quickly.
  - ❑ It allows the blood supply to the abdomen to equilibrate following the abrupt decrease in abdominal contents. If the fluid is emptied too quickly, blood will pool in the abdominal blood vessels and may result in circulatory shock and/or death of the mare.
- Administration of intravenous fluids is recommended during the acute phase of fluid drainage to maintain blood pressure.
- Uterine involution is typically normal following resolution of the pregnancy.
- There are reports of normal foals being born from hydropic conditions, but most are either grossly abnormal or nonviable. It has been suggested that hydrops may have a heritable component. Therefore, the mare should not be bred to the same stallion in future pregnancies to reduce the chances of the condition re-occurring.

Premature placental separation

Premature placental separation, also known as a 'red bag delivery', occurs when the placenta separates from the endometrium prior to the fetus breaking through the allantochorion by entering the pelvic canal.[25] The placenta (allantochorion) does not rupture at the cervical star region as would occur normally. The mare then attempts to deliver the entire fetoplacental unit intact through the vagina. As a result, instead of seeing the bluish white amniotic sac at the vulvar lips, the velvety red surface of the chorion is seen (Fig. 8.25). This complication is most commonly seen with:

- Fescue toxicosis, which induces placental edema.
- Stress in late gestation.
- Excessive nutrition in late gestation.
- Ascending infection (placentitis) or other pathology of the allantochorion, which may cause the initial separation at the cervical region.
- Induced parturition.

There may be a history of bleeding from the uterus in the last few days prior to parturition, which is indicative of the disorder in some cases. The chorioallantois is typically thickened and edematous.

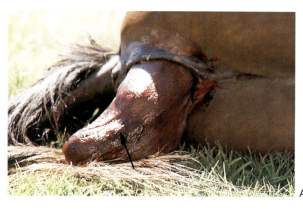
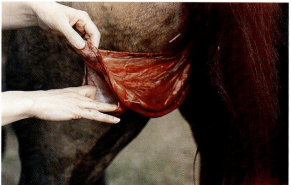

Fig. 8.25   Premature placental separation ('red bag delivery'). (A) Note the placental star (arrowed) and the chorionic surface of the placenta extruded more than normal (B).

Diagnosis

- The diagnosis is made by observing a red, velvety structure presented at the vulva prior to the amniotic sac (grayish-white sac which covers the fetus directly).
- There is usually no evidence of the water breaking in these cases.

Treatment

- This is a true emergency situation because the blood supply of the fetus is effectively lost as the placenta separates.
- The allantochorion should be opened as quickly as possible. As it is often impossible to break open the allantochorion manually due to the thickness of the placenta, a knife or scissors is often required (see Fig. 8.25b). Although in theory it is better to avoid cutting the major blood vessels in the membranes, they are usually impossible to see. If the cervical star is visible, this should be the site of the incision.
- The fetus should be extracted as quickly as possible and supplemental oxygen supplied until the foal is stable.

- It is common to have neonatal maladjustment following this condition in spite of the best attention.[53]

Depending of the cause of the abnormality of the placenta, the foal may be premature or dysmature.

Ventral rupture

Rupture of the prepubic tendon, the rectus abdominus musculature and the transversus abdominus muscle may occur in the pregnant mare.[25,54] These ruptures may occur singly or in combination, one after another, as a direct result of a previous rupture, a weakened body wall, and/or increased stress and pressure on the remaining abdominal wall from the enlarging pregnancy. Rupture of the prepubic tendon usually occurs in the last third of gestation as the fetus is growing at a rapid rate. It is more common in older, multiparous mares and draft mares, as age, multiple pregnancies and the increased weight of the fetus weaken the abdominal wall. Inactivity, twins and hydropic conditions may predispose to rupture.

Diagnosis

- The mare will usually display abdominal pain and a reluctance to walk.
- Often the first sign of impending rupture is a thick plaque of ventral edema (often >15 cm) due to reduced blood supply to the ventral abdominal wall.
- The abdomen will often appear dropped or bulging either along the entire abdomen or along one side (see Fig. 8.22).
- With complete prepubic tendon rupture the udder is pulled cranially and will appear to be in middle third of the abdomen, rather than between the back legs.[54]
- The ischial tuberosities will also appear elevated if rupture is complete.
- Rectal examination may identify the deficit at the cranial margin of the pubis but can be difficult due to the presence of the gravid uterus.

- Ventral rupture must be differentiated from hernias. Physical examination and ultrasonography will often aid in this differentiation.

Treatment

- Treatment consists of supportive slinging of the abdominal wall until term or induction of parturition if severe.
- Assistance during labor is invariably required due to the inability of the mare to sustain normal abdominal contractions. Therefore, if the mare is allowed to go to term, she must be monitored closely as her due date approaches. The cervix

will relax, but the mare often cannot strain effectively to get the fetus up in the birth canal.

- If labor is not noticed in its early stages, the placenta will separate and the fetus will die. If the pregnancy is beyond 340 days, induction is recommended, after checking for fetal maturity as described under induction of pregnancy (p. 279). Induction is also recommended if the mare becomes recumbent.
- Cesarean section with euthanasia before recovery is often the most humane way of dealing with the problem if surgical repair of the defect(s) is not economically feasible or the damage is too severe for repair to be successful (see Figs 8.21, 8.22).

Once foaling is over and edema diminishes, surgical repair of the rupture is sometimes possible using a mesh implant. If the cause of the previous rupture can be prevented during future foaling (i.e. twins or hydrops), these repairs may be successful. In cases where surgical repair is believed to be an unlikely success (i.e. the aged mare), embryo transfer can be employed to continue the reproductive capacity of these mares.

- If a viable foal is born, care should be taken to evaluate colostral quality, since there is often edema in the udder and rupture of blood vessels leading to the udder, resulting in blood in the milk.
- Colostral quality may be poor.
- If inadequate colostrum is found, colostrum supplement or replacement or hyperimmune plasma should be provided immediately after delivery of the foal.

Rupture of the middle uterine or utero-ovarian artery

Rupture of the middle uterine arteries, the utero-ovarian arteries or external iliac arteries may occur in the late gestational mare, during parturition or immediately after delivery (up to 24–48 hours).[25,55,56]

It is more common in older (>12 years of age) multiparous mares as their reproductive tracts and the associated blood vessels have been stretched with each successive pregnancy.

Hemorrhage may occur into the broad ligament (mesometrium) or directly into the abdomen. In some cases, bleeding may initially be restricted to the broad ligament, with subsequent rupture of the ligament, followed by uncontrolled hemorrhage into the abdominal cavity. Typically the mare shows signs of mild to moderate colic, but some bleed sufficiently rapidly to result in death within hours (Fig. 8.26).

Diagnosis

- Mares that are hemorrhaging may demonstrate the Flehmen response (upturned upper lip) for an unknown reason.

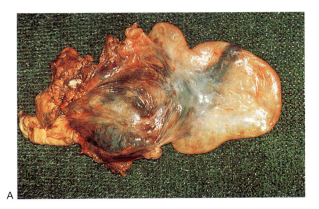

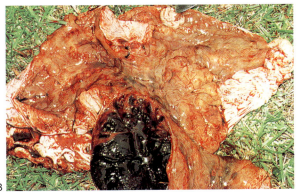

Fig. 8.26 (A) Broad ligament hematoma. (B) Uterine wall hematoma.

- If the hemorrhage into the broad ligament is not severe, or is slowed by the pressure of the two sides of the mesometrium around it, a hematoma may form and the bleeding may stop. The size of the hematoma may be small to large (golf ball/basketball) depending on the amount of hemorrhage that has occurred.
- Palpation of the broad ligaments often reveals the presence of the hematoma, usually with associated discomfort on palpation soon after the damage has occurred.
- Over-enthusiastic efforts to confirm the diagnosis per rectum can be harmful and may convert a potentially resolvable problem into a disaster.
- If the hemorrhage into the broad ligament subsequently ruptures and intra-abdominal hemorrhage occurs, the mare will show signs of shock with extreme pallor and a very high heart rate with a 'thready' pulse. Signs of trembling, sweating, shaking and unwillingness to rise are indicators of shock and possible hemorrhage, and medical attention should be provided immediately. If the hemorrhage is not curtailed, the mare will commonly exsanguinate in a matter of minutes to hours.

Treatment

Treatment consists of a combination of the following:

- Supportive care to avoid any extra stress or excitement in an effort to keep the blood pressure low. Stress should be minimized for several weeks post partum to reduce the chances of hemorrhage starting anew. Procedures such as teasing, breeding and episioplasty should be avoided during this time period.
- Intravenous naloxone has been found to be helpful but the reasons for this are not known.
- Intravenous formalin solution (50 ml of 10% formalin solution diluted in 1 liter of saline) may slow the bleeding.
- Blood transfusions have had mixed results but would seem a sensible measure. Measures that increase blood pressure may be life-saving but may also cause more bleeding.
- Sedation should be avoided, but if it is absolutely necessary care should be taken not to use drugs that exacerbate hypotension such as acepromazine. However, lowering of blood pressure could be viewed as an advantage in reducing blood loss.

Prognosis

- Most mares under the age of 14 years with hematomas that are restricted to the broad ligament will survive. Usually the hematoma will organize over time into a fibrous scar, although some hematomas remain palpable for years following the acute event.
- It is not known if the affected mare has an increased or lesser tendency to recurrences at subsequent pregnancies.
- Most mares with intra-abdominal hemorrhage will die from acute blood loss in spite of best efforts to support the circulation. Surgery has proved to be very unrewarding as it is virtually impossible to localize the source of the hemorrhage in the broad ligament to allow ligation.

Rupture of the uterus

Uterine rupture may occur spontaneously in an otherwise normal delivery or as a secondary consequence of hydropic conditions,[52] uterine torsion,[45] violent fetal movement, or from manipulations during a dystocia (mutation or fetotomy).[25,52,57] Uterine rupture occasionally occurs immediately preterm and a portion of (or the whole) foal may lie outside the uterus.[41] Uterine lacerations can be full-thickness or partial-thickness. Most tears in the uterine wall occur on the ventral or abdominal surface and are more prone to causing peritonitis if full-thickness (see Fig. 8.27) because gravity will allow fluid to pool near the laceration.

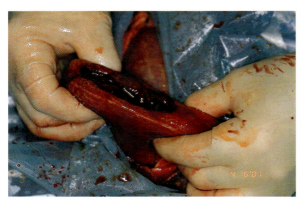

Fig. 8.27   Uterine tear caused by foal's foot.

Diagnosis

- In most cases there is a recent history of acute abdominal pain.
- There may or may not be significant hemorrhage into the abdomen from the rupture; in spite of the excellent blood supply to the gravid uterus, hemorrhage is usually very limited. If there is no (or little) hemorrhage, the fetus may remain free in the abdomen for some time before any other signs are noted. The uterus may involute and there may then be little indication of a problem until secondary signs of colic, etc. arise from adhesions of intestine to the dead fetus and membranes. Severe hemorrhage will inevitably result in shock and the mare may die before any signs are seen.
- Partial-thickness lacerations may not be diagnosed at all, or they may be diagnosed during the postpartum examination if a full vaginal/uterine examination is performed.
- Some partial-thickness and full-thickness tears will first be recognized when the uterus is lavaged routinely after foaling (especially during the first 12–24 hours). Fluid is pumped into the uterus and then cannot be retrieved as it has flowed from the uterine lumen into the abdomen. The inability to recover fluid lavaged into a mare should immediately alert the operator. No more fluid should be added to the uterus and it should be assessed carefully for a laceration. A partial-thickness tear may be turned into a full-thickness tear by distending the uterus so much that the tear increases in size and/or thickness. Some full-thickness tears can be repaired with vaginal suturing with a blind technique if they are within reach of the operator's arm.[58] However, abdominal exploration is preferred to allow for assessment of the degree of peritonitis and to determine if any other damage has occurred to the abdominal contents.
- A full-thickness tear might not result in any clinical signs; more commonly, however,

peritonitis may develop if fluid and debris leak into the abdominal cavity. Signs of peritonitis may include fever, depression, abdominal guarding, colic, diarrhea, and laminitis if septicemia or endotoxemia develop. In other cases, peritonitis will not develop unless some contamination from the uterus enters the abdomen before the rupture can heal.
- Urgent further examination of the reproductive tract is indicated in recently foaled mares that show temperature rise, increasing heart rate, increasing depression or diminished milk secretion.

Diagnosis may be confirmed by:

- Rectal palpation and transrectal ultrasound examination of the uterus.
- Transabdominal ultrasonography: the fetus may be seen on the floor of the abdomen, outside the uterine walls. Sometimes the rupture itself can be appreciated (especially when a fetal extremity is protruding through it).
- Peritoneal fluid analysis (free blood or blood-stained peritoneal fluid and/or high peritoneal fluid white cell count with prominent neutrophilia).
- Manual examination of the uterus per vaginum.
- Typically the foal is dead and no fetal heartbeat can be identified by ultrasonography or electrocardiography although some foals remain alive.[52]

Treatment

Most partial-thickness tears will heal on their own without treatment as uterine involution occurs. As the uterus decreases in size the edges of the laceration are held in close apposition allowing healing to occur by second intention. If the laceration includes the endometrium and myometrium without affecting the serosa, it may present as a partial-thickness tear, or it may ooze uterine secretions through the serosa and into the abdomen and present clinically as a full-thickness tear.

- Oxytocin is routinely administered to facilitate clearance of uterine contents and decrease uterine size. If a partial-thickness tear is diagnosed and is allowed to heal spontaneously, no uterine lavage should be performed for 60 days.
- Full-thickness tears that result in peritonitis require surgical repair and lavage of the abdomen. Treatment involves surgical repair of the laceration via ventral midline laparotomy.[59] A drainage tube may be left in the abdomen to allow lavage to be continued for a few days postoperatively.
- Affected mares should also be treated with intravenous fluids and broad-spectrum systemic antibiotics, nonsteroidal anti-inflammatory drugs (e.g. flunixin meglumine or

phenylbutazone), oxytocin (to facilitate uterine involution and evacuation of fluid from the uterus), heparin if indicated and prophylactic treatment for laminitis if it is not already clinically evident.

Prognosis

- Mares with any type of uterine laceration should not be rebred for a minimum of 60 days, and artificial insemination is the preferred method of breeding. If natural service is required and the mare is small or the stallion has a large penis, use of a breeding roll is recommended.
- The prognosis remains guarded. Although there are reports of successful breeding,[59] this depends heavily on the extent of the problem and the presence of complicating factors such as abdominal (serosal) or luminal adhesions and chronic uterine infections.

Cervical laceration

Cervical lacerations are usually associated with parturition and commonly result from the delivery of a fetus before complete cervical dilation has developed or by extracting a fetus without adequate lubrication.[60] Tears may also occur during resolution of dystocia by mutation or fetotomy. Lacerations sometimes occur spontaneously during apparently normal deliveries.

The problem is described on p. 175.

Lacerations of the caudal reproductive tract

Lacerations of the vulva and vagina are common in mares. They are usually classified according to their severity and the tissues that are involved. Although some occur in what otherwise appears to be a normal delivery, they are usually due to:

- Delivery of the foal before the caudal tract has had time to relax completely or without adequate lubrication.
- Delivery of a large foal, fetal malposture or malposition, or maiden mares with a small pelvic diameter or inadequate relaxation of the caudal tract prior to delivery.
- Failure to relieve a previously performed Caslick's vulvoplasty operation (see Fig. 8.4) prior to delivery of the foal. The force of the contractions will force the fetus through the vulvar lips resulting in tearing. This seldom occurs along the natural border of the vulvar lips, but rather in a 1 to 3 o'clock or 9 to 11 o'clock direction.

Injury to the vagina and vulva may result in hematoma formation and perineal edema. These conditions will resolve with time, although admin-

istration of nonsteroidal anti-inflammatory drugs may make the mare more comfortable until the injuries begin to resolve.

Treatment

- Some vulvar lacerations that are small and do not affect vulvar tone may be allowed to heal by second intention.
- Serious vulvar lacerations are best repaired immediately after foaling so that the mare does not develop a pneumovagina as a result of a poor vaginal seal and relaxed tissues in the vaginal and vulvar areas from foaling. Although some dehiscence occurs in severe injuries, much is salvaged due to excellent perineal blood supply assisting the healing process.
- Lacerations associated with significant vaginal hemorrhage are best repaired surgically immediately after foaling to prevent significant blood loss.
- Hemorrhage can be controlled with a tampon (made from rolled cotton and umbilical tape) that can be inserted into the vagina until the hemorrhage subsides.
- Adhesions may form across the vagina if the lacerations are severe or if there is significant inflammation in the vagina, either from manipulation during delivery or following retained placenta or metritis. These adhesions can sometimes be manually broken down, or surgically removed, although the prognosis for normal delivery in subsequent pregnancies is low if the vaginal adhesions are severe.
- Antibiotic creams containing corticosteroids applied 1–2 times daily intravaginally may significantly reduce the occurrence of adhesions.

Perineal lacerations

Perineal lacerations are a regular clinical and surgical challenge in breeding farm practice.

Primiparous mares are particularly susceptible to trauma of the perineum at foaling. This may be due to the prominence of the vestibulovaginal sphincter and possible remnants of the hymen. These anatomic features may direct the fetal foot upwards during delivery.

Alert observation by attendants at foaling may prevent serious vaginal and perineal injuries. If entrapment of the forefeet of the foal is suspected, immediate manual correction of the problem by repelling the foal cranially into the uterus and redirection of the limbs will allow normal delivery and prevent serious laceration.

Perineal lacerations typically occur during foaling as a result of fetal oversize or, more commonly, fetal malposition. The common malpresentation involved is when one or both fetal limbs are positioned over the top of the head and neck and are therefore at an abnormal angle upwards. The angle of the limbs is such that one (or both) penetrates the dorsal vaginal wall. As the mare strains, the limbs are forced dorsally to exit through the ventral perineal body and vulvar area, continue through the perineal body to exit just ventral to the anus, or continue on into the rectum to exit out of the anus. Most perineal lacerations occur in the dorsal vaginal vault. Very occasionally the foal's foot tears out the lateral vaginal wall into the caudal rectum and anal sphincter.

In all cases of perineal lacerations/injury, the mare must receive suitable immediate care to limit the damage to the tissues; her whole breeding future may depend on the measures taken immediately. A 4–6-week interval should pass before repair of perineal and rectovestibular lacerations is attempted. Edema, inflammation and necrosis of devitalized tissue are major causes of failure of the surgical repair of freshly lacerated tissues.

- Immediate care consists of administration of tetanus toxoid, systemic antimicrobials, and nonsteroidal anti-inflammatory drug therapy.
- The tissues are carefully assessed and debrided if necessary.
- Daily cleansing of the wound and application of antiseptic creams during the first week is beneficial and ensures repeated examination for developing complications.
- Most mares rid themselves of the fecal contamination of the uterus spontaneously after the defect is repaired.
- The prognosis for future fertility after successful surgical repair is good.

Perineal lacerations are classified as first-, second-, or third-degree tears according to the tissues involved and the extent of the damage.

First-degree perineal lacerations

A first-degree tear is the mildest perineal laceration and involves only the mucosa of the vestibule and the dorsal commissure of the vulva (Fig. 8.28).

Treatment

- Many first-degree perineal lacerations will heal without surgical repair, although they can be repaired either immediately after foaling or after a short delay to allow edema and inflammation to subside.
- The surgical repair is usually simple and follows the procedure for Caslick's vulvoplasty (see p. 184).

- Re-breeding may be undertaken as soon as the inflammation subsides if artificial insemination is used, but a healing period of at least 30 days should be allowed before natural service.

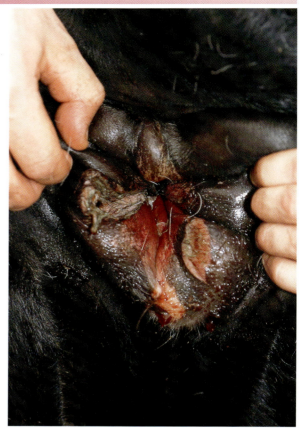

Fig. 8.28 First-degree perineal laceration. The mucosa of the vestibule and dorsal commissure are disrupted.

Second-degree perineal lacerations

These involve the mucosa and submucosa of the vestibule, the skin of the dorsal vulva and part of the perineal body musculature (Fig. 8.29). Second-degree lacerations may be of greater economic significance than third-degree lacerations because they are more inclined to be overlooked or left unrepaired and so have an insidious deleterious effect on fertility.

Failure to rebuild the perineal body will result in:

- Sinking of the anus and dorsal vagina, with resultant pneumovagina.
- Predisposition to ascending infection.

Treatment

- Some second-degree lacerations will heal on their own, although, if there is a significantly disrupted perineal body, surgical repair will re-establish more normal anatomy somewhat earlier.
- Healing in most cases does not result in reunion of the muscles and effective return of the constrictor function of the vulva. Air and feces can be aspirated into the vulva and vagina, causing chronic irritation, inflammation, and consequent infertility.

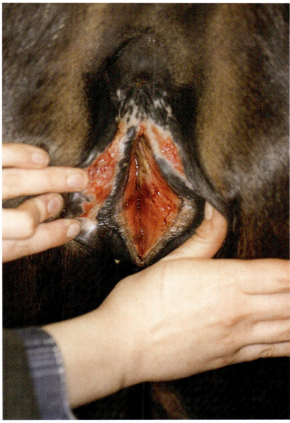

Fig. 8.29 Second-degree perineal laceration. The mucosa and submucosa of the vestibule, the skin of the dorsal vulva and part of the perineal body are disrupted.

- It is probably best to wait for inflammation to subside prior to surgical repair unless the damage is minimal and there is little inflammation and edema.
- Healing up to the stage of granulation should be allowed to occur. From this point careful repair of disrupted tissues is essential if normal fertility is to be restored.

Third-degree perineal lacerations

This is the most severe form of perineal injury and involves all layers of the vestibule, perineal body and the rectum, with disruption of the anus (Fig. 8.30).

Severe anterior tears that penetrate the peritoneal cavity can lead to rapid death as a result of massive peritoneal contamination, particularly when the extent of the damage is not recognized. Treatment at a late stage (after 4–6 hours) is invariably ineffective.

Mares with third-degree perineal tears that are presented immediately (within 4 hours of trauma) can be successfully treated by emergency reparative surgery. However, mares presented more than 6 hours post foaling carry a very poor prognosis for a complete repair as partial breakdown frequently occurs.

- If surgery cannot be undertaken immediately due to time, distance or facility constraints, the mare will require careful manual removal of feces three of four times daily until she can evacuate this for herself. Although this procedure may be effective for shallow tears, deeper injuries may require manual removal until reparative surgery can be performed.

Healing and granulation of the torn area takes between 4 and 6 weeks and surgery is usually delayed until this time so that all inflammation can subside.

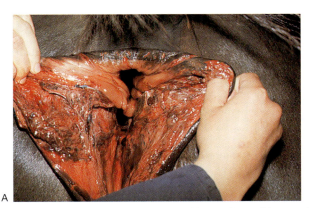

A

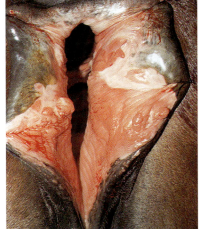

B

Fig. 8.30 (A) Third-degree perineal laceration. All layers of the vestibule, perineal body and vulva are torn, with entrance into the rectum and disruption of the anus. (B) The appearance of the healed lesion 8 weeks later.

- These injuries must be surgically repaired if the mare is to return to breeding soundness.
- Without repair, both third-degree perineal laceration and rectovaginal fistula result in persistent fecal contamination of the vagina. Inevitably this leads to a permanent state of vaginitis and endometritis, and there is little or no chance of conception while this problem remains.
- The results of surgery can be disappointing unless scrupulous care is taken. Good results are achievable in all but the most severe cases.
- In a mare with a live foal that has a severe tear it may be advisable to delay repair until weaning. However, this will probably mean loss of a whole breeding season.

Treatment

Dietary considerations

- Prolonged fasting is not recommended.

Fecal volume and consistency must be reduced. If this is not accomplished, postoperative pain leads to reluctance to defecate and causes rectal impaction, often leading to dehiscence of the suture line. A laxative diet is therefore essential.

Methods to achieve this include:

- Reduction of the concentrate bulk in the ration.
- Feeding lush green pasture grass.
- Pelleted rations.
- Danthron purges, laxatives (e.g. mineral oil and magnesium sulfate in feed or by stomach tube). Routine daily mineral oil drenches (by stomach tube) are sometimes used. Some care must be taken with the use of mineral oil as its presence in the 3–4-day postoperative period may actually cause breakdown of the suture line.
- Wet bran mashes.

A suitable preoperative dietary regimen that may be used for mares with normal hydration status:

- The grain ration is decreased from 1 week before surgery, so that the mare is receiving a 50/50 grain/wet bran mash meal 24 hours before surgery.
- Alfalfa chaff hay is added slowly to the diet so by the time of surgery the mare is receiving at least 50% alfalfa.
- A saline purgative is administered 48 and 24 hours before surgery (see Table 8.5).
- Feed should be withheld for 24 hours before surgery to reduce fecal passage during the operative and immediate postoperative period.

- Surgery should not be attempted until a satisfactorily loose fecal consistency is achieved.

Note:
- The administration by nasogastric intubation of up to 5 liters of mineral oil (liquid paraffin) 2–4 days before surgery has been used commonly but this cannot be recommended. Oil is very detrimental to the suture line and is better avoided prior to surgery and up to 4 days post surgery. It is far better to manipulate fecal consistency by other means.

Perioperative medications

- Regardless of when the procedure is to be performed, antibiotics are usually administered for 5–7 days after injury.
- Antibiotics are instigated 24 hours before surgery and maintained for at least 5 days post-operatively.
- Nonsteroidal anti-inflammatory drugs are instigated 12 hours before surgery and maintained for at least 7 days after surgery as indicated.
- Tetanus prophylaxis is mandatory.

Immediate repair

Serious perineal lacerations can sometimes be repaired immediately after foaling (i.e. within 4 hours). If immediate surgery is to be attempted there should be no inflammation or edema present; this is highly unlikely in most cases and recognition of this situation will dictate the future management of the case.

- Nonsteroidal anti-inflammatory drugs should be administered to minimize inflammation and edema if the procedure is performed immediately after the injury has occurred (within 4 hours).

Surgical procedure for the repair of perineal lacerations (4–6 weeks)

Prior to surgical repair a full breeding soundness examination (see p. 128) is recommended. This should include a uterine biopsy to ensure that the mare is likely to be adequately fertile after the surgery.

Clinical appraisal and its interpretation

- The position of the actual tear is important. Most occur dorsally between the rectum and vaginal roof (between 10 and 2 o'clock) in the perpendicular plane. Those so deviated give a 'lopsided' appearance to the area of injury.
- Simple third-degree tears have little if any serious loss of either rectal or vestibular tissue and the degree of difficulty is related more to the caudocranial length of the tear between the rectum and vagina.
- Where there is serious tissue loss such as portions of anal sphincter, vestibule, vaginal

Table 8.5 Pre- and postoperative measures that may improve the prognosis for effective repair of perineal lacerations

Measures undertaken 1–2 weeks before surgery
- The mare should be in good or improving condition
- The mare should be on green feed or high-energy soft chaff and some grain such as barley for 5–7 days prior to surgery

Measures undertaken 1 day before surgery
- Withhold feed from the mare for 18–24 hours prior to surgery
- It is helpful to administer a saline purgative drench by stomach tube 18 hours before surgery. A suitable solution is made up of:
  - ❑ 150 g magnesium sulfate (Epsom salt)
  - ❑ 150 g sodium sulfate (Glauber's salt)
  - ❑ 150 g sodium chloride (common salt)
  - ❑ 4 liters of water

Measures undertaken immediately prior to surgery
- Empty and clean the vagina
- Administer parenteral antibiotic
- Tranquilize the mare
- Bandage and 'bag' the tail
- Sterilize the perineum with surgical scrub
- Administer epidural anesthesia
- Perform surgery

Measures taken postoperatively
- Monitor mare every 3–4 hours for general clinical status
- Continue with full courses of antibiotics
- Administer analgesics (such as phenylbutazone or flunixin meglumine)
- Management of fecal consistency and avoidance of straining are vital
  - ❑ Feces are not normally passed in first 6 hours
  - ❑ Evidence of straining must be dealt with urgently
  - ❑ A light, laxative but nourishing diet, fed 3–4 times daily
  - ❑ Further saline drenches should be given sparingly.
- Remove sutures 10–14 days after surgery

and rectal wall, repair is much more problematical. Fortunately, loss of tissue is seldom so severe that repair cannot be achieved with careful technique.
- The combination of tissue loss and a tear that extends more than 10 cm cranially makes repair much more difficult.

The surgical procedure may be performed in one or two stages depending on the surgeon's preference.[37,61] There are many procedures described in surgical and obstetric texts and any of the described procedures can be used successfully to repair rectovaginal lacerations if a few basic principles are rigidly followed:

- Strong suture material that maintains its strength and tissue apposition for a minimum of 10–14 days must be used (e.g. 4 metric synthetic absorbable material or 2 metric nonabsorbable material).
- Tension on the suture line must be minimized by adequate dissection of tissues to allow for apposition without tension.
- Maximum apposition of tissues creates a thicker, stronger shelf between the rectum and vestibule after healing. It also ensures a seal between the rectum and vestibule to prevent fecal contamination and fistula formation.

- Suture placement is critical. Poorly or inappropriately placed sutures will increase the chance of wound disruption and further complication.

Restraint

Restraint in stocks is essential so that the surgeon can operate safely under good lighting conditions. The procedure should not be attempted without adequate restraint.

Sedation and anesthesia

Suitable tranquilization and epidural anesthesia are essential (the technique for epidural anesthesia in the mare is described in standard texts on anesthesia and surgery).

- Acepromazine (0.02–0.055 mg/kg intravenously) followed by xylazine (0.44–0.66 mg/kg) or romifidine (40–60 µg/kg) or detomidine (0.01–0.04 mg/kg) provides adequate sedation for standing procedures.
- If additional analgesia is needed, an opioid such as butorphanol (0.088 mg/kg) may be combined with either an α_2-agonist and/or acepromazine.

Preparation of the mare

i. The tail is wrapped.
ii. The epidural site is prepared aseptically. Successful epidural anesthesia is often the most difficult part of the surgery, especially if the epidural space has been entered previously.

- Analgesia can be achieved with 1.0–1.25 ml of a solution of 2% lidocaine per 100 kg. This will provide approximately 60 minutes of analgesia.
- Alternatively, a combination of xylazine and lidocaine may be injected into the epidural space. Anesthesia occurs in 3–5 minutes.
- Xylazine may be given alone but it may take 35–45 minutes before anesthesia is adequate.
- The benefits of xylazine epidural anesthesia include decreased motor weakness (compared with lidocaine) and prolongation of anesthesia up to 4 hours. The epidural dose for xylazine is 0.17 mg/kg, or 100 mg for a 450-kg mare, diluted either with 5 ml of lidocaine or with 10 ml of saline solution if used alone.
- When adequate epidural anesthesia cannot be obtained for rectovaginal surgery, sedation with xylazine (0.6–1.1 mg/kg) and morphine (0.6 mg/kg) can be given intravenously.
- Morphine must be administered slowly and should be given only after the full sedative effects of xylazine have developed.
- Repeated doses of xylazine may be needed 20–30 minutes after the administration of morphine because the sedative effects of xylazine wear off in 10–20 minutes and the effects of the opiate last approximately 45 minutes.
- The mucosa surrounding the affected tissue may have to be infiltrated with lidocaine.

iii. Thoroughly lavage the perineum, vaginal and rectal vault.
iv. Any excessive fluid remaining in the rectum or vagina should be sponged out.
v. The perineum is prepared for aseptic surgery.
vi. A rectal tampon made from a roll of cotton is placed in the rectum anterior to the surgery site to avoid fecal contamination of the operative field. Provided that the correct fecal consistency is present it should not be necessary to evacuate the rectum.

Surgical procedure

The fundamental initiation of the surgery is the same irrespective of the final procedure used.

i. The tail is wrapped and held to the side.
ii. Towel clamps are placed one on each side at the anal sphincter–vestibular junction and drawn outwards and backwards to tense the sides of the vestibule.

iii. An initial horizontal incision is commenced, starting at one anal sphincter–vestibular junction, cutting anteriorly, passing through the mucosa and underlying tissue forward to the rectovaginal shelf.
iv. This procedure is repeated on the other side.
v. The rectovaginal shelf is then split forward for 4–6 cm and laterally to join with the two lateral incisions.
vi. A vertical incision is made starting from the caudal end of the horizontal incision between the vulvar skin and vestibular mucosa extending downwards from the anal sphincter–vestibular junction to the original dorsal commissure of the vulva on each side.
vii. This creates two right-angled flaps which are carefully dissected from the lateral walls to form as thick a vestibular flap as possible.
viii. Sufficient lateral dissection is performed to allow the two sides of the vestibular flap to meet easily in the midline without any tension.
ix. Hemorrhage is usually insignificant if blunt dissection is used. However, it may be necessary to ligate any vessels that bleed persistently. Continued postoperative bleeding can lead to hematoma formation and failure of the reconstruction.

One-stage repair procedure

In this procedure the vagina, perineal body, and rectum are repaired at the same time. Many methods of repair are described in standard surgical texts; they vary in the timing of the phases of surgery and/or the suture pattern used:

- Six-bite suture pattern (see below) knotted on the vestibular side: dissection should create a thicker rectal flap than a vestibular flap.
- Four-bite suture pattern (see below) knotted on the rectal side: dissection should create a more substantial vestibular flap.
- Multilayer suture pattern: dissection should create flaps of sufficient thickness on both the vestibular and rectal sides to permit deep bites in the two submucosal lines.

1. Six-bite suture technique

A heavy, noncapillary, nonabsorbable synthetic suture material and a heavy Martin's uterine half-circle cutting needle are used in the six-bite vertical suture pattern for the reconstructive surgery.

i. The suture is passed through the left vestibular flap 3 cm from the edge, emerging in the dissected plane.
ii. A deep bite is taken in the left rectal flap starting 3 cm from the edge. The needle should not penetrate the rectal mucosa and should emerge from the submucosa at the edge of the flap.
iii. A deep bite is taken in the right rectal flap,

entering at the edge and emerging from the submucosa 3 cm from the edge in the dissected plane. Again, this should not penetrate the rectal mucosa.

iv. The suture is passed through the right vestibular flap 3 cm from the edge. A shallow bite is taken 0.5 cm from the edge, passing the suture from the mucosal surface of the flap back to the bisected surface.

v. The suture is passed through the left vestibular flap from the cut surface to the mucosal surface 0.5 cm from the cut edge; it is then pulled tight and knotted in the vestibule so that the rectal edges are everted.

vi. No suture should be palpable on the rectal surface. The suture is tied by hand to maintain tension in the suture, appose the rectal flaps, and invert the vestibular flaps into the vestibule.

vii. This pattern is started in the cranial pocket created in the rectovestibular septum by dissection and continued caudally to a point 4–6 cm from the cutaneous perineum.

viii. The ends are left 10 cm long to facilitate removal.

2. Four-bite suture technique

In this method, no attempt is made to suture the rectal submucosa or mucosa. Apposition of a thick vaginal flap and the clot that forms on the rectal surface seal the suture line and thus prevent leakage. As the wound heals, the rectal mucosa heals over the granulating bed.

i. Suturing is begun with a continuous horizontal mattress pattern of 4 metric polyglactin in the edge of the vestibular mucosa for 4–5 cm (or continue to caudal edge of flap).

ii. A purse-string suture of 5 metric polyglactin is placed in the space created by splitting the intact cranial shelf between the rectum and vestibulum.

iii. The pocket that tends to form at the beginning of the suture line is obliterated with two to three or more of these sutures placed 1 cm apart.
   - If this pocket is not obliterated, feces accumulate at this point and can lead to fistula formation.

iv. When the caudal margin of the surgical split in the intact rectovestibular septum is reached and apposition of the surgically created shelves is begun, a four-bite (modified Lembert) pattern is used.
   - A deep bite is placed in the perivestibular tissue of the thick vestibular flap on the right.
   - A shallow bite is placed in the vestibular submucosa on the right, and another shallow bite is placed in the vestibular submucosa on the left.
   - A deep bite is placed in the heavy connective tissue of the left vestibular flap.

- Tightening this suture causes the vestibular tissues to invert and the rectal mucosa to come into closer apposition.

v. When reconstruction reaches the end of the continuous horizontal pattern initially placed in the edge of the vestibular mucosa, this continuous suture pattern is continued caudally for another 5 cm.

vi. The main four-bite suture pattern can then be continued caudally also.

vii. These two suture lines are continued alternately to the cutaneous perineum.

3. Rectal 'pull-back' technique

This technique carries a high rate of success and is strongly recommended. It has the advantage of moving the intact rectal shelf as far caudally as possible; this reduces the likelihood of pocketing of feces in a less-accessible anterior position. Furthermore, the healing process is more rapid and more effective.

i. Suturing is begun with a continuous horizontal mattress pattern of 4 metric polyglactin in the edge of the vestibular mucosa to the caudal edge of the flap.

ii. Four long Allis tissue forceps are then placed in the rectal submucosa along the caudal margin of the dissected rectal shelf. Note that the dissection should be adequate to allow the rectal floor to be pulled caudally towards the level of the anal sphincter.

iii. The rectovestibular septum is reconstructed by placing 5 metric polyglactin in an interrupted purse-string pattern, starting at the most cranial aspect of the dissection and continuing caudally.
   - The tissue incorporated in each suture includes (in order): right perivestibular tissue, right vestibular submucosa, right rectal submucosa, left rectal submucosa, left vestibular submucosa, left perivestibular tissue.
   - With each suture, the rectal floor is retracted further caudally before the rectal submucosal bites are placed.
   - The suture does not penetrate the rectal or vestibular mucosa.

iv. The purse-string pattern is continued caudally until the caudal edge of the rectal shelf is reached.

v. A continuous horizontal mattress pattern is then placed in the edges of the vestibular flaps using 5 metric polyglactin.
   - This pattern inverts the edges of the vestibular flaps into the vestibule and is continued to the point at which the purse-string pattern ended.
   - It is then tied and the remainder of the suture is left in the vestibule until needed again.
   - In this manner, the two suture patterns are alternated to the point at which the

perineal body reconstruction (phase 2) is started.

vi. Occasionally, the intact rectal floor cannot be pulled caudally to the anal sphincter. If this occurs the purse-string pattern is continued past the caudal edge of the intact rectal floor, creating a floor by apposing the submucosa of the remaining left and right rectal flaps. The purse-string sutures are placed from the rectal edge and tied with long ends protruding out through the final repaired anal sphincter.

vii. The perineal body is then reconstructed.

- Surgical repair of the perineal body and anal sphincter resembles reconstruction of the perineal body after second-degree laceration and is completed immediately or at least 2–3 weeks after completion of phase 1.

> Note:
> - Careful closure is essential to prevent the repaired sphincter being too tight as it will greatly impede passage of even soft feces and so be a further cause of constipation and straining.

- Two triangular areas of mucosa and skin overlying the muscle of the perineal body and anal sphincter are dissected from the level of the external anal sphincter ventrally to the level of the dorsal commissure.
- The rectal and vestibular mucosae are apposed at the margin with simple interrupted sutures of 3 or 4 metric nylon or polypropylene.
- The freshened surfaces between the margins are apposed with simple interrupted sutures of 2 or 3 metric polyglactin or polypropylene.

Two-stage repair

Here, the vagina and perineal body are repaired and allowed to heal, then a second surgery is performed to repair the defect in the rectum.

Rectovaginal fistulas can be repaired in situ by performing a perineal body transection, or the fistula can be converted into a third-degree laceration and then repaired as such.

Postoperative care

Once surgical repair has been performed, 10 days of recovery time should be allowed prior to assessment of the surgery site.

- Postoperative examinations must be approached cautiously if breakdown of the surgery site is to be avoided.
- Antibiotics are usually administered continuously during the repair stages.

- The mare should be monitored at least every 3–4 hours.
- Feces are not normally passed in the first 6 hours postoperatively.
- Any sign of straining to pass feces must be dealt with urgently as straining is almost certain to disrupt the repair. It is vital, therefore, that the mare's feces are softened and maintained in a laxative state postoperatively so that the sutures are not torn out when the mare strains to defecate. This can be achieved through the use of:
  - ❑ Laxative administered by nasogastric tube (e.g. magnesium or sodium sulfate); further saline drenches should be given sparingly in response to fecal consistency.
  - ❑ Lubricants (mineral oils should not be used before the fourth postoperative day).
  - ❑ Feeding a complete pelleted ration, or allowing the mare a diet of lush grass pasture only.
  - ❑ Reduced soft feed three to four times daily; hay and other such roughage is not recommended.
  - ❑ Gentle rectal lavage with warm water administered through a small-gauge, soft rubber tube if fecal consistency becomes firmer. This technique is particularly useful in the early postoperative stages when the mare may be reluctant to pass feces because of the discomfort; any delays result in a drier fecal consistency and so progressive difficulty with defecation and increased straining.

> - Insert a 10-mm diameter hosepipe against the dorsal rectal wall and allow water to flow gently to soften the feces as the tube is inserted. This procedure will have to be carried out as aften as necessary to stop accumulation of feces and the instigation of straining, because straining with impacted fecal balls is more dangerous to the suture line.
> - This procedure may be necesary for up to 6–7 days after surgery.

- The exposed nonabsorbable sutures should be removed on the tenth day post surgery.
- A uterine culture and cytology should be performed to determine if uterine therapy is also required.
- The mare can be rebred by artificial insemination 2–3 weeks after surgery or 3 months postoperatively if natural service is used.

Complications

1. Total wound breakdown.
   - The procedure should be re-attempted after controlling infection and allowing a suitable healing period.
   - The prognosis will inevitably be worse for cases that have recurrent breakdowns.

- The most common causes of breakdown or failure are:
  - ❑ Insufficient thickness in the flaps.
  - ❑ Tension along the flap suture line.
  - ❑ Insufficient time interval from the original injury.
2. Fistula formation.
   - The perineal skin and most caudal part of the repair are healed but the suture line disruption occurs more anteriorly.
   - This can be retreated as for a rectovaginal fistula, but only where fistulated tissue is thick enough to be repaired in this way.
   - Reconstruction by third-degree repair allows for better and thicker flap reconstruction.
3. Infection/contamination.
   - This is almost inevitable to some degree, but scrupulous attention to surgical detail minimizes its significance.
4. Urine pooling.
   - This is difficult to treat and may require surgical attention to the urethral orifice.
5. Constipation.
   - This is a common sequela and MUST be prevented as far as possible for a successful outcome.
     - ❑ Straining almost inevitably causes dehiscence of the surgical site at any stage up to 2–3 weeks postoperatively.
     - ❑ Careful attention to fecal consistency throughout the postoperative period will improve the prognosis.

Surgical repair of rectovaginal fistulae

This is a clinical condition that exists when a communication opening is found between the rectal and the vaginal cavities with an intact anus and perineal skin (Fig. 8.31). The condition is usually caused by:

- Foaling accidents. These occur when the foal's foot leaves the vagina dorsally and penetrates the rectum, but is then retracted or repelled back into the vagina prior to delivery; the remainder of the perineal structures remain intact. This injury leaves the anal sphincter intact. A rectovestibular fistula has the same extent of rectal and vaginal damage but the anal sphincter is not damaged; the perineum may appear normal.
- Poor healing or repair of third-degree perineal tears.

Several methods have been described for repairing rectovaginal fistulae.

Method 1

Fistula repair by surgical excision of the anal sphincter and the perineal body, and repair of the resulting third-degree laceration by one of the methods described above.

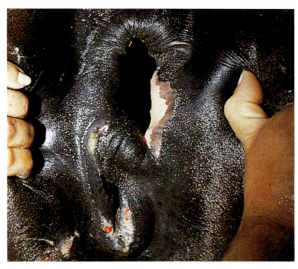

Fig. 8.31 Rectovaginal fistula. All layers of the vestibule, perineal body and the rectum are disrupted, leaving the vulva and anus intact.

- Repair of a fistula by this method is not recommended for novice surgeons.
- It allows the reconstruction of a stronger shelf than any other method
- The other advantage is good exposure for repair.

A major disadvantage initially is loss of support for the repaired tissue provided by the perineum and perineal body. This can be overcome by careful reconstruction of the perineal body either with the first repair, or at a stage 2 some 2–3 weeks after the initial repair.

Method 2

1. Fistula repair by splitting the perineum transversely so that the anal sphincter and perineal bodies are preserved

   i. The perineum is incised in the frontal plane and then bisected transversely so that the anus and rectum are separated from the vulva and vestibule. This dissection is continued cranially to the fistula and 3–5 cm beyond.
   ii. When the dissection is complete, two holes can be viewed in the dissected plane, communicating dorsally with the rectum and ventrally with the vagina.
   iii. These two fistulae are then closed using a modified Lembert pattern of 3 or 4 metric polyglactin or polypropylene.
   iv. This suture pattern is continued, placing the sutures 1 cm apart. This progressively apposes the submucosal tissues and everts the margin of the rectal fistula into the lumen of the rectum until the rectal fistula is closed.

2. Alternative repair

Because the peristaltic stress on the rectum is at right-angles to the long axis of the bowel, sutures placed parallel to the long axis (i.e. suturing the fistula in a transverse rather than a craniocaudal direction) have less stress on them and less tendency to fail.

i. The rectal repair is closed in a transverse manner using sutures oriented craniocaudally. This can be very difficult, however, given the limited exposure provided by the perineal dissection.

ii. Closing the rectal fistula with sutures oriented perpendicular to the long axis of the bowel can be successful despite the stress placed on them by rectal peristalsis if the sutures are close together and adequate bites in the connective tissue of the submucosa are taken. Suturing in this manner is much easier. In either method of suturing, the sutures should be placed approximately 1 cm apart.

iii. The vaginal fistula is closed next. The suture is passed into the vaginal submucosa 2 cm from the margin of the fistula, emerging near the margin of the fistula on the left. The suture is placed near the margin of the vaginal fistula on the right, emerging 2 cm from the fistula laterally. When the suture is tied, the vaginal submucosa is apposed and the fistula margin is inverted into the vagina.

iv. The dissection dead space between the two repairs is closed with simple interrupted sutures of no. 0 gut or polypropylene.

v. The skin of the perineum is then closed with nonabsorbable suture using a vertical mattress or simple interrupted pattern.

> **Note:**
> - Alternatively, if the rectovaginal septum is thin, the dead space created by dissection can be packed with gauze. In this case, the perineal skin is loosely sutured to hold the packing in place while the defect fills with granulation tissue. A thicker septum is obtained by healing the dissection in this manner. This technique, however, requires daily repacking and cleaning of the perineum until healing is complete.

Method 3

Fistula repair is by the transrectal approach.

> **Note:**
> - Methods 3 and 4 can only work as well as the exposure achieved to effect the repair.
> - Removal of some tissue allows nonmucosal surface contact when sutured.

> - All sutures must be securely, evenly and accurately placed for successful results to be achieved.

i. For the procedure to be successful, the anal sphincter must be sufficiently relaxed after epidural anesthesia to permit full dilation with either a Balfour retractor with 8.75- or 13.25-cm jaws or a modified Finochietto retractor.

ii. The fistula is dissected around its circumference for 4–8 cm and is then closed in three layers.

iii. The vestibular shelf is closed first with a continuous horizontal mattress pattern using 3.5 metric absorbable suture such that the edges of the vestibular flaps are inverted into the vestibule. This can be performed either through the rectum or through the vagina.

iv. The submucosa may be closed with a continuous four-bite suture pattern if the fistula is small, or with interrupted sutures placed either transversely or perpendicularly to the long axis of the bowel.

v. The rectal shelf is closed with 3.0 metric absorbable suture in a continuous horizontal mattress pattern.

Method 4

This method uses the transvaginal approach.

i. The vestibulum is dilated with Balfour retractors.

ii. The Balfour spoon is then placed in the dorsum of the vestibulum to lift the dorsal vestibular wall dorsally and cranially. This orients the fistula vertically, making it easier to dissect and suture.

iii. A stay suture of heavy nonabsorbable material may also be placed in the dorsal vaginal wall cranial to the fistula. Tension on this suture will increase vertical orientation.

iv. The fistula is dissected as described for the transrectal approach.

v. The fistula may be closed using either two or three layers of suture.

vi. If a three-layer closure is used, the rectal mucosa is closed first with a continuous horizontal mattress pattern.

vii. The submucosa is preferably closed with longitudinally placed sutures in an interrupted Lembert pattern using 5.5 metric absorbable suture material. This technique may be difficult, depending on exposure and the width of the mare's vestibulum.

viii. The submucosa may also be closed using either a continuous purse-string suture pattern if the fistula is small or with interrupted sutures placed perpendicular to the long axis

ix. The vestibular mucosa is closed with a continuous horizontal mattress pattern using 3 metric absorbable suture.

x. If nonabsorbable suture material has been used and the suture ends have been left exposed, sutures should be removed in 14 days.

- Continuation of the laxative diet is essential for 14 days after repair of a rectovaginal laceration or fistula.
- See above for methods that can be used to maintain soft fecal consistency.
- Natural breeding should be delayed for 2 months, but artificial insemination can be undertaken 3–4 weeks postoperatively.

Vaginal bleeding

Vaginal bleeding during pregnancy is seldom due to placental or uterine problems. Blood accumulating at the vulvar lips in a pregnant mare is more often due to varicosity of vaginal blood vessels or from vulvar trauma.

Vaginal varicosity usually occurs in the dorsal vaginal wall just cranial to the urethral opening. This is common in the vagina of older mares during pregnancy and sometimes during estrus. Once varicosity occurs it remains a problem, with intermittent slight hemorrhage during pregnancy. Increasing incidence or severity should be viewed seriously and may require surgical intervention after parturition.

Diagnosis

- It is important to eliminate urinary tract bleeding whenever postparturient hemorrhage is present.
- Observation of urination and a careful rectal, ultrasonographic and endoscopic examination will help to eliminate urinary tract bleeding as a cause of the hemorrhage.
- Examination of the vestibule, vagina and cervix with an illuminated vaginal speculum will usually locate the source of the problem.

Treatment

- No treatment is warranted if the extent of bleeding is insignificant.
- If more severe hemorrhage occurs or there is a recurring problem, laser or diathermy can be used to cauterize the region, or a small volume of 5% formalin can be injected into the varicosity under endoscopic guidance.

Retained placenta

This is probably the most common complication in the postpartum mare,[25,62] occurring in around 2–10% of all deliveries.[63] Normal placental release occurs within 3 hours of birth, but many wild mares retain the placenta for up to 24–48 hours without any difficulty or immediate or future complications.[41]

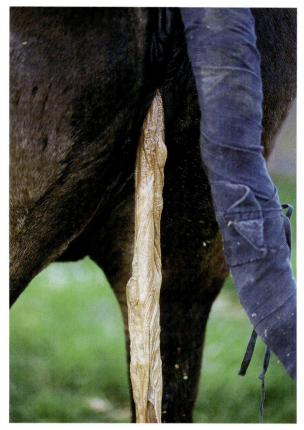

Fig. 8.32 Retained placenta.

However, many mares that retain the placenta for much less time in domesticated conditions have serious difficulties within 4–8 hours after foaling.

Retained placenta (Fig. 8.32) probably arises as a result of any factor that alters or interferes with uterine motility, but it can arise without any obvious cause in a delivery that is otherwise normal. Although it is likely that it has a multifactorial etiology, factors that have been suggested include:

- Uterine inertia and fatigue. Uterine inertia may be caused by hypocalcemia, hydropic conditions, twin pregnancy, inadequate exercise prepartum, and following dystocia or general anesthesia.
- Calcium/phosphorus imbalance.
- Selenium deficiency.
- Induced delivery.
- Dystocia (particularly cases requiring extensive mutation or fetotomy).[64]
- Cesarean section.

Other potential factors that have been incriminated include abnormal hormonal environment, physical mechanical intervention, and placentitis. Abnormalities in oxytocin release may result in retained placenta, although the reason for this is not known.

There is a higher incidence in:

- Draft mares.
- Fescue toxicosis.
- Cesarean section.
- Older, multiparous mares.
- Mares that have had retained placenta previously; they are more likely to suffer from this condition during subsequent pregnancies if an identifiable cause cannot be defined and treated. Injection of vitamin E 2 weeks prior to foaling is advised for mares with a history of repeat retained placenta.

Retained placenta is quite common following extensive obstetric manipulations such as fetotomy or prolonged mutation. There is considerable debate over what constitutes a 'retained' placenta.

- Placental delivery (stage 3 of labor) occurs because umbilical rupture arrests umbilical blood flow; this results in collapse of the fetal placental blood vessels.[65–67]
- Separation of the chorionic villi from the endometrial crypts results from simultaneous shrinking of the blood-deprived chorionic villi and relaxation of the opposing maternal crypts.
- Continued uterine contractions move from the tips of the horns towards the cervix resulting in the allantochorion being everted and it is finally passed 'inside-out' through the cervix.
- The weight of the placenta passing through the cervix adds to the pressure on the crypts and facilitates the continued expulsion of the fetal membranes.
- Retention more commonly involves the tips of the horns than other sites.
- Most reports suggest that the placenta in the nongravid horn is more often retained than the edematous one in the gravid horn.

Complications

Complications from placental retention are probably more common in large, heavy mares than in the lighter breeds and ponies. Most of the serious complications are attributable to a combination of bacterial replication in the uterus (both during the retained placenta episode and in the period immediately following during uterine involution) and autolysing enzymes released from the decaying membranes.

- *Streptococcus zooepidemicus* and *Escherichia coli* infections are most often implicated.
- Bacteria and endotoxin may be absorbed into the bloodstream resulting in bacteremia, septicemia, and endotoxemia.
- Uterine involution is inevitably delayed in mares that have significant placental retention.[68]

Common complications of retained placenta include:

- Metritis/endometritis.
- Septicemia.
- Endotoxemia.
- Laminitis (founder/laminar destruction with pedal bone sinking or rotation). Laminitis is more common in draft mares and in mares that develop fulminating metritis.
- Uterine prolapse. This can arise spontaneously (possibly from straining or uterine horn inversion) or if excessive tension is applied to the placenta in an attempt to remove it.

Diagnosis

In most circumstances the mare is considered to have a retained placenta if it remains attached for more than 3 hours post partum. However, a defined temporal approach to retention of fetal membranes is potentially misleading in the horse. Many mares retain the placenta for much longer without any harmful effect while others are seriously (dangerously) affected within much shorter periods.

- Usually the placenta is noted hanging from the vulvar lips. The amnion is often hanging outside while the allantochorion remains internally.
- Usually the mare displays little or no signs of abdominal discomfort (which is typical of normal placental passage).

Treatment

If the placenta is hanging below the hocks it should be tied up to prevent the mare from stepping on it and to prevent her from kicking at the placenta and injuring the foal by mistake.

- The hanging portion of the placenta should not be cut off and weights should not be tied to it.

Treatment is aimed at hastening the release of the placenta and the prevention of secondary conditions, any of which could be life-threatening within a few hours.[1,69,70]

In the early stages (first 24 hours):

i. Oxytocin (20–40 IU) is administered as a slow intravenous drip, or as an intramuscular bolus, or in multiple repeated intravenous or intramuscular injections.
ii. Oxytocin may be administered every 2 hours if given as a bolus. Intravenous bolus doses do, however, have less chance of success and may cause colic (this can be controlled with mild analgesics) and spasmodic contraction rather than a sustained milder involution. These signs are less significant if intramuscular bolus doses are used.
iii. If oxytocin therapy fails to release the placenta, uterine lavage, using large volumes of saline

solution, mild antiseptic solutions or even water are utilized.[71] Some practitioners fill the allantochorion with fluid in an attempt to stretch the uterus and placenta and facilitate detachment of the microvilli.

- A small amount of gentle traction in a twisting motion is acceptable if the placenta releases easily with this technique.
- The placenta should not, however, be manually forcibly removed as this may result in hemorrhage, uptake of endotoxin and bacteria from the uterus or fibrosis of the endometrium.[72] Permanent endometrial damage has been reported following manual removal.[62]
- Aggressive manual removal may result in invagination of the uterine horn.
- Additionally, aggressive manual removal may result in villi breaking off in the crypts or a small portion of the placenta remaining in the uterus. These retained villi or placental remnants may be a nidus for serious (and often life-threatening) infection.
- Separation of the placenta from the endometrium by placing the hand between the two structures and gently encouraging separation is an old method that has a high rate of complication and is not recommended in any situation.

Supportive care should be provided to the mare until the placenta is recovered and any resulting metritis is resolved. This may include any (or all) of the following:

- Antibiotics.
  - ❏ Broad-spectrum drugs are indicated because infections are usually mixed.
  - ❏ Gram-negative organisms are possibly the most serious and should be addressed specifically.
  - ❏ Anaerobic organisms are sometimes a serious problem and metronidazole or penicillin can be effective.
- Intravenous fluids if the mare becomes dehydrated or endotoxemic.
  - ❏ Fluids help to counter the effects of endotoxemia and reduce the chances of shock.
  - ❏ Maintenance of renal function is important in the excretion of endotoxin.
- Nonsteroidal anti-inflammatory drugs (particularly flunixin meglumine).
  - ❏ These are routinely used both for their anti-inflammatory effects and for the anti-endotoxic effects.
  - ❏ Affected horses are, however, seldom in any significant pain with this disorder.

- Sole supports to control or prevent pedal bone rotation, sinking (founder) and laminitis.
  - ❏ Laminitis is a particularly common consequence of retained fetal membranes and large breeds are more susceptible.
  - ❏ Support for the feet is probably essential.
  - ❏ Drugs to control laminitis: flunixin meglumine; acepromazine; nitroglycerine treatment (to improve digital circulation).
- Heparin therapy.
- Tetanus prophylaxis.
  - ❏ Vaccination (booster) in vaccinated mares.
  - ❏ Hyperimmune antiserum in unvaccinated mares.

Occasionally, the amnion tears away from the umbilicus and leaves the allantochorion inside the uterus with the remaining umbilical stalk. In these cases, there is no weight on the placenta from the exterior to facilitate release of the microvilli. If possible, a small, damp towel can be tied to the umbilical stalk or chorioallantoic body, using umbilical tape. This is then allowed to hang outside the vulvar lips. Care should be taken not to use too large (or wet) a towel such that excessive weight or pressure is applied to the retained placenta. It is also imperative that the material used to tie the towel to the placenta is not irritating to the vagina/vestibule/vulvar labia, or serious adhesions may result.

The placenta must be examined carefully following its retrieval to be sure it has released in its entirety. The standard method of examination is followed (see p. 328).

- If a missing piece is identified, immediate measures must be taken to retrieve it.
- Uterine lavage (using antibiotic-based solutions) and or video uteroscopy can be used.
- The uterus should be completely distended with fluid (saline or water) after placental passage to ensure that invagination of either horn has not occurred. If eversion has occurred and involution is allowed to progress, either necrosis of the tip of the horn or adhesions of the tip of the horn to the more distal uterus may result. If necrosis occurs, peritonitis and subsequent death of the mare is possible.
- The mare's uterus should be lavaged once to twice daily following placental expulsion to facilitate clearance of bacteria, endotoxin and debris/fluid from the uterus. Lavage should be continued until no further purulent or mucoid material is effluxed from the uterus.

Follow-up examination of the uterus including culture and cytology should be performed 25 days after foaling, even if the mare is apparently normal. If antibiotic therapy is indicated based on culture and cytology, it should be performed with vigor.

- The mare should not be bred prior to the second natural postfoaling cycle.

Prognosis

- Early intervention appears to be the most important aspect of therapy.
- Neglected and advanced cases carry a poor prognosis.

There is no difference in fertility between normal mares and appropriately treated mares with retained placenta, although mares that do not receive antibiotic therapy as part of the management have a poorer future fertility.[66]

Septic metritis

Acute (septic) metritis is a postpartum condition occurring within the first 10 days after parturition,[25] in which there is significant inflammation of the uterus and myometrium, making absorption of bacteria and their associated toxins into the systemic circulation more likely.

- The most common causative agents are *Escherichia coli* or other Gram-negative bacteria.
- Septic metritis is a very serious condition and is more common in large heavy mares than in light horse mares or ponies.
- It is a possible complication of dystocia involving extensive interference with the reproductive tract during foaling and is a frequent complication of a retained placenta or a retained tags/portions of placenta.
- When it is the result of (or associated with) retained placenta, the progression of the systemic consequences can be alarming and should always be treated as an emergency.

Diagnosis

- The onset can be very acute with a rapid and progressive deterioration in the physical and metabolic status of the mare.
- Affected mares are often systemically ill, showing:
  - ❑ Depression.
  - ❑ Fever.
  - ❑ Diarrhea.
  - ❑ Laminitis.
- Most commonly, a brownish-red, fetid vaginal discharge will be noted.
- Rectal palpation will reveal an enlarged, doughy and thickened uterus.
- Ultrasound examination will reveal fluid in the uterus that is echodense in nature. The endometrial folds are usually quite prominent. A portion of (or even the entire) placental membrane may be identifiable.

Complications

- Bacteremia.
- Septicemia.
- Endotoxemia.
- Laminitis.

Treatment

Septic metritis can be a life-threatening disease for the mare if it is not treated appropriately and aggressively. Timely and appropriate treatment will usually result in salvage of the reproductive potential of the mare. Although in theory bacterial swabs and culture/sensitivity should be established, treatment cannot wait for these results. The treatment is in any case rather basic and only demanding of time and effort.

Uterine lavage is the mainstay of treatment. It removes gross bacterial contamination (and so prevents or limits bacteremia) and flushes out residual endotoxin (thereby reducing the severity of endotoxemia).

i. One to three liters of warm sterile saline (possibly with broad-spectrum antibiotics/antiseptics) should be introduced into the uterus via a soft tube and siphoned off immediately (see p. 200, Fig. 5.70).

- If retained fetal membranes are present this flushing process can be difficult. The membranes tend to enter the flushing catheter, preventing efflux of fluid, and must be constantly moved off the end of the catheter whenever they become entrapped.

ii. The procedure is repeated several times and finally an antibiotic solution effective against Gram-negative organisms (such as *Escherichia coli*) should be infused into the uterus.

iii. The whole procedure is repeated every few hours, until all evidence of pus and placental debris is removed and the uterine exudate has cleared. This can be a very demanding procedure but without it the prognosis is much reduced.

Further treatment includes supportive care until the uterine infection is controlled:

- Timely administration of appropriate broad-spectrum systemic antibiotics (see p. 199).
- Oxytocin (see p. 201).
- Nonsteroidal anti-inflammatory drugs (flunixin meglumine is particularly helpful).
- Intravenous fluids if the mare is dehydrated or becomes endotoxemic
- Tetanus prophylaxis in unvaccinated mares.
- Affected mares are usually best managed in a veterinary hospital.
- Prophylactic or aggressive treatment of laminitis.

Prognosis

- The prognosis is heavily dependent on the speed of diagnosis and the intensity of treatment.
- Despite considerable effort some mares still die from this disorder, as result of endotoxemia or irreversible extreme, secondary laminitis.

Puerperal tetanus

Puerperal tetanus is a potentially very dangerous disorder that should not occur in properly vaccinated mares. If vaccination is not performed satisfactorily, tetanus may occur following either retained placenta and/or septic metritis. It is important to remember that, if the mare is unvaccinated, the foal will have no tetanus cover and this must be addressed also.

Diagnosis

Signs of tetanus include:

- A stiff, stilted gait often accompanied by tail elevation and a worried hyperalert facial expression.
- Hyperexcitability and hyper-responsiveness to noise.
- Flashing of the third eyelid in response to noise or facial stimulation, or continuous protrusion of the third eyelid.

Treatment

There are three basic objectives for treatment:

1. Eliminate the source of the toxin. Since the nidus of infection is the uterus in this case, uterine lavage is performed to remove the causative agent and is essential. Treatment is the same as for retained placenta and/or septic metritis (see p. 199). However, the choice of antibiotics may be different. High doses of intravenous or intramuscular penicillin are essential to ensure that the bacterium (*Clostridium tetani*) is eliminated.
2. Control the toxin already within the circulation (and the nervous system). Tetanus antitoxin and if necessary a toxoid vaccine may be administered. It is probably not possible to affect the toxin that is already bound within the central nervous system and so a single large dose (50,000–75,000 IU) administered intravenously, possibly repeated after 72 hours, should be sufficient if the toxin production is eliminated. Alternatively, where suitable surgical facilities exist, intrathecal injection of tetanus antiserum may help. Withdrawal of a volume of cerebrospinal fluid and replacement with hyperimmune tetanus antiserum carries a somewhat better speed of effect.
3. Control the consequences of the toxin. The toxins block the inhibitory mechanisms for upper motor neurons. Sedation with acepromazine is a standard approach, but more potent agents such as guaicolglyceryl ether can be used also.
   - Avoidance of any unnecessary stimuli (noise, light, etc.) will reduce the exhaustion of the muscles. The mare should be housed in a dark, quiet environment.
   - The specific circumstances will dictate the care of the foal: the mare may be more upset if the foal is removed but the foal may be in danger of starvation or trauma if it is left with the mare. It is usual to pen the foal in a protected area and supplementary feed it during the early stages of treatment.
   - High levels of nursing care are always required. Intravenous fluids and even total parenteral nutrition may be needed.

Further information on the treatment of tetanus is included in standard medical texts.

Prognosis

- Those mares that continue to eat and drink and remain standing have a much better prognosis than those that cannot eat or drink. Recumbency is a very poor prognostic sign.
- Full recovery may take over 4 weeks.

Uterine prolapse and eversion of the uterine horn

Uterine prolapse is an uncommon occurrence in the mare.[25] Identified circumstances that predispose to uterine prolapse include:

- Fetal extraction prior to complete relaxation of the reproductive tract.
- Too forceful an extraction.
- Too fast an extraction (especially if the foal is large).
- Prolonged/difficult dystocia or mare exhausted from foaling.
- Conditions in which the mare is straining after delivery, such as:
  - ❏ Retained placenta.
  - ❏ Vaginal or vulvar lacerations.
  - ❏ Uterine lacerations or rupture.
  - ❏ Rupture of mesorectum.
  - ❏ Abortion in mid- to late gestation.
  - ❏ Old mares in poor body condition.

Diagnosis

- Total uterine prolapse is obvious (Fig. 8.33).
  - ❏ The placenta may still be attached to the prolapsed, everted uterus. Initially, the mare may prolapse down to above the level of the hock.
  - ❏ This is usually unrelated to internal tearing of the broad ligament or ovarian ligament, and usually there is no resultant hemorrhage.
- Where a greater part of the uterus has prolapsed, there is the potential of serious tearing and significant (often life-threatening) internal hemorrhage.
- Mares with uterine prolapse will often rapidly develop signs of shock as a result of ischemia and necrosis with endotoxemia.
- The prolapsed uterus has a diminished blood

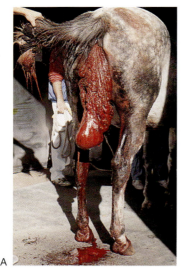

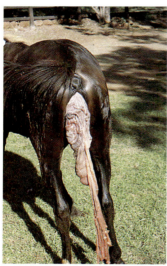

Fig. 8.33 (A) Prolapsed uterus, following prolonged dystocia. (B) Partial uterine prolapse, with retained fetal membranes still attached.

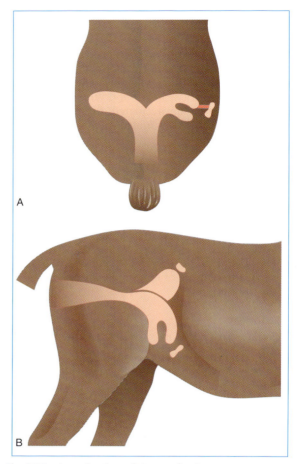

Fig. 8.34 Invagination of the uterine horn. Inappropriate use of traction or a fast delivery may result in invagination of the tip of the gravid horn. Also, attempts to remove the placenta manually may result in invagination of either horn.

supply and becomes friable very quickly; it is easily traumatized, especially if the mare is recumbent.
- Rupture of the ovarian arteries and rapid death can occur in a standing distressed mare.
- The tip of a uterine horn may become invaginated (Fig. 8.34) without subsequent prolapse. This state may be noted during routine postpartum examination, or at the first examination prior to re-breeding.
  - ❏ In the postpartum mare, colic that is usually nonresponsive to analgesics and sedatives is a common presenting sign.
  - ❏ As the horn invaginates further, traction on the ovary increases the degree of pain.

Treatment
- All cases require immediate attention.
- Restrain the mare and keep her quiet if possible until help arrives.
- Tranquilizers, especially those that lower blood pressure, should be avoided as they may cause the mare to collapse, with the subsequent possibility of more severe injury to the uterus. Nevertheless, there may be circumstances when some sedation is essential.
- The mare should be kept quiet and standing if possible; sedation with an α_2-agonist such as romifidine or detomidine is helpful. The uterus should be elevated (possibly on a tray) to the level of the vulva to decrease the gravitational effects on the uterus and thereby improve the blood flow to and from the prolapsed organ. This procedure is physically demanding and may require at least two assistants.
- Replacement of the uterus is performed under epidural anesthesia using a combination of 2%

lignocaine hydrochloride (or mepivicaine) and xylazine to provide longer-term pain control during both the replacement procedure and the immediate post replacement period.

- The uterus should be cleaned and carefully examined to identify any lacerations or serious damage. It should then be carefully cleaned with warm water followed by copious irrigation with normal saline. Application of an obstetric lubricant may help to protect it during reduction.
- If hemorrhage continues, the uterus can be bandaged with sheeting to maintain pressure on the bleeding area.
- If the uterus is very friable, it can be helpful to place it in a plastic bag before making any attempt to replace it. This decreases the chances of tearing the uterus while it is replaced.
- Removal of the placenta may be attempted if it is significantly detached already, but, if hemorrhage begins increases, no further traction should be applied and the procedure abandoned.
- Lacerations should be repaired using sterile surgical instruments and absorbable suture materials, before the uterus is replaced.
- A logical treatment progression should be followed. Initially the vaginal prolapse is replaced (reduced), followed by the cervix; finally, the uterus is replaced through the cervix.
- Cupped hands and gentle pressure should be used when manipulating the uterus back into position so that punctures or lacerations to the friable tissue are not caused by the fingertips.
- Once the uterus is returned to its abdominal position, the tips of the uterine horns should be assessed to ensure that they are completely reduced. If the arm of the operator is not long enough to reach to the end of the affected horn, filling the uterus with water or saline will help to evert the tips of the horns completely.

> - Failure to return the tips of the horn to a normal position may result in re-prolapse of the uterus or the tip remaining inverted as the uterus involutes, with subsequent occlusion of one oviduct and a decrease in total uterine volume and possibly subsequent necrosis of the invaginated tip or adhesion to the remaining uterine horn.

- Low doses of oxytocin are used to facilitate rapid uterine involution after reduction is complete.
- Systemic antimicrobials are essential. It is common practice to instill an antibiotic solution into the uterine lumen to prevent the development of metritis. (The treatment of metritis has been discussed previously.)

- Nonsteroidal anti-inflammatory drugs (such as phenylbutazone and particularly flunixin meglumine) serve to counteract endotoxemia and help prevent the onset of laminitis.
- If the placenta is retained after replacement of the uterus, treatment is as described in the previous section.
- A properly repositioned uterus usually remains in situ. Recurrence is usually indicative of failure to effect full reduction or straining for some other reason.
- Reduction of the uterus is much easier if the mare is standing with her hindquarters elevated (30 cm) by a bank or in a loading race.

Invagination of the tip of a uterine horn is not usually an emergency.

- In the early stages, the invaginated uterine horn may be replaced by distending the uterus with water or preferably saline. If myometrial spasm has already occurred, then firm manual pressure in a sustained manner will usually result in resolution. It is important to remember the dangers of aggressive uterine manipulations and experience is usually required to effect this procedure without serious mishap.
- Sedation and analgesia may facilitate the replacement and, in cases where this is inadequate, general anesthesia may be required.
- In chronic cases the uterine horn may fibrose, or scar, in this position. Surgical removal of the ovary and the tip of the affected horn may be effective in treating the problem, as long as enough uterus remains to allow maternal recognition of pregnancy.

Prognosis
- Death following prolapse is not uncommon, and it often occurs before help arrives.
- If the mare survives the process of replacement of the uterus, metritis is a common sequel and therefore supportive prophylactic treatment is essential.
- Uterine prolapse is no more likely to occur in a subsequent pregnancy than it was at the time it initially occurred, and is not a reason to discontinue breeding a mare.

Bladder eversion or prolapse

Bladder eversion and bladder prolapse are rare conditions in the mare.[25,73,74] Both conditions are more common in draft mares, possibly due to increased urethral size and decreased urethral tone. Straining post partum as a result of vulvar and vaginal injury, dystocia, retained placenta or fecal constipation may occur and predispose the mare to eversion or prolapse.

- Bladder eversion (Fig. 8.35) occurs as a result of a tear in the ventral vaginal floor, and with

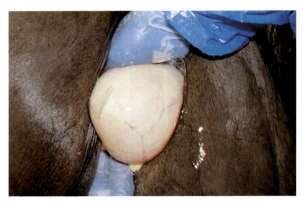

Fig. 8.35 Bladder eversion. Note the exposed serosal surface of the bladder. The bladder prolapsed through a vaginal tear following dystocia and assisted delivery.

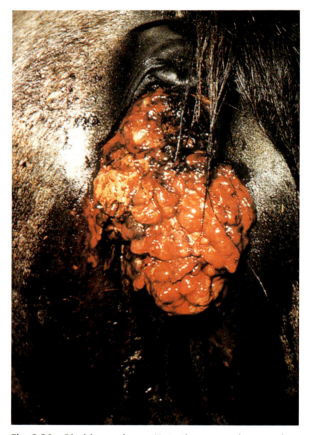

Fig. 8.36 Bladder prolapse. Note the exposed mucosal surface of the bladder and vesico-ureteral openings which continued to produce urine.

abdominal contractions or straining the bladder is forced through the opening.
- Bladder prolapse (Fig. 8.36) is due to straining during or after delivery and results in the bladder being everted through the urethral opening to appear in the vagina and/or vulva.

Clinical signs
- In bladder eversion, the smooth, vascular serosa of the bladder and (usually) the ureters (but not of course the ureteral openings) are visible to the observer.
- In bladder prolapse, the mucosa of the bladder and the ureteral openings (through which pulses of urine may be noticed) are visible.

Treatment
Epidural anesthesia is required for treatment of both conditions.

1. Bladder eversion.
   i. The bladder should be cleaned and emptied and then replaced into the abdominal cavity.
   ii. The hole in the vaginal floor must be surgically repaired so that eversion does not recur. Placement of a Foley catheter in the urethra prior to closure of the vaginal defect prevents inclusion of the urethra in the closure of the vaginal floor.
2. Bladder prolapse.
   i. Initially the bladder must be completely emptied.
   ii. If it is edematous it should be wrapped, with pressure, in a cool soft cloth, soaked in dextrose solution to facilitate removal of edema fluid.
   iii. It can then usually be carefully and slowly replaced through the urethral opening.
   iv. If the bladder is too large to be returned, the urethral opening can be enlarged surgically and, once the bladder is inverted, the resulting surgical wound is closed to provide a normal urethral orifice.

It is important in both cases to prevent the mare from continued straining, once the bladder is replaced.

- Repeated epidural anesthesia using combinations of analgesics and anesthetics, or morphine epidural can be used.
- Alternatively, a nasotracheal tube can be placed for 24 hours to prevent the mare from closing her glottis and straining.
- If the cause of the straining can be controlled this is ideal.

Prognosis
There is an increased incidence of urinary incontinence in mares that have had a prolapsed bladder.

Rupture of the mesocolon/mesorectum or cecal infarction

These conditions are rare and are more often found in postparturient mares. The etiology is presumed to be trauma from the fetal extremities, but prolonged

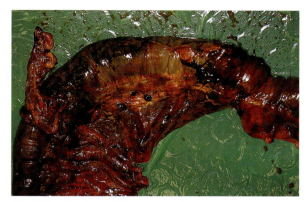

Fig. 8.37   Rupture of the mesorectum.

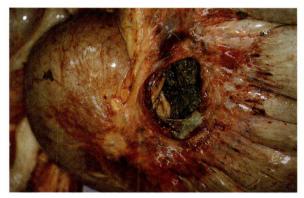

Fig. 8.38   Colon infarction.

or unsympathetic delivery can be responsible. Most mares with these conditions are presented for postparturient colic, sometimes several days after apparently uncomplicated or assisted delivery. Rupture of the mesorectum (Fig. 8.37) results in postparturient colic and usually peritonitis. Colonic infarction (Fig. 8.38) is of uncertain etiology but circulatory obstruction may be involved.

Clinical signs

- Initially, signs of low-grade colic are presented.
- The colic may be partially responsive to analgesics.
- The mare is usually febrile and produces little milk; the foal may be thin and hungry.
- Peritoneal fluid is invariably turbid with a neutrophil pleocytosis suggestive of peritonitis.
- Abdominal guarding is suggestive of parietal pain.
- Rectal examination is sometimes useful but can be dangerous if the disruption is in the distal rectal wall.
- There is a rapid progression to endotoxemia and shock.

Treatment

Surgical intervention is essential but can be extremely difficult because of the inaccessible cecal lesions and the extent of rectal wall and mesocolonic disruption.

- Enterectomy of the affected small colon/mesocolon is invariably needed.
- The peritoneum is lavaged copiously with warm saline and suction and antibiotics introduced before abdominal closure.
- High-intensity intravenous antibiotics are required, including penicillin, an aminoglycoside, and metronidazole.
- Intensive care is essential following the surgery if the mare is to survive.

Prognosis

Without skilled surgical intervention these conditions are invariably fatal. There is a serious risk of rectal or small colon stricture following the end-to-end anastomosis of the small colon.

MANAGEMENT OF THE PERIPARTURIENT AND FOALING MARE AND THE NEWBORN FOAL

Routine preventive medicine

Antibiotics

In some studs, antibiotics have been routinely administered to both mare and foal. There is debate about the value of this, but if hygiene is of significantly poor quality it would seem to be a sensible precaution. A single injection of a long-acting form of penicillin (benzathine and procaine G penicillin) should NEVER be used because this promotes bacterial resistance to the drug and may result in resistant super-infections. A full course of 5 days should always be given if antibiotics are to be used at all. It is unlikely that treatment of every mare and neonate with a 5-day course of antibiotics can be justified either medically or economically on any stud. Therefore it is recommended that only specific cases be administered postpartum antibiotics.

In cases where hygiene surrounding the birth is such that infection of the mare or foal is imminent and likely, prophylactic antibiotics may be justified. This may afford some protection against the most likely pathogens during the first 12–36 hours when colostral immunity is developing to its maximum. In one study, blood cultures from newborn foals revealed Gram-positive organisms, but neonatal septicemia is far more commonly due to Gram-negative bacteria.[75] In reality, therefore, simple penicillins alone might not be the most appropriate choice.

If a foal is delivered in poor conditions, or if there is a history of the mare having a vaginal discharge or when the placenta shows overt evidence of bacterial infection, immediate broad-spectrum antibiotics are warranted. All foals that have failure of passive transfer should/must receive appropriate antibacterial cover until other protection can be provided (see p. 362).

Prophylactic antibiotics can not replace good hygiene and proper periparturient care of the mare or the foal and cannot possibly on their own substitute for effective passive (colostral) transfer of antibody (see p. 374).

Multivitamin injections

Routine injections of vitamins A, D and E and selenium are sometimes administered but the value of this procedure is very contentious. In general, unless the mare can be shown to be deficient or unless vitamin deficiency is clinically suspected, there is probably no need to administer any supportive vitamin injections to newborn foals. In any case, overt clinically significant deficiencies are very rare. Excessive doses of vitamins A and D can cause serious toxic effects, but vitamin E is probably innocuous in excess (there are suggestions that it can enhance immune mechanisms when given in high doses[76]).

Vaccination/tetanus cover

Protection of the foal against the common environmental bacteria and viruses should be afforded by efficient passive transfer (see p. 374). This should be particularly effective if:

- The mare has been in the same environment for the last 3–4 weeks of pregnancy (she will hopefully have encountered all the pathogens in the environment and have had time to develop antibodies to these).
- The mare has been vaccinated during the last 3–4 months of pregnancy.

If the mare's vaccination history is uncertain, 6000 IU of tetanus antiserum should be administered at birth to the foal by subcutaneous injection.[77] Under these conditions there is some value in vaccination at an early age (see p. 362). Although totally unvaccinated mares are uncommon on well-managed farms, it is routine practice to give 1500 IU of hyperimmune serum to the foals immediately at birth. Under such management, cases of tetanus are extremely rare.

REFERENCES

1. Rossdale PD, Ricketts SW. Equine stud farm medicine. 2nd edn. Philadelphia: Lea & Febiger; 1980.
2. Vandeplassche MM. Delayed embryonic development and prolonged pregnancy in mares. Current therapy in theriogenology. 2nd edn. Toronto: WB Saunders; 1986:685–692.
3. Howell CE, Rollins WC. Environmental sources of variation in the gestation length of the horse. Journal of Animal Science 1951; 10:789–796.
4. Arthur GH. Veterinary reproduction and obstetrics. 4th edn. London: Baillière Tindall; 1975.
5. Ousey JC, Dudan F, Rossdale PD. Preliminary studies of mammary secretions in the mare to assess foetal readiness for birth. Equine Veterinary Journal 1984; 16:259–263.
6. Ousey JC, Delclaux M, Rossdale PD. Evaluation of the three strip tests for measuring electrolytes in mare's prepartum mammary secretions and for predicting parturition. Equine Veterinary Journal 1989; 21:196–200.
7. Cash RSG, Ousey JC, Rossdale PD. Rapid strip test method to assist management of foaling mares. Equine Veterinary Journal 1985; 17:61–63.
8. Brook D. Evaluation of a new test kit for estimating the foaling time in the mare. Equine Practice 1987; 9:34–37.
9. Pashen RL. Maternal and fetal endocrinology during late pregnancy and parturition in the mare. Equine Veterinary Journal 1984; 16:233–238.
10. Haluska GJ, Currie WB. Variation in plasma concentrations of oestradiol-17β and their relationship to those of progesterone, 13,14-dihydro-15-ketoprostaglandin $F_{2\alpha}$ and oxytocin across pregnancy and at parturition in pony mares. Journal of Reproduction and Fertility Supplement 1988; 84:635–646.
11. Ginther OJ. Reproductive biology of the mare: basic and applied aspects. Cross Plains, WI: Equiservices; 1979.
12. Ammons SF, Threlfall WR, Kline RC. Equine body temperature and progesterone fluctuations during estrus and near parturition. Theriogenology 1989; 31:1007–1019.
13. Stewart DR, Stabenfeldt GH, Hughes JP. Relaxin activity in foaling mares. Journal of Reproduction and Fertility Supplement 1982; 32:603–609.
14. Barnes RJ, Comline RS, Jeffcott LB, et al. Foetal and maternal plasma concentrations of 13,14-dihydro-15-oxo-prostaglandin F in the mare during late pregnancy and at parturition. Journal of Endocrinology 1978; 78:201–215.
15. Shaw EB, Houpt KA, Holmes DF. Body temperature and behaviour of mares during the last two weeks of pregnancy. Equine Veterinary Journal 1988; 20:199–202.
16. Doarn RT, Threlfall WR, Kline R. Umbilical blood flow and the effects of premature severence in the neonatal horse. Proceedings of the Society of Theriogenology 1985:175–178.
17. Hillman RB, Lesser SA. Induction of parturition. Veterinary Clinics of North America: Large Animal Practice 1980; 2:333–344.
18. Jeffcott LB, Rossdale PD. A critical review of current methods for induction of parturition in the mare. Equine Veterinary Journal 1977; 9:208–215.
19. Ley WB, Hoffmann JL, Crissmann TN, et al. Daytime foaling management of the mare. 2: Induction of parturition. Journal of Equine Veterinary Science 1989; 9:95–99.
20. LeBlanc MM. Induction of parturition. In: McKinnon AO, Voss JL, eds. Equine reproduction. Philadelphia: Lea & Febiger; 1993.
21. Leadon DP, Jeffcott LB, Rossdale PD. Mammary secretions in normal spontaneous and induced

premature parturition in the mare. Equine Veterinary Journal 1984; 16:256–257.

22. Ousey JC, Dudan FE, Rossdale PD. Mammary secretions in normal spontaneous and induced premature parturition in the mare. Equine Veterinary Journal 1984; 16:256–259.

23. Rossdale PD, Pahen RL, Jeffcott LB. The use of synthetic prostaglandin analogue (fluprostenol) to induce foaling. Journal of Reproduction and Fertility Supplement 1979; 27:521–529.

24. Alm CC, Sullivan JJ, First NL. Induction of premature parturition by parenteral administration of dexamethasone in the mare. Journal of the American Veterinary Medical Association 1975; 165:721–722.

25. Perkins NR, Fraser GS. Reproductive emergencies in the mare. Veterinary Clinics of North America: Equine Practice 1994; 10:643–670.

26. Vandeplassche M. The pathogenesis of dystocia and fetal malformation in the horse. Journal of Reproduction and Fertility Supplement 1987; 35:547–552.

27. Vandeplassche M, Simeons P, Bouters R, et al. Aetiology and pathogenesis of congenital torticollis and head scoliosis in the equine foetus. Equine Veterinary Journal 1984; 16:419–424.

28. Fraser GS, Perkins NR, Blanchard TL, et al. Prevalence of fetal maldispositions in equine referral hospital dystocias. Equine Veterinary Journal 1997; 29:111–116

29. Youngquist RS. Equine referral hospital dystocias. Proceedings of the Society of Theriogenology 1988:73–84.

30. Vanderplassche M. Embryotomy and caesarotomy. In: Oehmes FW, ed. Textbook of large animal surgery. 2nd edn. Baltimore: Williams & Wilkins; 1989:598–622.

31. Vandeplassche M, Bouters R, Spincemaille J, et al. Caesarean section in the mare. Proceedings of the American Association of Equine Practitioners 1977; 23:75–79.

32. Vandeplassche M. Operative interventions: the caesarean operation. In: Arthur GH, Noakes KE, Pearson H, eds. Veterinary reproduction and obstetrics (theriogenology). 6th edn. Philadelphia: Baillière Tindall; 1989:318–322.

33. Edwards GB, Allen WE, Newcombe JR. Elective cesarean section in the mare for production of gnotobiotic foals. Equine Veterinary Journal 1974; 6:122–126.

34. Stashak TS, Vandeplassche M. Cesarean section. In: McKinnon AO, Voss JL, eds. Equine reproduction. Philadelphia: Lea & Febiger; 1992:437–443.

35. Juzwiak JJ, Slone DE, Santschi EM, et al. Caesarean section in 19 mares: results and postoperative fertility. Journal of Reproduction and Fertility Supplement 1990; 19:50–52.

36. Vandeplassche M, Bouters R, Spincemaille J, et al. Cesarean section in the mare. Proceedings of the American Association of Equine Practitioners 1977:75–79.

37. Vaughan JT. Equine urogenital system. In: Jennings PB, ed. The practice of large animal surgery. Philadelphia: WB Saunders; 1984:1145–1147.

38. Madigan JE. Manual of equine neonatal medicine.

Woodlands: Live Oak Publications; 1997:29–30.

39. Hillman RB, Loy RG. Estrogen secretion in mares in relation to various reproductive states. Proceedings of the American Association of Equine Practitioners 1969:111–119.

40. Pascoe JR, Meagher DM, Wheat JD. Surgical management of uterine torsion in the mare. Journal of the American Veterinary Medical Association 1981; 179:351–354.

41. Sertich PL. Periparturient emergencies. Veterinary Clinics of North America 1994; 10:20–36.

42. Vasey JR. Uterine torsion. In: McKinnon AO, Voss JL, eds. Equine reproduction. Philadelphia: Lea & Febiger; 1993:456–460.

43. Bowen JM, Gabory C, Bousequet D. Nonsurgical correction of a uterine torsion in the mare. Veterinary Record 1976; 99:495–496.

44. Guthrie RG. Rolling for correction of uterine torsion in the mare. Journal of the American Veterinary Medical Association 1986; 181:66–67.

45. Wheat JD, Meagher DM. Uterine torsion and rupture in mares. Journal of the American Veterinary Medical Association 1972; 160:881–885.

46. Wichtel JJ, Reinertson EL, Clark TL. Nonsurgical treatment of uterine torsion in seven mares. Journal of the American Veterinary Medical Association 1988; 193:337–338.

47. LeBlanc MM. Multifactorial diseases: dystocia. In: Colahan PT, Merritt AM, Moore JN, Mayhew IG, eds. Equine medicine and surgery. St Louis: Mosby; 1999:1153.

48. Allen WE. Two cases of abnormal equine pregnancy associated with excess foetal fluid. Equine Veterinary Journal 18:220–222.

49. Blanchard TL. Hydrallantois in two mares. Equine Veterinary Science 1987; 7:222–225.

50. Lofstedt RM. Hydrops of the fetal membranes. In: McKinnon AO, Voss JL, eds. Equine reproduction. Philadelphia: Lea & Febiger; 1993:596–597.

51. Vandeplassche M, Spincmaille J, Bouters R. Dropsy of the fetal sacs in mares: induced and spontaneous abortion. Veterinary Record 1976; 99:67–69.

52. Honnas CM, Spensley MS, Laverty S, Blanchard PC. Hydramnios causing uterine rupture in a mare. Journal of the American Veterinary Medical Association 1988; 193:332–336.

53. Asbury AC, LeBlanc MM. The placenta. In: McKinnon AO, Voss JL, eds. Equine reproduction. Philadelphia: Lea & Febiger; 1993:513.

54. Hanson RR, Todhunter RJ. Herniation of the abdominal wall in pregnant mares. Journal of the American Veterinary Medical Association 1986; 189:790–793.

55. Rooney JR. Internal haemorrhage related to gestation in the mare. Cornell Veterinarian 1964; 54:11.

56. Pascoe RR. Rupture of the utero-ovarian or middle uterine artery in the mare at or near parturition. Veterinary Record 1979; 104:77.

57. Brooks DE, McCoy DJ, Martin GS. Uterine rupture as a postpartum complication in two mares. Journal of the American Veterinary Medical Association 1985; 187:1377–1379.

58. Perkins NR, Robertson JT, Colon LA. Uterine torsion and uterine tear in a mare. Journal of the American Veterinary Medical Association 1992; 201:92–94.

59. Fischer AT, Phillips TN. Surgical repair of a ruptured uterus in five mares. Equine Veterinary Journal 1986; 18:153–155.

60. Aanes WA. Cervical laceration(s). In: McKinnon AO, Voss JL, eds. Equine reproduction. Philadelphia: Lea & Febiger; 1993:444–449.

61. Stickle RL, Fessler JF, Adams SB. A single-stage technique for repair of rectovestibular laceration in the mare. Veterinary Surgery 1979; 8:25–27.

62. Held JP. Retained placenta. In: Robinson EN, ed. Current therapy in equine medicine. 2nd edn. Philadelphia: WB Saunders; 1987:547–550.

63. Vandeplassche M, Spincemaille J, Bouters R. Aetiology, pathogenesis and treatment of retained placenta in the mare. Equine Veterinary Journal 1971; 3:144–147.

64. Vandeplassche M, Spincemaille J, Bouters R, et al. Some aspects of equine obstetrics. Equine Veterinary Journal 1972; 4:105–109.

65. Vandeplassche M, Spincemaille J, Bouters R. Aetiology, pathogenesis and treatment of retained placenta in the mare. Equine Veterinary Journal 1971; 3:144–147.

66. Provencher R, Threlfall WR, Murdick PW, et al. Retained fetal membranes in the mare: a retrospective study. Canadian Veterinary Journal 1988; 29:903–910.

67. Steven DH, Jeffcott LB, Mallon KA. Ultrastructural studies of the equine uterus and placenta following parturition. Journal of Reproduction and Fertility Supplement 1979; 27:579–586.

68. Gygax AP, Ganjam VK, Kenney RM. Clinical, microbiological and histological changes associated with uterine involution in the mare. Journal of Reproduction and Fertility Supplement 1979; 27:571–578.

69. Burns SJ, Judge NG, Martin JE, et al. Management of retained placenta in mares. Proceedings of the American Association of Equine Practitioners 1977:381–390.

70. Arthur GH, Noakes DE, Pearson H. Veterinary reproduction and obstetrics. 5th edn. London: Baillière Tindall; 1982.

71. White TE. Retained placenta. Modern Veterinary Practice 1980; 61:87–89.

72. Threlfall WR, Immegart HM. Postpartum period: retained fetal membranes. In: Reed SM, Bayly WM, eds. Equine internal medicine. Philadelphia: WB Saunders; 1999:782–784.

73. Hackett R, Vaughan J, Tennant B. Prolapse of the urinary bladder. In: Mansmann R, McAllister E, Pratt P, eds. Equine medicine and surgery. Santa Barbara, CA: American Veterinary Publications; 1982:920–921.

74. Nyrop K, DeBowers R, Cox J, et al. Rupture of the urinary bladder in two postpartum mares. Compendium of Continuing Education for Practicing Veterinarians 1984; 6:S510–513.

75. Madigan JE, Wilson WD, Spensley MS, et al. Reliability of blood culture findings in normal and septicaemic neonatal foals. Equine Veterinary Journal Supplement 1988; 5:57–58.

76. Blanchard TL, Varner DD, Schumacher J. Routine management of the neonatal foal. Manual of equine reproduction. Philadelphia: Mosby; 1998:104–105.

77. Liu IKM, Brown SL, Kuo J, et al. Duration of maternally derived immunity to tetanus and response in newborn foals given tetanus antitoxin. American Journal of Veterinary Research 1982; 43:2019–2022.

Chapter 9
THE PLACENTA

Reg Pascoe,
Derek Knottenbelt

THE NORMAL PLACENTA

The placenta comprises the chorioallantois, the amnion, and the placental vasculature that constitutes the umbilical cord. All of these tissues are of fetal origin, and, although there are very significant effects upon the mare consequent upon failure to expel all or part of the placental membranes, examination of all the placental tissues is vital for the foal. Indeed, it is suggested that examination of the placenta provides as much information about the pregnancy and the foal itself as almost any other procedure. A considerable amount of information can also be gleaned about the status of the endometrium, which might have implications for subsequent pregnancies.

The equine placenta can be defined as diffuse, microcotyledenary and epitheliochorionic in character. The structure of the placenta and its relationship with the maternal endometrium are illustrated in Fig. 9.1.

This placental arrangement has a number of significant implications:

- Placental transfer of nutrients to the foal is relatively poor; only one foal can be fully supported.
- The entire endometrial surface is required to provide adequate nutrition and gas exchange for a single fetus.

- Twins are therefore always dysmature to some degree at least (see p. 242).

(see p. 242)

- Areas of scarring on the maternal endometrium do not have the normal structure that allows placental attachment and transfers, and are avillous. The result of endometrial scarring or other avillous areas is the loss of effective transfer capacity. The extent of the deficits is reflected in deficiencies of growth or maturation in the foal. Minor placental inadequacy as a result of endometrial scars or cysts may have no detectable effect on the foal's well-being, but more extensive ones will have an increasing influence. Thus, a foal born to an affected mare may be less developed than it should be.
- If twin pregnancies are present, the problem of avillous areas of endometrium is relatively minor. The problem here is that the two placentas will abut each other and so the placental surfaces will reflect avillous areas that do not correspond with endometrial damage (Fig. 9.2). This may perhaps explain the significant number of abortions or stillborn foals and the widely held belief that twins are usually disastrous. However, it is also important to realize that a very small percentage (<1%) of twins are born relatively normal and can also grow well and mature into normal adults. More commonly one foal is better than

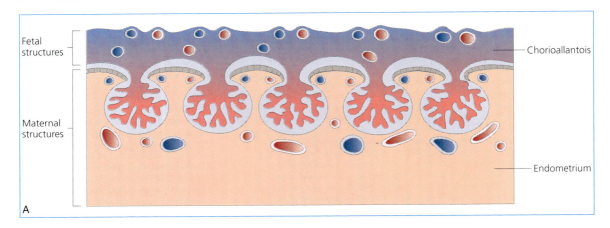

Fetal structures — Chorioallantois

Maternal structures — Endometrium

A

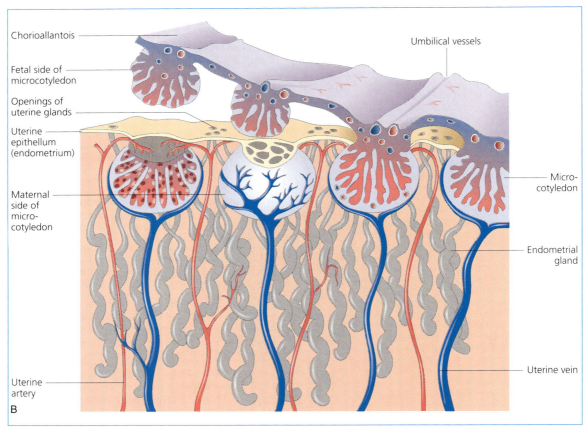

Chorioallantois

Fetal side of microcotyledon

Openings of uterine glands

Uterine epithellum (endometrium)

Maternal side of micro- cotyledon

Uterine artery

B

Umbilical vessels

Micro- cotyledon

Endometrial gland

Uterine vein

Fig. 9.1 (A) The macroscopic structure of the mare's placenta, illustrating microcotyledonary structures. (B) The mature equine placenta, showing the nature of the cotyledons. (C) The vascular arrangement of an equine placental microcotyledon.

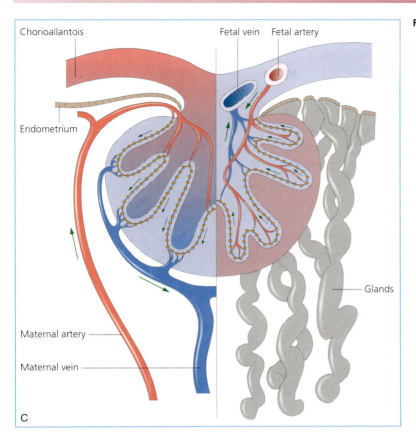

Fig. 9.1 *cont'd*

Chorioallantois

Fetal vein   Fetal artery

Endometrium

Glands

Maternal artery

Maternal vein

C

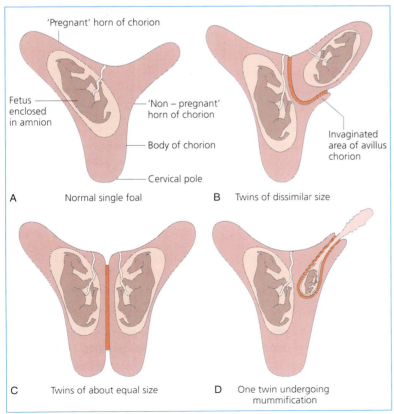

'Pregnant' horn of chorion

Fetus enclosed in amnion

'Non – pregnant' horn of chorion

Body of chorion

Cervical pole

A   Normal single foal

Invaginated area of avillus chorion

B   Twins of dissimilar size

C   Twins of about equal size

D   One twin undergoing mummification

Fig. 9.2 Various types of twin placentation. (A) One twin occupies the uterine body and one horn and possesses 70% of the functional surface area. Where the two chorions abut there is usually a degree of invagination of the smaller into the other. (B) The chorion of one twin almost totally excludes the other, occupying the uterine body, one horn and most of the other. (C) Equal division of surface area with no invagination of one chorion by the other. (D) One twin undergoing mummification.

the other and the large majority of twin births result in poorly grown foals that do not adapt well to extrauterine life. A mare that is known to be carrying twins or has previously had twins is therefore classified as high-risk (see p. 252). Proper management of a twin pregnancy at an early stage can reduce the risks of twinning (see p. 242).

- Placental transfer of large protein molecules is not possible. There is no effective/significant acquisition of immunoglobulins before birth. Consequently, the newborn foal is best regarded as immunologically naive.
- There is little chance for transfer of infective organisms to the foal without concurrent placentitis, and abortion will commonly ensue in such cases. Even minor placental inflammation can result in rapid abortion or significant compromise in the development of the foal. Therefore the health of the pregnant mare is critical for the delivery of a healthy foal at full term. Serious infections carry a significant danger of early termination of the pregnancy.
- Endometrial bleeding, such as is seen in the human hemochorionic placentation, is not possible. Significant blood loss at parturition usually means maternal (cervical, uterine or vaginal) trauma or premature rupture of the umbilical cord. Fresh bleeding after delivery of the foal (and the placenta) is usually a result of uterine, cervical, vaginal or vulvar damage.
- Premature separation of the umbilical cord is a relatively frequent event in mares foaling under disturbed conditions. In this situation, the foal can be deprived of up to 1.5 liters of blood.[1] This can result in considerable problems with metabolic acidosis and failure to adapt quickly to the free-living state.[2] There is debate about the significance of the early separation of the cord and the importance of the blood remaining in the placenta.[3] However, it seems reasonable that a foal will be slower to adapt and may be more susceptible to infection if it is deprived of the maximum amount of blood.
- Any factor that adversely affects the intimate relationship of the placenta with the endometrium has the potential to cause serious problems, such as abortion, fetal reabsorption, deformity, or neonatal infection or compromise.

Abnormalities of the placenta are extremely important and allow the attending clinician to make a rational and often life-saving assessment of the viability of the foal before any clinical abnormality becomes apparent.

Note:
- Examination of the placenta (fetal membranes) is a vital part of the assessment of the newborn foal. It is important to recognize the normal placenta and the normal variations that have no significance on fetal viability. The clinical appearance of the placenta changes quickly after delivery and these normal changes may easily be over-interpreted.
- A careful placental examination should be used to investigate failed pregnancies and abortions and may in fact be more useful than examination of many of the other fetal tissues.
- Recent research suggests that placentitis is a common feature with mares showing (heavy) prepartum lactation.

The problems associated with placental retention in the mare are described on p. 313.

EXAMINATION OF THE PLACENTA

- Early examination of the placenta provides the clinician with valuable and potentially life-saving information for the foal (as well as the mare). It should never be ignored in any foaling.

The stud manager/owner should place the unwashed placenta carefully into a plastic bag immediately it is passed, and store it in a cool place (not a freezer) until examination. The placenta should be examined within 12–24 hours; usually this will conveniently coincide with the primary (2–6-hour) examination or the second routine examination of the foal (at 24 hours).

The stud manager or groom should be asked to write down the findings as the clinician dictates them. It is unwise to rely on memory. An examination form can be useful in ensuring that nothing is omitted and that the results are recorded correctly. (An example of a suitable form is shown in Fig. 9.25 at the end of this chapter.) In an increasingly litigious society, a meticulous record of events should be kept.

Step 1: Prepare by appropriate dress with protective coveralls, gloves, and boots

i. Remember that the placenta may carry infective organisms.
   - Do not be responsible for the transmission of infective agents from stud to stud.

ii. Leave protective boots and overalls on the stud to be washed.

iii. Perform normal hygiene precautions (hand-washing and changing of overalls, etc.) before and after examining the placenta.

iv. Always examine the healthy prepartum mares first, then the foals and other mares, and finally the placenta.

Step 2: Prepare all equipment required

- Disposable gloves/apron/mask.
- Scissors.
- Scalpel handle and blade (preferably disposable).
- Sterile swabs with bacterial and viral transport medium.
- Sampling bottles:
  - ❏ 10% formal saline.
  - ❏ Michelle's medium.
  - ❏ Plain (Carnoy's) tubes.
- Disinfectant for washing up afterwards.
- Notepad and paper; record findings as they are identified (it is often useful to dictate to the stud groom as the procedure is performed or use a tape recorder). A suitable protocol is shown at the end of this chapter (pp. 340–342).
- A refrigerator and freezer are also useful, but potentially infected specimens must never be stored in a freezer or fridge that also contains other material such as colostrum or plasma.
- If there is a possibility that viral agents are involved, a pack of dry ice is often useful as many specimens deteriorate markedly unless cooled quickly.

Step 3: Weigh the placenta

It is useful to encourage stud managers to weigh the placenta and record the weight routinely before storing it prior to examination. This limits errors arising from drying, predation, contamination, etc.

- The normal fresh (wet) weight is about 10–11% of the foal's body weight[4] (e.g. the placenta of a foal born to a multiparous Thoroughbred mare should weigh 4.8–5.5 kg).
- A placenta that is heavier than expected may signify edema or inflammatory changes, or the presence of an abnormal amount of fetal blood (suggestive of possible early cord separation).
- A placenta that is lighter than normal is usually immature, incomplete or has significant avillous areas.

Step 4: Examine the placenta

It is essential to examine the placenta thoroughly from both sides (chorionic and allantoic) and to examine the amnion and the cord. Failure to do this could result in failure to recognize vital clues that might impact on the foal and/or the mare.[5]

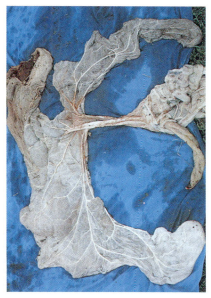

Fig. 9.3 Laid-out placenta viewed from the allantoic side with amnion and cord attached, showing the normal distribution of the chorionic vasculature. It is important to recognize these so that abnormal and missing portions can be identified.

i. Place the placenta on a clean dry surface (e.g. concrete floor) well away from any area where other horses might make contact with it (it might carry infectious agents).

ii. Lay the placenta out in the shape of an 'F', the way in which it was delivered (see Fig. 9.3). The smooth gray, shiny allantoic surface of the allantochorion is exposed (this is the inside of the chorioallantois; it should not be confused with the thinner, tough, smaller amnion, which should be identifiable as a separate entity).

iii. The bottom leg of the 'F' is the cervical end; the cervical star and rupture line should be situated here. The vertical part of the 'F' corresponds to the uterine body. The larger upper (longer, wider and thicker) side-arm of the 'F' corresponds to the pregnant horn, and the lower, smaller and narrower side-arm corresponds to the nonpregnant horn.

iv. The whole visible allantoic surface should be examined carefully, then turned over to inspect the other side. Particular care must be taken to examine any area that may indicate uterine injury from the foal's feet or legs. This may be the only outwardly detectable indicator of trauma to the uterine wall.

v. The integrity of the blood vessels that lie on the allantoic surface should be examined: missing portions of the placenta are characterized by blood vessels that do not correspond; tears in the membrane can be recognized when the vessels can be re-aligned accurately.

vi. The placental blood vessels are examined in detail for the presence of any inflammatory margin, which is characteristic of some bacterial infections (particularly those that are liable to cause septicemia in the foal such as *Escherichia coli* and *Klebsiella* spp.).

Examine the umbilical cord and the amnion

The umbilical cord should be examined closely for evidence of abnormal twists and bruising or other damage. The normal cord has a number of regular nonobstructive twists and shows no evidence of hemorrhage at any point (Figs 9.4, 9.5).

i. If the placenta is very fresh it sometimes useful to collect a sample of blood from the free end of the umbilical vessels.

ii. The umbilical vessels should be checked for defects or areas of bruising or other changes.

iii. The cord in the Thoroughbred is normally less than 84 cm in length.[6] An abnormally long cord may be associated with a higher risk of cord torsion and allantochorionic necrosis at the cervical pole, and therefore with a higher rate of abortion. Abnormally short cords are probably

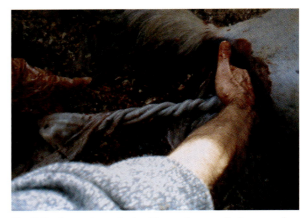

Fig. 9.5   A newborn foal with an abnormally long cord. Note the even, regular and nonobstructive twists in this case.

more liable to early (sometimes prepartum) cord rupture/separation and consequent fetal asphyxia.[7] There is a great deal of variation in the amount and type of twisting that occurs in the normal cord; cord torsion is commonly blamed for fetal death but this may be unjustified. Normally there are about 6–8 even twists (although these are usually obliterated by fetal separation and handling of the placenta and so are not always visible in normal delivered placentas).

iv. Aborted fetuses within the membranes provide a better opportunity for assessment of umbilical torsion when up to 12 uneven and distorted twists can be present.

v. The presence of unequal twists, abnormal edema or gross varicosity of the umbilical veins in particular should be noted.

Examine the chorionic surface

i. Turn the placenta inside out by pulling it through the cervical-star tear to expose the chorionic surface of the chorioallantois; this is the fleshy brown-red granular (villous) surface. The amnion and the cord are now enclosed within the chorioallantois and are in any case of lesser importance at this stage.

ii. The membranes are spread out in the same 'F' shape.

iii. The chorionic surface should be uniformly covered by small villi and is usually a dark red-brown in color (see Fig. 9.6). The color and appearance will differ markedly with the state of freshness of the placenta. By 24 hours it is often a dark red-brown color and the surface structure may not be discernible.

• This is the surface that will show the avillous areas.

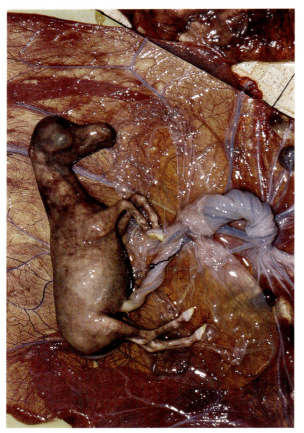

Fig. 9.4   A normal pony fetus showing a normal cord (with regular, nondilating twists and no obvious urachal dilations).

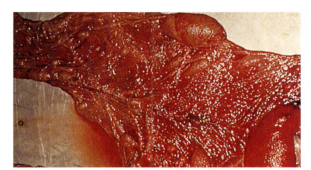

Fig. 9.6 The chorionic surface of the placenta. The appearance of this surface varies with the freshness of the placenta and its storage. If the placenta is passed within minutes of delivery of the foal it has a fleshy villous appearance. However, storage and delays in delivery of the membranes result in a brown, slimy appearance, which can easily be mistaken for infection. Histological examination will establish if this is normal or not.

Normally, avillous areas only appear:

- At the cervical star (Fig. 9.7a).
- At the 0.5-cm diameter sites corresponding to the papillae of the fallopian tubes at the apex of each horn (Fig. 9.7b).
- At sites of folding of the allantochorion (Fig. 9.7c).
- At sites of endometrial cysts (Fig. 9.7d).

Some placentas may show scars of the remnants of the endometrial cup sites (Fig. 9.7e).

Obtain samples

i. Samples such as swabs or tissues should be taken from the area around the cervical star and any other suspicious-looking locations. In particular, any area that varies in color, thickness or consistency should be sampled.

ii. A sample of blood can usually be expressed from the free end of the umbilical vessels of a fresh placenta. This should be collected into a plain sterile tube for transmission to the laboratory if needed. The blood contained in the placental vessels is of course foal's blood; if a very fresh sample can be obtained it may be possible to collect it into an anticoagulant tube (EDTA) and so avoid the need for jugular sampling of the foal. However, placental blood clots within 5 minutes and then only a clotted sample can be obtained. Nevertheless, this is sometimes very useful.

Normal incidental findings of no significance

- Occasionally, chorionic endometrial out-pouchings are present (Fig. 9.8); these probably arise as a result of corresponding endometrial scarring. They have a pouched appearance with a stalk on the allantoic side and are sometimes termed chorioallantoic vesicles. Some contain remnants of endometrial cups.

- A single hippomane, which is a flat rubbery, brown-yellow, oval-shaped structure (see Fig. 9.9) found floating freely in the allantoic fluid, is a 'normal' finding and is passed during second-stage delivery. Its size is variable (around 14 × 1.5 cm). It is composed of complex minerals and desquamated cells from the foal and fetal membranes. Similar material can sometimes be found adhering to the chorioallantoic vesicles but has no clinical significance. The earliest stages of development of a hippomane can be detected at 75–80 days. Its shape is determined by its location in the dependent part of the allantoic sac.

- Small granular deposits possibly deriving from urinary salts are sometimes found in the amnion (Fig. 9.10). They are of no known significance.

- Remnants of the yolk sac may be found in the infundibulum (Fig. 9.11). These can resemble abnormal tissue structures but can be treated as insignificant.

Histopathologic examination of the placenta

Significant histological abnormalities can be detected, even if the appearance of the placenta is normal. Unfortunately, histopathologic examination is very infrequently performed. Of 124 placentas examined in one study, the histopathologic findings correlated more accurately with the outcome of the pregnancy than the gross ones did.[8] This study identified inflammatory and infarctive processes as being of significance. Long-standing changes in the placenta might be expected to have a considerably different effect on the fetus than those that develop at or around parturition/abortion; the estimated duration of the pathological changes is therefore important.

- Placentitis primarily affects the villous layers of the chorion and may be diffuse or localized, and the pattern of inflammatory responses relative to the anatomical features might be instrumental in establishing the likely portal of entry. For example, localized placentitis around the cervical star might reasonably be supposed to originate in the vagina or vulva as an ascending infection and may suggest cervical incompetence or inflammation. Inflammatory changes detected along vessel walls might derive from hematogenous infections.

- Chronic changes are reflected in a significant reduction in the efficiency of the microvilli. Shorter and thicker villi might reasonably be expected to cause long-term alterations in placental efficiency, thereby compromising the long-term development of the foal.

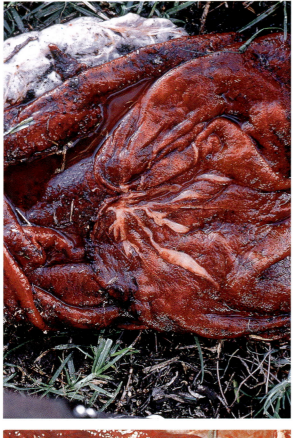

A

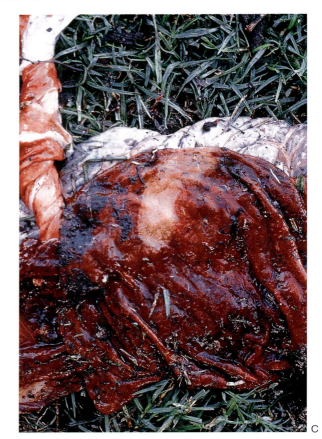

C

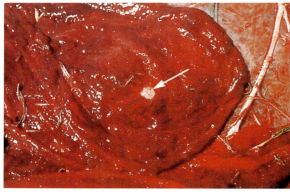

B

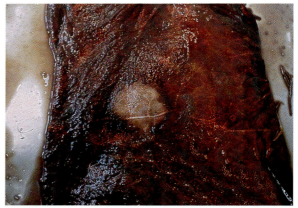

D

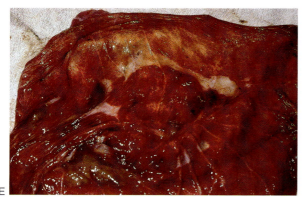

E

Fig. 9.7 (A) The normal avillous area at the cervical end of the placenta reflecting the avillous cervical star. In this case the placenta has not been torn by delivery; more usually, of course, the tear occurs at this point allowing the foal to be delivered. If this is identified intact during delivery it constitutes an emergency indication of early placental separation (see p. 299). (B) The normal avillous area at the fallopian papilla. This is small and round and situated at the tip of each horn. (C) A normal, incidental, linear avillous area resulting from a fold in the chorion. Such areas can be recognized by their very smooth but thin appearance. (D) An avillous area derived from contact with an endometrial cyst. These are of little or no significance to the pregnancy even when they are extensive and multiple. Routine prebreeding checks will usually have identified them and so the location of the avillous area can be defined. (E) Avillous areas derived from contact with the endometrial cups. These are totally insignificant.

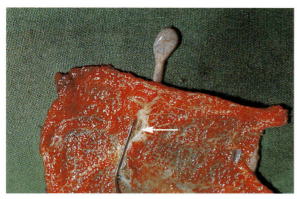

Fig. 9.8   Chorionic out-pouching (often termed 'cysts'). These are probably of no significance.

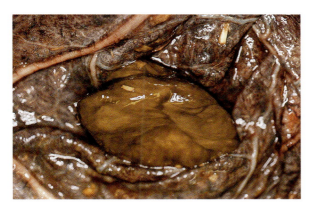

Fig. 9.9   A normal placenta with normal hippomane.

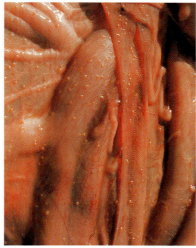

Fig. 9.10   Amniotic granules (these are probably of no significance).

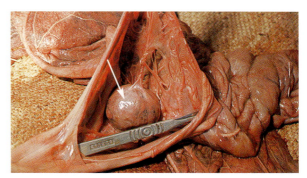

Fig. 9.11   Yolk sac remnants (arrow).

Note:
- Studies on the equine placenta are sparse and further study needs to be encouraged; veterinarians should therefore submit samples from apparently normal and suspect placentas for pathological examination at every opportunity.

ABNORMALITIES OF THE PLACENTA

PHYSICAL DISORDERS OF THE PLACENTA

Avillous areas

These are areas that do not have the normal fleshy red-brown character of the chorionic surface with well-developed villi. Avillous areas are most often associated with twin pregnancies (even if a second twin is not found, or is very small, or is mummified), and correspond to areas of abutment of the two placentas (see Figs 9.2, 9.12).

Pathological avillous areas include those with:

- Endometrial scarring: this is an important finding, but the significance will vary depending on the extent. Scars vary in size and shape; for example, a linear avillous area may reflect an endometrial scar from a previous cesarean section but may also resemble a fold in the chorion.
- Linear folds (folding of the placenta causes linear avillous areas): usually of little significance (see Fig. 9.7c).
- Endometrial cysts: usually of little consequence, appearing as roughly circular areas 1–3 cm in diameter (see Fig. 9.7d).

The pathological avillous areas should not be confused with naturally occurring avillous areas (see p. 332) at the cervical star and at the uterine papillae/fallopian tube opening at the end of each horn.

Placental edema

Placental edema is always significant, although the normal full-term placenta may show some evidence

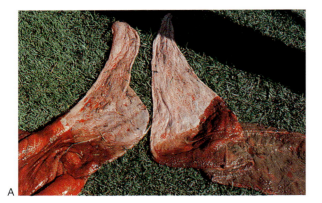

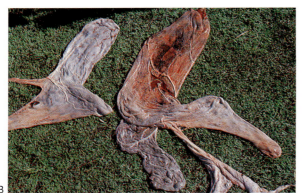

Fig. 9.12 (A) Placenta of a twin pregnancy, viewed from the chorionic (fleshy) side, showing a large avillous fibrous area of apposition of the placentas from the two twins (arrow). (B) The same placenta viewed from the allantoic (smooth) side.

of mild edema at the tip of the pregnant horn when examined histologically. The placenta is fetal tissue and edema is indicative of circulatory disorder or inflammation (or both). Any edema will necessarily affect placental transfer both ways.

- The edema may be obvious (see Fig. 9.13) and/or reflected by increased weight.
- It occurs in generalized or focal forms. Localized placental edema can easily be overlooked in a casual examination and is no less significant than edema affecting wider areas.
- Histological examination may be required for definitive identification.

Note:
- The normal pregnant horn is commonly mildly edematous and thicker than the nonpregnant horn. Occasionally, with twin placentas, both horns are similar to the normal thickened pregnant horn from a single fetus.

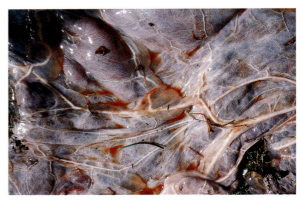

Fig. 9.13 Gross edema of the placenta.

Placental hemorrhage/bruising

This is usually obvious as a focal localized or diffuse area of darkening that is also visible on the (shiny, smooth) allantoic surface (Fig. 9.14). This is always significant, but mild localized very fresh bruising may occur at a stage when it has no material effect on the foal (i.e. during delivery).

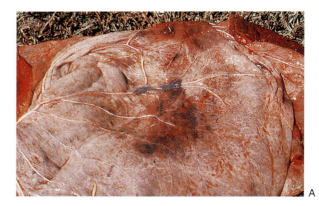

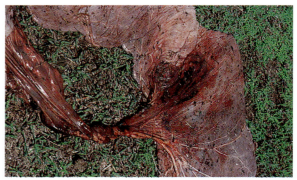

Fig. 9.14 (A) Focal intramural hemorrhage probably derived from direct trauma by a fetal foot. (B) Severe placental hemorrhage that was probably caused early in the delivery process. The extent of hemorrhage indicates that the blood pressure in the placental vessels was still high when it occurred and that it possibly involved arterial damage. Damage to the mare's uterus can be suspected and investigated.

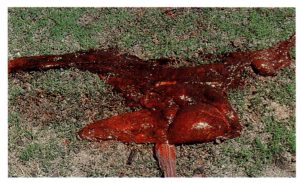

Fig. 9.15   Placental hematoma viewed from the chorionic surface showing a large blood clot in the chorioallantois.

Placental hematoma

Placental hematomas are rare but are suggestive of trauma during parturition. They are often accompanied by endometrial damage/bruising and occasionally by more severe uterine hematoma (see Fig. 9.15) or even rupture, most being due to the impact of fetal limbs. Of course, the endometrial damage can only be inferred from the placental examination but the benefit of this information is obvious.

> Note:
> * Remember to also consider hemorrhagic
>   diatheses/hemophilia if the umbilical vessels
>   continue to bleed.

Meconium staining of placenta (and foal)

The placenta takes on a yellow-orange color, affecting the amnion in particular and to a lesser extent the allantoic surface. This is suggestive of fetal stress and may involve inhalation of meconium, which is a serious problem, particularly if extensive and solid pieces are involved (see Fig. 9.16).

* Frequently the foal will also be stained by the meconium.
* Examination of the medial canthus of the eye and the skin of the foal may reveal meconium staining. This may be subtle but it is always an important indicator of fetal stress.
* Meconium aspiration is a very serious disorder that can easily be fatal.

Umbilical torsion

The normal umbilical cord usually has about 6–8 twists, which are normally evenly distributed. There should be no edema or varicosity/congestion of

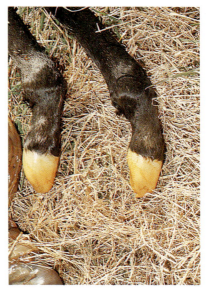

Fig. 9.16   Meconium staining of the foal, which was particularly obvious on the feet.

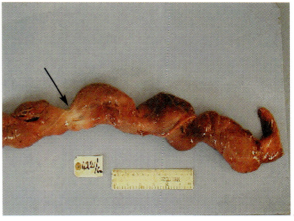

Fig. 9.17   An abnormally long umbilical cord that included several abnormal twists. Note the tightly constricted zone (arrow). (Slide courtesy K. Whitwell.)

vessels. Abnormal cord twists are uneven, edematous and often associated with hemorrhages and vascular congestion (see Figs 9.17, 9.18).

* The cord may encircle the limbs or neck of the foal, resulting in strangulation of the affected portion (often leading to abortion) (Fig. 9.19).

Urachal cysts

These fluid-filled, irregular, thin-walled sacs are sometimes seen in the amniotic part of the cord and are local distentions of the urachus (Fig. 9.20). They are of dubious/unknown significance and appear to have no obvious relationship with the survivability

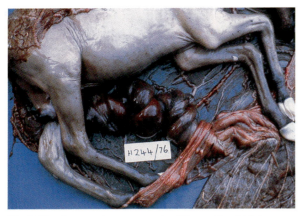

Fig. 9.18 A severely compromised 7-month-old fetus with an abnormally twisted cord that resulted in severe fetal compromise and death with subsequent abortion. (Slide courtesy K. Whitwell.)

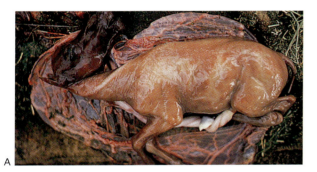

A

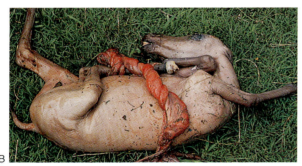

B

Fig. 9.19 Torsion/alterations in the umbilical cord: (A) cord strangulation of the neck of the foal; (B) cord strangulation of hindlimb. Both resulted in abortion.

of the foal. They tend to occur in foals with longer cords that have fewer twists, but are not associated with either the lymphatic or vascular components of the cord.

Chorionic cysts

One or two of these cysts are relatively common and probably of little significance. In some cases there may be many larger or smaller cyst-like structures or 'tags'.

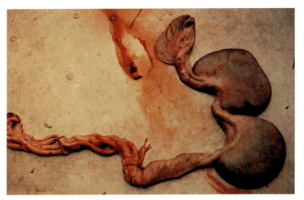

Fig. 9.20 Urachal cysts.

Hypoplastic villous areas (villous atrophy)

These are pale, thin shiny, plaques in the chorion and vary in size from small (possibly insignificant) to large (certainly significant). They are most common in old mares and particularly those with a history of endometritis/scarring and endometrial cysts. Significant endometrial hypoplasia may result in infertility or an unstable pregnancy.

Their occurrence probably reflects the corresponding endometrial microanatomy.[7] Usually the areas affected are visible and multiple, with paler areas with short, poorly developed villi reflecting areas of endometrium with no, or small, endometrial glands (often due to scarring). The pattern and distribution will usually mirror abnormalities on the endometrial surface. Large areas are associated with fetal growth retardation due to poor/inadequate placental exchange.

- A diagnosis of villous hypoplasia may rely on histological examination because they may resemble a totally avillous area in a placenta that is not absolutely fresh.
- Hypoplastic villi may result in a poorly developed fetus, commonly associated with prolonged gestation (>365 days) and dysmaturity (see p. 372).
- Mares showing these changes are to be regarded as high-risk at all subsequent pregnancies as the changes in the endometrium are not usually reversible. There will inevitably be some compromise to the fetus[9] and possibly early fetal death with abortion.[10]

Missing portions

The identification of missing portions of the placenta is a critical stud procedure.

- Even very small, retained pieces may be life-threatening for the mare.

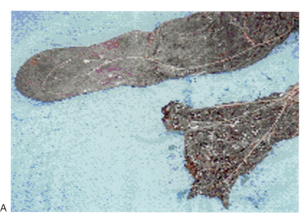
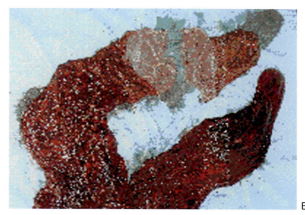

A   B

Fig. 9.21   (A) Allantoic view of the placenta passed by a mare during an apparently normal delivery. The tip of the pregnant horn is missing and the blood vessels are obviously disrupted. Careful examination of the mare revealed the missing portion, which was then removed without difficulty. (B) Chorionic view of the placenta after retrieval of the missing section.

Usually the missing portions of the placenta are the nonpregnant horn or parts of the end of the nonpregnant horn (see Fig. 9.21), but portions may be missing at other locations.

- If a piece of the chorioallantois is missing, the mare must be manually examined very carefully. The manual examination may even be performed without gloves to improve the possibility of locating the pieces and determining the integrity of the endometrial surface.
- Other procedures such as an endoscopic examination may be indicated.

> Note:
> - The specific problems associated with placental retention or retained portions of placenta in the mare are described in Chapter 8 (p. 278)

Pregnancy in the uterine body

This is fortunately a rare finding.[7,11] Careful examination of the relative sizes of the two horns of the placenta and the body will identify that the horns are relatively equal in size and both will be smaller than a normal pregnant horn (Fig. 9.22). The body portion of the placenta corresponding to the body of the uterus will be obviously larger than normal. Growth of the fetus is inevitably retarded in this condition and there is a high risk of abortion when the nutritional needs of the fetus cannot be met.

INFECTIOUS DISORDERS OF THE PLACENTA

Viral placentitis

- Equine herpesvirus 1 (abortion strain), or less commonly herpesvirus 4 cause placentitis.

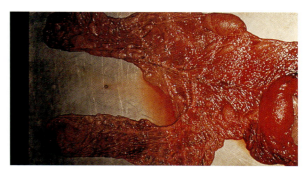

Fig. 9.22   Body pregnancy placenta. Note the abnormal size of the body portion of the placenta and the roughly equal size of the two horns. This placenta derived from an aborted foal.

- The most prominent signs in the mare involve the respiratory tract in the early stages of infection.
- Rapid abortion with early placental separation ('red bag delivery') is common.
- Foals born alive are usually weak and nonviable (see above).
- The placenta may be normal but may show chorionic edema (this can only be detected histologically).
- The chorion usually shows an edematous red appearance and is much thickened.
- The placenta is seldom if ever retained under these conditions ('clean abortion') (see p. 253).

> Note:
> - The significance of the neurological syndrome of equine herpesvirus infection in the mare should not be forgotten.
> - Aspects of equine herpesvirus abortion are described on p. 253.

Bacterial placentitis

- Specific features are recognizable in placentas that have been infected by Gram-negative bacteria (*Escherichia coli*, *Klebsiella* spp. and others) and Gram-positive bacteria (*Streptococcus equi*, *Streptococcus zooepidemicus*, *Streptococcus faecalis* etc., *Staphylococcus* spp. etc.) (Fig. 9.23).
- Abortion and/or placentitis due to bacterial infection is usually 'dirty', with significant edema of the placenta, mucopurulent change over the surface of the placenta and maternal cervical/vaginal discharges.
- Placentitis is a common feature with mares showing heavy prepartum lactation.
- Any purulent or fetid vaginal discharges prior to or following foaling must be regarded as significant. Discharges occurring within 12 hours of parturition should arouse suspicion of possible sepsis in the foal. The foal should immediately be classified as high-risk (see p. 355) and blood culture should be instigated at birth (see p. 364). Prior suspicion of a problem means that a fetal blood sample from the cord can be obtained during delivery or immediately afterwards; this should be subjected to both immediate blood culture and full hematological examination.

Fungal placentitis

Fungal placentitis is a very rare event. However, it can be a major cause of abortion and/or delivery of poorly grown, dysmature and septic foals as well as of stillborn foals.

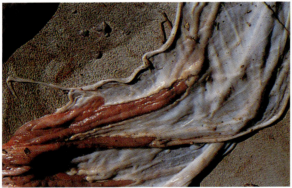

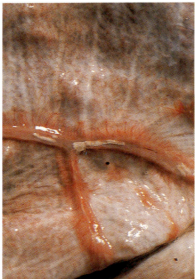

Fig. 9.23 Placentitis due to (A) *Klebsiella pneumoniae* and (B) β-hemolytic streptococcus. Note the difference in the distribution of the inflammatory changes and that they are centered along the blood vessels suggesting a hematogenous origin.

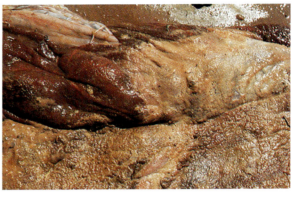

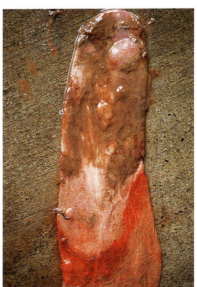

Fig. 9.24 (A) Diffuse fungal placentitis with a leathery appearance characteristic of fungal placentitis. (B) A rare case of fungal placentitis at the tip of one horn. The diagnosis was confirmed from histological sections and it is likely that the infection had been present from the start of the pregnancy.

Fungal infections of the placenta usually gain access via the cervix. Most cases arise from ascending infection from the vagina/cervix, so the most severe changes are at the cervical star end of the placenta and spread from there (Fig. 9.24a). Although the region of the placental star is therefore most often involved, in some cases the terminal regions of the nonpregnant horn may be more involved (Fig. 9.24b).

- Placentitis may be focal (limited and discrete areas) or generalized.
- Rarely fungal placentitis may affect other focal areas of the placenta and endometrium and then it may be possible to conclude that the primary endometrial infection was long-standing (possibly even before conception).
- The placenta is usually overweight and the chorion shows proliferative and exudative pathology, with areas of diffuse thickening and edema.
- The chorion mostly has a tan color and a leathery texture in affected areas.
- There is usually little or no mucoid/purulent material on the surface or there may be obvious surface exudate.
- Histological examination is a very useful method of detecting fungal infections.
- Fungal abortion is a rare event in horses. Most foals born under these circumstances are in an advanced stage of decay at the time of abortion.

Note:
- Fungal infections (most frequently *Aspergillus* spp.) are much less common than bacterial infections.
- Foals may have fungal infections of both gut and lungs at birth. These are very difficult to diagnose unless the placenta has been examined carefully.
- Differentiation between fungal and bacterial placentitis is not always easy without culture and histopathologic examination.
- All forms of placentitis may result in partial placental separation with consequent premature delivery and premature lactation.
- There is a very high incidence of sepsis in foals delivered to mares that have had premature lactation over some days or even weeks before delivery.

Summary
- Every available source of information should be used in every case. This will enable the clinician to be forewarned of potential hazards.
- If any placental deficiency or abnormality is recognized, the mare must be examined in detail, including ultrasonographic, manual, vaginoscopic, and, if possible, endoscopic examination of the reproductive tract, including the uterus. The foal should immediately be classified as 'high-risk' and all sensible measures should be taken to monitor its health over the ensuing 12 weeks.
- Examination of the reproductive tract of the mare should be performed routinely at 24 hours post delivery. There may be significant signs of bacterial or fungal infection, which might affect the viability of the foal.
- It is very easy to forget to examine the mare when the foal is clearly sick and the mare is apparently well.
- All foals delivered with any evidence of placentitis and/or premature lactation should immediately be classified 'high-risk'.
- Beware of premature lactation. It is never insignificant and is often associated with placentitis, and/or placental or fetal compromise.

REFERENCES

1. Rossdale PD, Mahaffey LW. Parturition in the Thoroughbred mare with particular reference to blood deprivation in the newborn. Veterinary Record 1958; 70:142–152.
2. Rose RJ, Leadon DP. Severe metabolic acidosis manifested as failure to adapt in a newborn Thoroughbred foal. Equine Veterinary Journal 1983; 15:177–179.
3. Madigan JE. Manual of equine neonatal medicine. Woodland: Live Oak Publications; 1997:3–6.
4. Madigan JE. Manual of equine neonatal medicine. Woodland: Live Oak Publications; 1997:29.
5. Whitwell KE, Jeffcott LB. Morphological studies on the fetal membranes of the normal singleton foal at term. Research in Veterinary Science 1975; 19:44–55.
6. Whitwell KE. Morphology and pathology of the equine umbilical cord. Journal of Reproduction and Fertility Supplement 1975; 23:599–603.
7. Whitwell KE. Investigations into fetal and neonatal losses in the horse. Veterinary Clinics of North America 1980; 2:213–331.

8. Cottrill CM, Jeffers-Lo J, Ousey JC, et al. The placenta as a determinant of fetal well-being in normal and abnormal equine pregnancies. Journal of Reproduction and Fertility Supplement 1991; 44:591.

9. Doig PA, McKnight JD, Miller RB. The use of endometrial biopsy in the infertile mare. Canadian Veterinary Journal 1981; 22:72–76.

10. Kenney RM. Cyclic and pathologic changes of the mare endometrium as detected by biopsy, with a note on early embryonic death. Journal of the American Veterinary Medical Association 1978; 172:241–262.

11. Rooney JR. Autopsy of the horse. Baltimore: Williams & Wilkins; 1970.

Placental examination form

Note:
- Specialized diagnostic tests and examinations identified in this form require specialized reports – attached where needed.
- Ensure that a copy of this form is included with specimens submitted for laboratory analysis.
- Photographic records of lesions/abnormalities with identification / date are useful.

Case No: Date:

Mare's name: Breed: Age: Parity:

Foal's name (or stallion's name if unnamed)

Owner's name: Telephone No:
Address:

Date of foaling: Time of call out:

Date of placental examination: Time of examination:

Bodyweight of foal: kg   Gestational age: days   Dystocia: Yes / No

Sex: Breed:

Condition at birth: normal / premature / dysmature / comatose / dead

Comments:

Condition of foal at time of placental examination: normal / sick / comatose / dead

Comments:

Condition of placenta at time of examination:
- normal-fresh / frozen / decayed / necrotic / predated / intact / partially-completely macerated

Contamination:
- negligible / obvious / severe / extreme

Comments:

Notes:

Fig. 9.25 Placental examination form.

Placental weight: kg
  • Proportion of fetal weight: (%) (normal 10–12% of foal's weight)

Physical appearance of placenta (obvious abnormalities):

Photograph: Yes / No

Hippomane identified: Size / volume: ml   Weight: g

Amnion:

Photograph: Yes / No

Cord and Vessels:
      Engorged / empty / edematous

Photograph: Yes / No

   Number of twists (if determinable)

   Any gross dilatations: Yes / No   if Yes state location, size and number

   Oedema: Yes / No   if Yes extent: mild / moderate / severe

   Haemorrhage: Yes / No   if Yes extent: mild / moderate / severe

---

Allantochorion: Photograph: Yes / No

         Cervical star-ruptured / not ruptured
            If not ruptured location of delivery tear:

Avillous areas seen: tick if located

☐   Papillary spots (end of each horn corresponding with fallopian tube)

☐   Cervical star:

☐   Other: describe size, shape and extent (approx. area in square cm)

☐   Appearance:

☐   Obvious abnormalities (specify):

Allantoic surface of chorioallantois:
         Appearance:

         Obvious abnormalities:

Photograph: Yes / No

Chorionic surface of chorioallantois:
         Appearance:

         Obvious abnormalities:

Photograph: Yes / No

Fig. 9.25   Placental examination form (*cont'd*).

Samples obtained (tick if present)

tissue/location	smear	swab VT	BT	PL*	fresh tissue (ice)	formol saline	other fixative
chorion							
preg horn							
non preg horn							
avillous area							
allantois							
preg horn							
non preg horn							
avillous area							
allantoic fluid							
amniotic fluid							
amnion							
cord							
cord blood							

* VT = virus transport medium   BT = bacterial transport medium   PL = plain swab

Samples submitted to: (name of laboratory): _____ Laboratory

Laboratory reports: Attached.
(Reference numbers and dates to be listed here)

Telephone preliminary results to be written here:

Fig. 9.25 Placental examination form (*cont'd*).

Chapter 10
THE MAMMARY GLAND

Derek Knottenbelt

The mammary gland is a vital part of the reproductive anatomy of the mare. There is no doubt that milk is the ideal food for the very young foal, and under natural conditions continues to provide important nourishment for the growing foal up to natural weaning (often at about 8–9 months of age). Furthermore, the mammary gland plays a vital role in providing early immunological protection for the foal through the production of immunoglobulin-rich colostrum. Without effective production of high-quality colostrum containing appropriate antibody IgG, the foal has a dramatically reduced chance of survival[1] (see p. 374). Of all the domestic species, the foal is probably the most reliant upon colostral intake for its survival in the first few weeks of extrauterine life.

In spite of the significance of mammary gland function to the survival of the foal, little is known about the specific features in the mare. Diseases and disorders of the mammary gland are usually manifest by changes in size and texture of the gland and alteration in the natural secretions.

ANATOMY

The mammary glands are located high in the inguinal region. Their relatively small size and protected position reduce the risks of trauma, sunburn, and infections. In the dry (nonlactating) mare, the glands are small (except that, in older multiparous mares, the teats may be long and the udder skin rather slacker than in young mares) and have an almost insignificant blood supply; the lactating gland is somewhat larger and the blood supply is greater. Inflammatory and other disease conditions invariably increase the blood supply.

The mare has two mammary glands separated completely by a facial sheet. There is one teat per gland.[2] Each teat usually has two openings (Fig. 10.1), but occasionally there are three, reflecting the number of mammary lobes present. This has implications for mammary disease and the use of intramammary therapy.

Milk is secreted into the teat sinus from specialized cells that form the bulk of the gland. The glandular tissue itself is generously supplied with myoepithelial cells that have the ability to contract in response to oxytocin in particular.

MAMMARY GLAND DEVELOPMENT AND MILK PRODUCTION

The mammary gland of the horse is relatively small and the foal feeds frequently during lactation. This provides a significant protection mechanism against infection.

Mammary gland development and the production of milk is a highly complex process requiring fine

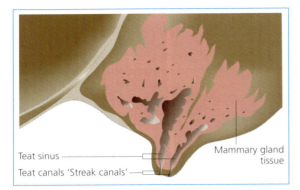

Fig. 10.1 Anatomy of the mammary gland. Cross-section showing major anatomical structures (lactating mare).

Table 10.1 Variation in milk composition during lactation[9]

Weeks of lactation	Energy (kcal/100 g)	Protein (%)	Fat (%)	Lactose (%)	Total solids (%)
0–4	58	2.7	1.8	6.2	10.7
5–8	53	2.2	1.7	6.4	10.5
9–21	50	1.8	1.4	6.5	10.0

control and coordination of birth and mammary development; milk production needs of course to be coordinated closely with delivery of the foal. The process of the manufacture of milk is demanding of energy and requires a fully functional mammary cell structure free of inflammation. The process is largely governed by the interrelationships between the hypothalamus, the anterior pituitary gland, the ovaries, and the placenta. Several hormones are responsible for individual aspects of the development of the mammary gland and the change from a quiescent nonsecretory structure to a highly specialized secretory function which, in the first instance, produces colostrum and then quickly shifts to produce milk.

Mammary development begins around 1 month before foaling. This process is believed to be instigated by ovarian and adrenal steroids, prolactin, growth hormone, insulin, thyroid hormones, and oxytocin:

- Estrogen causes development of the duct system.
- Progesterone stimulates the development of the milk-producing cells but inhibits milk production.
- Prolactin concentration increases dramatically in the last week of gestation and remains elevated until some 3 months after parturition.[3] This increase is probably instigated by the cessation of release of an inhibitory factor in the hypothalamus.[4]
- The decline in progesterone at the end of gestation and the rise in prolactin over the last few days are probably the basis of the trigger for milk production to begin.
- Oxytocin is secreted from the neurohypophysis of the pituitary glands in response to stimulation of the udder (usually by nursing).[5] Oxytocin causes contraction of the myoepithelial cells and ejection of milk into the duct system and eventually into the teat sinus. Circulating oxytocin released during labor will also have an effect on the mammary glands, so milk may be ejected from

the teats during later stages of labor. This may have implications for the quantity and quality of colostrum available to the foal. The so-called 'milk let-down' response can also occur in the absence of any detectable oxytocin in the circulation.[6]

During the last 2 weeks of gestation, the mammary gland actively concentrates immunoglobulin from the blood. This abstraction from the mare can sometimes be detected by a fall in immunoglobulins in the blood of the mare during this time. The protein-rich secretion that is produced first (colostrum) is high in IgG but it is only produced once; once the colostrum has been removed from the udder no more is produced in that lactational period. Within 12–14 hours of birth the IgG concentration falls dramatically. The other immunoglobulins (IgM and IgA) are at low levels in colostrum but are sustained for weeks in normal milk.

Milk contains more calcium and potassium and less sodium than blood, and as parturition approaches these changes become more apparent in the mammary secretion.[7] The concentrations of the various electrolytes in mammary secretions are used to provide information on readiness for birth[8] (see p. 270).

Milk is an ideal food material for the newborn and very young foal but becomes an inadequate total feed within a few weeks of birth (see Table 10.1). Low levels of iron and some other trace elements mean that a totally milk-based diet will result in significant metabolic deficiencies, and the energy requirement for the growing foal cannot be met solely by the volume of milk produced by the mare.

Lactation is maximal at around 2 months postpartum, the average production in a Thoroughbred mare being around 10–12 kg/day. This production is roughly equivalent to 2–3% of bodyweight and should enable the foal to grow at a rate of around 1 kg/day. In order to produce this amount of milk the mare needs to be fed additional food value of 1.5 times the normal requirements for energy and protein. Mares that are deprived of food or which do not eat for other reasons will inevitably produce less milk in response to the deprivation and negative energy balances. In some cases (ponies in particular) the negative energy balance results in the mobilization of fat and hyperlipemia can develop. This condition carries a poor prognosis and is a relatively common occurrence in late pregnancy or early lactating overweight pony mares. Any overweight mare that is subjected to a reason for negative energy balance may precipitate hyperlipemia. The disease is not the sole preserve of overweight pony mares.

WEANING

Under natural conditions weaning occurs at around 7–9 months, but most management systems wean foals at around 5–6 months of age. The weaning process is usually done abruptly by separating the mare and foal out of sight and hearing for 2–3 days. After a few days the foal will have forgotten the mare and can then be grouped with other weanlings in a small paddock. There are numerous variations in the weaning process, including gradual weaning or housing mares and foals together and gradually removing individual mares from the group, leaving an old experienced mare in the group for company.

Management of the mare is at least as important as management of the foal. The mammary secretions will, of course, continue to be produced and so the glands invariably become mildly or moderately engorged with milk. This accumulation induces a suppression of activity in the glandular cells and so milk production is gradually 'turned off'. This mechanism can also be instigated by lack of nursing in a younger foal, so it is important to examine the udder of nursing mares regularly to identify foals that are off suck at an early stage so that lactation is not inhibited.

Normally, the glandular distention that develops at weaning subsides gradually over a few days without evidence of inflammatory response, but occasionally mastitis develops. Failure to detect mastitis can have serious repercussions both immediately and at a future lactation. Therefore, regular attention should be paid to postweaning mares for 2 weeks after weaning. It is probably not advisable to milk-off the mare even if the udder is grossly distended, for fear that either infection will be introduced or because release of the pressure may reinstate lactation. Any serious oversupply of milk and associated congestion may respond best to restriction of food and water for a few days.

DISORDERS OF THE MAMMARY GLANDS

Eclampsia/hypocalcemia

Profile

This is not really a disease of the mammary gland but is supposedly due to rapid falls in serum ionized calcium associated with the onset of lactation. It is a relatively rare disorder of lactating mares and occurs within 10 days of foaling or 1–2 weeks after weaning.[10] Stress (such as transportation) and mammary development together are particularly dangerous.

Clinical signs

- A variable increase in muscular tone, stiff stilted gait with hindlimb ataxia. Trismus (lockjaw) can be seen.
- Muscle fasciculation (especially of the temporal, masseter, and triceps muscles).
- Profuse sweating.
- Dysphagia.
- Cardiac dysrhythmia.
- Synchronous diaphragmatic flutter (abrupt spasm of the diaphragm at each heart beat, noticeable as hiccoughs or thumps in the costal margin).
- Convulsions, coma, and death.

- Usually, excitement is the only sign when serum Ca^{2+} concentrations are between 2 and 2.5 mmol/l.
- The normal reference range is around 2.7–3.5 mmol/l (corresponding to 10.5–13.5 mg/dl).
- Concentrations below 2 mmol/l usually induce tetanic spasms and convulsions.
- Below 1 mmol/l the horse will usually be recumbent and possibly comatose.

Diagnosis

The signs are similar to those of:

- Tetanus.
- Cranial (or major body) trauma.
- Viral encephalitis.
- Hepatoencephalopathy.
- Herpesvirus myeloencephalopathy.
- Equine protozoal myeloencephalopathy.
- Bacterial meningitis.
- Verminous encephalitis.
- Laminitis.
- Colic (particularly catastrophic abdominal accidents).
- Hyperkalemic periodic paralysis (Quarterhorses).

Diagnosis can be confirmed by measurement of serum Ca^{2+} concentration. Hypomagnesemia and hypophosphatemia may accompany the condition and may be part of the syndrome.

Treatment

Slow intravenous administration of 250–500 ml of 20% calcium gluconate diluted in glucose saline (1:4) is rapidly curative. The response to treatment confirms the diagnosis.

Note:
- The solution must be administered slowly with continuous cardiovascular monitoring.
- The initial stages of the treatment are often difficult because of the added stress that the mare suffers.
- Supplementation with small amounts of phosphate and magnesium may help to correct the underlying physiological imbalances.

- Treatment should be repeated as indicated from clinical and laboratory information.
- Supplementary feeding of the foal for a day or two may be helpful in reducing the calcium drain.
- Oral calcined magnesite may be used to supplement the dietary calcium. Alfalfa hay has a high calcium content and thus can be an effective high-calcium feed material. Stimulation of the parathyroid can sometimes be encouraged around parturition by feeding a low-calcium diet prior to the last 3–5 days before delivery and then increasing the availability of dietary calcium.

Agalactia

Common causes
- Premature birth/abortion.
- Periparturient illness:
  - Fever.
  - Anemia.
  - Endotoxemia.
  - Septicemia.
- Malnutrition.
- Mammary hypo(a)plasia.
- Mastitis.

Less common causes
- Endocrine dysfunction.
- Fescue toxicity.
- Trauma.
- Nutritional deficiencies/starvation.
- Neoplasia:
  - (Malignant) melanoma.
  - Pituitary adenoma (Cushing's disease).

Profile
- Poor body condition; physiological or psychological stress.[11]
- Early parturition/abortion.
- Fescue toxicosis.[12] This pasture grass is associated with a high incidence of agalactia, thickened placenta, prolonged gestation, stillbirths, and occasionally abortion. Infertility at subsequent breeding is also reported.[13,14]
- Secondary to systemic illness including strangles.
- Specific udder diseases such as mastitis and mammary neoplasia.

Clinical signs
- Absence of milk production when it is expected.
- Secondary effects through lack of colostrum intake by the foal and consequent immunological compromise. Foal starvation may also be significant (even if lactation is suppressed rather than absent).
- If a foal is dull and apparently malnourished or ill and the udder of the mare is empty and remains so, agalactia can be suspected.

Diagnosis
- Clinical absence of lactation at a time when milk should be present.
- Prolactin concentration is lower than that in normal lactating mares.[15]

Treatment (see Table 10.2)
- Thyrotropin-releasing hormone stimulates prolactin production.[16] Lactation can therefore be instigated by administration of this hormone.[17]
- Drugs such as phenothiazine ataractics and metaclopramide also cause an increase in prolactin by reducing the inhibiting effects of dopamine.[18]
- Avoidance of fescue grasses in the last 3 months of pregnancy is advised because of the known risks associated with it.

Enlarged mammary gland

Common causes
- Udder edema.
- Precocious or inappropriate lactation.
- Mastitis (acute or chronic).

Table 10.2 Drugs used to stimulate lactation[9]

Drug	Dose (mg)	Route	Frequency (hours)
Thyrotropin-releasing hormone	2.0	Subcutaneous	12
Reserpine	0.5–2.0	Intramuscular	48
Perphenazine	0.3–0.5 (per kg)	Oral	12
Human chorionic gonadotropin	3000–5000 IU	Intravenous	Within 24 hours of birth

- Abscessation.
- Weaning/failure of feeding in foal.

Less common causes
- Trauma.
- Excessive carbohydrate before parturition.
- Avocado poisoning.
- Neoplasia:
  - ❏ Sarcoid.
  - ❏ Melanoma.
  - ❏ Adenocarcinoma.

Udder edema

Profile
- Ventral edema is very common in heavily pregnant mares in the last weeks of gestation (particularly in maiden mares). The development of edema has been used as an indicator of imminent parturition but this may be misleading.
- The swelling may involve the mammary gland and affect milk production.

Clinical signs
- Obvious ventral edema (that pits on pressure).
- Mild discomfort and reluctance to move.
- Pain on nursing (resentment to the foal's attempts to suckle).

Diagnosis
- The condition is easily appreciated.
- It should be differentiated from:
  - ❏ Ventral rupture.
  - ❏ Rupture of the prepubic tendon.
  - ❏ Edema due to other causes.

Treatment
- Encouragement to move gently and frequently.
- Hydrotherapy with cold running water played over the ventral abdomen is simple and helpful.

Premature/inappropriate lactation

Profile
Premature lactation in a pregnant mare is never insignificant. No matter how little milk is produced it must be taken seriously. Normal mares show the first signs of mammary development at around 2 weeks prepartum.

Premature lactation is usually a sign of:

- Impending abortion.
  Fetal stress.
- Intrauterine death of the foal (or one of twins).
- Early placental separation (whatever its cause; see p. 299).
- Placentitis (viral, bacterial, or fungal).

Premature lactation has serious implications for the survival of the foal (independent of the significance of the etiology of the lactational onset). Colostrum will be lost and will not be replaced, no matter how early the lactation or how much effort is taken to treat the cause.

- Mares with equine Cushing's disease (pituitary adenoma) often show inappropriate lactation (i.e. the mare is not pregnant at all).
- Occasionally foals are born in a stage of lactation. They have grossly large mammary glands and the secretion is clearly milk ('witch's milk'). It is thought to result from high concentrations of lactogenic hormones derived from the mare's circulation.[19]
- Regular and sustained stimulation by suckling can induce a low level of lactation in some mares, but this is not an exploitable method of creating a wet nurse mare.

Clinical signs
- Early lactational secretion at an unexpected time in late gestation.
- Lactation and mammary development in an older, nonpregnant mare is usually indicative of a hypothalamic–pituitary disorder. The affected mare may have other clinical signs of the disease such as hirsutism, polydipsia, weight loss, and fat redistribution.

Diagnosis
- A careful clinical examination of the pregnant mare MUST be undertaken to establish the primary cause of the problem.
- Cushing's disease can be confirmed by a number of functional and static blood tests, including resting blood glucose and cortisol, thyrotropin-releasing hormone stimulation and an overnight dexamethasone suppression test. Insulin assay is also useful. These tests are described in standard medical texts.

Treatment
- There is no specific treatment for premature lactation because it is invariably secondary to other serious conditions. Many attempts have been made using progestogen, etc., but these methods are not well established and there are no certain protocols for successful restoration of lactational function.
- Treatment for Cushing's disease with pergolide and or cyproheptadine controls the production of pituitary or hypothalamic hormones and so can reduce the inappropriate lactation. Cases of Cushing's disease are invariably immunologically suppressed or compromised and so mastitis is, at least in theory, more likely in these cases.

Mastitis (Figs 10.2–10.5)

Profile

Mastitis is rare in horses (far less than in cattle). It is usually restricted to adult horses and in particular lactational or postweaning mares. Mastitis can, however, occur in nonlactational mares[20] and on occasion even in foals.[21]

- Most cases occur in summer months[22] (corresponding with lactation).

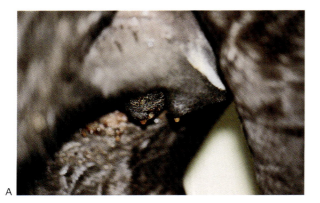

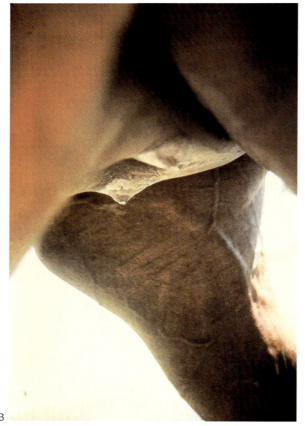

Fig. 10.2   Acute mastitis. (A) Serosanguinous discharge from both teats. (B) An udder with acute mastitis with agalactia.

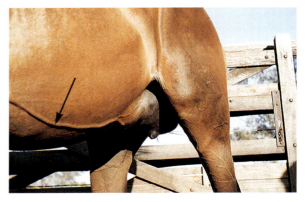

Fig. 10.3   The engorged mammary vein of a mare with acute mastitis.

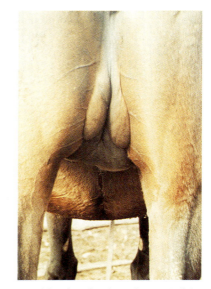

Fig. 10.4   Mastitis. The gland was hot, painful, and had stringy milk without clots. Note edema above the gland.

- Infectious causes include primary bacterial infections.
  - ❏ Nearly 50% of cases involve *Streptococcus equi*.[9]
  - ❏ Gram-negative bacteria such as *Escherichia coli* or *Pseudomonas* spp. and Gram-positive *Corynebacterium* spp. or staphylococcal organisms may be involved.
- Noninfectious causes such as trauma are much less common.

Clinical signs

- A warm/hot, swollen and painful udder is characteristic.
- Ventral edema may be extensive and the mammary vein may be very prominent on the affected side.

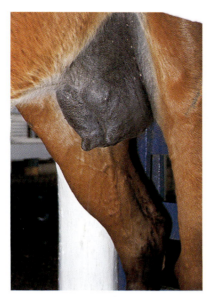

Fig. 10.5 Chronic mastitis. The udder is grossly enlarged on both sides and is indurated and 'knobbly'. Lactation was severely reduced and the mare's foal required supplemental feeding from birth.

- Systemic signs such as pyrexia, depression or anorexia may be present, but the mare may show none of these, even with severe localized infection.[23]
- Hindlimb lameness or stiffness can be present.
- The mammary secretions are invariably abnormal (Fig. 10.2a), but the extent of this may be masked by the production of normal secretions from the normal parts of the affected gland.
- Occasionally agalactia is present and such a gland may be very hard and hot although no secretion can be expressed (Fig. 10.2b).
- Mares with chronic mastitis develop fibrosis and scarring within the mammary gland and it takes on a 'knobbly' firm texture (Fig. 10.5).

Diagnosis
- Clinical examination and examination of mammary secretions.
  - ❏ Mastitis tests for cattle using soaps or indicators (California Mastitis Tests, for example) can be used in mares also. These tests detect high cellular (DNA) content and changes in acidity.
  - ❏ Mastitic milk is usually salty and either patently purulent (with clots and strings) or pale and watery (often with a sanguineous appearance).
  - ❏ Cytology: large numbers of neutrophil leukocytes, and possibly identifiable bacteria.[24] Normal milk has almost no cellular content.[25]
  - ❏ Culture and sensitivity: these are important for logical therapeutic intervention.

- Blood samples are often unremarkable but there may be a leukocytosis with neutrophilia and hyperfibrinogenemia.
- It is important to differentiate mastitis from neoplasia. Fortunately, the latter is rare and most are benign (see below). However, some neoplastic masses can be secondarily infected and so have a concurrent mastitis.

Treatment
- Frequent stripping of the infected udder provides essential drainage.
- Hot compresses.
- Systemic antibiotics.
- Local intramammary antibiotics must take account of the two or three separate glands with separate teat openings. It is relatively easy to damage the teat openings by this method and only a short-nozzle intramammary preparation should be used.
- Nonsteroidal anti-inflammatory drugs (e.g. phenylbutazone or flunixin meglumine) are helpful in controlling the fever and the pain. They also improve the mare's well-being and so the mare may continue to eat and drink. If fluids are not taken by mouth, they should be administered intravenously.
- Furosemide diuretic can be used to reduce edema but may not be very effective.
- The response to treatment is usually rapid and, provided that the condition is brought quickly under control, the long-term impact is usually minimal. Treatment should be continued for a day or two after resolution.
- Only rarely do cases develop fulminating gangrenous mastitis; if this develops the mare's life is seriously in jeopardy.
- Management of chronic mastitis is very difficult and in some cases mastectomy is indicated.

Mammary abscess

Profile
- Usually solitary but sometimes multiloculated or miliary abscessation occurs.
- Most cases are caused by *Streptococcus equi* or *Corynebacterium* spp.
- May be part of a disseminated infection, or be a solitary occurrence if the route of infection is direct via the teat canal or a wound.

Clinical signs
- Single, circumscribed, slowly expanding mass in the udder with associated inflammatory response in surrounding tissues.
- Local lymph nodes are usually enlarged but may be difficult to palpate effectively.
- Some systemic effects such as pyrexia, anorexia

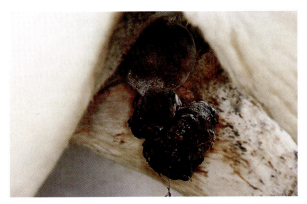

Fig. 10.6 A mixed fibroblastic and nodular invasive sarcoid in the mammary gland of a mare.

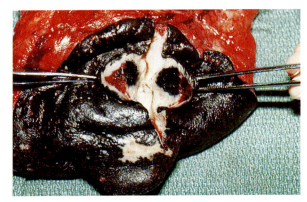

Fig. 10.7 Mammary melanoma (gray mare). Note melanosarcoma and melanin deposits in mammary tissue above lactiferous sinus.

and depression may be seen (especially if part of a generalized septicemic condition).

- Some local discomfort to palpation or movement (may be lame).

Diagnosis

- Aspiration (cytology/culture and sensitivity).
- Ultrasonography shows a fluid-filled structure containing flocculent material.
- Can be mistaken for tumor or mastitis.

Treatment

- Local drainage and flushing of the site (possibly requiring general anesthesia).
- Antibiotics may not be required for a single localized mammary abscess.

Tumors of the mammary gland

Profile

Fortunately, genuine neoplastic diseases are rare.[26–28] A prevalence of around 0.2% has been reported.[29]

- Viral papilloma frequently affects the udder and teats in particular, but this is a transient disorder of no material importance.
- The equine sarcoid is by far the most common tumor involving the mammary gland (Fig. 10.6).
  - ❑ Nodular sarcoids (types A and B) are found deep in the subcutaneous tissue of the udder or teat skin.
  - ❑ Verrucose or fibroblastic sarcoid lesions are common on the skin of the teats and udder.
- Melanoma is also a common tumor in gray horses. They are often embedded in the mammary tissue (Fig. 10.7). Most are benign and well demarcated but occasionally they can be large and invasive.
- Mammary adenocarcinoma has occasionally been identified (Fig. 10.8). These tumors have a strong tendency to metastasize to local inguinal and iliac

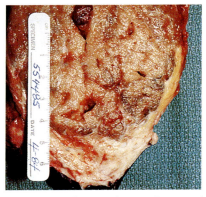

Fig. 10.8 Mammary adenocarcinoma. Cross-section of gland after surgical removal showing loss of lactiferous sinus.

lymph nodes and via the blood to the lungs.[30,31] The tumors appear as multifocal, cutaneous deep nodules that may ulcerate. Often they are easier to palpate than to see. Ultrasonographic examination is helpful.

- Generalized lymphosarcoma or localized lymphomas may also occur in the mammary gland.
- Ulcerated tumors may exude and drip plasma or blood-stained fluid and may predispose to mastitis.

Clinical signs

- Viral papillomatosis is distinctive but can easily be confused with verrucose sarcoids. They are transient and self-limiting and are commonest on young horses at grass. Usually there will be other typical papillomata at other sites (e.g. the face).
- Sarcoids are usually obvious, but the nodular form can be confused with melanoma in a gray horse. The presence of sarcoids at other sites may support (but not confirm) the diagnosis.

- The ultrasonographic and aspiration characteristics are distinctive to each type of tumor. The presence of other tumors at different sites may be supportive but some mares have both tumor types at the same time.
- Melanomas that have pink (nonpigmented) areas are probably highly malignant and should be managed with considerable caution.
- Adenocarcinoma is usually less well defined and highly aggressive.
- Secondary tumors occurring in the mammary glands are usually relatively insignificant in the overall condition of the animal.

Diagnosis

- Mammary masses should be subjected to careful clinical and ultrasonographic examination.
- Rectal examination must be performed to assess the iliac lymph nodes.
- Biopsy by fine-needle aspiration or column biopsy can be helpful, particularly in identifying the major tumor types in the gland. The procedure is relatively simple.
- Cytological examination of mammary secretions can be helpful but may also be misleading, particularly if secondary infection or bleeding is present.

Treatment

- Viral papilloma is a benign self-limiting condition that will spontaneously resolve after some months. Autogenous vaccines can be effective but are not usually necessary.
- All mammary tumors are difficult to treat.
- Equine sarcoid can be treated by a combination of topical cytotoxic drugs, or intralesional cisplatin injections. Teletherapy or interstitial radiation brachytherapy are useful if they are available. Surgical removal carries a high rate of failure.
- Melanomas can be surgically removed if they are troublesome.
- Adenocarcinoma requires mastectomy but even then there is a high risk of extension metastasis. Fortunately these tumors are very rare.
- Ultimately a decision must be taken with all tumor types to perform radical mastectomy but this procedure can be very difficult. The detailed technical aspects of mastectomy are described in current surgical texts.

MAMMARY SURGERY

Mastectomy

Indications

Surgical removal of one or both mammary glands is indicated when:

- There is serious neoplastic invasion of the gland(s).
- There is intractable and nonresponsive abscessation or mastitis.
- There is traumatic damage that precludes repair.

Procedure

The procedure is far easier when the gland is not lactating because the blood supply is reduced and the volume of tissue that needs to be removed is usually less in nonlactating mares.

 i. Preoperative antibiotics are administered with suitable nonsteroidal anti-inflammatory drugs and analgesics.
 ii. The surgery is performed under general anesthesia in dorsal recumbency with full aseptic precautions.
iii. After the initial elliptical skin incision is made (in such a way that the minimum of skin is removed), the gland is undermined by blunt dissection. Blood vessels are ligated carefully to minimize bleeding.
 iv. Specific surgical details are provided in advanced surgical texts. Particular attention is paid to the condition of the mammary lymph nodes (located at the base of the udder).
 v. Surgical drains are inserted to minimize fluid accumulation and undue pressure on the incision.
 vi. The surgical wound is closed in such a way as to reduce dead space to an absolute minimum. The value of stent pressure compresses is considerable.
vii. Recovery should be as quiet as possible to avoid the possibility of immediate wound dehiscence.
viii. Antibiotics and analgesics are maintained for 3–7 days.
 ix. The stent sutures are removed after 2–3 days and the skin staples or sutures removed at 7–10 days.
 x. In the event of wound breakdown, the wound can be allowed to heal by second intention.

Removal of localized tumors

 i. The mare should be prepared as above.
 ii. General anesthesia, with lateral or dorsal recumbency according to the precise location, is required. It is probably unwise if not impossible to attempt surgery in this area under local anesthesia and sedation alone.
iii. The overlying skin (unless it is involved in the pathology) should be preserved.
 iv. Surgical excision of a melanoma is usually feasible with little risk, but an occasional case has been highly malignant. In general, it is best to avoid any interference with the tumor itself as far as possible.

v. Sarcoid tumors are particularly difficult to remove surgically. The tumor tissue itself should not be traumatized and scrupulous hemostasis is essential for successful removal.

vi. All excised tissue should be carefully identified (location and stage) and submitted for histological examination by a skilled pathologist. Removal of tumors requires total excision but this may not be feasible and the owner may need to know this.

REFERENCES

1. McClure JJ. The immune system. In: McKinnon AO, Voss JL, eds. Equine reproduction. Philadelphia: Lea & Febiger; 1992:1003–1016.
2. Getty R. Sisson and Grossman's anatomy of the domestic animals. Philadelphia: WB Saunders; 1975:296–297.
3. Worthy K, Escreet R, Renton JP. Plasma prolactin concentrations and cyclic activity in pony mares during parturition and early lactation. Journal of Reproduction and Fertility Supplement 1986; 77:569–574.
4. Forsythe IA, Rossdale PD, Thomas CR. Studies on milk composition and lactogenic hormones in the mare. Journal of Reproduction and Fertility Supplement 1975; 23:631–635.
5. Sharma OP. Release of oxytocin elicited by suckling stimulus in mares. Journal of Reproduction and Fertility Supplement 1974; 37:421–423.
6. Ellendorf F, Schams D. Characteristics of milk ejection, associated intramammary pressure changes and oxytocin release in the mare. Journal of Endocrinology 1988; 119:219–227.
7. Schryver HF, Parker MT, Daniluk PD, et al. Lactation in the horse: the mineral composition of mare milk. Journal of Nutrition 1986; 116:2142–2147.
8. Ousey JC, Dudan F, Rossdale PD. Preliminary studies of mammary secretions in the mare to assess foetal readiness for birth. Equine Veterinary Journal 1984; 16:259–263.
9. McCue PM. Lactation. In: McKinnon AO, Voss JL, eds. Equine reproduction. Philadelphia: Lea & Febiger; 1992:589–984.
10. Hintz HF. Eclampsia. In: Robinson NE, ed. Current therapy in equine medicine. Philadelphia: WB Saunders; 1983:111.
11. Cowles RR. Lactation failure in the mare. Proceedings of the Society of Theriogenology 1983:222–233.
12. Green EM, Loch WE. Fescue-induced agalactia in mares: management and treatment. Proceedings of the American College of Veterinary Internal Medicine Forum 1990:551–553.
13. Riet-Correa F, Mendez MC, Schild AL, et al. Agalactia, reproductive problems, and neonatal mortality in horses associated with the ingestion of *Claviceps purpurea*. Australian Veterinary Journal 1988; 65:192–193.
14. Henton JE, Lothrop CD, Dean D, et al. Agalactia in the mare: a review and some new insights. Proceedings of the Society of Theriogenology 1983:203–221.
15. Lothrop CD, Henton JE, Cole BB, et al. Prolactin response to thyrotropin-releasing hormone stimulation in normal and agalactic mares. Journal of Reproduction and Fertility Supplement 1987; 35:277–280.
16. Johnson AL, Becker SE. Effects of physiologic and pharmacologic agents on serum prolactin concentrations in the non-pregnant mare. Journal of Animal Science 1987; 65:1292–1297.
17. Caudle AB. Effects of thyrotropin releasing hormone in agalactic mares. Proceedings of the Society of Theriogenology 1984:235.
18. Loch W, Worthy K, Ireland F. The effect of phenothiazine on plasma prolactin levels in non-pregnant mares. Equine Veterinary Journal 1990; 22:30–32.
19. Roberts SJ. Veterinary obstetrics and genital diseases (theriogenology). 3rd edn. Woodstock; 1986:528–531.
20. Roberts M. *Pseudomonas aeruginosa* mastitis in a dry, non-pregnant pony mare. Equine Veterinary Journal 1986; 18:146.
21. Pugh D, Magnussen R, Modransky P, et al. A case of mastitis in a young filly. Equine Veterinary Science 1985; 5:132.
22. McCue PM, Wilson WD. Equine mastitis: a review of 28 cases. Equine Veterinary Journal 1989; 21:351–353.
23. Perkins NR, Threlfall WR. Mastitis in the mare. Equine Veterinary Education 1993; 5:192–194.
24. Freeman K. Cytological evaluation of the equine mammary gland. Equine Veterinary Education 1993; 5:212–214.
25. Freeman K, Roszel J, Slusher S, et al. Cytologic features of equine mammary fluids: normal and abnormal. Compendium for Continuing Education 1988; 10:1090–1094.
26. Acland HM, Gillette DM. Mammary carcinoma in a mare. Veterinary Pathology 1982; 19:93–95.
27. Moulton JE. Tumors of domestic animals. Berkeley: University of California Press; 1961.
28. Martel H. Cancer in horses. American Veterinary Review 1913; 44:299–300.
29. Schmahl VW. Solides Karzinom der Mamma bei einen Pferd. Berliner und Muenchener Tieraerztliche Wochenschrift 1972; 85:141–142.
30. Surmont J. l'Epitheliome mammaire de la jument et ses metastases pulmonaires. Bulletin of the French Cancer Association 1926; 15:98–101.
31. Foreman JH, Weidner JP, Parry BW, et al. Pleural effusion secondary to thoracic metastatic mammary adenocarcinoma in a mare. Journal of the American Veterinary Medical Association 1990; 197:1193–1195.

Chapter 11

THE NEWBORN FOAL

Derek Knottenbelt

NEONATAL PHYSIOLOGY

The changes that the newborn foal must make at birth are very profound, involving to a lesser or greater degree almost all the body systems.

CARDIORESPIRATORY ADAPTATION

The transition from a fetus that is protected and nourished within the uterus to the free-living neonatal foal is probably the most profound change the foal will have to face. Airway clearance and the establishment of a normal respiratory function are vital. This is integrally coordinated with the cardiovascular adaptations that need to occur. Passage of the foal through the birth canal provides significant beneficial thoracic compression to drive excess fluid from the airway. Foals delivered by cesarean section do not have this mechanism and so need extra care for a clear airway to be established.

At the moment of birth the lungs must expand and the pulmonary circulation 'switched-on' to ensure a perfect ventilation–perfusion match between the two sides of the circulatory system. The change to pulmonary breathing and the circulatory adjustments that must accompany such a change within minutes of birth must be perfect if the foal is to survive and be able to move quickly to ensure safety.[1] Up to this point the blood from the pulmonary artery is shunted via the ductus arteriosus into the aortic circulation as a result of the high resistance afforded by the collapsed lungs and the relatively low aortic pressure. Oxygen-saturated blood arriving in the caudal vena cava from the placental vessels passes through the foramen ovale to the left atrium so that the brain receives freshly oxygenated blood. This pathway is obliterated within the first few weeks of life.[2]

At the moment of birth the lungs expand in response to a dramatic rise in PCO_2. This reduces the pressure in the pulmonary artery to below that in the aorta and so blood is directed into the lungs, with some being shunted by the relatively high aortic pressure into the pulmonary artery. At the same time there is no further need for the foramen ovale. The highly elastic nature of the ductus arteriosus means that some shunting one way or the other is present for up to 48–72 hours, but thereafter the ductus closes and becomes a fibrous band.

In the newborn foal respiration is often gasping in character and necessarily rapid as the foal attempts first to ensure full insufflation of the lungs and then to correct the acid–base imbalances that have arisen during the birth process. The efficiency of oxygenation of the blood is profoundly affected by the breathing pattern and any decrease in ventilation can alter the blood oxygen severely (and possibly dangerously).

The position the foal adopts also influences the oxygenation of blood. A foal in lateral recumbency may have a markedly lower partial pressure of arterial oxygen than one in sternal recumbency. This forms one of the most important principles of the management of neonatal foals. Also, the chest wall of the newborn foal is very compliant and so any respiratory disorder may have a disproportionate adverse influence on lung efficiency.[3]

Cardiac murmurs in foals

Although congenital defects of the heart and great vessels are rare, up to 90% of newborn foals have obvious continuous murmurs associated with a patent ductus arteriosus that are audible over the left base of the heart for the first 15–30 minutes of life.[4] In most cases the murmurs will not be audible by 72 hours, but some may persist for some weeks.[5] Murmurs are also commonly associated with sepsis, fever, anemia, etc.; these may vary from day to day.

> Note:
> - A ventricular septal defect presents a persistent, severe, systolic murmur associated with left–right shunt that increases with exercise. The murmur is usually more audible on the right side of the chest but may be inaudible or left-sided.

If cyanosis is present with a murmur it may indicate:

- Respiratory distress syndrome or pneumonia with functional murmur.
- A significant congenital heart lesion resulting in pulmonary overcirculation/edema.
- Complex heart defects with right–left shunting, causing systemic arterial desaturation.

Arrhythmia, including atrial fibrillation, atrial tachycardia and ventricular depolarization, is also common in newborn foals within the first 15–30 minutes of life. However, although such events could be alarming they are almost invariably due to high vagal tone and will resolve spontaneously over a short period.[6] It may be unwise to perform an electrocardiographic examination on a very new foal because the results may be misleadingly alarming. Differentiation of the abnormal is the challenge for the clinician.

LOCOMOTION

The foal needs to rise quickly to its feet and to move with certainty. This means that the muscles and skeleton also need to adapt quickly to new forces and functions. This also involves the nervous system, which has to perform a vast range of functions that have been only 'tested' in utero. It would be a major disadvantage if a full-term foal were to practice and develop the full range of muscular activity in utero. There is some evidence that in utero movement of the foal becomes progressively more limited in the last months of pregnancy. Owners might therefore report that the foal's movements have reduced or may even have apparently stopped altogether, suggesting that there may be a problem with the pregnancy. The limited movement in the later stages of pregnancy may predispose the relatively long-legged foal to abnormalities of growth and discrepancies between bony growth (over which there is almost no control) and tendon/ligament growth (which is probably coordinated by movement, posture and forces applied during their development).

ALIMENTATION

The next obvious major adaptation is the change from placental nutrition to alimentation. In order for the foal to feed effectively it must first have a perception/instinct to rise and then to seek the teat. Sight may be less important than would be expected but it obviously helps. Having once located the teat it must be in a position to suckle effectively and to swallow. Once swallowed, the milk must be delivered to the gastrointestinal tract and then digested efficiently. The gut must be fully patent to the anus and there should be no physical, neurological or other obstruction. The waste material from the digestive processes, which have also been going on during gestation (the meconium), have to be passed shortly after birth. The residues from digestion of colostrum support this by a laxative effect.

Milk is the source of nutrients for the neonatal mammal and the composition of the mammary secretion changes considerably with time.[7] In the first hours after birth the milk is rich in immunoglobulins (colostrum). It is tempting to assume that milk provides all the nutritional requirements for the foal. However, in the longer term this is not necessarily so; foals need to supplement the milk feed with other ingesta within weeks of birth and will often be seen to take grass or hay within days of birth. Although natural mare's milk is used to provide the formula for the preparation of artificial milk supplements, it does contain a delicately balanced variety of essential nutrients, including vitamins, minerals and enzymes, and artificial milk replacers are unlikely ever to match the gold standard of normal milk for any particular species.

The normal foal has a defined demand for food materials, but the abnormal or sick foal will inevitably have an increased demand for all the components. The demand for energy is often at least 50% above normal and can be much higher. The same applies to protein and fats as well as minerals and vitamins. Premature foals require extra food to complete organ maturation, but infection, fever, etc. place extreme demands on the foal's ability to ingest enough raw materials. In reality, a sick foal often has a reduced appetite and so can easily fall into a downward spiral.

The specific requirements of the normal newborn foal are:

- Energy: 120–150 kcal/day.
- Protein: 5.5–6.0 g/kg/day.

Normal feeding should result in a normal growth rate (weight gain) of around 1.25–1.5 kg/day in a Thoroughbred foal.

- The normal birth weight of a Thoroughbred foal is 46–52 kg (42–48 kg for primiparae).

NEUROLOGICAL FUNCTION

The nervous system has an additional role in the adaptive period with the employment of the senses and mentation, including maternal imprinting/recognition and behavior. Survival will clearly depend on these as much as the ability to stand and breathe.

RENAL FUNCTION

Urinary excretion begins during gestation, with passage of urine into the bladder and then into the allantoic space. A smaller volume of urine will pass into the amniotic fluid via the urethra. The mean urine production in a neonatal foal is around 145–155 ml/kg bodyweight per day.[8] This figure is far higher than in mature horses. These factors can be explained simply by the fact that the neonatal kidney is not functionally mature at birth and so renal concentration of urine is much less efficient than in adult horses. Foal urine is frequently more dilute than that of adult horses. The naturally high fluid intake and the lack of concentrating ability means that a foal's urine has a naturally low specific gravity. The inability to concentrate urine means that it may remain relatively dilute in the face of dehydrating conditions that might otherwise be expected to cause urinary concentration. Foals also often have a relatively high urinary protein concentration[9] and this can be significant, even in the normal foal. Furthermore the ability of the kidney to withstand toxic insult and to excrete some drugs etc. efficiently may be very immature. Therefore, drugs and chemicals that damage renal tissue might be expected to have an enhanced toxicity in foals.

The first passage of urine is an important event with respect to neonatal assessment (see p. 371). Colt foals usually pass their first urine at around 5–6 hours of age. By contrast, filly foals may delay their first micturition up to 10–11 hours. Observation of the first and subsequent micturition is an important stud procedure and the timing of the first natural urination has implications for those foals that have urinary tract defects such as patent bladder or ruptured ureters.

ENDOCRINE FUNCTION

The development of the endocrine system is very complex, but again maturation should coordinate with the change to outside life. Reliance upon the endogenous homeostatic mechanisms for almost all biochemical functions of the body is paramount. Unfortunately, we are uncertain of the specific changes that occur in the foal. Most statements related to endocrine adaptation are extrapolated from other species, particularly man. Although the relevance of these is probably minimal, in any mammal there will clearly be similarities that are justifiably assumed to operate.

THERMAL REGULATION

The neonatal foal is born wet and even in the best of circumstances will have to withstand a thermal shock at the time of birth. The ambient temperature is rarely high enough to overcome heat lost by evaporation or by direct loss into the cold undersurface. The considerable muscular effort that foals exert at the time of birth will compensate for some of this, but there is almost inevitably a fall in body temperature at birth.[10] Body temperatures below 37°C are regarded as hypothermic and can precipitate a shock-like state. Significantly, hyperthermia can also have serious effects on the foal and temperatures above 40°C can cause convulsions and coma.

ASSESSMENT OF A FOAL'S RISK CATEGORY

The concept of a risk category for foals[11] has been used for many years and has been instrumental in saving many lives. A system involving three broad categories, in which the foal is classed as high-risk, moderate-risk or low-risk, is most widely used.[12] This is simple and serves the purpose well. A two-category classification is a simpler method that avoids the equivocal moderate category and has the advantage that more foals will be classified as high-risk and are therefore likely to be monitored more closely. The recognition that a problem might be present will enable the clinician to take pre-emptive measures to minimize any clinical consequences. On the basis that prevention is better than cure, the system has much to commend it. The concept should be used to guide the level of supervision and interference for a newborn foal. All management strategies for pregnant mares should be directed towards detection of potential or actual problems before they are so advanced that therapy may not be effective.

Why is risk categorization useful?

An assessment of the likely risk category of the foal will be of considerable benefit to its survival. A predesignated high-risk foaling provides a good chance of improving the survival rate by taking suitable planned measures in advance. Some factors can be predicted (particularly those relating to the mare and her breeding history) but others become significant as the pregnancy and parturition advance. In considering these factors the reproductive and general history of the mare and the pregnancy is paramount. Furthermore, it is important to regularly assess both mare and the unborn foal during gestation so that potential problems can be identified early.

It is virtually impossible to categorize mares without any historical information and in this case they should probably be classified as high-risk immediately. The major problem here is that those with no history are probably those that are of less importance to their owners and their classification may be less significant.

High-risk mares are therefore those in which possible complications can be expected. This means that parturition can be monitored closely and completely. In this way a higher foal survival rate can be expected. An additional benefit is that the survival rate of mares can also be improved and in most such cases their future fertility can be supported.

- Risk factors can be predicted from an accurate history of the mare and the pregnancy.
- Some of the factors that direct the classification of risk category of the foal will arise during the delivery or immediately afterwards. Therefore, while a foal could fit into the low-risk category until delivery it could be reclassified into a higher risk category as a result of events during or immediately after delivery. The clinician will need to be flexible in the classification and take appropriate steps to ensure that the foal has the best possible chance of survival.

- For example:
- If during a routine late-gestation check in a low-risk mare significant udder development is observed and there is ultrasonographic evidence of placental edema or separation, the pregnancy can immediately be classified as high-risk. Repeated examinations at sensible intervals may then allow this to be monitored up to and including delivery.
- A foal that is born to a low-risk mare could be exposed to traumatic events or infection at the time of birth; it should then immediately be reclassified as high-risk.

High-risk foals

These are cases in which there is a significant danger to the life of the foal as a result of:

- Maternal circumstances and conditions.
- Events occurring around and during parturition.
- Conditions and circumstances arising immediately after delivery of the foal.

Maternal conditions

Factors that are present at any stage before birth may have a profound effect on the prognosis for the pregnancy (see Table 11.1). In particular, any factors that influence placental nourishment of the foal or subsequent colostrum production are of major importance.

Table 11.1 Possible consequences of maternal conditions on the foal

Maternal status	Consequence on foal
• Virus/bacterial infection	• Infection (sepsis) • Poor-quality/quantity of colostrum • Placentitis/abortion/sepsis
• Uterine torsion • Hydrops allantois	• Placentitis • Neonatal maladjustment • Dysmaturity
• Colostral leakage • Placental insufficiency	• Failure of passive transfer
• Isoantibodies (anti-A/ anti-Q) in serum	• Neonatal isoerythrolysis
• Anemia • Toxemia • Cardiovascular compromise	• Dysmaturity • Stillborn • Abortion
• Weight loss	• Dysmaturity • Weakness • Slow adaptation
• Transport/stress	• Dysmaturity • Prematurity • Abortion • Infection
• Intercurrent disease • Drug treatments of any sort	• Poor growth • Hypothyroidism • Fetal depression • Slow delivery • Gastric ulceration syndrome • Toxemia • Infection
• Surgery/anesthesia	• Abortion • Hypoxia • 'Red bag' delivery • Infection

- Prolonged or shortened pregnancy.
- Discrepancy between size of foal and size of mare and her birth canal.
- History of problem foals (e.g. dysmature/premature, neonatal isoerythrolysis, neonatal maladjustment/asphyxia syndrome, congenital defects).
- History of previous uterine torsion in present or previous pregnancy.
- History of colostral leakage or premature lactation prior to delivery.
- Purulent vaginal discharge or vaginal bleeding.
- Disease/injury with or without drug administration.
- Pelvic injuries (fresh or long-standing), or space-occupying lesions that might alter the dimensions and congruity of the birth canal.
- Lameness or neurological disorders that prevent normal behavior and posture prior to and during delivery.
- Pyrexia/toxemia/septicemia/endotoxemia.
- Poor bodily condition/poor nutritional status (primary or secondary).
- Hydrops amni (very rare).
- Colic/colic surgery/other surgery (cesarean section or uterine torsion)/anesthesia.
- Primiparous delivery (especially if suspect behavior) or history of aggression.
- Twin pregnancy.
- Transport prior to delivery (last 4 weeks of gestation).

Parturition conditions

Factors affecting the process of parturition would necessarily have a profound effect on the viability of the foal (see Table 11.2). Any factor that affects the ability of the foal to adapt (e.g. loss of blood from early cord separation may cause a slow adaptive period and inability to rise) will have significance:

- Prematurity (gestational age <320 days) (see p. 372).
- Prolonged gestation (overdue foal).
- Prolonged labor/dystocia.
- Perineal laceration/rectovaginal fistulae.
- 'Red bag' delivery (early placental separation).
- Premature rupture of fetal membranes.
- Induced parturition.
- Colostral leakage/early lactation.
- Early (premature) cord separation.
- Uterine bruising/tearing.
- Vaginal blood loss from mare.
- Cesarean section.

Factors involving the foal itself or becoming apparent in the foal at delivery

- Obvious congenital abnormalities (in any organ system).
- Weakness or 'small for breed' foals.
- Meconium staining of foal or fetal membranes.

Table 11.2 Possible consequences of parturition conditions on the foal

Parturition disorders	Consequence on foal
Prematurity	• Poor adaptation • Poor respiratory function • Poor feeding
Prolonged gestation	• Poor size • Adrenal insufficiency • Limb abnormalities • Neurologic abnormalities
Prolonged labor/dystocia	• Fetal hypoxia • Neonatal maladjustment • Sepsis
Perineal lacerations/fistulation	• Slow delivery • Early placental separation • Blood loss
Early placental separation/'red bag' delivery	• Hypoxia • Neonatal maladjustment • Death
Induced parturition	• Hypoxia • Poor maturation • Slow adaptation
Colostral leakage	• Failed passive transfer • Infection/sepsis
Early cord separation	• Hypoxia • Weakness • Secondary consequences such as inability to feed
Cesarean section	• Hypoxia • Poor colostral intake • Poor maturity
Uterine bruising/bleeding/hematoma	• Depressed mare with poor mothering

- Trauma/predation.
- Potential infection (poor hygiene or management).
- Low or no colostral intake (either because of disability or lack of natural behavior).
- Twin foals.
- Death of dam.

Low-risk foals

A foal can be classified as low risk if:

- There are no maternal factors that might adversely affect survival of the foal.
- Gestation is of normal duration and there have been no complications with the health of the mare during pregnancy (or any previous pregnancy).

Note:
- Mean gestation length is 340 days (range 330–350 days). However, normal gestation can be well in excess of 350 days and there are many reports of pregnancies of over 365 days resulting in a normal foal).

- Delivery of the foal is normal and without complication or delays.

> Note:
> - Parturition should in this classification take no more than 20–30 minutes from start to finish.
> - No manipulation or interference is required either to the foal or to the mare.

- The adaptive period should be normal with the foal standing within 2 hours and suckling by 3 hours.
- Colostral intake is effective and raises the foal's IgG concentration to over 8–10 g/l.
- The placenta is normal and is passed freely.
- There are no external dangers (such as infections in other horses, inclement weather, predators, etc.).

Moderate-risk foals

A foal is classified as moderate-risk if only one of the factors that increase its risk is present. Such factors could involve either the mare or the foal itself. In this respect, it is important to remember that the placenta is derived entirely from the foal; there is no component of the placental membranes that belongs to the mare.

> Note:
> - In practical situations a classification of high-risk or low-risk is an effective compromise because a moderate risk may serve only to over-emphasize minor problems or under-emphasize the more major ones.

EVENTS FOLLOWING DELIVERY IN THE NORMAL FOAL (THE ADAPTIVE PERIOD)

The adaptive period is the time during which the foal must adjust from the uterine environment to the 'independent dependence' of extrauterine life.

It is important to recognize the normal events that take place (see Table 11.3) so that any abnormal events can be quickly recognized and appropriate corrective action taken. Unfortunately, there are wide variations in the normal pattern of delivery and neonatal adaptation, thus making the decision to interfere difficult. The extent of veterinary intervention will often depend heavily on the experience of the

Table 11.3 Events occurring in foals during the first 72 hours of life

Time (age)	Body temperature (°C)	Pulse (per minute)	Respiration (per minute)	Notes
0–1 minute	37.5	70–80	70	<ul><li>Hypoxia</li><li>Metabolic and respiratory acidosis</li><li>Breaks amnion by limb/head movement</li></ul>
2–30 minutes	38.0	120–140	50	<ul><li>Cord rupture</li><li>Shivering</li><li>Righting reflex</li><li>Sucking movements</li><li>Attempts to stand</li></ul>
1–12 hours	38.0	140–150	40	<ul><li>Coordination</li><li>Auditory/visual responses</li><li>STANDING <2 hours</li><li>Teat-seeking</li><li>EFFECTIVE FEEDING <3 hours</li><li>PASSAGE OF FIRST MECONIUM</li><li>FIRST URINATION</li><li>Acidosis ↓</li><li>Lactate ↓</li></ul>
12–18 hours	38.0	110–120	35	<ul><li>Maternal bonding</li><li>End of colostrum feeding/absorption</li><li>Meconium passing</li></ul>
24–48 hours	38.0	90–100	30	<ul><li>Increasing muscular activity</li><li>Last meconium passed</li></ul>
48–72 hours	38.0	60–80	20	<ul><li>Full coordination</li><li>Environmental exploration</li><li>Closure of ductus arteriosus</li><li>Urine/feces normal</li></ul>

owner/handler or groom. More experienced grooms may not need anything like as much support and will also often recognize problems earlier than less experienced grooms. Furthermore, the value of the foal and any complications during pregnancy will often dictate the role of the veterinary surgeon. Probably the majority of foalings attended by veterinarians are recognizably abnormal in some respect.

The recognition of abnormalities can be more difficult than would appear. Intervention needs to be limited but sensible. There is little point in leaving an obviously abnormal situation to sort itself out; conversely, interfering when there is no need to do so can do harm.

- The foal is delivered during second-stage labor. Usually the foal is within the amnion, which usually breaks spontaneously as a result of opposing movements of the forelimbs and head.
- The foal takes its first breaths with chest and abdominal movements (usually within 30 seconds of delivery of the chest). There may be a series of initial gasps with neck arching.
  - ❏ This is not a signal for intervention unless the cord has separated.
- The normal respiratory pattern is rapidly established. The newborn foal will show fast and deep breathing; this is accompanied by a dramatic rise in arterial blood oxygen (PaO_2) which progressively increases with increasing muscular effort. There are significant other signs for a similar increase in respiration rate (see below).
- The mare will usually undergo a period of tranquility (lasting up to 40 minutes), during which time the foal shakes its head and gains sternal recumbency with 'righting reflex'. Throughout this the mare remains quiet (usually in sternal recumbency) and will often vocalize to the foal.
  - ❏ This is not a sign for intervention.
- The foal may show strong blinking reflexes as hearing and vision are established. It may whinny on its own or in response to the mare. The foal's head bobs up and down markedly, and suckling responses with lips and mouth are present with increasing strength.
- The foal struggles and moves to the side of the mare. Usually the cord ruptures at this time, either because the foal moves or because the mare stands up. The cord usually ruptures about 6–8 minutes after delivery at a predetermined site (3–5 cm from the umbilicus). Shorter ruptures may have serious consequences, including internal hemorrhage. Severe tension on the cord at the umbilicus may also cause serious internal bleeding (although this is very rare). Premature rupture of the cord may compromise the foal (up to 25–30% of the foal blood volume can be lost).

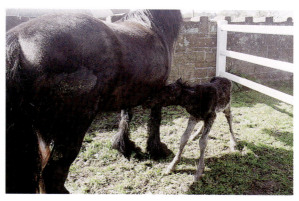

Fig. 11.1 Foal seeking the teat.

- The mare nuzzles, licks and encourages the foal. In response, the foal makes its first attempts to stand, usually within 30 minutes of delivery.
- Normal foals will stand by around 45–90 minutes after delivery (often with apparent incoordination); they may fall several times before establishing a steady stance and the ability to move. A normal foal may take up to 2 hours before standing, but the longer it takes the greater the likelihood of a problem being present.
- The foal then seeks the mare's udder (Fig. 11.1). This is often aimless at first but increases in accuracy. Once the teat is located a strong suckling reflex is established. The first effective suckling takes place within 60–90 minutes of delivery. In response, the mare will 'let down her milk' and the colostrum will be seen to stream from the teats.
- After about 30–60 minutes (especially if a feed has been successfully obtained) the foal will lie down again. The foal may make its first energetic steps on rising again, may jump up and down, and may then fall again. All foals have an inherent incoordination and may seem to be ataxic for the first 24 hours.

Note:
- The amnion must be distinguished from the chorioallantois and bladder.
- The correct time of interference needs to be recognized; minimal interference is desirable.
- Cutting the amnion is sometimes a desirable safety precaution; the foal's nose can be uncovered and there is then less risk of asphyxia. However, it is important not to disturb the mare if at all possible while this is done.

- Cord rupture usually causes slight blood flow, most often from the placental end (venous flow at low pressure). Severe arterial blood loss from the umbilical end of a ruptured cord requires immediate attention: clamp with sterile artery forceps or umbilical clamp (plastic bag clamps are useful). The cord should not be tied with string, etc.

- Dress the navel (e.g. with teat dip or povidone iodine solution, chlorhexidine or antibiotic spray) within 30 minutes of delivery. Recent work suggests that the best results are obtained with chlorhexidine and that povidone iodine may not be as effective as was first thought.[13] Ensure thorough soaking of the navel but avoid over-handling. Aerosol sprays may give a false impression of their effectiveness because they are under mild pressure and their cover is more defined and can be seen, but the antibacterial effects are probably poor and nonpersistent. The antibiotic may not be effective against the organisms present (many significant Gram-negative bacteria, including *Escherichia coli*, are tetracycline-resistant).

- Full hygiene measures are imperative for anyone handling the foal. It is remarkable how few stud personnel have any concept of cleanliness when handling foals and parturient mares.

- It is advisable to wear gloves and overalls that can be changed frequently on every occasion when dealing with neonatal foals (preferably protective clothing should be changed between different foals). Washing hands and changing overalls frequently also minimizes cross-contamination between mares foaling at the same time.

- All reasonable hygiene precautions should be in effect at all times, including the provision of freshly washed or disposable aprons/gowns for each mare/foal and for each stud. It is best to advise the stud to maintain a stock of these for their own personnel and for visiting veterinarians.

EVALUATION OF THE NEWBORN FOAL

Evaluation of the newborn foal is very important as it provides the first and earliest opportunity to assess its potential viability. It also allows a veterinarian to assess whether there is anything that needs to be addressed immediately, such as provision of oxygen, artificial (positive-pressure) ventilation, blood transfusion, antibiotics, etc.

Foals are best scored at 1–3 minutes of age. Note, however, that foaling mares exhibit a natural period of tranquility following the expulsion of the foal (the foal usually still has its hind legs in the birth canal). During this stage the foal's umbilical circulation is still very active (a pulse is still palpable in the umbilical artery) and the uterus is actively contracting. This causes a progressive arterial resistance and an active return of the foal's venous blood into its systemic circulation. This is a very important stage of delivery and disturbances to assess the foal at this stage may be counterproductive. Early rupture of the cord resulting from early disturbance of the mare may result in significant deprivation for the foal. Up to 1 liter of circulating blood may be left in the placental circulation when rupture is rapid. Adaptation must under these circumstances be abrupt and this allows little scope for interference in the event of a problem.

The APGAR scoring system[14]

The APGAR system is a scoring system that is used to assess Appearance, Pulse (rate), Grimace (response), Activity (muscle tone), and Respiration (rate). It is a simple method that can be used for the immediate assessment of the foal during the first 3 minutes of birth (see Table 11.4). A more complex system in which muscular activity parameters carry a higher loading can be used in specialist hospitals for older foals (up to 2 hours) (see Table 11.5).

- Provided problems are recognized early, even some seriously depressed foals can be saved with effective intensive care. Some conditions arise before birth, so accurate history and careful clinical assessment is vital. Owners can be taught to assess the foal at birth; this does not reduce the necessity for a full examination as soon after birth as possible.

- Many high-risk foals look relatively normal at birth and up to 12–18 hours of age. Once problems develop, deterioration is usually rapid. This makes early recognition of problems an important management procedure.

- Newborn foals that are high-risk or that show any evidence of respiratory or neurological (or other) compromise, should be subjected to APGAR scoring at regular intervals over the first 30 minutes. Apparently normal foals should be scored only once and then left alone.

ROUTINE VETERINARY AND MANAGEMENT PROCEDURES FOR A NEWBORN FOAL

In performing the following procedures, the groom/ veterinarian must balance the need to interfere against the possible disturbance that this creates. If a foal is delivered in a safe clean environment, little

Table 11.4 APGAR scoring method for the assessment of a foal within 3 minutes of birth

	Score		
	0	1	2
Heart rate (per minute)	Undetectable	<60	>60
Respiratory rate (per minute)	Undetectable	Slow/irregular	Regular, >60
Muscle tone	Limp	Extremity flexion	Sternal recumbency
Nasal stimulation	No response	Grimace/movement	Sneeze/active rejection

Score: normal, 7–8; moderately depressed, 4–6; markedly depressed, 1–4; 0, dead.

Table 11.5 Advanced APGAR score sheet for foals (at 10 minutes of age)

	Score		
	0	1	2
Pulse (per minute)	Absent	<60 or irregular	>60 or regular
Respiration (per minute)	Absent	<60, irregular	>60, regular
Muscle tone	Flaccid	Sluggish attempts to sit up	Sternal recumbency
Ear tickle	No response	Slight head shake	Shakes head/moves head away
Nose stimulus	No response	Moves head	Grimace/sneezes/moves away
Rump scratch	No response	Moves/no attempt to stand	Attempts to stand
Mucous membrane color	Gray/blue	Pale pink	Pink

Interpretation and actions: 11–14, normal (continue to monitor; avoid interference); 7–10, moderate depression (administer nasal oxygen; stimulation by external rubbing; encourage sternal recumbency); 2–6, severe depression (administer doxapram, nasal oxygen; external stimulation; encourage sternal recumbency); 0–2, dead or almost dead (administer artificial respiration and full cardiopulmonary resuscitation for limited time only; do not waste time on these foals).

interference should be required and routine procedures can be delayed until the foal is standing and has bonded with the mare.

1. Establish a clear airway

- Gravity can be used to help; slope the foal down from the tail end. Lifting the foal by the back legs can be used, but is difficult and very disturbing to the mare.
- If necessary use aspiration (short sharp aspirations are better than prolonged suction). Suitable suction/aspiration systems are available in disposable form.
- Ventilation can be encouraged by gently blowing into the nose or by using a mask system fitted to a pressure-limited pump.

2. Umbilical care

- Ideally the navel should be immersed in a 0.5% solution of chlorhexidine (this should be repeated every 6 hours for the first 24 hours).
- The use of povidone iodine for this purpose has been called into question.[15] Strong solutions of iodine or tincture of iodine can cause burning and necrosis of the umbilical stump.
- Aerosolized antibiotic sprays (e.g. tetracycline) are useful in that they dry the moist stump while applying a dose of antibiotic but have very limited efficacy and short duration.

3. Administration of colostrum by nasogastric tube

- At birth, oral nutrient intake becomes the sole source of nutrition and the importance of colostral antibody transfer cannot be overstated.

Note:
- It is routine practice on many stud farms to administer 250–300 ml of good-quality colostrum to newborn foals. The merits of this are viewed as greater than the unwanted consequences of disturbance or stress.
- Many practitioners and stud owners believe that this measure is essential for the health of the newborn foal. Not only does it ensure good colostrum intake but it is also suggested to be an important measure for encouraging passage of meconium.
- Foals receiving immediate colostrum probably have a higher overall survival rate than those that are left to their own devices.

- Newborn foals can easily be intubated. A soft rubber tube (diameter <1 cm) is best and can be passed up the ventral meatus of the nose. Passage up the middle meatus is more difficult and tends to induce significant ethmoidal damage and bleeding.

- Always use as small a tube as possible that is consistent with requirements. Enteral feeding tubes are very much smaller and well tolerated, even allowing normal feeding to take place with the tube in situ.
- Usually the act of swallowing can be felt and the tube advanced gently but swiftly.

Note:
- Do not introduce any material down the tube until it is certain that the tube is in the esophagus.
- If you can blow and suck on the end of the tube, it is likely that it is in the trachea.
- If you cannot blow or suck, it is likely that the tube is kinked over itself and must be carefully withdrawn. Severe trauma can occur when this happens.
- If you can blow but cannot suck, the tube is most likely in the esophagus.
- The passage of the tube down the esophagus can usually be seen in the left jugular furrow.
- The tube can usually easily be palpated in the neck.
- There is usually some resistance to the passage of the tube in the esophagus.
- There is no resistance to the tube in the trachea and it may be 'rattled' within it.
- If the foal coughs it is likely that the tube is in the trachea.
- Aspiration of stomach contents means that the tube is correctly placed.

Long-term enteral nasogastric tubes can be introduced through a wider tube, which can then be removed. Enteral feeding tubes are commercially available (Nutrifoal Tubes®). These tubes have a bag attachment for feeding up to 3 liters of liquid feed. It is essential to measure the length required before insertion; there have been occasions when extra length inserted into the stomach has caused the tube to tie itself into a knot, making removal impossible. The end of the tube should preferably be in the distal esophagus. Suture the end of the tube into the nostril or glue are tape to head collar (foal slip) to prevent rub removal. When using a long-term tube there is no need for the tube to reach the stomach; there is a slight risk of knotting if too much length is introduced. Wide tubes make for easier insertion but have a higher incidence of pharyngeal damage (including necrosis, abscessation, and inflammation); thin tubes are more inclined to blockage and can be rejected from the esophagus.

Once the tube is in position it should be briefly flushed with warm water and the end plugged. Aspiration of air can be a serious complication of long-term stomach tubes if the tube is left open.

Larger tubes can be left in situ for 24–36 hours (not longer), but enteral feeding tubes are well-tolerated for up to 4 days. Indicators for removal and replacement of the tube include:

- Pain.
- Coughing.
- Dysphagia and/or repeated swallowing.
- Nasal bleeding.

It is important to remember that a foal needs very small feeds repeated at regular intervals to try to mimic the natural state of feeding.

Nasal oxygen tubes are well tolerated by sick foals but less so as the foal gets better. The tube should be inserted so that the tip lies just within the internal nares. If the tube is advanced further it may induce repeated swallowing and less induces repeated sneezing/rejection.

4. Vaccination

Many studs routinely administer 3000–6000 IU tetanus antitoxin at, or soon after, birth regardless of the vaccination status of the mare. Tetanus vaccination (toxoid) can, in theory, be administered at birth but it is common practice to delay this for 2–3 weeks even in foals delivered to unvaccinated mares.

5. Antibiotics

A routine injection of a long-acting formulation of benzathine/procaine penicillin is commonly administered at birth or shortly afterwards. A full 3–5-day course of antibiotics is essential and best practice. Although the choice of penicillin would not seem to be the most appropriate as a prophylactic measure for neonatal septicemia (most such infections are Gram-negative against which simple penicillin has little or no effect), the occasional staphylococcal or streptococcal infection may be prevented by this.

6. Laboratory

The foal should be blood sampled (see below) at 12–16 hours for estimation of colostral transfer (IgG) and for routine hematology and biochemistry (see Table 11.6). At this stage the earliest evidence for impending problems can often be detected. If there is any suspicion of a problem, blood culture should be set up immediately. Cultures routinely take over 24 hours to yield any useful results. Although this can be a valuable prophylactic measure, it is an expensive procedure.

Blood sampling

Venous sampling

Foals are very liable to venous/jugular thrombosis and thrombophlebitis and every care needs to be taken to ensure that:

- The minimum number of venepunctures consistent with requirements are performed.

Table 11.6 Changes in a foal's hematology and biochemistry parameters over the first 7 days of life

	Birth	24 hours	7 days
Hemoglobin (g/l)	120–160		100–160[a]
Hematocrit (l/l)	0.32–046		0.28–0.44
Mean cell hemoglobin concentration (%)	32–40		34–36
Leukocyte count (×10⁹/liter)	5–12		6–13
Neutrophils (×10⁹/liter)	3.5–10.0		6.0–12.0
Eosinophils (×10⁹/liter)		0–0.2	
Lymphocytes (×10⁹/liter)	1.2–2.2		1.5–3.0
Monocytes (×10⁹/liter)		0.05–0.5	
Platelet count (×10⁹/liter)	100–250		150–400
Bilirubin (total) (μmol/l)		25–50	
Bilirubin (unconjugated) (μmol/l)		4–15	
Cholesterol (mmol/l)		2.5–3.5	
Triglycerides (μmol/l)		0.1–0.2	
Glucose (mmol/l)	3.0–3.5	4.0–5.0	4.0–5.5
Urea (mmol/l)	3.5–4.0		2.4–4.0
Total protein (plasma) (g/l)	45–47		60–62
Albumin (g/l)	25–28		22–25
Total globulin (g/l)	9–12		20–22
α-Globulin (g/l)	4–5		6.5–7.5
β-Globulin (g/l)		5.0–6.0	
γ-Globulin (g/l)	0	8.0–12.0	10–14
Fibrinogen (g/l)		1–3	
Serum amyloid A (U/l)		0–20	
Calcium (mmol/l)		2.5–4.0	
Inorganic phosphate (mmol/l)		2.2–5.2 (i.e. 2–3× adult levels)	
Sodium (mmol/l)		134–143	
Potassium (mmol/l)		3.5–5.5	
Chloride (mmol/l)		90–105	
Magnesium (mmol/l)		0.6–1.0	
Bicarbonate (mmol/l)	23	27	24
PCO₂ (mmol/l)		37–43[b]	
PO₂ (mmol/l)	77	83–98[c]	85–106
pH	7.36		7.39
Base excess (mmol/l)		0.9±1.0	
Cortisol (plasma) (nmol/l)	1.9–2.2	2.0–3.3	1.5–1.7
T₄ (thyroxine) (nmol/l)		12–18	
T₃ (tri-iodothyronine) (nmol/l)	3.5–12.6		4.0–18
Insulin (IU/l)	12–16		20–25
Alkaline phosphatase (IU/l)	<450 (up to 5× adult to 4 weeks, then 2× adult to 1 year)		
Creatine kinase (IU/l)		<50	
Aspartate transferase (IU/l)		<250	
Lactate dehydrogenase (total) (IU/l)		200–450	
Prothrombin time (seconds)		9.5–12.7	
Activated partial thromboplastin time (seconds)		29–59	

[a]Changes more quickly if cord ruptures early.
[b]Samples taken in lateral recumbency may be significantly higher: ±50 mmol/l.
[c]Samples taken in lateral recumbency may be significantly lower: ±75 mmol/l.

- Full aseptic precautions are taken, especially if blood cultures are to be performed.
- As small a needle as possible is used.

Note:
- Very fine needles may result in damage to cells, etc.
- Usually a 20/21-gauge needle is adequate.
- 16/18-gauge needles are unnecessary and traumatize the vein significantly.

Suitable venepuncture sites, which can also be used for catheter placement, include:

- Jugular veins (do not damage both).
- Cephalic veins.
- Lateral thoracic veins.

The umbilical vein(s) can be used in foals less than 24 hours of age but this carries a significant risk of navel infection/septicemia.

The placental vessels provide a good source of blood without the need to interfere with the foal at all immediately after delivery (within 2 minutes). The samples will need to be taken from the ruptured placental vessels immediately the foal is delivered so that the breaking of the cord can be directly observed. Sampling from the intact umbilical vessels before cord separation is simple but may disturb the mare. Placid, experienced mares may allow this to be performed without making any attempt to rise.

Note:
- Vacuum tubes are not generally regarded as good for collection of horse blood. The erythrocyte fragility is such that significant variations, damage and errors can be induced by their use.
- It is better to use a syringe and needle, and after removing the needle introduce the blood into the opened tube.

Samples for blood culture should be placed immediately in biphasic blood culture medium in full aseptic manner. Other samples collected in conventional blood collection vials are of no value for blood culture. Swabs are even worse and should not be taken for culture purposes.

Note:
- It is important to consider the exact type of samples that might be required before they are obtained.
- Calculate the volume required for the containers to be used.
- It is not correct to put 1–2 ml into a 10-ml tube containing EDTA or other anticoagulant; smaller containers should be used when only limited volumes of blood are required. Most laboratories now need only a few milliliters of blood, serum or plasma to perform extensive ranges of hematology and biochemistry. A specific test may require specific anticoagulants, so it is worth checking what the best sample is.

For example:
A platelet count can only be reliably estimated from a citrated sample, whereas blood glucose should be performed on a fluoride–oxalate sample.

Arterial sampling

Arterial blood can be obtained from:

- The tarsal artery (best).
- The transverse facial artery behind the eye.
- Femoral or carotid arteries.

Alternative sites include the median artery, the facial artery and the umbilical artery (in foals less than 24 hours old). The umbilical artery can easily be located by close examination of the navel. It is sometimes necessary to cut across the very end of the severed cord to reveal the three major structures. The artery is obvious and can be cannulated easily; a long catheter needs to be used (at least 30 cm). The risk of infection is very high.

- Full aseptic precautions must be taken and pressure applied to the site of puncture for at least 10 minutes after sampling is completed.
- Use specially prepared syringes (with heparin) and needles (Pulsator®, 3 ml with 0.7 mm × 25 gauge needle, single use arterial blood sampling system; Concord Laboratories, UK).
- Entry into the artery is indicated by the syringe self-filling.

CLINICAL EXAMINATION OF THE NEWBORN FOAL

It is impossible to perform a clinical examination of the foal without reference to the history relating to the dam, the pregnancy, and the foaling. The use of a proforma makes the examination simpler and the recording of the findings is important for subsequent examinations. Such a form helps ensure complete examination without serious omissions or errors. Events can change rapidly in foals and so repeated examinations are important to detect trends in physiological and pathological processes.

- The equine neonate can be difficult to examine effectively particularly when compromised or when very energetic.
- Some foals that are severely compromised by respiratory deficiencies can show considerable resistance to being handled and any attempt to forcibly restrain the foal may be counterproductive or dangerous.
- A detailed clinical examination should be performed on every foal; it is very easy to miss early signs of diseases that can progress rapidly beyond the point of recovery.

Disease is easily spread from stud to stud by fomites (fomites are substances, such as clothing, that are capable of absorbing and transmitting the contagium of disease) and contamination, so appropriate care needs to be exercised and demonstrated to lay persons. This has a beneficial effect upon the disease status of the studs in general and emphasizes the need for hygiene to the owners themselves.

PROTOCOL FOR EXAMINATION OF THE NEWBORN OR NEONATAL FOAL

The objective of a clinical examination (including the history) (see Fig. 11.2) is to establish:

- A diagnosis.
- A prognosis.
- A logical treatment plan to maximize the chances of a full recovery.

Symptomatic treatments for unknown conditions that have no identifiable diagnosis are commonplace and almost inevitable in practice. However, if a full history is obtained and a thorough clinical assessment performed it should be possible to establish at least a list of the problems that are present. From this list a presumptive diagnosis may be possible, although further diagnostic tests may be needed to eliminate some of the differential diagnoses. The main problem with many foal diseases is that delays in waiting for the results of tests may be harmful and could in some cases be too long to save the foal. Therefore, there are few opportunities for short cuts or presumptive tests. In every case, regardless of the possible diagnosis, the IgG concentration in the foal's blood must be established.

History

The history of the stud farm, the mare and the foal are very important features of the investigation of disease. It is very easy to be drawn into the problems of the foal, but there may be helpful factors from a carefully derived history, including:

- Previous disease history of the property.
- Disease history of in-contact animals.

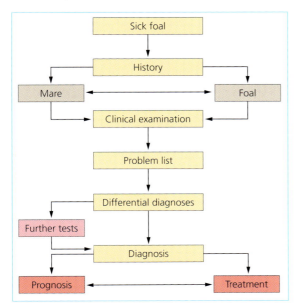

Fig. 11.2   Examination of the newborn or neonatal foal.

- Previous reproductive history of dam.
- Gestational age.
- Duration of parturition duration.
- Time taken to rise and to nurse.

Examination of the environment

The environment of the foal is important and the clinician needs to be aware of the implications of dirty versus clean stables, contact with other foals and/or adult horses and/or other species of animal.

- Foals born at the end of the stud season can be subjected to significantly increased challenge by infectious organisms than early foals. By contrast, the weather conditions and feeding of the mares can be more problematic in the early season.
- Many mares foaling in the early parts of the year are required to foal inside; this may add potential challenges to the foal and to the mare.

Examination of behavior

The behavior of the foal vis à vis the dam and its environment should be assessed early and certainly before any disturbances to either the dam or the foal.

> Note:
> - Maternal affinity and the presence or absence of any overtly abnormal behavior (e.g. convulsions, ataxia, colic or lethargy).
> - The suckle enthusiasm and ability should be observed.

- Does the foal recognize the dam and is teat-seeking direct and effective?
- Does the foal appear to see normally? (Does it bump into walls, etc.?)

> Note:
> - Newborn foals are normally clumsy and may sometimes appear to be severely ataxic. It is often difficult to separate the normal state from pathological ones.

- Is feeding normal?
- Is there milk on the foal's face (indicating that the foal has at least been in the right vicinity)?
- Is the mare's udder full or empty, and is there evidence of milk loss over the lower hindlimbs?
- Is there evidence of nasal reflux of milk during or after feeding?
- The respiratory rate should be measured before handling the foal if at all possible.

- Is there any evidence of abnormal breathing pattern, rate or is there a nasal discharge?
- Observe and assess restraint (e.g. 'flop' reflex) (see Fig. 11.3).

Examination of vital signs

The vital signs should be recorded early, as they are likely to alter significantly with handling.

- Respiratory rate and character can be measured and should be assessed before restraint. After the foal has been restrained the chest should be auscultated carefully with a stethoscope.
- Heart and pulse rate/quality should be measured (it is wise to check multiple arteries if possible). An abnormally low heart rate is usually a serious indicator of compromise; a very high rate can indicate anemia, pain, infection, or toxemia.
- Mucous membrane color and capillary refill time should be measured and recorded. Normal mucous membranes are a uniform salmon-pink color, and the capillary refill time is normally less than 2 seconds. Again it is wise to use all the mucous membranes available as some may be misleading (e.g. a bruised eye). Furthermore, the mucous membrane color may not be a good indicator of the oxygenation status of blood. The mucous membranes may be pale as a result of loss of blood, or icteric if internal hemorrhage, red cell destruction or liver disease is present. The presence of petechial hemorrhage is usually significant and can indicate toxemia or serious septicemic infection.
- The rectal temperature is an important parameter for the foal. Subnormal temperatures can be serious but can be the result of errors of technique. Ideally, a digital thermometer should be used and it should be pressed gently against the rectal mucosa. Any abnormal temperatures should be repeated to test the accuracy. The extremities (feet/limbs and ears, nose, tail) should be palpated to detect altered temperature.
- Bodyweight should be obtained routinely, but this is unfortunately not commonly done. The weight of a foal can usually be obtained simply by deduction from the total of a handler and the foal on normal bathroom scales.
- The body condition score may be very difficult to assess in a newborn foal as the usual parameters are not easy to identify. However, it should be possible to establish if the foal is reasonably covered with muscle and the extent of fat can sometimes be assessed.

A logical anatomical or systems approach is essential for the clinical examination, and the examination should always be performed in the same way. This will ensure that nothing is missed out. With experience some short-cuts can be taken but even then this may be unwise. There is much to commend the 'body systems' type of examination technique because, although it is more time-consuming, it does ensure that every system is examined carefully and, in the process, allows every anatomical site to be examined more than once.

> Note:
> A proforma for clinical examination is a very useful aid to both the examination and the subsequent clinical assessment. Recording the results of the clinical examination in an understandable form is important so that:
> - Progress (or otherwise) can be assessed.
> - A colleague or referral center can make a true assessment of progression of signs.

DETAILED EXAMINATION OF THE BODY SYSTEMS

Cardiovascular system

- The heart rate should be 40–80 immediately after delivery, with rises up to 130–150 while attempting to stand. Over the first 7 days the rate should gradually fall to 60–70. Foals are easily excited or stressed, so handling may cause increases in the heart rate.
- Sinus arrhythmia may be present in the first few hours but should then stabilize. Murmurs are common. The ductus arteriosus frequently remains patent for up to 48–72 hours; a characteristic 'machinery murmur' (often grade 3–4/5) may be heard predominantly at the level of the base of the heart (i.e. around the mid-point

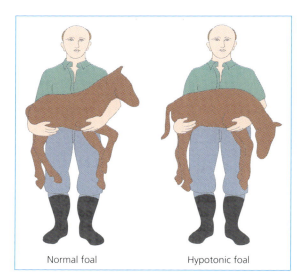

Normal foal   Hypotonic foal

Fig. 11.3 Normal and hypotonic foals.

of the chest at the level of ribs 4–5). [The machinery murmur is a continuous, often vibratory, sound that increases and decreases with the changes in arterial blood pressure but which does not disappear at any stage in the cardiac cycle.]

- Serious heart defects may or may not have accompanying murmurs, and the associated signs may be subtle or dramatic.
- The normal pulse in a peripheral artery is usually only just palpable. Usually the facial, metatarsal and median arteries can be felt with the fingertips. It may be possible to feel the carotid pulse fairly easily deep in the lower quarter of the jugular groove.
- Normal blood pressure (measured from a tail cuff applied with the foal in lateral recumbency) is 35–45/85–90.
- The distal extremities such as the ears and feet should be warm.
- A jugular pulse is not normal. The distensibility of the jugular vein should be assessed; it should fill briskly unless the foal is hypovolemic.
- There are few palpable lymph nodes in the normal foal. Enlarged glands may be significant directly or they may be more noticeable if the foal is in poor bodily condition.
- As blood is also a part of the cardiovascular system, the color of the mucous membrane and the specific characteristics of a blood sample can be important aspects of the examination.

Respiratory system

> Note:
> - Because auscultation of the chest and upper airways alone is not a reliable means of assessing the respiratory function of newborn foals, all the associated features (including mucous membrane color, respiratory behavior and airflow) should be examined carefully.

- The resting respiratory rate and regularity of rhythm are best observed from a distance, without restraint or excitement. Thoracic/respiratory function should be very carefully assessed to ensure that nothing is missed.
- Immediately after birth the respiratory rate is normally >60 breaths/minute, but this falls after 1–2 hours to 20–40 breaths/minute.
- Breathing should require minimal effort, and should be smooth with passive elastic recoil during expiration. There should be equal airflow from both nostrils.
- Rapid respiration can be the result of many systemic conditions, including:
  - ❑ Blood loss.
  - ❑ Sepsis.
  - ❑ Fever.
  - ❑ Pain.
  - ❑ Shock.
- Significant respiratory difficulty can also arise from congenital deformity of the airway (choanal atresia, subepiglottic cyst formation, laryngeal deformity or functional disability, tracheal collapse).
- During rest and sleep, respiration can become irregular and there may be some snoring/stertor.
- Beware of paradoxical chest patterns (the chest moves in and the abdomen moves out during inspiration). Excessive chest or abdominal movement is best regarded as abnormal and should be investigated. The patency of the airway MUST be assessed in any foal showing respiratory difficulty.
- Auscultation of the chest is much easier in the foal than in the adult horse, but even in severe pathology (e.g. *Rhodococcus equi* abscessation) there may be few abnormal sounds. The dependent lung of a recumbent foal may be almost silent.
- Percussion of the chest is very useful and under-utilized.
- Absence of sounds is possibly more sinister than obvious adventitious noises.
- Foals seldom cough or have nasal discharges even in severe disease.
- Too few foals are subjected to blood gas studies, ultrasonography, endoscopy and radiography.
  - ❑ Arterial blood gas estimations provide the best index of respiratory efficiency in foals (see p. 364 for blood sampling technique).
  - ❑ The partial pressure of oxygen (PO_2) reflects the respiratory status; the PCO_2 reflects the ventilation efficiency.
- Congenital defects that cause changes in respiratory function include: stenotic nares, choanal atresia (narrowing), hypoplasia of the palate, pharyngeal/epiglottic cysts, guttural pouch tympany, tracheal narrowing (scabbard/spiral deformities), diaphragmatic hernia, fetal respiratory distress syndrome, atelectasis, surfactant deficits, etc.

Alimentary system

- The mouth should be examined carefully for the bite, cleft palate or for evidence of pharyngeal paralysis. Abnormalities such as cleft palate, brachygnathism, etc., may be obvious, but there may be no clinical evidence in some cases. The newborn foal will not usually have any erupted teeth.
  - ❑ The central incisors and the first three cheek teeth (premolars 2–4) on the upper and lower

arcades will usually erupt within or around the first 2 weeks.

❏ The lateral (second) incisor usually erupts at around 2–3 weeks and the corner at around 7–10 months.

❏ Normally there are few adverse consequences of normal tooth eruption.

- The oropharynx is difficult to examine orally; palpation is possibly as helpful.
- The foal should be observed during nursing. It may be possible to identify nasal regurgitation of milk or loss of suckle. In order to suckle, the foal must adopt a characteristic posture; foals that are unable to do this (either for musculoskeletal or other reasons) cannot feed effectively.
- The abdomen can be examined by palpation and auscultation.

❏ Normally some borborygmi can be heard over all four quadrants of the abdomen. Splashing fluid sounds may herald diarrhea; tympanic sounds may suggest obstruction.

❏ Meconium impaction can sometimes be felt.

❏ Abdominal distention can be appreciated directly. A measuring tape may be useful to assess changes arising from accumulation of gas, urine/blood or fluid within the abdomen.

  i. Fluid distention can be a sign of impending enteritis or ileus and is commonly seen in premature or dysmature foals that have been overfed.

  ii. Gas distention/abdominal tympany can indicate intestinal obstructions such as strangulating lesions.

  iii. Nonstrangulating obstructions such as meconium impaction or congenital atresia of the intestine can also cause gas distention but are usually a combination of gas and fluid.

  iv. Most of the above cases will show overt colic signs associated with abdominal pain.

❏ Ballottement can be used to detect fluid thrills. Fluid distention should then be noticeably different from gas or fluid intestinal distention. Uroperitoneum from rupture of the urachus or from a patent bladder is the most common cause of fluid distention of the abdominal cavity.

❏ Extensive peritonitis may also cause a combination of gas and fluid distention of the abdominal cavity. In this case palpation of the abdomen will be resented and reflex boarding of the abdomen will be detectable. The foal will probably be reluctant to move.

- Rectal examinations should be avoided if possible, especially in colt foals.

❏ Rectal probing may be useful to test intestinal continuity; a dry rectum with no evidence of meconium is suggestive of an incomplete tract or of a serious long-standing obstruction.

- Radiography and ultrasonography are useful aids in the diagnosis of abdominal disorders of the foal.

❏ Both techniques may be particularly useful in cases of impaction, colic, or uroperitoneum.

❏ The contents of hernial sacs can easily and safely be appreciated by even the simplest ultrasonographic techniques.

- Abdominocentesis is easy in the standing foal but is difficult if the foal is recumbent.

❏ The newborn foal's intestines may be rather more fragile than those of adult horses and ultrasonography can be very useful in identifying pockets of fluid that can be sampled safely.

❏ Collect samples into EDTA and plain tubes and observe character (appearance, volume, sediment, etc.) and tendency to clot.

❏ Specimens should be submitted to the laboratory for detailed examination.

Urogenital system

- The external genitalia can easily be examined for evidence of congenital abnormality.
- The vulva is a mucous membrane that is useful in assessing cardiovascular function (color, hemorrhages, edema, etc.).
- A protruding vulva may be suggestive of ureteral rupture and retroperitoneal accumulation of urine.
- Scrotal hernia is common in the first 24–48 hours and should be differentiated from fluid accumulations in the scrotum (uroperitoneum, ascites, inflammation, and infections).
- Urination is a very important clinical event and should be observed.

❏ Foals should pass a full flood of urine within 8 hours of birth.

❏ Colts foals usually urinate earlier (by 1–2 hours) than filly foals.

❏ The specific gravity of foal urine is low and, unlike the urine of adult horses, is not cloudy or mucinous in character.

❏ A transient proteinuria is common in all foals but may be particularly high following an effective colostral feed.

❏ Some glycosuria is commonly encountered in normal foals but this should not persist nor should it be markedly elevated.

- The umbilicus should be examined in detail with washed, gloved hands.

❏ Any swelling or abnormal thickening should be subjected to ultrasonographic examination.

❏ The urachus may remain patent for 12–24 hours in normal foals, but all foals with a patent urachus should be assessed for possible sepsis. A patent urachus may be obvious during urination but sometimes it

only shows as a few damp hairs at the umbilicus.
- ❏ There is a higher incidence of primary urachal patency in foals whose cords have been clamped and cut rather than broken naturally.
    - i. Excessive tension from ill-advised pulling and tearing of the cord can also cause serious urachal damage and bleeding.
    - ii. Substantial hemorrhage from the umbilical stump is serious; remember that intra-abdominal bleeding can be serious without outward sign.
- ❏ Examination of the placental part of the umbilical cord might provide helpful information about the location of the rupture of the umbilical vessels (see p. 330).

Musculoskeletal system

- The conformation of the foal can easily be examined by direct inspection, but it is wise to avoid making judgments for the first 24–48 hours. Many foals appear to have serious conformational problems only to be normal a few days later.
- The newborn foal is often poorly coordinated; the joints and ligaments are notably slack and may seem to be weak.
    - ❏ In some cases the flexor tendons in particular are tight and 'contracted'; they commonly improve dramatically over the first week of life, so beware of over-emphasizing their importance.
    - ❏ However, do not under-estimate the truly weak foal or one with serious and prolonged tendon or ligamentous disabilities.
- Premature foals will often exhibit an inordinate laxity of joints with an increased range of motion. As long as they are otherwise healthy, well nourished and are carefully managed to minimize trauma to the foot, many of these cases improve remarkably over a week or two. The problematic cases remain slack or fail to improve sufficiently to prevent damage to the skin.
- Examine the skull, axial skeleton and limbs for congenital deformities and disease.
- Examine the chest for possible fractured ribs, pneumothorax or hemothorax.
- Radiographs should be taken of the carpus and tarsus of every premature or dysmature foal to establish the degree of mineralization of the small carpal and tarsal bones.
- Examine the limbs and joints during weightbearing, and if possible with the foal recumbent, to test for range of movement and angular and flexural deformities.
- Swollen, hot or painful joints must be explored immediately using every available means. It is important, of course, to observe the necessary precautions when examining or sampling joints.

- Test limb reflexes (see neurological examination, p. 370).
- The gait should be assessed.
    - ❏ Lameness in foals may be difficult to identify, as they are often mildly uncoordinated and can seldom be made to walk in a straight line under restraint.

Ophthalmic system

- An ophthalmoscopic examination is compulsory in all foals subjected to clinical examination.
- Foals may be difficult to examine because the eyes may not be fully mature at birth.
    - ❏ Foals appear to have weak corneal and palpebral reflexes.
    - ❏ Iris reflexes are sometimes slow in normal foals, especially if the foal is excited or in pain.
    - ❏ Examination may be made difficult by movement.
- The eyelids must be examined carefully for entropion; this can be primary or secondary.
- Both eyes must be examined directly (size, integrity and possible entropion/loss of symmetry); cataracts, uveitis and retinal hemorrhages are very important signs.
- The surface integrity of the cornea MUST be tested in all examined foals less than 7 days of age. There is some suggestion that many suffer from corneal ulceration without showing any outward sign of pain or discomfort. Routine use of fluorescein dye is common practice and is a wise precaution.
    - ❏ Compromised foals (and some normal ones) may have extensive corneal ulcers, sometimes without any obvious outward discomfort or lacrimation.
    - ❏ The cause of an ulcer should be established and, if possible, corrected as a matter of urgency.
- Sight can be difficult to assess with foals being uncoordinated and having particularly poor menace reflex.
    - ❏ Intact pupil light reflexes do not mean that there is vision.
- Both pupils should be the same size and respond equally to the same light challenge.
    - ❏ The swinging light test is a useful means of establishing the visual function of individual eyes.

Method
- i. The test is performed in subdued light or dark conditions.
- ii. A bright light is shone into one eye. After the eye has adapted fully (by pupillary constriction), the light is immediately transferred and shone into the other eye.

iii. The test should be repeated for each side on several occasions.

iv. Note that there may be a blink response to a very bright light; this does not necessarily equate with vision. It is sometimes useful to get the foal accustomed to the swinging light before trying to perform the test.

Interpretation

i. The pupil of the second eye should constrict further when the light impacts the retina.

ii. If the pupil of the second eye dilates rather than constricts, the eye is probably blind.

iii. A bound-down iris will not move in response to darkness or to bright light.

> Note:
> - Rare congenital defects of the iris musculature may be misleading.
> - Uveitis resulting in spasm of the iris (miosis) is an important sign of sepsis.
> - The lens can be examined for the presence of a cataract.

Integumentary system

- The skin of the normal foal is normally soft and pliant.
- The hair should be of approximately uniform length and consistency.
- Mane and tail hairs are also soft and may be short.
- Skin tenting can be used to assess the hydration status.
  - ❏ A skin tent formed by lifting a fold of skin on the side of the neck should return to its normal position within 2–5 seconds.
  - ❏ Skin tenting can be deceptive because very young foals may show prolonged tenting with normal hydration.
  - ❏ Prolonged tenting suggests dehydration and loss of skin turgor and elasticity.

Endocrine system

- The only endocrine gland that can easily be assessed physically is the thyroid gland.
- Foals born with bilaterally enlarged thyroid glands (goiter) may or may not have abnormalities of metabolic function. In some cases the consequences of this are profound.
- Abnormalities of the adrenal glands can reflect significant difficulties with the neonatal adaptive period. Affected foals are usually premature or dysmature (see p. 371) and often have serious

respiratory difficulties as a result of poor surfactant function.

Neurological examination

Examination of the newborn foal is rendered difficult by its inherent incoordination and the normal apparently ataxic state. Because this persists for up to 2 or 3 days in some cases, the difference between normal and abnormal neurological function is of great importance in the diagnosis of many neonatal disorders.

The protocol for neurological examination of the newborn foal is considerably different from that for the adult horse.[16] Different individuals often report very different results from the same foal, so it is important to maintain continuity of personnel when dealing with foals, especially if they are abnormal (e.g. neonatal maladjusted foals and convulsive foals). It is also important to record the findings at each examination; the use of a proforma form is useful to ensure that nothing is missed.

The most important features of the clinical assessment of the neurological status include:

- Affinity to, and recognition of, the mare. Loss or absence of maternal recognition/affinity is often the earliest sign of neurological problems. This should not be confused with the mare's disinterest in the foal, which may have other implications and other reasons.
- Reflex relaxation. When a newborn foal is restrained by chest–buttock grasp, the normal foal will 'flop' (i.e. become relaxed in an almost catatonic state). It may also show the Flehmen reaction (the foal lifts its upper lip and nose) and jaw relaxation. Hypotonic foals 'flop' inordinately (see Fig. 11.3). The normal floppiness should not be confused with an inordinate reduction in muscle tone. Critically ill neonatal foals are often inordinately floppy. Generalized floppiness is associated with:
  - ❏ Neonatal sepsis/septicemia.
  - ❏ Prematurity/dysmaturity.
  - ❏ Metabolic disorders.
  - ❏ Collagen disorders.
  - ❏ Neuromuscular problems.
  - ❏ Hypoxic/ischemic encephalopathy (neonatal asphyxia syndrome).
- Behavior. Normal foals are usually mildly resentful of restraint and appear to be 'rather nervous'. This is a normal behavioral response.
  - ❏ Foals should remain bright and alert and able to respond to all external stimuli.
  - ❏ Alterations in mentation are usually a result of cerebral dysfunction.
  - ❏ Coarse, exaggerated movements, and an intention tremor strongly implicate cerebellar disease.

- Limb position and pastern axis. Abnormal positions can be normal, but these should change rapidly with development of nervous control of the limb muscles. In some cases they are associated with abnormal/disease states.
- Gait examination. Gait is difficult to examine exactly because the foal cannot easily be restrained and will not usually walk in a straight line under restraint. Gait is therefore best observed when the foal follows the mare.
  - ❑ Few (if any) will react normally to a head collar/foal slip.
  - ❑ Sway tests are very unreliable indicators of weakness due to the uncoordinated responses and the relative size/strength of the tester compared with the foal.
- Cranial nerve examination. This is similar to that in the adult horse, but normal foals will often have very poor withdrawal reflexes.
  - ❑ The menace reflex is normally weak but should be normal by 7–14 days of age.
  - ❑ The 'slap test' should be carried out, but its interpretation is equivocal. It is, however, at least one detailed complex reflex that can easily be tested by palpation.
  - ❑ Cervicofacial reflex is usually well developed in young foals and tests ipsilateral cervical and facial nerve integrity.
  - ❑ Careful testing of each cranial nerve is a wise precaution because, although some signs suggest cranial nerve dysfunction (e.g. a flaccid hanging tongue), the responses can be used to establish that the sign is not significant.
- Limb reflexes. These are tested with the foal recumbent.
  - ❑ Extending all limb joints and then exerting sudden pressure on the sole of the hoof to extend the toe further tests the extensor recumbent thrust reflex. The normal response is limb extension with a jerk. The hindlimbs normally show a better response than the forelimbs. This reflex should have disappeared by 24 hours of age.
  - ❑ In young foals flexor or withdrawal reflexes cause extension of the contralateral limb. This reflex usually disappears by 3–4 weeks of age.
  - ❑ Normal patella and triceps reflexes remain exaggerated for up to 10–14 days.

Note:
- The newborn foal has an inherently high level of limb elasticity and it is usually possible to flex the forefoot and limb so that the foot reaches the shoulder joint. This range of flexibility is a combined product of tissue slackness and poor neural limitation of the movement range and is not a reflection of poor muscle/nerve tone.

- The problems of neurological examination of premature foals are even greater than with full-term foals.
- The differences between neurological deficit and neural immaturity have not been established for the horse. The clinical expression of neurological damage depends largely on the stage at which the original insult occurred and what was happening at the time. Damage occurring before 50 days of gestation is frequently severe enough to cause abortion/fetal death or produces major organogenesis deficits (e.g. anophthalmia/microphthalmia, cardiac deformities and limb defects).
- Foals showing convulsions at or soon after birth may have subtle signs, lip-smacking, irregular breathing, random nystagmus and blinking being the most obvious.
- Overt seizures are usually manifest by odontoprisis, bruxism, chewing/salivating, sneezing, paddling of limbs and opisthotonus.

RECOGNIZING THE POTENTIALLY ABNORMAL FOAL

Following a detailed clinical examination, the clinician should be able to establish the normality or otherwise of the foal. The importance of early recognition of significant problems that are likely to affect the viability of the foal cannot be over-emphasized. Early recognition of compromised or sick foals provides the best opportunity for successful treatment regimens. Useful early information may be gained from an immediate examination of the placenta and this opportunity should never be wasted. The major problem with the horse is that many foals are delivered without supervision and many mares are somewhat (or largely, in some cases) ignored during pregnancy in the expectation that 'all will be well'.

Establishing the risk category of a foal (see p. 355) provides the clinician and the owner with some indication of the likely problems that may develop. Of course any such system has major pitfalls in that a pregnancy may be classified as low-risk but may have major problems, and a high-risk foaling may proceed without any detectable problem.

One of the most significant diagnostic decisions that the veterinarian has to make is the recognition of prematurity or dysmaturity. The premature or dysmature foal has added demands on nutrition and care and without these the foal is most unlikely to survive. Developments in equine neonatal intensive care have resulted in significant improvements in the survival of foals, but the most significant factor still remains the overall health status of the foal at birth (whether it is premature or dysmature or neither).

Recognition of prematurity/dysmaturity

Most Thoroughbred and Purebred mares have certified service dates and when this information is available the length of the gestation can usually be accurately calculated. Length of gestation in paddock or naturally bred mares is more difficult (or impossible) to predict and every effort should be made to identify dates of service by careful observation and recording of estrous behavior.

It is important to assess both the gestational age and the clinical appearance together as the normal gestational length is variable in the horse and foals may be obviously abnormal at full or even extended gestational age. This makes for very unpredictable results from induced parturition.[17] Generally, an induced delivery should not be regarded as normal even when the induction is performed for purely elective reasons in a full-term mare. A 365-day gestation can be normal in some horses, whereas in others it is the result of persisting placental insufficiency and the results of the pregnancy are equally unpredictable.

Although the terms prematurity and dysmaturity are applied to different circumstances relating to the duration of gestation, the clinical signs of the two states are for all practical purposes the same and the two 'conditions' can be grouped together under the term 'unreadiness for birth'.[18,19] Survival rates for premature or dysmature foals is lower than normal in spite of the extra effort that can be brought to bear. Premature foals have a 70–75% survival rate.[20] For the most part, foals that do not establish normal righting reflexes and a normal suck reflex will die. Those that show normal righting and a strong suck reflex will often progress satisfactorily until 24 hours and then will rapidly fade and die unless strong intervention is applied. If the foal can stand and suckle within 2–3 hours of birth the prognosis is better, but such a foal will need intensive care if it is to survive normally.

A foal born before 320 days of gestation is classified as premature.

Note:
- The accepted limit of viability for foals is taken to be 300 days of gestation. This has sometimes been exceeded, but the survival of any foal with a gestational age <320 days has a poor chance of survival even in the best circumstances.
- Most very early foalings are best regarded as abortions.
- For the most part, it is unwise to offer a better prognosis than is realistic.

A foal born within the normal gestational range (320–345 days) but showing the signs normally associated with prematurity is classified as dysmature. These foals are often termed 'immature' or 'unready for birth' in that they apparently have little ability to maintain body homeostasis and show slow adaptation to extrauterine conditions.

- Foals may even have a prolonged gestational age (<350 days).

Prematurity/dysmaturity can be recognized by:

- Underweight for type (small body size for age/type). Although many foals are not weighed accurately, most of these foals are clearly small and underweight. They may be obviously dehydrated at birth, which adds to the weight deficit. Twins are invariably underweight and small.
- Bulging prominent forehead and eyes (especially noticeable in twins). This common sign can be misleading because some breeds (notably the Welsh pony and the Arabian) have naturally prominent foreheads.
- Weak musculature and slack/lax flexor tendons (front limbs in particular), with a noticeably long pastern angle. Most of these shortcomings will correct fairly quickly.
- Collapsed tarsal or carpal bones due to poor/delayed ossification, with consequent angular and flexural deformities.
- Tongue that often has a prominent red/orange color rather than the normal salmon-pink color.
- Coat that has a fine, silky texture; the nose/ears are soft and pliant.
- Dehydration, which is relatively common either at birth or develops shortly afterwards.
- Postprandial colic. This has several causes, including poor/absent (ileus) or uncoordinated excessive intestinal activity, gas accumulation, or overfeeding.
- Uncoordinated limb movements, reflecting neurological and muscular dysfunction.
- A slow respiratory rate or an abnormal respiratory pattern, reflecting the likely fetal atelectasis (failure of lung expansion and maturation with surfactant deficits).
- Slow respiration, which is particularly indicative of a poor prognosis; as the central respiratory centers are deprived of oxygen, the control becomes even less effective.
- Progressive deterioration in environmental awareness and maternal recognition; this is a common feature. Abnormal mentation reflects failure of neurological adaptation or the results of progressive oxygen starvation in the central nervous system. Affected foals may be, or become, blind.

- Immature foals that are born emaciated and dehydrated. Sometimes this is a result of diarrhea but more often reflects serious metabolic derangement of the adrenal glands and kidneys.
- Diarrhea; premature and dysmature foals are much more susceptible to infection than normal foals are.
- Biochemical signs:
  - ❑ Evidence of hypoventilation: reduced PaO_2 (which responds to 100% oxygen by rising to normal; withdrawal of the oxygen results in a rapid fall again); increased $PaCO_2$.
  - ❑ Acidosis (venous pH 7.25 and tendency to become more acidotic).

Note:
- Normal foals are acidotic at birth but their trend is towards normality.

  - ❑ Leukopenia due to a profound neutropenia ($<1.0 \times 10^9$/liter) with lymphocytosis ($>4.0 \times 10^9$/liter). A neutrophil:lymphocyte ratio <1.0 is accepted as being significantly abnormal; the normal ratio is >2.0.
  - ❑ Low blood glucose. Values less than 2.5 mmol/l at 2 hours and a decreasing trend are significant findings.
  - ❑ Low colostral absorption with a high tendency to infection. The reasons for this could include poor colostral quality in a mare that foals very early (or late), failure to ingest the colostrum, or failure to absorb immunoglobulins adequately as a result of poor intestinal function.
  - ❑ Blood insulin and cortisol very low for the first 24 hours (at least) with no response to endogenous or exogenous adrenocorticotropin.
  - ❑ Reduced plasma cortisol (<30 ng/ml; normally >100 ng/ml).

Note:
- Glycogen stores are depleted or have failed to develop.
- Lung surfactant may be abnormal and result in significant respiratory difficulties (impaired compliance with failure to expand at birth and consequent hypoxia).

Note:
- Prematurity and dysmaturity are virtually the same problem and should be treated in the same way.
- The theoretical differences are insignificant and the approach and therapy are the same.

Remember:
- There is no transplacental transfer of immunoglobulin, so the foal is immunologically naive at birth.
- Passive transfer is the most significant (only) source of immunoglobulin in the newborn foal.
- The fetus has some immunological competence from 6 months of gestation but only starts to produce significant antibodies at birth. It takes >14 days to produce any effective active humoral protection, and the establishment of normal cellular responses may take longer than this.
- The mare concentrates IgG in the udder during the last 3 weeks of gestation in preparation for colostrum production.

- Very rapid loss of IgG occurs when the mare starts lactating. During the first 6 hours there is at least a 75% fall in the IgG concentration in the mammary secretion and by 24 hours there is no effective IgG in the milk.
- There is only one effective colostral production. Leakage of colostrum is therefore very significant in terms of the reason for it and the subsequent loss of colostral quantity and quality for the foal.
- Milk contains only small amounts of IgM and IgA, but these are important, especially if the foal has diarrhea. Artificial milk has neither of these immunoglobulins, so mare's milk should be used whenever possible.
  - ❑ Intestinal closure is effectively complete at 12 hours of age.
- Foals must have had an adequate volume of good-quality colostrum by 4 hours (6 hours maximum). Local effects are maintained within the gut after closure but these are inefficient and unreliable means of disease prevention and last only as long as the provision of colostrum.
- It is likely that a foal that is totally deprived of colostrum will retain its ability to absorb colostrum for longer than one that receives adequate or inadequate colostrum shortly after birth. It therefore seems wise to administer a full dose of colostrum rather than very small amounts repeatedly (such as arises when a mare is milked repeatedly). It is better to accumulate the colostrum and administer it in one dose when it is of sufficient volume. However, this may delay the immunological protection afforded by the colostral IgG.
  - ❑ The presence of the mare during colostral feeding has a significant benefit on the absorption of colostrum (even when this is administered by stomach tube). This is a poorly understood phenomenon, but certainly

foals that feed properly on normal-quality colostrum have a high absorption rate and rapidly develop an effective passive immunity.

- Orphaned foals and those fed on artificial colostrum or stored colostrum may have a more problematical start in this respect with poorer absorption and a slower development of an effective passive immunity.
  - ❏ Foals raised on artificial replacements for colostrum and milk (whether this involves artificial milk replacers or milk from other species) appear to have a higher incidence of allergic disorders in later life. Some develop food allergies that result in recurrent urticarial episodes in response (usually but not invariably) due to cereal feeds.
  - ❏ Passive immunity lasts 6–8 weeks but varies with individual antibodies; some last longer than others.
  - ❏ Vaccination of the mare 3–4 weeks before parturition with the available and relevant vaccines provides maximum passive protection.
- Vaccination for tetanus may not be sufficiently reliable to protect the foal and so in all cases where the vaccination status of the mare is uncertain, or where she has been vaccinated over 6 months previously, the foal should receive a suitable dose (6000 IU) of tetanus antitoxin at birth. This is a routine procedure on many studs regardless of the vaccination status of the mares.
- Vaccination or prior exposure to infection may not result in transferable immunity in every disease or infection.

Prevention of prematurity

In order to limit the devastating effects of premature delivery, it is important to attempt to prevent it developing in the first place. This is easier said than done. Measures that result in a reduction in placental insufficiency will result in an improved chance of a normal gestation and a normal foal. By far the best method of prevention of prematurity is obviously to prevent early delivery. However, it is important to balance the threat of a deteriorating placental environment with the risks of early delivery. Repeated careful prenatal assessment of the foal by combinations of ultrasonographic, electrocardiographic and clinical assessment (of fetal movement and size) can be helpful. It is probably a sensible precaution to make these assessments in all high-risk mares.

- An abnormal placenta can sometimes be detected by transabdominal ultrasonographic examination.[21]
- Other aspects of the fetus that are suggestive of fetal stress include heart rate and size, fetal movement, and the volume and character of the allantoic fluid.

UNDERSTANDING IMMUNITY IN THE FOAL

Survival against infectious disease depends upon adequate host–defense mechanisms, which include the complex of immune processes and natural barriers to the invasion of pathogenic organisms. Skin and mucosal surfaces are effective barriers, acting largely in a physical manner, but they also contain enzymes, fatty acids and secretions which limit the penetration of microbes.

Innate or natural resistance is a very complex procedure, which is poorly understood. These aspects do not require prior exposure to the pathogen.

Adaptive immunity/resistance originates in the interaction between antigens and the lymphoreticular system. This produces a state in which the antibody/resistance is directed specifically at the antigen.

There are two significant types of immunity that are responsible in combination (to a lesser or greater extent mutually) for the protection of the foal (or any other animal) from infections:

- Humoral immunity.
- Cellular immunity.

Each is responsible for a different type of response and affords resistance in different ways. The deficits of each process are manifest in a variety of clinical syndromes, which are significant in foals. However, the two systems are interactive and in most protective mechanisms both are necessary.

As illustrated in Fig. 11.4, significant immunodeficiency disorders can arise at various points in the immune system:

1. Combined immunodeficiency. There is a complete break in the production of stem lymphocytes and neither humoral nor cell-mediated immunity can occur.
2. Agammaglobulinemia. The absence of B lymphocytes results in no production of γ-globulins; however, cell-mediated immunity is active.
3. Specific IgM deficiency. A specific cell deficit occurs, resulting in normal globulins except for IgM.
4. Transient hypogammaglobulinemia. A temporary immaturity of any or all of the cell types is theoretically possible but are seldom diagnosed.

- Fell pony syndrome. The true nature of this has not yet been established. Normal or near-normal lymphocyte counts are found but with obvious evidence of immunocompromise. The condition is not the same as the severe combined immunodeficiency syndrome of Arabian foals.

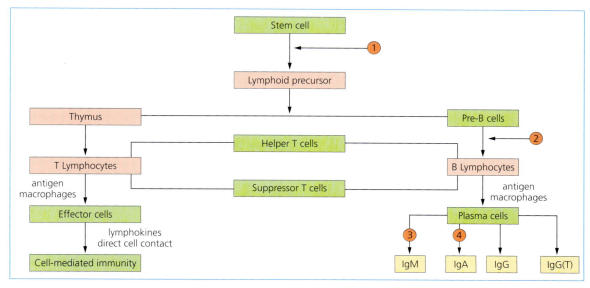

Fig. 11.4 Schematic description of the functional aspects of the equine immune system. The encircled numbers indicate various points at which significant immune disorders can arise (see text for full explanation).

THE ROLE OF COLOSTRUM IN IMMUNITY

> • It is probably impossible, or at least it is unwise, to consider immune processes of the neonatal foal without reference to the importance of colostral/passive immunity.

The most important single factor in the humoral immunity process in the newborn foal is the transfer of passive immunity via the colostrum.

The actual amount (weight) of immunoglobulin absorbed in the intestine of the foal depends on the:

1. Quality of the colostrum.[22]
   • Colostral quality is affected by the age of the mare (those over 15 years of age produce colostrum of a lower quality).
   • Mares producing early foals have colostrum of lower quality.
   • The quality of the colostrum depends on the health of the mare and the conditions under which she foals.
   • Certain breeds (e.g. Standardbred) have lower colostral quality than others.
2. Volume of colostrum available.
   • Primiparous mares may produce less colostrum than multiparous mares.
   • Stressed, injured or diseased mares will certainly produce less colostrum than those not so affected.
   • Previous (or concurrent) mastitis or other damage to the udder will result in less colostrum production.

3. Volume of colostrum ingested.
   • This depends heavily on the ability of the foal to nurse effectively and the production of quality colostrum by the mare. Clearly the two should coincide.
   • If a mare leaks colostrum from one teat while the other is being suckled, the overall volume of colostrum available to the foal will be reduced; although this may be insignificant, an adequate volume of good quality colostrum is produced.
   • Prior lactation or colostral leakage will reduce the amount of colostrum available (even though the foal may feed well).
4. Timing of the ingestion of colostrum.
   • Ingestion within the first 4–6 hours of life results in the best absorption.
   • Delay in ingestion will usually result in reduced absorption (and a greater risk of infection gaining access to the bloodstream).
5. Health status of the foal (ingestive and absorptive efficiency).
   • A healthy foal ingesting a good quantity of good-quality colostrum within 4 hours of birth has the best chance of good passive transfer of immunoglobulins.
   • Stressed, sick or injured foals will inevitably have reduced appetite and will also probably have a delay in ingestion of colostrum unless intervention is available.
   • Stressed, sick or injured foals also appear to have a significantly reduced absorptive ability.

What is colostrum?

- Colostrum is a complex of electrolytes, carbohydrates, fats, and proteins.
- Mammary development in the mare accelerates in the last 2 weeks of pregnancy, during which there are significant physical and structural changes in the secretions of the mammary glands.
- The mammary glands themselves do not synthesize any immune proteins except IgA; rather, under hormonal influences, it selectively aggregates the IgG molecules from the blood over the last 2–3 weeks of gestation (this change can sometimes be detected in the mare).
- In multiparous mares the average rate of secretion of colostrum is about 300 ml/hour and the total available secretion averages 5 liters (range 3.2–7.0 liters).
- Colostrum with high levels of immunoglobulins is replaced by milk with a low immunoglobulin level within 24 hours of parturition.
  - ❏ Colostral quality should, if possible, be measured before the foal suckles.
- Colostrum is only produced once.
- At foaling the mean IgG concentration is 166 g/l (range 30–120 g/l). This level falls rapidly after 2–3 hours to below 5 g/l at 24 hours.
- 80% of the protein in presuck colostrum is IgG and IgG(T), with only very small amounts of IgA and aggregating immunoglobulin. Secretory IgA levels rise as lactation advances but levels of other immunoglobulins decline rapidly.
- The loss of significant volumes of colostrum before or during delivery of the foal therefore has a dramatic effect on colostral quality. Reduction of the overall volume of colostrum available to the foal inevitably results in a reduction of the immunological protection it affords.

How is colostrum absorbed into the blood of the foal?

Fig. 11.5 provides a schematic description of the mechanisms involved in intestinal colostral absorption.[23]

1. Specialized cells (enterocytes) in the mucosa of the small intestine selectively absorb immunoglobulins by pinocytosis (the process of actively engulfing a liquid into minute vesicles by enclosing liquid droplets). This process is enhanced by the presence of low-molecular-weight proteins in normal colostrum.
2. Immunoglobulin molecules then travel via lymphatic vessels to the bloodstream.
3. Following ingestion of a good volume of good-quality colostrum, IgG is detectable in the blood at around 6 hours. However, there is no point in sampling the foal to establish IgG levels before 12–24 hours as it is only possible to establish the

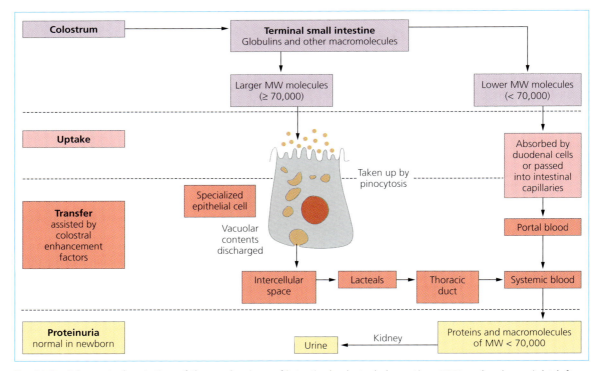

Fig. 11.5 Schematic description of the mechanisms of intestinal colostral absorption. MW, molecular weight (after Jeffcott[23]).

true IgG concentration after the gut has lost its ability to absorb the globulins delivered to it. At this point the blood IgG concentration will be maximal.

4. More mature cells without the capacity to absorb IgG replace the enterocytes 12–24 hours after birth. There is considerable debate as to the mechanism for this; it may be that the presence of high levels of endogenous corticosteroids is responsible for the 'closure'.

5. Absorption declines with time to reach almost zero by 12–24 hours after birth. There is some doubt as to whether a foal that receives no colostrum has a longer potential time for absorption. If this is the case, a single small feed of colostrum can be regarded as potentially harmful as it will allow the absorption of a small amount of IgG followed by early/normal closure of the absorptive mechanisms. However, while the intestinal absorption remains 'open', there is a higher risk of penetration of bacteria and therefore a higher risk of septicemia. Molecules of lower molecular weight, which are absorbed at the same time, commonly leak into the urine through immature glomeruli and commonly produce a transient proteinuria. This should not be misinterpreted, because the neonatal kidney is probably not capable of functioning at full adult capacity for some weeks and thus some protein loss is commonly present in normal foals.

NUTRITION OF THE FOAL IN HEALTH AND DISEASE

NORMAL REQUIREMENTS

From the point of birth, enteral nutrition becomes the only source of food for the foal. The need for food may drive the desire to rise quickly and to feed as soon as possible. The foal appears to make feeding the second major priority after breathing,[24] and nutritional compromise develops quickly in those foals that fail to feed effectively (for whatever reason) soon after birth.[25]

A healthy full-term foal will stand and suckle strongly from the dam within 2–3 hours of birth.[18] Thereafter it quickly develops a regular feeding pattern. Milk provides all the necessary nutrients, enzymes, hormones, minerals and vitamins that the very young foal requires. Milk is regarded as the gold standard for early nutrition for young mammals and artificial feeding regimens are based around the analysis of milk. Many of the nutrient components of milk are important in the development of normal intestinal function,[26] which will need to adapt quickly to the increasing demands and the change to a more complex digestive physiology. The demands on milk as a source of nutrition are considerable. Not only

does it need to provide for high-energy expenditure, but growth and final organ development also add to the demands. Although a healthy foal will utilize almost 100% of the available energy from milk,[27] milk alone is not nutritionally sufficient beyond the first few weeks of life. Furthermore, milk alters significantly through the course of lactation to correspond with the changing role of milk in the nutrition of the foal.[28] Young foals are commonly given a creep feed or access to grass to help balance out the dam's milk. There are no useful means of manipulating the content of mares' milk (e.g. by manipulation of dietary fiber or roughage). The volume and nutritional value of the milk ingested means that there is a significant oversupply of energy; this results in a significant daily weight gain which over the first few weeks should be in the region of 1.5 kg/day (for a Thoroughbred foal).[29]

Any alteration in the health of the foal or of the milk supply from the mare will have a disproportionately deleterious effect on the nutritional status of the foal. The failure of milk supply as a result of maternal problems can be difficult to identify; the udder may give the impression of being empty and it is easy to conclude then that the foal is being fed fully. The first indications of a problem may be slow to appear and the foal may lose weight and vitality. It may be seen to be suckling more often than expected or may drink water to compensate. If the foal is ill, the problem is often more obvious; the mare's udder will be seen distended and milk may drip almost constantly. By the second or third day these signs may be less obvious. A sick or stressed foal has a much higher nutritional requirement than a healthy one and usually a depressed appetite serves to exaggerate the discrepancy between demand and supply. Foals that cannot feed because of congenital defects are usually obvious from an early stage.

- A normal foal will nurse up to 7–8 times per hour throughout the day,[30] taking about 80 ml per feed and a total of about 450 ml/hour.[25]
- A healthy Thoroughbred foal (50 kg bodyweight) requires about 300 kJ/kg bodyweight per day.[31] Normal ingestion of milk by a healthy foal from a healthy mare will provide up to 600 kJ/kg/day. The excess is diverted to weight gain and growth.
- Premature or convalescent foals may need over 180 kcal/kg/day.
- A healthy newborn foal raised on its mother (or by hand) should gain 1–2 kg bodyweight per day and should be weanable by 3 months of age.

In order to obtain its minimum requirement a healthy foal must drink 12–13 liters of milk per day (10–15% of bodyweight daily for the first 2 days then up to 25% of bodyweight).[32] It is clearly impossible to mimic the natural feeding behavior of foals under artificial conditions. Total colostrum/milk consumption within the first 24 hours is about 15% per kg bodyweight; for a Thoroughbred foal of 50 kg this is around 8 liters. Of this total volume 2.5–3.5 liters will be colostrum.[33] Thereafter there is a steady increase in the volume of milk ingested; the maximum is usually achieved at around 3 months when the foal will be ingesting around 18 liters of milk per day.[34]

FEEDING THE ORPHAN FOAL

Nutritional status is critical to the survival of sick as well as healthy foals.[28] Feeding the orphan foal is very labor-intensive; it requires strict hygiene and very careful, full-time care. Hand-reared foals should always have access to fresh water and salt but particular care must be taken to monitor intake. Engorgement on salt can be dangerous and some foals will develop habitual drinking (psychogenic polydipsia).

Sepsis can increase the demand for energy by over 100%. Inadequate nutrition causes poor growth in the long term, but impaired immunological (T cell) function, complement levels, etc. make infection more likely.

An undernourished foal has a greater tendency to decubital (pressure) sores and poor wound healing, and secondary infections can develop if the immune system is compromised by poor nutrition.[35]

The most common mistake is to underestimate the requirements for calorific intake and nutritional support. The gastrointestinal tract of sick foals will often not tolerate some foods in excessive amounts, making continuous accurate and detailed clinical assessment critical.

> Note:
> - Remember that placental insufficiency (dysmaturity/prematurity) results in a similar state with similar demands; neonatal examinations therefore are critical to survival.

Decision 1: Does the foal warrant the effort required?

Foals of little or no commercial value or those with other serious complications (such as fractures or congenital deformities) may not be worth the effort that it takes to raise it up to weaning. Hand-reared foals may develop serious behavioral problems that make the effort a waste of time.

Decision 2: Is there sufficient money, time and manpower available to ensure that the procedures are performed correctly?

A feeding regimen that mimics natural feeding habits is almost impossible to sustain, but the nearer it is the better the outcome with the least number of complications.[36] Regimens that provide between five and 12 feeds per day are usually tolerable for both

the carers and the digestive tract of the foal. Feeding regimens involving four feeds a day have proven successful and have the advantage that foals are hungry at the time of feeding.[37]

There are clear advantages in feeding ad libitum,[38] but hygiene and the stability of the replacement mixture is important. There is also a high tendency for foals to overfeed under ad libitum conditions, so this should probably be avoided if alternatives can be established. Moreover, orthopedic or intestinal disorders may develop.

- Compromises in feeding regimens (number of feeds, volume of feeds) are almost always less effective than the normal situation.

Decision 3: Is fostering a viable alternative?

A safe fostering is highly satisfactory, and there are few (if any) problems once the procedure is safely established.

Decision 4: Choosing between bottle-, tube- or bucket-feeding

> Note:
> - Boredom and obesity must be prevented.
> - It may be useful to rear the foal with an old pony.
> - Do not allow foals to become 'cute' with rearing, striking or biting.
> - Mixing an orphaned foal with other mares and foals is an unwise management system. 'Intruders' are seldom tolerated or allowed to suckle by mares; if the foal does attach itself to a mare it should be removed from contact.

Bottle-feeding

- This is very time-consuming.
- Lamb nipples are suitable for foals (calf nipples are often too large).
- The foal should be standing during feeding as this prevents aspiration.
- It is easy to provide multiple feeds and this can more effectively mimic the natural state. However, although it is easier to avoid overfeeding, it may encourage underfeeding.
- Hygiene can be excellent if bottles are sterilized between feeds.
- Bottle-feeding increases human–foal bonding. This is probably not advantageous because many hand-reared foals have serious behavioral problems later in life and some become impossible to handle.

Tube-feeding

- This is a short-term measure and should be limited to foals whose suckling reflexes are poor/absent. Most foals that need tube-feeding are those under intensive care and may be better starting on partial parenteral nutrition (see p. 385).

- Tube-feeding is an intensive care procedure and the foal should be referred or hospitalized.
- Owners can be taught to insert a nasogastric tube, but there are significant inherent dangers that can have fatal consequences.
- If prolonged tube-feeding is likely, feeding with an indwelling nasogastric tube or fine tube with constant flow can be considered.

Bucket-feeding

- This is convenient, but foals are inclined to overfeed at each feed and it is more difficult to mimic the natural state. There is a strong tendency to feed 3–4 times daily rather than 12 or more.
- Diarrhea and hygiene problems (enteric infections) are more common.
- On balance, bucket-feeding is preferred over bottle-feeding for ease of management and fewer bonding/behavioral problems associated with human imprinting.

Decision 5: Choosing an artificial diet

It is essential that both owner/handler and veterinary surgeon are aware of the amount of food that is required for the foal. Furthermore, there are very important considerations for feeding of colostrum to the orphaned foal (see p. 375). The need for both colostrum and nutrition from milk may be higher in sick, compromised or orphaned foals under stress than in normal healthy foals.

- Abrupt changes of feeding and management must be avoided. Every effort should be made to mimic the natural state and regularity of content and frequency is essential for successful artificial rearing of foals.

- Colostrum is essential.
  - ❏ 1–2 liters of good-quality colostrum must be fed in the first 6 hours.
  - ❏ A frozen store of colostrum is a very useful safety measure for any stud veterinary surgeon.
  - ❏ Artificial colostrum is now available commercially (e.g. Equicol®, Nu Wave Health Products, Warton, UK) and is of a standard good quality; such products are usually based on bovine colostrum and are expensive. Bovine, sheep and goat colostrum have also been used effectively; they do have limitations, but can be used if there is no more natural option. The relevance of the antibodies may be questionable.
- Proprietary mare's milk replacements are available commercially.[28,39] Mare's milk replacers

should contain ±22% protein and 1.5% fat (on a dry matter basis) with <0.5% fiber. The manufacturers' dietary instructions must be followed meticulously if problems are to be minimized.
- Cow's milk (see Table 11.7) can be made to resemble mare's milk more closely by adding two teaspoonfuls of honey (or 20 g of dextrose) per liter of semi-skimmed milk (2% fat).
- Goat's milk is well tolerated and seems very palatable. Nanny goats have often been reported to serve well as surrogate milk suppliers. No alterations to the milk are needed and it could be viewed as the preferred choice.[40] However, it may be expensive and difficult to obtain in some places.

- Human milk substitutes are not suitable.

Decision 6: Decide when and how to wean the foal onto fiber and supplemental feed

- There are clear merits in an early transition to adult-type enteral feeding, but care must be taken that all feeds are introduced slowly.
- Introduce creep feed from 1 week and good-quality hay immediately.
- Access to the fresh droppings of healthy horses should be encouraged.
- Wean at 3–4 months.

Points to note/remember in feeding orphan foals

1. Hygiene is vital (e.g. sterility of buckets, bottles and teats).
   - It is important not to forget that a foal that has to be artificially fed will be more liable to infections. Environmental and dietary hygiene is paramount.
   - The stable should be sterilized with suitable disinfectants and in any case should not have been occupied by any other horse (or other large animal species) in the last 4 weeks.
   - There should have been no history of enteric disorders associated with any animal in the loose box at any time.

Table 11.7 Nutritional constituents of cow's and mare's milk

Constituent	Cow's milk	Mare's milk
Protein (%)	3.8	2.4
Fat (%)	4.4	1–1.5
Lactose (%)	6–6.5	4.5–5.0

- All equipment used for the feeding should be sterilized with hypochlorite soaks or with another approved (harmless) agent.
2. Frequent small feeds are best (4–6 feeds per day is the accepted minimum), particularly in the early stages.
    - Large milky feeds often cause diarrhea by allowing proliferation of enteric pathogens in an excessively acidic gut.
    - It is important to mimic natural loading of the stomach (i.e. no more than 500 ml at any feed and up to 15 times per day).
3. The normal meal intake (i.e. 500 ml maximum for a 50-kg foal) should not be exceeded at any meal. The total daily requirement can be calculated and divided into a feasible number of feeds.
4. If diarrhea occurs, oral rehydration electrolytes with glucose (e.g. Lectade® Smithkline Beecham Animal Health; Ion-aid®, Rhone Merieux) for 36–48 hours should be used (e.g. one sachet of electrolyte replacement powder dissolved in 4 liters of water, or normal water intake if this is sufficient), with a gradual return back to milk.
    - It is possible and feasible to administer the food by stomach tube if the foal will not feed itself.
    - Water should be available after administration of medication.
5. All changes in feeding should be made gradually (over 24–48 hours).

FOSTERING THE ORPHAN/REJECTED FOAL

Success depends on both the foal and the dam. It is unwise to attempt to foster a second foal onto a mare; this can be very dangerous and rarely works.
   There are various points to note:

- Mares that have lactated for a few days are more likely to accept a foal than those that have not.
- A longer time between the death of a foal and offer of a foster foal gives worse results (the mare is most likely to accept fostering on the same day).
- A significant size discrepancy between the dead foal and the foster foal gives poorer results.
- A strong enthusiastic foal gives a better chance of a successful fostering. Foals that have learned to suck from a mare are more inclined to adapt to the new mare than those that have not suckled at all (e.g. bucket- or bottle-fed foals).
- A hungry foal is often more enthusiastic and less likely to be put off by a mare's reluctance, so it is possibly better not to feed the foal before it is introduced to the mare.
- The mare's temperament is very important. Some are gentle and maternal, whereas others may be vicious, aggressive or 'sullen'. The latter are

particularly difficult because handlers may get the impression that the mare has accepted the foal only to find that she becomes aggressive when left alone with the foal.

- Fostering to a goat (or cow) is possible and has been known to produce good strong foals. Goat's milk may not be as good as supposed, but many foals have been raised on it without significant problems.
- The weight of the foal should be recorded at regular intervals; it should not be committed to memory.

Methods of fostering foals

Direct fostering

- This only works for certain mares with a strong maternal instinct.
- Rearing two foals is sometimes possible but places inordinate strains on the mare and it is seldom successful.
- 'Wet-nurse' mares (those that lactate for long periods without necessarily having had a foal and will tolerate nursing any foal) are very rare and expensive. However, in some countries they are commercially available and the mare is generally loaned for the duration of lactation with the hirer being obliged to return the mare pregnant when the foal is weaned.
- It is useful to remove the foster mare from the stable where her own foal died.
- Foals can sometimes be fostered to a nanny goat. However, the volume of milk available usually becomes inadequate quickly. There are logistical problems, of course, both in frequency of feeding and management.
    - ❏ A 50-kg foal needs 11–13 liters/day. Normal feeding patterns require numerous feeds (7 per hour) during the day (500 ml/hour) and the goat (obviously) has to be presented on a table to allow the foal to nurse.

Deception

- This depends upon the inability of the mare to recognize the foal.
- The usual way to achieve this is to use the mare's own dead foal's skin and to cover the foster foal (Fig. 11.6). However, this is a troublesome and very unhygienic method. It should not be used if at all possible. The weight of the skin is considerable, and the developing smell and discomfort (heat and possible infection) are not generally acceptable.
- The same effect can sometimes be achieved using the fetal membranes from the mare's own foal, but this carries the same limitations as the skin method.
- Odor deception using strong odors on the mare's nose and over the foal (e.g. aniseed, peppermint

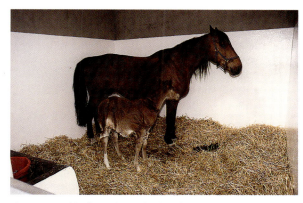

Fig. 11.6 Skin fostering. This has been used widely but is unhygienic and unpleasant for both foal, mare and handlers.

or perfume) is definitely worth trying and can work simply and rapidly.

Tranquilizers/sedation

- The mare can be tranquilized (sometimes heavily) so that she does not mind the new foal nursing.
- Repeated doses may be needed and the mare should never be left alone with the foal (even for a few minutes) until bonding is definite and solid (sometimes days later).

Physical restraint

- The mare and foal can be physically restrained and introduced to each other across a board or door first and then, with persistence, the mare may accept the foal after several days.

Note:
- All fostering must be performed with care and sympathy.
- The mare and foal should never be left alone until fostering has certainly been successful.
- A successful fostering is highly satisfactory for all parties.

FEEDING THE SICK FOAL

Foals that cannot obtain enough energy and protein from enteral intake, either for reasons of poor suckle reflexes, inability to feed and/or those that require to be starved for treatment reasons, require parenteral nutritional supplementation.

- Starvation for more than 24–36 hours makes parenteral nutrition compulsory.[41]

Feeding the foal on the dam's milk is a very time-consuming and frustrating business.

- Milking mares is difficult and the rewards are poor.
- Milk let-down can be encouraged by the intravenous injection of very small doses (1 IU) of oxytocin.
- A milking machine or modified 60-ml syringe can help.
- Once lactation has ceased it is almost impossible to restart it.

Nevertheless, because mare's milk is nutritionally ideal for foals it should be supplied as far as possible (within the constraints of the illness).

- Wherever possible enteral feeding should be continued (even in small volumes) (minimal enteral feeding) because it supports normal intestinal function and reduces the tendency to gastric ulceration.[42] It also makes the transition back to normal enteral feeding easier.
- Continued milking of the mare also encourages and maintains lactation so that once the foal is able to feed naturally it can revert to natural suckling.

Artificial feeding of the premature foal is more complex than for normal foals and a sick premature foal has very complex nutritional needs.

- Organ immaturity results in extra nutritional demands and this is complicated by inefficient organ function.[43]
- Although little is known about the composition of milk produced by mares that deliver prematurely, it is likely that it is less nutritious than normal milk and it may contain little or no IgG (i.e. it may not be classifiable as colostrum). Both these factors make the nutritional management of premature foals difficult at best. The premature foal requires the provision of certain nutrients that would ordinarily be obtainable from metabolic processes; these are called conditionally essential nutrients.
- Foals that are unable or unwilling to suckle do not make good candidates for bottle-feeding.
- The nutritional demand (particularly for energy and protein) of sick foals (no matter what the illness or disability) will be considerably higher than that of an equivalent normal healthy foal (although the extent of this has not been established).

Parenteral nutrition of the foal

Total or partial parenteral nutrition has become more-or-less standard procedure for neonatal foals in high-quality equine practice.[44] Its theory and clinical applications are being increasingly understood, as knowledge is gained of the physiological demands of young foals. There are still large gaps in our understanding of the newborn foal, and much of the current information has been extrapolated from other species (including man). However, we do know that:

- Foals have few energy reserves at birth.
- Their requirements/needs are much greater weight-for-weight than those of adult horses.
- Their glycogen reserve will probably only supply their energy needs for 2 hours after birth.[33]
- Mobilization of lipid reserves from which energy deficits are normally satisfied is inefficient in foals.

Because it may take several days to achieve a normal energy balance, parenteral nutrition should be instituted early in the course of disease. This will invariably result in better responses and higher success rates for therapy of some difficult disorders.

- A successful outcome is satisfying to both veterinarian and the owner and is ample reward for the effort.

The primary objective of parenteral nutrition is to provide all (total parenteral nutrition) or some (partial parenteral nutrition) of the nutritional needs (in terms of energy and protein in particular) of the foal when normal enteral nutrition is either impossible or inadequate.[45] Although all the theoretical needs can often be met over the short term, most intensive care specialists rely on a mixture of parenteral and enteral nutrition (i.e. partial parenteral nutrition).

Total parenteral nutrition should be capable of producing significant weight gain in the foal; this involves a very high-intensity feeding regimen with specially formulated materials. Regular accurate weighing of foals on total or partial parenteral nutrition should be undertaken.

Total parenteral nutrition is usually instituted and run for 3–4 days with a slow 'weaning' period. Partial parenteral nutrition can be maintained for longer, but for the most part is applied to foals that will respond earlier and hopefully return to normal enteral nutrition quickly.

Clinicians involved in equine neonatal care should be fully conversant with the application, procedures and management of parenteral nutrition. The procedure is inevitably expensive and labor-intensive but its advantages far outweigh the problems and many foals can be saved.

- Fluid requirements can also need to be met using saline or Hartman's solution if indicated. A basic maintenance volume of 100 ml/kg/day should be provided, but this can be reduced if enteral fluids are being given. Repeated checks on hydration status must be made.
- Most of the required solutions are compatible with each other, but should be delivered

individually from their containers into fluid lines; this will ensure that they are not held in contact for long periods. If mixing of solutions is essential, compatibility needs to be established and aseptic precautions need to be taken during the preparation of the mixture.

- Unless specifically contraindicated, oral feeding should be maintained as far as possible alongside parenteral nutrition. Partial parenteral nutrition makes the transition back to normal enteral nutrition simpler and encourages normal gut function. It makes the best use of the normal physiological mechanisms of the intestinal tract and can regulate aspects of nutrition that are not possible to calculate.

Solutions

The clinician can construct suitable parenteral nutritional fluids but precautions need to be taken during their preparation. The foal will necessarily be compromised and liable to sepsis in particular,[46] so sterility and continued hygiene precautions need to be maintained throughout the procedure.

Glucose solutions

Glucose provides the basis for calorific supply. It has a strong protein-sparing effect even at low doses, but in the absence of protein it may cause hepatic damage and stresses on the cardiorespiratory system. Glucose solutions alone cannot provide sufficient energy for a normal foal, let alone a sick one. They are not suitable on their own for parenteral nutrition and are best regarded as immediate sources of energy.

- 5% glucose saline will provide 170 kcal/l against a basal maintenance requirement (in a normal foal) for 7000 kcal/day; it would thus take over 40 liters of this solution to meet the requirements.

A sustained slow administration of a low concentration of glucose, calculated to supply the needs, is far better than giving a bolus of a strong concentration (much of which will be excreted via the urine). Also, changes in glucose concentrations should be made slowly to avoid the effects of rebound hypoglycemia that arise from insulin release. Although stronger concentrations of glucose can be given, they become significantly hypertonic. Concentrated glucose solutions can also be irritant to veins and cause catheter problems. Glucose should always be used in low concentrations, as high concentrations will likely cause phlebitis.

- Osmotic diuresis with glycosuria and hepatic lipid deposition are possible secondary effects.
- Septic and injured foals tend to hyperglycemia, whereas premature or dysmature foals tend to be hypoglycemic. Laboratory support is essential to establish the needs for each individual.

- Glucose can also increase the demands on the respiratory system and so should be used sparingly in foals with respiratory distress.

> Note:
> - Many sick foals have a paradoxical hyperglycemia ('hyperglycemia of stress') and an insulin resistance. They may therefore show abnormal/unexpected responses to glucose infusions.

Lipid emulsions

The net energy supply from lipid is far greater than from other sources. Lipid emulsions provide between two and three times the calorific value of glucose or protein (38 kJ/g compared with 14 kJ/g for glucose and 17 kJ/g for protein).

- Lipids provide high-energy levels with relatively small volumes and few side-effects.
- A 10% emulsion can provide up to 9–10 kcal/ml; many preparations also contain essential fatty acids, which is advantageous.
- However, sick foals may not be able to metabolize lipids effectively, so no more than 60% of the calorific requirements should be given via this means.

Commercially available lipid emulsions are usually specially formulated for human parenteral feeding but can be useful in foals also. Most of them contain amino acids as well (see below) and are therefore ideally suited for parenteral nutrition.

Administered at a rate of 1 g/kg/day these emulsions provide 10 kcal/kg bodyweight daily; the rate can be increased slightly if the needs are greater. The blood should be regularly checked for hyperlipemia, when it is obvious the rate should be reduced, although the foal is usually tolerant of some circulating lipid. Lipid supplies of 3.5 g/kg bodyweight daily are often the maximum tolerated and needs beyond this should be supplied by glucose.

Amino acid solutions

The amino acid solutions that are available for human parenteral nutrition can provide a good basis for feeding the neonatal foal over the short term. The conditionally essential amino acids (i.e. those that are only essential for abnormal foals) are not known; thus longer-term use can lead to deficits and consequent organ compromise.

A variety of veterinary solutions containing amino acids (usually with electrolytes and glucose) are available commercially. The exact requirements for these are largely unknown, but a slow continuous drip feed will provide suitable support to enhance the protein-sparing effects of glucose. These solutions are designed to cater for the protein needs of the foal and are assumed to mimic the natural variations occurring in normal foals.[47] Specific parenteral protein/amino acid and vitamin solutions are available (8.5% amino acid solutions), but for the most part are never capable of providing even the most basic of maintenance requirements. Some of these solutions are combined with electrolytes, but even the 10% solutions do not meet the total requirements for the foal.

The solutions should be administered at a rate of around 2 g/kg/day; this may be adjusted as needed. There is little information about the specific needs of foals, but as proteins are vital for tissue repair and function this aspect cannot be ignored even for 1–2 days.

Electrolyte solutions

Electrolyte balance is vital to the well-being of any sick or compromised young animal. They are less tolerant of variations than adults. Furthermore, the newborn foal has an immature renal development and so has less ability to compensate for errors and variations in fluids.

Potassium, sodium and calcium are the major anions; chloride and bicarbonate are the major cations. Serum potassium is probably the single most critical electrolyte in compromised foals and must be monitored carefully and regularly. Part of the intensive care equipment must therefore be a means of measuring blood electrolytes and gases.

During administration of intensive care fluids it is easy to forget the importance of the total volume of fluid administered. Volume overload places intolerable burdens on the cardiorespiratory system and the renal and hepatic functions. The normal volume of fluid administered to a sick foal is about 100–200 ml/kg/day. This is lower than the total volume ingested by a normal healthy foal (about 250 ml/kg/day), but fluid overload is a very dangerous event and must be avoided. Provided that renal function is sustained and has some concentrating ability, the reduced overall volume should not affect the foal significantly.

Vitamin and trace element solutions

Many complex amino acid and vitamin/mineral fluids are made commercially, but although they can provide useful additions to fluid therapy they cannot be relied upon to provide all the needs. Fortunately, reductions in the dietary supply/absorption of most vitamins and minerals are tolerated reasonably well for the duration of total parenteral nutrition (usually 2–3 days maximum).

Preparation of parenteral nutrition solutions

Many commercial solutions are available, although most are not prepared specifically for foals. They are usually available in pre-prepared or ready-to-mix formulations. Premixed preparations have the advantage of sterility without compromise but are less flexible in their use. For example, as the foal is weaned off total parenteral fluid, it is wise to reduce the lipid component first and then the amino acids. This would be impossible with the use of a single mixed solution.

Individual component solutions, on the other hand, mean that calculations of volumes and flow rates need to be made carefully to ensure the correct final drip balances. Premixing of individual solutions can solve many of these problems, but compatibility and sterility may be significant problems.

- Infusion pumps can be used to make calculations exactly but are not widely used in equine practice.
- Repeated monitoring of the metabolic and clinical status of the foal is essential for success.
- Suitable solutions for parenteral feeding for total and partial nutrition can be made relatively easily from individual solutions. Typical examples are shown below.

Partial parenteral solution
- 1500 ml of 50% dextrose.
- 100 ml of 8.5% amino acid solution.

This provides about one-third of the maintenance requirement for energy (50 kcal/kg/day).

- Begin with 50 ml/hour, increasing to 100 ml/hour over 12–24 hours; the rate is then gradually reduced during the 'weaning-off' period.
- Regular monitoring of urine output and content, hydration and plasma electrolyte status is needed. Urea should be estimated daily.

Total parenteral solution
- 1000 ml of 50% dextrose.
- 1000 ml of 20% lipid emulsion.
- 1500 ml of 8.5% amino acid solution.
- Electrolyte solutions (saline or Hartman's); these should not be mixed with other solutions but should be administered via a separate line to the catheter.

This provides 85 kcal/kg at 145 ml/hour.

- Start at 90 ml/hour and increase to 145 ml/hour over 12–24 hours.
- Monitor weight, hydration and electrolyte, urea and protein status.
- Monitor urine output and content.

Administration of parenteral nutrition

Indications[48]
- Undernourished foal. These animals do not maintain their birth bodyweight in the first 24–36 hours of life. This may be due to poor feeding, extra demands or dehydration. A normal foal should consume 10% of its bodyweight in the first 24 hours and should gain weight at about 1 kg/day from birth.
- Premature or dysmature foal. These foals have reduced or absent suckle reflexes and impaired intestinal absorption. Glycogen stores are severely depleted. Total or supportive parenteral nutrition should be started immediately to ensure that the foal does not lose weight. It is not helpful to delay parenteral nutrition until signs are obvious. Supportive parenteral nutrition is instrumental in improving the prognosis for these foals.
- Sick or compromised foal, especially if coupled with significant gastric reflux. Parenteral nutrition should be instituted immediately and only reduced when intestinal motility is capable of progressive/normal activity. The energy demand of a sick (febrile) or severely compromised foal may be far higher than that of a normal healthy foal of similar size. In certain circumstances it may be impossible to administer the total needs. The benefit of provision of nutritional support and, if needed, antibody supplementation, cannot be over-emphasized.
- Severe diarrhea/sepsis/ileus. These conditions may be complicated by an underlying failure of passive transfer.
- Surgical and medical cases. It is often wise to pre-empt problems with early parenteral nutritional support, especially in foals recovering from gastrointestinal surgery.
- Postoperative care that precludes normal feeding (e.g. cleft plate or esophageal stricture repair).
- Colic (for whatever reason).
- Botulism (shaker foal syndrome).
- Gastroduodenal ulceration syndrome with or without surgery.
- Dysphagia/pharyngeal disorders/surgery (e.g. epiglottic/pharyngeal cysts).
- Septicemia.

Method

A dedicated intravenous line should always be used, not one that is also used for blood samples and drug administration. However, veins are often at a premium and this may not be practical. If the same line is to be used for other purposes ensure that total parenteral nutrition is switched off and that the catheter and the line itself it are flushed with heparin saline before and after sampling or drug administration. Absolute asepsis is obligatory at all times during parenteral medication.

- A nonthrombogenic, central venous catheter (16G, 15–25 cm long) should be placed with full aseptic precautions.

Note:
- In the event that a catheter develops any problem at all it must be removed and if necessary replaced immediately. **This is an emergency procedure.**
- Replacement of a catheter in the same site is probably unwise. A new site in another vein is best.
- Delays in removing a problem catheter and sudden withdrawal of parenteral nutrition can be catastrophic and will negate all the previous hard work.

- A flexible 'Susi' administration set is useful when the foal can walk; indeed movement should be encouraged and not hindered.
- Fluid should always be administered at blood temperature (heated wrappers and bag warmers) may be very useful.
- Adjust flow rates carefully in the light of clinical and laboratory assessments.
  - Drip calculations are useful and practical.
  - Dedicated peristaltic and infusion pumps are very useful.
- Flow rates can be adjusted to within milliliters per day.

Complications/problems

- Too fast or too slow rates of flow.
  - Measured and monitored by the hydration status of the foal.
  - Bodyweight can also be an effective monitor of hydration.
- Hyperglycemia
  - Glucose concentrations up to 8 mmol/l are common during both total and partial parenteral nutrition. This should subside to 6–8 mmol/l at 24–36 hours.
  - Sustained high concentrations coupled with glycosuria can cause dehydration, fatty liver and predisposes to sepsis.
  - Glycosuria is common under normal circumstances in foals and this can increase markedly during infusion.
  - Metabolic consumption of glucose can be affected significantly by the underlying disease.
  - There is often an imbalance between glucose and insulin (insulin resistance) when the insulin is high without reducing the glucose.
  - Flow rates for glucose are usually adjusted empirically starting at 10 g/kg bodyweight administered daily at 7 mg/kg/minute. Increased or reduced rates are used according to laboratory results and clinical judgment.
  - To correct problems of hyperglycemia, reduce the flow rate of combined solution and increase the rate of saline administration to

make up the fluid deficit. It is far easier to adjust the glucose with fewer metabolic effects if separate solutions are used and manipulated independently.
  - Glucose should be used carefully – its benefits are not as obvious as the disadvantages.
- Hyperlipidemia.
  - Patent lipemia is undesirable. It is most common if simultaneous intake of milk is high.
  - Flow rates are adjusted to reduce the level of lipid in the blood but it is fairly well tolerated.
- Hypokalemia.
  - Loss of potassium ions into urine occurs in the face of hyperglycemia as a result of osmotic diuresis. Losses also occur via diarrhea.
  - Use oral supplementation of potassium chloride or parenteral administration of 10–20 meq/l solutions to provide 1 meq/kg/hour.
  - Monitor heart (rate/rhythm) and plasma potassium regularly.
- Acidosis (metabolic).
  - Usually from excessive chloride ions. Reduce chloride by slowing the fluid solution.
- Infection.
  - Maintain scrupulous asepsis/hygiene and continuous antibiotic therapy (even if these are only prophylactic).
  - Change/manage catheter.
  - The free end of the catheter should always be subjected to culture on removal whether or not there has been a detectable problem
  - Monitor plasma fibrinogen and white cell count.

- Total parenteral nutrition should probably not be used when it is clearly hopeless and the foal is dying; it merely wastes time and the owner's money.
- The procedure is both expensive and time-consuming, so careful case selection needs to be made.
- Nevertheless, some very ill foals will respond remarkably well to a well-managed and well-constructed protocol for parenteral nutrition (whether partial or complete).

CONGENITAL DISORDERS OF THE FOAL

Congenital disorders are those that are present at birth. They may or may not be inherited; indeed, most congenital disorders are not inherited. Nevertheless, it is important to remember that inherited disease takes many forms (see Table 11.8). Recessive genes are

Table 11.8 Conditions known or thought to be inherited

Condition	Breed(s) affected	Age when disorder is manifest
Ileocecal aganglionosis	Overo-Paint	Immediate (<24 hours)
Brachygnathism	Thoroughbred	Immediate
Interventricular septal defect	Welsh Section A	Immediate
Cataract	Shire	Immediate to later
	Quarterhorse	
	Thoroughbred	
	Morgan	
Hemophilia	Thoroughbred	Immediate
Severe combined immunodeficiency	Arabian	4–16 weeks
Lavender foal	Arabian	Immediate
Fell pony immunodeficiency	Fell pony	1–12 weeks
Hyperkalemic periodic paralysis	Quarterhorse	6 months to mature
Cerebellar hypoplasia/abiotrophy	Arabian	Immediate to 48 hours
Narcolepsy	Appaloosa	1 day to 3 months
	Fell pony	
Scabbard/spiral trachea	Shetland	Later/never
Patella luxation (lateral)	Shetland	Variable
Atlantoaxial malformation	Arabian	Immediate

carried unnoticed, while some disorders have a complex genetic origin in which environmental and genetic factors combine to produce clinical disease.

REFERRAL OF A FOAL TO A SPECIALIST CENTER

Many diseases and conditions can be effectively treated on the farm, but this will depend on:

- The facilities available for nursing both mare and foal.
- The number of support staff available and their ability and experience (enthusiasm is seldom in short supply, at least in the early stages of the nursing).
- The experience and facilities of the clinician.
- The condition of the foal and the mare and their tolerance of transportation (e.g. some mares may not tolerate transport and so might jeopardize the foal and its handlers).
- The specific needs of the parent (e.g. splinting of a fractured leg, control of seizures, correction of hydration and electrolyte status).
- The distance to the center and the time the journey is likely to take.

Considerations prior to referral of a sick foal to a specialist unit[49]

- An early decision to refer is clearly better than undue delay. There is little rationale in sending a dying foal, which has little or no hope of surviving the journey, let alone the rigors of an intensive care regimen. The mare and the foal

should be considered together and individually, not just the condition that is of most concern (e.g. has the foal got 'bent' legs or a septic joint) which might influence the prognosis markedly.

- Referral should be considered seriously. A journey may make the condition worse. It is wise to seek advice from the referral hospital early if there are doubts about the necessity to transport the foal. The referral center will be grateful for continued contact in the early stages; they may be able to give advice and avoid transporting the foal unnecessarily. This will also give the center useful information before the arrival of the foal.
- Consider whether proper care can be given on the farm. Drugs and equipment (including laboratory support) may be essential to the survival of the foal in some cases, but in others minimal supportive equipment may be needed. The environment should be conducive to maintenance of body temperature and hygiene for example.
  - ❑ Are the correct drugs, fluids and catheters available?
  - ❑ Is a suitable stomach tube or foal feeding tube available?
  - ❑ Can oxygen be administered easily and safely over the full 24-hour day?
  - ❑ Is a respirator available?
  - ❑ Assuming that all the equipment for the particular foal is present, does the clinician have experience in its use/administration?
  - ❑ Is there suitable experienced help available to maintain the effort after the clinician leaves the premises?

- If the answer is no to any of these, refer immediately and expedite departure.

- The likely cost of the procedure must be discussed with the owner/stud manager. Foal intensive care is a very expensive affair and the implications (win or lose) need to be considered before starting out.
- The nearest referral center with known expertise and the facilities to cope should be selected. There is no point in sending the foal to another similarly equipped or experienced practice just to shift responsibility for the foal to someone else.
- Phone and discuss the case early (preparation is maximized and guidance can be given which might save the foal's life or may prevent an unnecessary journey).
- A written record of all clinical findings and any procedures (including the timing and doses of any drugs given) should be sent with the foal. The letter should be signed by the clinician and it should include contact numbers and addresses.
- All specimens taken (e.g. peritoneal fluid, blood or joint fluid) should be packed accordingly and sent with the foal.
- The placenta should be sent if available (packed on ice in a clean, sealed plastic bag).
- If the mare is not accompanying the foal, some milk/colostrum should be obtained and sent with the foal.
- Any interested insurance company should be informed; this is often forgotten in the heat of the moment and failure to comply with policy procedures may create difficulties later on.
- As soon as laboratory results become available these should be sent by fax or e-mail to the referral center.

Transportation of the sick or injured foal

The most significant aspects are:[50,51]

1. Restraint and protection from self-inflicted or other trauma.
   - If the mare and foal cannot be safely transported together, consider sending the foal first and follow with the mare in another transporter.
   - Physical support helps if the foal is amenable to this. Sternal recumbency is the best physiological supportive position and this should be maintained during recumbency as far as possible.
   - If the foal is in pain and thrashing or convulsing, suitable medication to control pain and seizures should be given.

   - ❏ Seizure control is usually best effected with diazepam at 5–20 mg administered in 5-mg increments.[52]
   - ❏ Do not use acepromazine or xylazine.
   - ❏ Handlers may be instructed to administer repeat doses during travel via an intravenous catheter.
   - ❏ It is always wise to check the blood glucose of any convulsing neonatal foal prior to and during transportation (if possible).
2. Prevention of hypothermia.
   - Take rectal temperature before starting and take appropriate measures to restore to normal (e.g. blankets, bottles and rectal gloves filled with warm water and tied).
   - Do not put the foal onto hot surfaces; application of direct heat can harm the circulation and cause skin damage/thermal necrosis.
   - It is sometimes possible to have the foal in the heated cab and still within sight of the mare.
3. Maintenance of blood glucose and prevention of nutritional depletion.
   - Energy, fluids and electrolytes are the earliest and most significant requirements.
   - Maintenance of normal blood glucose is particularly important for recumbent or weak foals.
     - ❏ Blood glucose should be checked before departure with a dextrose stick.
     - ❏ If blood glucose is less than 2.5 mmol/l and the journey is likely to be longer than 1–2 hours, it is wise to place an intravenous catheter and administer warm 5% glucose solution at 4 ml/kg/hour. It is probably unwise to administer a large bolus of glucose intravenously at the start of the journey as this might easily induce a rebound hypoglycemia.
   - Administration of 200–250 ml mares' milk or colostrum by stomach tube is helpful if the foal has not been feeding and if there is no nasogastric reflux.
4. A sample of the colostrum should be sent with the foal so that the specialist center can assess its quality. This will be particularly helpful if the foal is less than 18 hours old.
5. If the foal has any respiratory compromise[53] it should not be left in lateral recumbency. Sternal recumbency is very helpful to normal lung function.
   - Oxygen should be administered if:
     - ❏ The respiratory rate is <30/minute or >80/minute.
     - ❏ The mucous membranes are pale or cyanotic.
     - ❏ There is any evidence of respiratory tract infection.
     - ❏ A nasopharyngeal tube is easy to insert and is well tolerated by foals. A direct oxygen

line into the trachea that can be inserted percutaneously is also available.

❑ Oxygen can be administered directly via a normal cylinder with a pressure-limiting valve. A demand valve can also be used.

Note:
- A normal E-size cylinder will provide a flow rate of 5 liters/minute for 1 hour.
- If a facemask is used, ensure that it has a release/overflow valve or that the fit is loose enough to avoid the foal rebreathing.

- If sternal recumbency cannot be sustained, the foal should be held in sternal recumbency for at least some of the time and should be turned from side to side at 30-minute intervals.

6. Unless the foal is already known to be infected, it is probably wise to delay the administration of antibiotics. However, if there is any suspicion of sepsis, a suitable broad-spectrum antibiotic may be administered.
   - It may be useful to discuss choice of antibiotic with the referral center.
7. The dose and time of all drugs and procedures used prior to departure and during transport should be recorded and sent with the foal. It is unwise to rely on memory.
8. If the placenta is available send it with the foal, in a sealed plastic bag packed with ice.
9. Do not forget the needs of the mare if she is traveling with the foal or if she is to be left behind.

Management of the mare and foal in transit

Confine the foal and mare in a quiet, safe area with (preferably) no opportunity for self-inflicted trauma. Size is very important as mares may become disturbed in a close confined area and traumatize the foal. A mare that will not settle should be placed in a separate stall so that she can see and smell the foal, which should then be held all the time by an experienced handler. Sedatives can be used to calm the mare but should not be used for the foal unless there is no option. A properly fitting foal slip should be used with suitable padding if necessary.

- Foals inclined to convulsions or uncoordinated movement need to be fully bandaged with protective padding on limbs and head to prevent injuries.
- The mare should have leg bandages applied, if only to protect the foal from damaging itself and her.

Body heat should be maintained by appropriate rugging and bandaging. This is vital when ambient temperatures are below 25°C.

- 'Space blankets' are a useful emergency measure and are extremely efficient at heat retention. Sweating is very 'cooling' and where present an appropriate undersheet made of absorbent cotton or wool is desirable.
- Toweling the foal dry before starting the journey is useful.
- In an emergency, sleeping bags, sweaters (foal's front legs through the arms and head through the neck) are good, simple measures.
- Hot water bottles and electrically heated pads can be valuable but they can cause serious skin burns especially in compromised recumbent foals.

Note:
- The direct application of heat to the outer surface can be harmful rather than helpful.
- Beware of lying a sick foal on an electrically heated pad. Extensive skin necrosis can occur as the circulation is poor and compressed by the bodyweight of the foal. Moreover, the skin is more liable to burn when the cutaneous circulation is impaired.
- Do not transport a sick foal in an open pick-up truck; heat loss and/or sunburn can be critical.

Prepare the box with adequate bedding over a rubber floor.

- An overlay of carpeting provides good insulation, reduces draughts and provides a clean surface.
- Shavings, sawdust or peat should not be used for young foals as these materials may harm the respiratory tract and the eyes in particular.
- 'Vetbed' artificial fiber blankets are excellent as they allow fluid to pass while still maintaining thermal insulation and dryness in contact with the skin.
- If the foal is standing do not make the bed too deep (6–12 cm is enough).

Trailers are less desirable than boxes and estate cars.

- Do not put a sick foal in the boot of a saloon car.
- It is illegal, irresponsible and dangerous to travel in a trailer with the foal (use closed circuit television if necessary).
- Equine ambulances are excellent but may not be equipped to transport a mare and foal.
- The greater the space and contact with handlers the better.
- Always have at least two people with the transporter; it is unreasonable and dangerous for the driver to have to cope with every demand.

- Avoid draughts in the transporter, but also avoid a steamy moist atmosphere by ensuring adequate ventilation.

Stop at regular intervals unless separate staff are looking after the animals. Some foals will not nurse when moving so it may be necessary to stop to allow feeding.

Load the foal before the mare and guide it carefully. If the foal can stand and coordinate normally, the mare and foal should be separated in the box. It is not necessary or wise to tie the foal, but a foal slip suitably padded is sometimes helpful with restraint.

If the foal has respiratory disease or compromise, oxygen cylinders and possibly an indwelling nasal tube with continuous oxygen should be used.

- Fluid therapy may need to be maintained for the duration of the journey, so suitable arrangements need to be made using a 'Susi' flexible, extendable intravenous administration set.
- The foal should be placed in sternal recumbency but should never be forced to adopt this position (it is better to leave it comfortable than to stress it).

It is often helpful to make written records of any measures taken before and during transportation so that the referral center is aware of these.

- The vital signs, feeding regimen and frequency, rectal temperature, fecal and urinary output, details of birth and any subsequent relevant details can usefully be supplied.

REFERENCES

1. Rose RJ. Cardiorespiratory adaptations in neonatal foals. Equine Veterinary Journal 1988; Suppl 5:11–13.
2. MacDonald AA, Fowden AL, Silver M, et al. The foramen ovale of the fetal and neonatal foal. Equine Veterinary Journal 1988; 20:255–260.
3. Koterba AM, Kosch PC. Respiratory mechanisms and breathing patterns in the neonatal foal. Journal of Reproduction and Fertility 1987; 35:575–586.
4. Rossdale PD. Clinical studies on the newborn Thoroughbred foal: II. Heart rate, auscultation and electrocardiogram. British Veterinary Journal 1967; 123:521–531.
5. Livesey LC, Marr CM, Boswood A, et al. Auscultation and two-dimensional M-mode, spectral and colour flow Doppler findings in pony foals from birth to seven weeks of age. Journal of Veterinary Internal Medicine 1998; 12:255–267.
6. Yamomoto K, Yasuda J, Too K. Arrythmias in newborn Thoroughbred foals. Equine Veterinary Journal 1992; 23:169–173.
7. Oftedal OT, Henz HF, Schryver HF. Lactation in the horse: milk composition and intake by foals. Journal of Nutrition 1983; 113:2196.
8. Brewer BD, Clement SF, Lotz WS, et al. Renal function in neonatal foals and their dams: a comparison of inulin, para-aminohippuric acid and endogenous creatinine clearance. Journal of Veterinary Internal Medicine 1990; 5:28–33.
9. Kohn CW, Strasser SL. 24-hour renal clearance and excretion of endogenous substances in the mare. American Journal of Veterinary Research 1986; 47:1332–1333.
10. Wennberg RP, Goetzman BW. Temperature regulation. Neonatal intensive care manual. London: Year Book Publishers; 1985:27–30.
11. Rossdale PD, Rickets S. Equine stud farm medicine. London: Baillière Tindall; 1980:220–276.
12. Madigan JE. Manual of equine neonatal medicine. 3rd edn. Woodland: Live Oak Publishing; 1997:1–12.
13. Madigan JE. Post foaling procedures: care of umbilicus. In: Manual of equine neonatal medicine. 3rd edn. Woodland: Live Oak Publishing; 1997:29–30.
14. Vaala WE, Sertich PL. Management strategies for mares at risk for periparturient complications. Veterinary Clinics of North America 1994; 10:237–265.
15. Madigan JE. Manual of equine neonatal medicine. 3rd edn. Woodland: Live Oak Publishing; 1997: 29–31.
16. Adams R, Mayhew IG. Neurologic examination of newborn foals. Equine Veterinary Journal 1984; 16:306–313.
17. Leadon DFP, Jeffcot LB, Rossdale PD. Behavior and viability of the premature neonatal foal after induced parturition. American Journal of Veterinary Research 1986; 47:1870–1874.
18. Rossdale PD, Ousey JC, Silver M, et al. Studies on equine prematurity. 6: Guidelines for assessment of foal maturity. Equine Veterinary Journal 1984; 16:300–302.
19. Rossdale PD, Silver M. The concept of readiness for birth. Journal of Reproduction and Fertility Supplement 1982; 32:507.
20. Leadon DFP, Jeffcot LB, Rossdale PD. Behavior and viability of the premature neonatal foal after induced parturition. American Journal of Veterinary Research 1986; 47:1870–1874.
21. Adams-Brendermuehl C, Pipers FS. Antepartum evaluations in the equine foetus. Journal of Reproduction and Fertility Supplement 1987; 35:565.
22. LeBlanc MM, Baldwin JL, Pritchard EL. Factors that influence passive transfer of immunoglobulins in foals. Journal of the American Veterinary Medical Association 1992; 220:183–197.
23. Jeffcott LB. Some practical aspects of the transfer of passive immunity to newborn foals. Equine Veterinary Journal 1975; 6:109.
24. Borum PR. Nutrient requirements of the critically ill neonate. Equine Veterinary Journal 1988; Suppl 5:14–16.
25. Koterba AM, Drummond WM. Nutritional support of the foal during intensive care. Veterinary Clinics of North America 1985; 1:35–40.
26. Wilson JH. Plasma amino acid concentration in neonatal foals fed defined enteral formulae or goats milk. Proceedings of the International Society of Perinatology 1990:223–224.
27. Ousey JC. How to feed the sick foal. Proceedings of the BEVA Specialist Day on Equine Nutrition, Harrogate 1999:91–96.
28. Doreau M, Boulot S. Recent knowledge on mare milk production: a review. Livestock Production Science 1989; 22:213–235.

29. Pagan JD, Jackson SG, Caddel S. A summary of growth rates of Thoroughbreds in Kentucky. Second European Conference on Horse Nutrition 1996.

30. Wilson JH. Feeding considerations for neonatal foals. Proceedings of the American Association of Equine Practitioners 1988:823–829.

31. Ousey JC, Holdstock NB, Rossdale PD, et al. How much energy do sick foals require compared with healthy foals? Proceedings of the Second European Conference on Horse Nutrition 1996:231–237.

32. Wilson JH. Feeding considerations for neonatal foals. Proceedings of the American Association of Equine Practitioners 1988:823–829.

33. Ousey JC. Thermoregulation and the energy requirement of the newborn foal with reference to prematurity. Equine Veterinary Journal Supplement 1997; 24:104–108.

34. Martin RG, McMeniman NP, Dowset KF. Milk and water intakes of foals sucking grazing mares. Equine Veterinary Journal 1992; 24:295–299.

35. Green SL. Feeding the sick or orphan foal. Equine Veterinary Education 1993; 5:274–275.

36. Ousey JC, Prandi S, Zimmer J, et al. Effects of various feeding regimes on the energy balance of equine neonates. American Journal of Veterinary Research 1997; 58:1243–1251.

37. Davis JL, Boero JA, DiPietro JA, et al. Practical aspects involved in raising the orphan foal. Equine Veterinary Journal 1988; Suppl 5:61.

38. Knight DA, Tyznik WJ. An artificial rearing method to produce optimum growth in orphaned foals. Journal of Equine Veterinary Science 1985; 9:319–322.

39. Ullrey DE, Struthers RD, Hendricks DG, et al. Composition of mare's milk. Journal of Animal Science 1966; 25:217–222.

40. Kent Carter G. Supplemental feeding of the normal foal. Proceedings of the American Association of Equine Practitioners 1990; 36:95–98.

41. Spurlock SL, Ward MV. Parenteral nutrition in equine patients: principles and theory. Compendium for Continuing Education 1991; 13:235–244.

42. Sanchez LC, Lester GD, Merritt AM. Effects of ranitidine on intragastric pH. I: Clinically normal neonatal foals. Journal of the American Veterinary Medical Association 1998; 212:1407–1412.

43. Mauer AM, Dweck HS, Finberg L, et al. Nutritional needs of low birth weight infants. Pediatrics 1985; 75:976–986.

44. Cudd TA. Parenteral nutrition support in foals. Compendium for Continuing Education 1993; 15:1547–1550.

45. Hansen TO. Nutritional support: parenteral nutrition. In: Koterba AM, Drummond WH, Kosch PC, eds. Equine clinical neonatology. Philadelphia: Lea & Febiger; 1990:747–778.

46. Madigan JE. Field applications of aggressive treatments. Proceedings of the 14th Bain-Fallon Memorial Lectures 1992.

47. Zicker SC, Rogers QR. Temporal changes in concentrations of amino acids in plasma and whole blood of healthy neonatal foals from birth to two days of age. American Journal of Veterinary Research 1994; 55:1012–1019.

48. Madigan JE. Parenteral nutrition. Manual of equine neonatal medicine. Woodland: Liveoak Publications; 1997:102–106.

49. Geiser DR, Henton JE. Transportation of the equine neonatal patient. Equine Practice 1986; 8:19–24.

50. Geiser DR, Henton JE. Transportation of the equine neonatal patient. Equine Practice 1986; 8:19–24.

51. Cudd TA. Neonatal transport. In: Koterba AM, Drummond WH, Kosch PC, eds. Equine clinical neonatology. Philadelphia: Lea & Febiger; 1990:763–769.

52. Madigan JE. Transport of the critically ill equine neonate. Manual of equine neonatal medicine. Woodland: Live Oak Publications; 1997:67–69.

53. Kosch PC, Koterba AM. Respiratory support for the newborn foal. In: Robinson NE, ed. Current therapy in equine medicine. Philadelphia: WB Saunders; 1987:247–253.

INDEX